Rick Pye

NEUROLOGIC COMPLICATIONS OF CANCER

CONTEMPORARY NEUROLOGY SERIES AVAILABLE:

19 THE DIAGNOSIS OF STUPOR AND COMA, EDITION 3
Fred Plum, M.D., and Jerome B. Posner, M.D.

26 PRINCIPLES OF BEHAVIORAL NEUROLOGY
M-Marsel Mesulam, M.D., *Editor*

29 ADVANCES IN CONTEMPORARY NEUROLOGY
Fred Plum, M.D., *Editor*

31 SEIZURES AND EPILEPSY
Jerome Engel, Jr., M.D., Ph.D.

32 CLINICAL NEUROPHYSIOLOGY OF THE VESTIBULAR SYSTEM, EDITION 2
Robert W. Baloh, M.D., and Vicente Honrubia, M.D.

33 SPINAL CORD COMPRESSION: DIAGNOSIS AND PRINCIPLES OF MANAGEMENT
Thomas N. Byrne, M.D., and Stephen G. Waxman, M.D., Ph. D.

34 GUILLAIN-BARRÉ SYNDROME
Allan H. Ropper, M.D., Eelco F.M. Wijdicks, M.D., and Bradley T. Truax, M.D.

35 THE NEUROLOGY OF EYE MOVEMENTS, EDITION 2
R. John Leigh, M.D., M.R.C.P. (U.K.), and David S. Zee, M.D.

36 DISORDERS OF PERIPHERAL NERVES, EDITION 2
Herbert H. Schaumburg, M.D., Alan R. Berger, M.D., and P.K. Thomas, C.B.E., M.D., D.Sc., F.R.C.P., F.R.C. Path.

37 PRINCIPLES OF DRUG THERAPY IN NEUROLOGY
Michael V. Johnston, M.D., Robert L. Macdonald, M.D., Ph.D., and Anne B. Young, M.D., Ph.D., *Editors*

38 PRINCIPLES OF GERIATRIC NEUROLOGY
Robert Katzman, M.D., and John W. Rowe, M.D., *Editors*

39 CLINICAL BRAIN IMAGING: PRINCIPLES AND APPLICATIONS
John C. Mazziotta, M.D., Ph.D., and Sid Gilman, M.D., *Editors*

40 DEMENTIA
Peter J. Whitehouse, M.D., Ph.D., *Editor*

41 INFECTIOUS DISEASES OF THE CENTRAL NERVOUS SYSTEM
Kenneth L. Tyler, M.D., and Joseph B. Martin, M.D., Ph.D., *Editors*

42 MIGRAINE: MANIFESTATIONS, PATHOGENESIS, AND MANAGEMENT
Robert A. Davidoff, M.D.

43 NEUROLOGY OF CRITICAL ILLNESS
Eelco F.M. Wijdicks, M.D., Ph.D., F.A.C.P.

44 EVALUATION AND TREATMENT OF MYOPATHIES
Robert C. Griggs, M.D., Jerry R. Mendell, M.D., and Robert G. Miller, M.D.

NEUROLOGIC COMPLICATIONS OF CANCER

JEROME B. POSNER, M.D.
George C. Cotzias Chair in Neuro-Oncology
Chairman, Department of Neurology
Memorial Sloan-Kettering Cancer Center
New York, New York
and
Professor of Neurology and Neuroscience
Cornell University Medical College
New York, New York

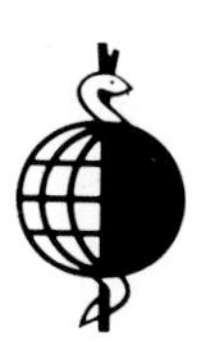

F.A. DAVIS COMPANY · Philadelphia

F. A. Davis Company
1915 Arch Street
Philadelphia, PA 19103

Printed in the United States of America

Last digit indicates print number: 10 9 8 7 6 5 4 3 2 1

Medical Editor: Robert W. Reinhardt
Medical Developmental Editor: Bernice M. Wissler
Production Editor: Roberta Massey
Cover Designer: Louis J. Forgione

As new scientific information becomes available through basic and clinical research, recommended treatments and drug therapies undergo changes. The author and publisher have done everything possible to make this book accurate, up to date, and in accord with accepted standards at the time of publication. The authors, editors, and publisher are not responsible for errors or omissions or for consequences from application of the book, and make no warranty, expressed or implied, in regard to the contents of the book. Any practice described in this book should be applied by the reader in accordance with professional standards of care used in regard to the unique circumstances that may apply in each situation. The reader is advised always to check product information (package inserts) for changes and new information regarding dose and contraindications before administering any drug. Caution is especially urged when using new or infrequently ordered drugs.

Library of Congress Cataloging in Publication Data

Posner, Jerome B., 1932-
Neurologic complications of cancer / Jerome B. Posner
p. cm.—(Contemporary neurology series; 45)
Includes bibliographical references and index.
ISBN 0-8036-0006-2
1. Neurologic manifestations of general diseases. 2. Cancer--Complications. 3. Nervous system—Physiology. 4. Nervous system--Pathophysiology. I. Title. II. Series
[DNLM: 1. Neoplasms—complications. 2. Central Nervous System Neoplasms—secondary. 3. Central Nervous System Diseases--complications. W1 C0769N v. 45 1995 / QZ 202 1995]
RC347.P67 1995
616.8—dc20
DNLM/DLC
for Library of Congress 94-45924

PREFACE

This book is intended for clinicians who care for patients with cancer when that cancer or its treatment secondarily affects the nervous system. The material in the book reflects my experiences as a neurologist working in a cancer hospital. Neurologic complications of cancer are occurring with increasing frequency as oncologists become more effective in treating the systemic disease, but many oncologists lack the understanding of nervous system physiology to allow appropriate clinical diagnosis and sometimes even appropiate interpretation of nervous system images. Neurologists, on the other hand, often lack sufficient specific knowledge of the behavior of individual cancers and of the side effects of specific treatments to assist the oncologist in making an accurate diagnosis and prescribing appropriate treatment. This book is intended to help both, although I recognize that the neurologist may find in it too much oncology and, especially because I am a clinical neurologist, the oncologist may find too much arcane neurology.

I have had a great deal of help in writing this monograph. Nevertheless, the book reflects my own personal biases; I use the first person singular to express my personal opinions. Furthermore, although my colleagues helped correct many errors and misconceptions that appeared in the original drafts of this book, I alone bear responsibility for any that remain.

Help in writing this monograph has been of several types. The first is technical and editorial support. Judy Lampron typed so many drafts of this manuscript that she is now a qualified neuro-oncologist. Brenna Nichols reviewed the entire manuscript and bibliography in detail and put many of my neologisms into straightforward English. Carol D'Anella proofread most of the chapters, identifying many errors of grammar, syntax, and, at times, concepts. She also proofread the galleys. Christine Schaar, Biomedical Illustrator at Memorial Sloan-Kettering, prepared Figures 2–1, 2–6, and 2–7.

Several colleagues read all or parts of the monograph and made extremely valuable suggestions, as well as corrected errors. Lisa DeAngelis and Robert Darnell, faculty colleagues, as well as Peter Forsyth, Susan Weaver, and David Schiff, neuro-oncology fellows, read the entire manuscript and were exceedingly helpful. Dr. DeAngelis also read the galleys. Zvi Fuks, Steven Leibel, Donald Armstrong, Russell Portenoy, Louisa Thoron, Ronald Blasberg, and Josep Dalmau read individual chapters and made valuable suggestions.

More indirect, but still important support has come from physician-administrators at Memorial Sloan-Kettering Cancer Center. Joseph Simone, Physician-in-Chief, and Paul Marks, President of the Center, gave me a period of leave from administrative responsibilities, which allowed me to finish the monograph. I hope they find this book worth their support.

Finally, a special thanks to Fred Plum. He read the entire monograph and gently made appropriate and valuable suggestions. But my gratitude is for more than that. Over the years that we have worked together, since my medical student days, he has been an unfailingly supportive mentor, giving me far more credit in our joint efforts than I ever deserved. He has been, as well, a model to which I, and indeed any academic neurologist, can aspire.

This book is dedicated to Gerta, Roslyn, Stanley, Cara, Joel, Tina, and PJ, with love.

Jerome B. Posner

CONTENTS

PART 1

General Considerations

CHAPTER 1

OVERVIEW

Neuro-oncology is a medical discipline that deals with the diagnosis and treatment of: (1) primary central nervous system (CNS) neoplasms, (2) metastatic and nonmetastatic neurologic complications of cancer originating outside the nervous system (i.e., systemic cancer), and (3) pain associated with cancer. This monograph addresses only the second aspect.

This chapter has two sections; the first describes the rationale for a discipline called neuro-oncology and the second establishes a working classification of neurologic complications of systemic cancer that is followed in subsequent chapters.

NEUROLOGIC COMPLICATIONS OF CANCER: WHY STUDY THEM?

Neurologists, oncologists, and internists must give special attention to neurologic complications of cancer for several reasons[2064,2065] (Table 1–1).

Nervous System Complications of Cancer Are Common

Cancer is the nation's second leading cause of death; for individuals 35 to 64 years old, it is the leading cause.[2527] Data indicate that in 1994, more than 1 million persons will develop a new cancer (excluding carcinoma in situ and nonmelanotic skin cancer) and more than half a million will die of cancer[274] (Table 1–2).

Autopsy data from Memorial Sloan-Kettering Cancer Center (MSKCC)[2073] identified intracranial metastases in 24% (572) of 2375 patients with cancer. If the prevalence of intracranial metastases in patients dying from specific cancers at MSKCC is similar in the rest of the nation and one multiplies by the American Cancer Society's national figures, one obtains a rough estimate of the number of patients dying with intracranial metastases in the United States each year. The 1994 figure is over 125,000. A clinical analysis of patients dying with brain metastases[363] sug-

Table 1–1. **NEUROLOGIC COMPLICATIONS OF CANCER: WHY STUDY THEM?**

1. Nervous system complications of cancer are common.
2. Neurologic complications of cancer are increasing.
3. Neurologic complications of systemic cancer are serious.
4. Diagnosis is often difficult.
5. Treatment helps.
6. Problems in neuro-oncology are unique.
7. Research is essential.
8. Relationships between the brain and systemic cancer are biologically important.

gests that two-thirds or 80,000 will have had significant neurologic symptomatology during life. Even if these data are overestimated by 100%, more than 40,000 patients die with symptomatic intracranial metastases each year, making the disorder almost 2½ times as common as primary CNS malignancies (17,500) and five times as common as Hodgkin's disease (7900).[274]

Intracranial metastases, however, are only one neurologic complication of systemic cancer; other brain lesions are also common. When Posner and Chernik[2073] (Table 1–3) examined the brains of patients dying of cancer over a 4-year period (1970 to 1973), they found lesions within the brain of potential clinical significance in 36% of patients; 16% had brain metastases (lower than the 24% *intracranial* metastases because lesions of the dura and leptomeninges were not considered); 8% had vascular lesions (see Chapter 9); and 4% had CNS infections (see Chapter 10). In other studies, epidural spinal cord compression, a major cause of disability in patients with cancer, was found in about 5% (37) of 704 patients at autopsy[151] (see Chapter 6).

Neurologic complications of systemic cancer are as common in the clinic as they are at autopsy. At MSKCC, in the first 10 months of 1994, 1,195 patients were seen in consultation on the Medical and Surgical Wards, and 650 patients were admitted to the Neurology/Neurosurgery Ward. These figures exclude consultations placed directly to the Pain or Psychiatry Services of the Depart-

Table 1–2. **FREQUENCY OF INTRACRANIAL METASTASES FROM SYSTEMIC CANCERS**

Primary Tumors	New Cases USA 1994[274]	No. of Deaths USA 1994[274]	% with Intracranial Tumor at Autopsy MSKCC[2073]	Estimated Total No. of Deaths with Intracranial Tumor
Lung	172,000	153,000	34	52,020
Breast	183,000	46,300	30	13,890
Colon and rectum	149,000	56,000	7	3920
Urinary organs	78,800	21,900	23	5037
Melanoma	32,000	6900	72	4968
Prostate	200,000	38,000	31*	11,780
Pancreas	27,000	25,900	7	1813
Leukemia	28,600	19,100	23†	4393
Lymphoma (non-Hodgkin's)	45,000	21,200	16†	3392
Female genital tract	75,300	25,200	7	1764
Brain and CNS	17,500	12,600	100	12,600
ALL SITES	**1,208,000**	**538,000**	**24**	**129,120**

*Largely skull and dura.
†Largely leptomeningeal.
CNS = central nervous system; MSKCC = Memorial Sloan-Kettering Cancer Center.

Table 1–3. **BRAIN LESIONS IN 1905 AUTOPSIES AT MSKCC: 1970–1973**

Brain Lesions	Number	% Total	% Brain Lesions
	687	36	—
Metastases	310	16	45
Vascular lesions	151	8	22
Infections	80	4	12

MSKCC = Memorial Sloan-Kettering Cancer Center.

ment of Neurology. Despite these exclusions, the most common complaint was pain, followed by mental status changes and muscle weakness[461] (Table 1–4). These data indicate that about 15% of patients with cancer suffer a symptomatic neurologic complication at some time during the course of the disease. For many patients, the neurologic disorder may occur late when the cancer is already widespread, but for many others, the neurologic symptoms may be the first evidence of cancer.

Other studies yield even higher figures. Gilbert and Grossman[920] from the Johns Hopkins Cancer Center report that, with the exception of planned admissions for chemotherapy, neurologic problems were the most common reason for admission to the Solid Tumor Service at their Center (Fig. 1–1). The major problems were changes in mental status, epidural spinal cord compression, and brain metastases. Collectively, neurologic problems represented more than 50% of the admissions. Sculier and colleagues[2349] report that of 641 patients with small-cell lung cancer, 29.5% (189) had at least one symptomatic neurologic disorder during the course of the disease. A survey from a Netherlands cancer hospital[1216] reports that among 7004 new adult patients during 2 years, 1105 were referred for neurologic evaluation. Breast cancer was the most frequent primary tumor, followed by lung, ovarian, head and neck, and non-Hodgkin's lymphoma. Pain was the most common complaint, with nerve root, plexus, and spinal cord problems being the most common final diagnosis.

Table 1–4. **MAJOR NEUROLOGIC COMPLAINTS IN 1,195 PATIENTS WITH CANCER[461]**

Back pain	155
Altered mental status	146
Headache	131
Pain in a limb	112
Leg weakness	84
Ataxia or gait disturbance	75
Sensory disturbance	53
Visual disturbance or diplopia	49
Arm weakness	47
Seizures	46
Speech or language disturbance	36
Hemiparesis	32
Movement disorder	24
Neck pain	23
Syncope	21

Neurologic Complications of Cancer Are Increasing

Autopsy data from MSKCC show a steady increase in the postmortem incidence of intracranial, brain, and leptomeningeal metastases from 1970 through 1979.[2073] Although these data may be contaminated because patients with neurologic disorders are likely to be referred to this hospital and no epidemiologic data are available for comparison, other autopsy reports support our findings. Pickren and associates[2037] (Fig. 1–2) report a steady increase in brain metastases encountered at autopsy between 1959 and 1979. Several clinical reports support these autopsy observations. Espana, Chang, and Wiernik[735]; Danziger and colleagues[560]; and Lewis[1551] report an apparently increasing incidence of brain metastases in sarcoma patients whose survival has been prolonged by systemic chemotherapy. Mayer, Berkowitz, and Griffiths[1713] note the same phenomenon with ovarian cancer. Nugent and associates[1906] report both an increasing frequency and a changing pattern of CNS metastases in patients with small-cell lung carcinoma. Prophylactic brain irradiation decreased the incidence of brain metastases, but leptomeningeal metastases increased. CNS metastases from non-Hodgkin's lymphoma also appear to be increasing.[413]

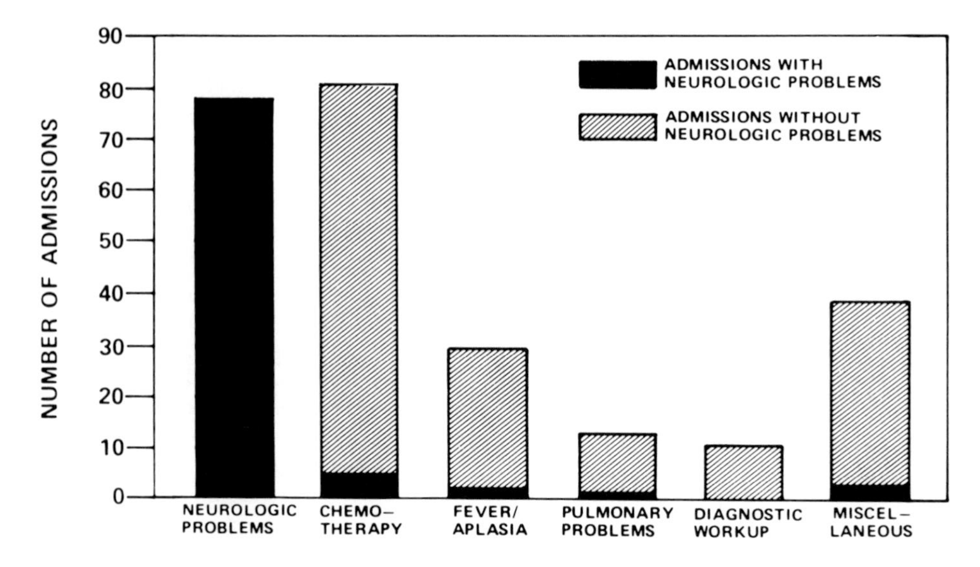

Figure 1–1. Reasons for hospital admission of 252 evaluable patients to Johns Hopkins Oncology Center during a 3-month period in 1984. The incidence of neurologic problems in those patients admitted for other reasons is indicated within each diagnostic group. (From Gilbert and Grossman,[920] p 953, with permission.)

Trivial reasons may be offered to explain this apparent increase in intracranial metastases: (1) A greater interest in the diagnosis and treatment of brain and leptomeningeal metastases, coupled with the availability of computed tomographic (CT) and magnetic resonance (MR) scanning, has led to more accurate diagnoses and, thus, an apparently increased incidence. (2) Because of improved supportive care, many patients with cancer live longer, allowing time for wider dissemination of metastases to all organs, including the CNS.

However, a nontrivial explanation is more likely; that is, that the CNS is a sanctuary for neoplastic cells when the systemic tumor is controlled by chemotherapy or immunotherapy. According to this view, the increased

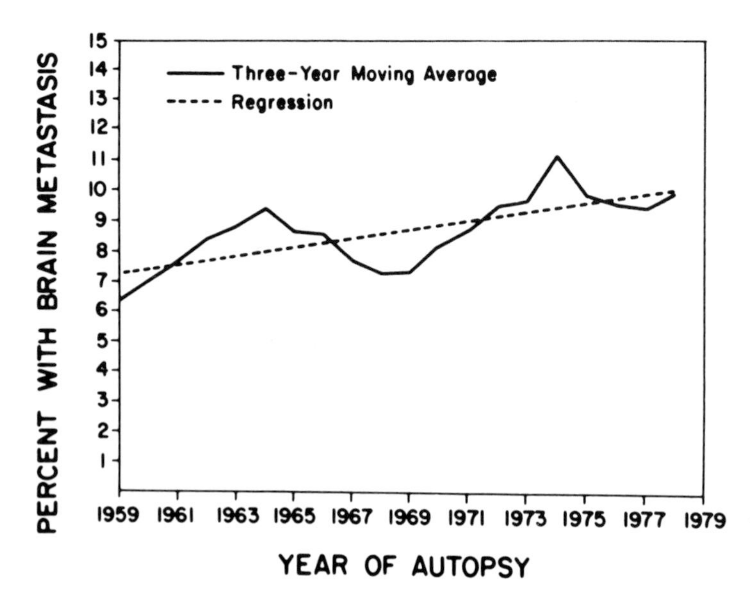

Figure 1–2. This graph illustrates an increase in the percentage of brain metastases at Roswell Park Memorial Institute from 1959 to 1979. Autopsies were performed on 95% of the deaths at that institute; almost all autopsies included a study of the brain. A statistically significant increase was observed in the percentage of patients with brain metastases, either for all cancers together or for individual cancers, with the exception of breast cancer. (From Pickren et al,[2037] p 310, with permission.)

incidence of CNS complications recapitulates the experience with acute lymphoblastic leukemia. Leptomeningeal leukemia was an uncommon clinical problem before effective chemotherapy for the systemic illness was developed.[1803] Beginning in the 1950s, as systemic treatment improved survival, the incidence of symptomatic meningeal leukemia increased rapidly until 50% of children developed that complication during the course of their illness.[1870] Leptomeningeal leukemia developed because leukemic cells found sanctuary behind the blood–brain barrier and were inaccessible to chemotherapy with parenteral water-soluble agents. The solution was to treat the CNS prophylactically. The situation has now come almost full circle as oncologists try to reduce CNS toxicity associated with intrathecal drugs by using parenteral drugs that cross the blood–brain barrier.[139] A situation similar to the early days of leukemia is now occurring in patients with breast cancer. In patients receiving adjuvant systemic chemotherapy, the first site of relapse is more likely to be the brain than it is in those not receiving systemic chemotherapy.[267,1995] A similar situation has been reported in patients with testicular cancer.[905a]

Nonmetastatic complications of systemic cancer may also be increasing. Although no epidemiologic data are available, nervous system complications of radiation therapy (RT) and chemotherapy (see Chapters 9 and 13) seem to be more frequent as these therapies become more vigorous and patients survive longer.

With respect to primary CNS tumors, recent epidemiologic studies report an increasing incidence of "brain and other central nervous system cancer" in the elderly,[286,994] young adults, and children.[570] Although these results may be biased by better ascertainment with modern imaging techniques, some observers believe the data reflect a true increased incidence.[570] Lymphomas originating in the brain are certainly increasing in incidence,[706,1173,1622a] as are other extranodal lymphomas.[620,1969a] The epidemiologic data are supported by the clinical impression of most neuro-oncologists that they are encountering many more immunocompetent patients with primary CNS lymphoma than previously. At MSKCC, primary CNS lymphomas, once representing about 1% of primary brain tumors, now represent about 15%.[577]

Neurologic Complications of Systemic Cancer Are Serious

Many patients suffering from systemic cancer, even some with widespread metastases, can, with appropriate therapy, function normally for prolonged periods. For example, a woman with breast cancer and also widespread bone metastases may with pain medication and perhaps a back brace lead a virtually normal life. However, if a vertebral metastasis compresses the spinal cord, then pain increases, neurologic disability develops, and her functional state worsens dramatically. Disorders of the brain and spinal cord, with their attendant symptoms of paralysis, incontinence, dementia, and seizures, often render a previously functional patient bedridden or hospitalized for the remainder of his or her life.[365]

Diagnosis Is Often Difficult

The neuro-oncologist is equipped by training and experience to handle difficult neurologic problems because the discipline combines familiarity of neurologic disease with knowledge of the common causes of neurologic disability in patients with cancer. Different disorders often present similar clinical signs, requiring meticulous and sophisticated clinical and laboratory evaluation to reach a definitive diagnosis. Many oncologists may be unaware, for example, that painless epidural spinal cord compression can clinically mimic a midline cerebellar syndrome[1060] (see Chapter 6) or that headache and syncope can be a sign of a recurrent neck tumor[1635] (see Chapter 8). Conversely, common neurologic syndromes often have uncommon causes when they occur in patients with systemic cancer, so that neurologists unfamiliar with the spectrum or complications of cancer may miss the diagnosis. For example, strokes are more likely to be due to nonbacterial thrombotic endocarditis than to hypertensive or arteriosclerotic cerebrovascular disease (see Chapter 9). CNS infections are usually caused by organisms different from those that the neurologist encounters in a general hospital population (see Chapter 10). Finally, about 20% of patients with cancer referred for neurologic consultation suffer from a neurologic disorder not related to their cancer (potentially treatable), such as migraine, neurocardiogenic syncope, and herniated disc.[461,1216] Thus, an accurate diagnosis, required to prescribe appropriate therapy, demands knowledge not only of the nervous system, but also of the cancer from which the patient is suffering, the treatment the patient is receiving, and the patient's likely neurologic complications. Failure to make the correct diagnosis often has tragic consequences.

Treatment Helps

Patients with neurologic complications of systemic cancer suffer persistent and/or progressive problems that require special management. Once a correct diagnosis is made, appropriate therapy directed at the nervous system complication frequently relieves symptoms and either prolongs life or improves its quality. Evidence presented in Chapter 6 indicates that, in patients suffering from epidural spinal cord compression, early diagnosis and vigorous treatment maintain the patient's ability to walk, often for the remainder of his or her life. Patients who are not treated inevitably become paraplegic or quadriplegic and spend the remainder of their life bedridden and incontinent. The same is true for patients with metastatic brain tumors. About 75% can be rendered symptom-free by appropriate treatment.[363] Many patients remain free of neurologic symptoms for the remainder of their life; death usually occurs from systemic disease. Prevention or effective treatment of paraplegia or hemiplegia considerably enhances the quality of a patient's remaining life and makes him or her less of a burden on loved ones. Similar therapeutic considerations also apply to nonmetastatic complications of cancer.

Problems in Neuro-oncology Are Unique

Several neurologic complications of cancer occur because of the unique anatomy and physiology of the nervous system; similar complications do not occur when cancer affects other organ systems (Table 1–5).

Table 1–5. **UNIQUE ASPECTS OF NEUROLOGIC COMPLICATIONS OF CANCER**

- The brain and spinal cord are enclosed in bone.
- Small lesions can cause "large" symptoms.
- The blood–brain (blood–nerve) barrier excludes many chemotherapeutic agents.
- The CNS lacks lymphatics, making removal of edema and detritus difficult.
- The CNS does not possess the capacity for clinically significant regeneration.
- Occult cancers can destroy nervous tissue ("remote effects") without direct contact.

CNS = central nervous system.

For example, the brain and spinal cord are enclosed in nondistensible bone. Small tumors that grow in the abdomen might simply move the normal organs aside and remain asymptomatic. In the brain or spinal cord, these tumors often cause severe and sometimes irreversible or lethal symptoms by compression and distortion of tissue that cannot move aside. Also, the CNS is heterogeneous; different small areas have different functions. A tumor must destroy a large fraction of liver, lung, or kidney tissue to cause organ failure, but in some areas of the nervous system such as the brainstem or spinal cord, severe disability may be caused by tumors too small to be visible on CT scan (although usually identified on MR scan). Anatomic and physiologic barriers (see Chapter 3) separate the nervous system from the rest of the body. These barriers often exclude water-soluble chemotherapeutic agents that might otherwise kill tumor cells sequestered behind it. On the other hand, when the blood–brain barrier is disrupted, as often occurs with brain metastases and other forms of brain injury, water-soluble molecules, some of which may be neurotoxic, can enter and spread into surrounding normal brain. The barrier disruption causes edema that, by its mass effect, often produces more brain dysfunction than the tumor itself (Fig. 1–3).

Another problem is that damaged CNS lacks the ability to regenerate meaningfully.

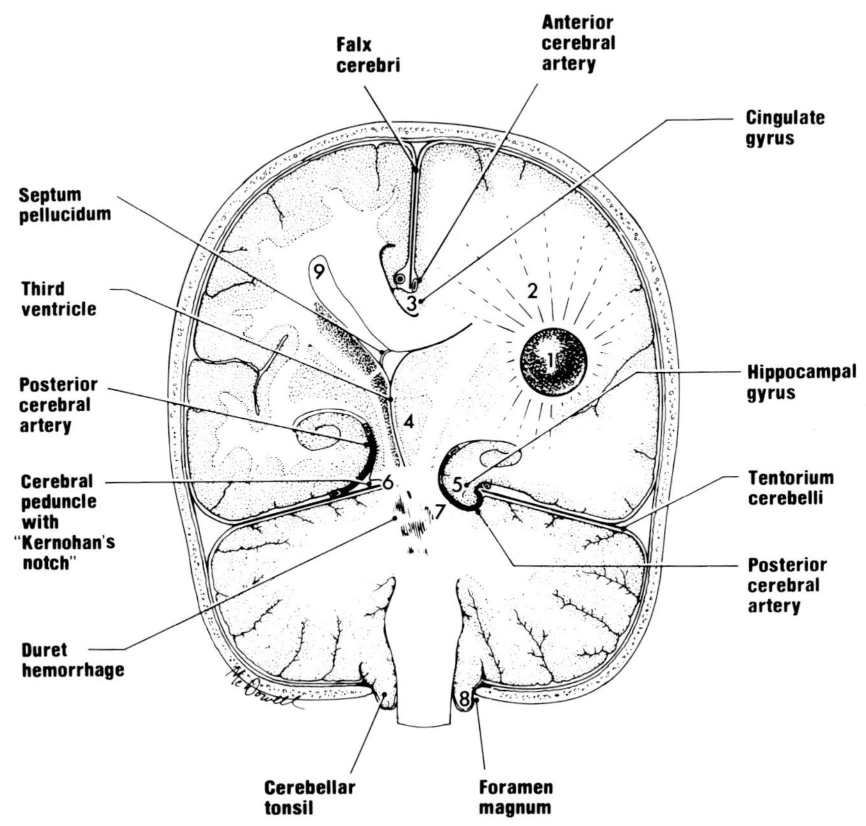

Figure 1–3. This schematic coronal section of the brain enclosed in the skull illustrates the changes caused by a large brain metastasis and why neuro-oncologic problems are unique. The lesion itself (1 [black sphere]) underlies the arm area of the motor strip and causes weakness of the contralateral arm. The edema (2) surrounding the metastasis involves most of the motor area and is likely to cause a contralateral hemiplegia. Because of the size of the brain metastasis and the surrounding edema, the normal brain shifts, compressing itself and other normal brain areas. Herniation of the cingulate gyrus (3) under the falx cerebri compresses not only the contralateral frontal lobe but also the anterior cerebral arteries. Such herniation can cause bilateral frontal ischemia, with weak legs, urinary incontinence, and mental changes. The diencephalon (4) shifts toward the contralateral side, compressing itself, the third ventricle, and the opposite diencephalon. The resulting diencephalic dysfunction causes diminished consciousness. Herniation of the uncus and hippocampal gyrus (5) of the temporal lobe into the tentorial notch compresses the posterior cerebral artery, leading to infarction in the ipsilateral occipital lobe. Uncal herniation also stretches the ipsilateral oculomotor nerve and compresses the brainstem and diencephalon, causing changes in the state of consciousness. Compression of the opposite cerebral peduncle (6) against the tentorium causes a hemiparesis that is ipsilateral to the side of the lesion (a false localizing sign). Downward displacement of the brainstem (7) alters consciousness and may cause midbrain and pontine hemorrhages (Duret hemorrhages). Herniation of the cerebellar tonsils (8) through the foramen magnum compresses the lower brainstem and may cause respiratory arrest. Hydrocephalus (9) occurs in the contralateral lateral ventricle as a result of obstruction of the third ventricle and Sylvian aqueduct by compression. Any combination of the mechanisms illustrated in this figure may play a role in producing the symptoms caused by a brain metastasis. (Adapted from Cairncross and Posner,[365] p 75.)

The clinical implication is that nervous system damage by metastatic cancer or by its treatment (see Chapters 12 to 14) may be irreversible, even if the treatment effectively destroys the tumor. This failure of the damaged nervous system to regenerate puts the onus on the physician to make the diagnosis early and to treat vigorously, while the nervous system can still be salvaged.

Research Is Essential

As I indicate in this book, even though diagnostic and therapeutic endeavors in neuro-oncology have advanced, treatment is still mostly unsatisfactory. In every area of neuro-oncology, treatment needs major improvements, which are likely to come only through research.

This book is concerned primarily with the diagnosis and treatment of neurologic complications of cancer and is addressed to the clinician, not the scientist. However, clinicians play an important role in fostering research.[715,917] Controlled trials of promising treatments are still the major hope for progress. These trials should be coupled with laboratory programs that investigate the biology of neuro-oncologic problems at the cellular and molecular levels. Such therapeutic research is difficult and often frustrating. Too few patients enter into investigative treatment protocols even when they are available. Farrar[755] estimates that only 2.5% of patients with systemic cancer are currently entered into therapeutic protocols, and Mahaley and colleagues[1648] estimate that only 8% of patients with malignant gliomas are enrolled in protocol studies. These percentages are low despite the evidence that patients who are entered into protocol treatments generally live longer and do better than patients who are not[1648,2499,2499a] and, while doing better, they advance the field and provide therapeutic answers. We physicians make an ethical judgment about clinical research every time we see a patient,[166] even when we choose not to offer a research program. As Eisenberg[715] points out, "not to act is to act."

Relationships Between the Brain and Systemic Cancer Are Biologically Important

Recent evidence indicates a reciprocal relationship between systemic cancer and brain function, a fascinating area for neuro-oncologic investigation. The field of psychoneuroimmunology provides evidence for the effect of the nervous system on the cancer and its metastases[305] and on the treatment of cancer.[282] In experimental animals, appropriately delivered stress can increase the incidence, growth rate, and likelihood of metastases,[924] presumably through alterations of immune system function. In humans, no substantial evidence is available yet to support the belief that patients can either prevent cancer or treat an established cancer effectively by the psychological or behavioral techniques of relaxation, biofeedback, and imagery. Reports that such techniques prolong life in patients with cancer are conflicting.[124,897,2470] Alterations of behavior, such as cessation of smoking and improvement of diet, are another matter. The widespread belief among laypersons that depressive symptoms predispose to cancer appears to be without merit.[2905]

The brain also may interfere with the treatment of cancer. Anticipatory nausea and vomiting is an obvious example of classic conditioning in human beings. The phenomenon, which affects about 20% of patients on chemotherapy, can be severe enough that the patient becomes nauseated and may begin to vomit upon entering the hospital, smelling alcohol, or beginning an intravenous infusion, even before the chemotherapeutic agent is added.[282] Because some patients are so severely affected, they abandon therapy.

An opposite relationship—that is, the effect of cancer on the nervous system—is the focus of this book. The literature abounds with examples of small and occult cancers that cause major changes in behavior and neurologic function by mechanisms that are not clearly established. Limbic encephalitis (see Chapter 15) associated with small-cell lung cancer causes severe memory loss when the cancer is small and restricted to the lung and mediastinum and is often not detectable by diagnostic techniques including CT scans.

CLASSIFICATION OF NEURO-ONCOLOGIC DISORDERS

The list of reasons given above dictates that neurologic complications of systemic cancer deserve the serious attention of physicians, both neurologists and nonneurologists who manage patients with cancer, and of neuroscientists interested in the effects of the body on the brain and the brain on the body. The first step in studying neurologic complications of cancer is to classify the ways in which a cancer may affect the nervous system (Table 1–6). This classification also serves to outline the detailed presentation of neurologic complications of systemic cancer in the subsequent chapters of this book.

Table 1–6. **CLASSIFICATION OF NEUROLOGIC COMPLICATIONS OF CANCER**

I. SPREAD OF CANCER TO THE NERVOUS SYSTEM (Metastatic or Direct Effects of Cancer)
   A. Intracranial
   B. Spinal
   C. Leptomeningeal
   D. Nerves (cranial nerves, peripheral nerves, nerve plexuses, or nerve roots)
   E. Muscle (rare)
II. INDIRECT NEUROLOGIC COMPLICATIONS OF CANCER (Nonmetastatic or Paraneoplastic)
   A. Vascular disorders
   B. Infections
   C. Metabolic and nutritional disorders
   D. Side effects of therapy
      1. Chemotherapy
      2. Radiation therapy
      3. Surgery and other diagnostic or therapeutic procedures
   E. "Remote" or paraneoplastic syndromes

Nervous system complications can be divided into two groups: (1) those caused by direct spread of cancer to the nervous system and (2) those in which the symptoms are an indirect effect of the cancer (nonmetastatic or paraneoplastic effects).

Spread of Cancer to the Nervous System (Metastatic or Direct Effects of Cancer)

The direct neurologic complications of systemic cancer can be subdivided into the anatomic area affected: intracranial (see Chapter 5), spinal (see Chapter 6), leptomeningeal (see Chapter 7), nerve root or plexus (see Chapter 8), and muscle (see Chapter 8). A given patient can, of course, have metastases to more than one region of the nervous system, often complicating both the diagnosis and the therapy.

The classification by anatomic area is useful because the diagnostic evaluation, the therapeutic approach, and even the pathophysiology of signs and symptoms are different for each area. For example, most intracranial metastases occupy the brain parenchyma, causing symptoms partly by replacing brain tissue and partly by shifts of brain structures caused by the tumor and its surrounding edema. By contrast, most spinal metastases are extradural and do not invade the substance of the spinal cord. Instead, they cause symptoms primarily by compression. Leptomeningeal metastases often appear as a microscopic sheet of tumor cells within the leptomeninges, neither invading nor compressing the parenchyma of the brain or spinal cord. Symptom production sometimes results simply from obstruction of cerebrospinal fluid pathways, leading to hydrocephalus. Cranial and peripheral nerve dysfunction caused by extradural tumors is usually compressive, whereas intradurally, the nerves are more likely to be invaded.

The laboratory evaluation also differs among the groups. For example, lumbar puncture is unhelpful and sometimes dangerous in the evaluation of intracranial or spinal metastases (see Chapter 14), whereas it is vital to the evaluation of leptomeningeal disease (see Chapter 7). Conversely, CT and MR scans are more helpful to diagnose intracranial and spinal metastases than leptomeningeal disease.

The therapy of metastatic disease obviously depends on an accurate diagnosis of the anatomic area involved. Not only must the radiation oncologist know where to draw the radiation portals, but also he or she must know that the principles of treatment vary with the locus of the lesion. For example, delaying RT of brain metastases for 48 to 72 hours after diagnosis to allow steroids to effect dramatic improvement will make the patient better able to tolerate RT. On the other hand, except for pain relief, steroids have been only modestly effective in ameliorating the symptoms of spinal cord compression. Although high-dose steroids are used at MSKCC for spinal cord compression, RT is begun immediately as an emergency measure (see Chapter 6).

Indirect Neurologic (Nonmetastatic or Paraneoplastic) Complications of Systemic Cancer

Indirect neurologic complications of systemic cancer can be divided into five subgroups based on etiology. The pathophysiology, diagnosis, and management of these subgroups will be considered consecutively in Chapters 9 through 15.

VASCULAR DISORDERS

Cerebral vascular disease frequently complicates systemic cancer. Most patients with cancer have measurable coagulation disorders (see Chapter 9). Intracranial or spinal hemorrhage can occur when patients become thrombocytopenic or if other clotting disorders develop. An intracranial subdural hematoma represents a potentially lethal but treatable complication of thrombocytopenia found occasionally in patients with cancer. Hemorrhage into a metastatic brain tumor may be the first symptom of cancer or the first symptom of brain disease in a patient known to have cancer. Certain metastatic tumors, such as melanoma and choriocarcinoma, are frequent causes of intracerebral hemorrhage, but any metastatic tumor may bleed. Cerebral infarction occurs in patients with cancer, but the causes of cerebral infarction in the cancer population differ from those in the general population. Atherosclerotic cerebral thrombosis and emboli from atherosclerotic plaques in the carotid are common causes of stroke in the general population. They are less common in patients with cancer because cerebral atherosclerosis is less pronounced in these patients than in the general population. In patients with cancer, nonbacterial thrombotic endocarditis or tumor emboli are more common sources of emboli than a carotid plaque. Small-vessel occlusion is more likely to occur as a result of hypercoagulability than of atherosclerosis. Occlusion of the dural sinuses is a more common cause of symptoms in patients with cancer, particularly those with leukemias and lymphomas, than it is in the noncancer population.

INFECTIONS

The organisms that cause CNS infections differ from those encountered in a general hospital and occur in patients with cancer whose immune responses are abnormal as a consequence of the malignancy or its chemotherapy (see Chapter 10). The most common causes of meningitis are *Listeria monocytogenes* and *Cryptococcus neoformans*. Pneumococcal meningitis is less common, and meningococcal or *Haemophilus influenzae* meningitis is rare. Brain abscesses are usually caused by fungi, such as mucormycosis or aspergillosis; by parasites, such as toxoplasmosis; or by unusual bacterial organisms, such as nocardia, rather than by the bacterial organisms that cause infection in the general population. Viral encephalitis is more likely to be caused by herpes zoster or JC virus (progressive multifocal leukoencephalopathy) than by the more common herpes simplex virus. In patients with CNS infections related to cancer, knowledge of the underlying primary tumor and of the patient's immune status often allows the physician to predict not only whether CNS infection is causing the symptoms, but also which organism is most likely to be involved.

METABOLIC AND NUTRITIONAL DISORDERS

Metabolic encephalopathy is a common cause of neurologic symptoms in patients with widespread cancer (see Chapter 11). Many individual causes of metabolic encephalopathy in patients with cancer, including hypoxia, vital organ failure, and electrolyte abnormalities (particularly hypercalcemia), are similar to those found on a general hospital ward. Other causes, such as iatrogenically induced opioid overdose, are not usually encountered on general hospital wards. Some unusual causes of metabolic brain disease, such as radiation-induced thyroid failure, must always be considered in appropriate patients to avoid overlooking a treatable illness.

SIDE EFFECTS OF CANCER THERAPY

The increase in CNS metastatic disease, which some observers believe has occurred as a result of effective systemic chemotherapy and immunotherapy, can be considered a complication of cancer treatment. More direct complications include those that arise from surgery around the head, neck, or spine (see Chapter 14); those that are caused by irradiation of the brain, spinal cord, or peripheral nerves (see Chapter 13); and those that result from chemotherapy, whether given systemically or intrathecally (see Chapter 12). New chemotherapeutic agents, with new and differing nervous system toxicity, seem to appear almost monthly. RT combined with certain chemotherapeutic agents may lead to synergistic toxicity even when the doses of the individual agents are delivered within a safe range.

"REMOTE EFFECTS" OR PARANEOPLASTIC SYNDROMES

Although all nonmetastatic complications of cancer can be considered "paraneoplastic," the term "paraneoplastic syndrome" is usually reserved for a rare but interesting group of disorders that may have an autoimmune pathogenesis (see Chapter 15). Even though they are rare, paraneoplastic syndromes are important for two reasons: (1) In

Table 1–7. **NEUROLOGIC COMPLICATIONS BY SITE IN PATIENTS WITH CANCER**

Site	Neurologic Problem
Brain	Metastasis
	Leptomeningeal metastasis
	Metabolic and toxic encephalopathy
	Infection (meningitis, brain abscess)
	Radiation encephalopathy
	Cerebral hemorrhage or infarction
	Paraneoplastic (limbic encephalopathy)
Spinal cord and cauda equina	Epidural compression
	Leptomeningeal metastasis (intradural compression, cord infiltration, root infiltration)
	Intramedullary metastasis
	Epidural abscess or hematoma
	Radiation myelopathy
	Myelopathy following intrathecal chemotherapy
	Paraneoplastic myelopathy
Cranial and peripheral nerve	Extrinsic compression by tumor or other mass (e.g., hematoma)
	Direct infiltration by tumor
	Drug toxicity
	Varicella zoster infection
	Radiation plexopathy
	Paraneoplastic neuropathy
Neuromuscular junction	Drugs (aminoglycoside antibiotics)
	Paraneoplastic disorders (Eaton-Lambert myasthenic syndrome, myasthenia gravis)
Muscle	Corticosteroid-induced myopathy
	Cachectic myopathy
	Paraneoplastic polymyositis or dermatomyositis

Source: Adapted from Henson and Posner,[1141] p 2269.

one-half to two-thirds of affected patients, neurologic symptoms develop before the cancer is apparent and, if recognized, particular neurologic syndromes may lead to a fruitful search for an occult and potentially curable cancer. (2) Although their etiology is presently unknown, they hint at a relationship between the brain and cancer which, if explored, may enhance knowledge of the biochemistry both of the brain and of the cancer.

CLASSIFICATION BY SITE OF LESION

Many patients with disorders described above present with clinical symptoms that are similar to each other. For example, parenchymal brain metastases, leptomeningeal metastases, and metabolic encephalopathy can all appear as delirium, pointing to the brain as the site of the lesion but giving no clue as to the nature of the lesion. Similarly, patients with epidural spinal cord compression, radiation-induced myelopathy, and paraneoplastic myelopathy can all present with similar symptoms, pointing to spinal cord dysfunction. Because such situations arise commonly in neuro-oncology, it is often useful for the physician first to determine the site of the lesion and then to consider the various neuro-oncologic disorders that may cause such a lesion. This approach is outlined in Table 1–7, which lists the common causes of neuro-oncologic disorders localized to specific portions of the central and peripheral nervous system.

CHAPTER 2

PATHOPHYSIOLOGY OF METASTASES TO THE NERVOUS SYSTEM

Many neurologic complications of cancer occur when tumor invades or compresses the nervous system. In our own studies of 851 neurologically affected patients with cancer, symptoms were a direct result of tumor involving the nervous system in 383 (45%); the other 468 (55%) suffered from either nonmetastatic complications of cancer or neurologic problems unrelated to the cancer.[461]

As shown in Table 2–1, cancer reaches the nervous system either by *metastasis* or by *direct extension*. Metastasis has three mechanisms: hematogenous dissemination (the usual mechanism of brain metastases), lymphatic dissemination (because the CNS does not contain lymphatics, this mechanism applies primarily to peripheral nervous structures), and dissemination through body fluids such as the cerebrospinal fluid (CSF) (the mechanism for leptomeningeal dissemination of tumor). By direct extension, a skull tumor, for example, may grow to compress or invade the nervous system; a breast tumor may metastasize to a lymph node that, in turn, may compress neural structures; a metastasis to the skull or vertebral body may compress the brain or spinal cord; or certain neurotrophic tumors may invade nerves of the organ in which the primary tumor arose and grow within the perineural sheath.[463]

Table 2–1. **HOW CANCER SPREADS TO THE NERVOUS SYSTEM**

Mode	Example
Metastasis	
• Hematogenous	Brain metastasis
• Lymphatics	Perineural lymphatics → leptomeninges
• Body fluids	Leptomeningeal metastasis ("drop metastases") from brain metastasis
Direct Extension	
• From tumor itself	Pancoast tumor → brachial plexus
• From lymph node	Breast cancer nodes → brachial plexus
• From a metastasis	Skull metastases → brain
• Perineural growth	Neurotropic tumor → leptomeninges

Metastases are a major cause of neurologic disability in patients with cancer and are often a direct cause of death when they affect the CNS. Unlike primary brain tumors (e.g., glioblastoma), which cause death as a direct result of local tumor growth, most primary cancers elsewhere can be locally controlled by surgery or other therapy; death occurs only if the tumor metastasizes.

PATHOPHYSIOLOGY OF THE METASTATIC PROCESS

Metastasis is a complicated pathophysiologic process that is not yet completely understood. Table 2–2 presents an overview of this process, which requires cells to behave substantially differently from normal cells to circumvent several bodily defenses. So many steps are involved in metastasis that only a small number of tumor cells ever complete this difficult and arduous process. Indeed, it is surprising that any cells possess the necessary multifaceted capacity for metastasis, each step of which, according to current evidence, is controlled by more than one gene.[108,2507] This chapter describes certain aspects of the metastatic pathogenesis relevant to neuro-oncology. Recent reviews* detail the complex processes involved in metastatic spread.

*References 108, 242, 776, 779, 1102, 1575, 1891, 1893, 2115, 2507.

Transformation and Growth

The development of a cancer is a complicated process involving a series of steps in which tumor suppressor genes are down-regulated or deleted and oncogenes are activated.[108,2507] Multiple mutations induce metastatogenic clones that are phenotypically and functionally distinct from nonmetastatic but transformed (i.e., cancer) cells.[1680] Cancers are heterogeneous; about 15% of cancer cells have metastatic potential, but most do not. Furthermore, metastatic clones probably arise from nonmetastatic tumor clones, indicating that the metastatic phenotype develops later than transformation. Among the many factors determining metastatic potential are aberrant expressions of dominant and regulatory genes, including:

1. Increased expression of the oncogene products N-*myc*, L-*myc*; eosinophil chemotactic factor receptors C-*myc*, C-*jun*; and HER-2/*neu*.[1182,2707a]
2. Ectopic expression of enzymes involved in the metastatic cascade,[1058] including heparinase, collagenase, proteases, and plasminogen activation.
3. Suppression of class I major histocompatibility complex (MHC) protein.[501,2656a]
4. Mutations in suppressor genes, such as *p53*, *Rb*, and *nm23*.[2479] The gene *nm23* encodes proteins with nucleoside diphosphate kinase enzymatic activity, and the presence of *nm23*-H1 allelic deletions correlates with the likelihood of distant metastases in colorectal

Table 2–2. **SEQUENCE OF EVENTS IN THE METASTATIC CASCADE**

Metastatic Cascade Event	Potential Mechanisms
Premetastatic Steps	
Tumor initiation	Carcinogenic insult, oncogene activation
Promotion and progression	Genetic instability, gene amplification
Uncontrolled proliferation	Autocrine growth factors, hormone receptors
Metastatic Steps	
Angiogenesis	Angiogenin; heparin-binding proteins; other growth factors
Invasion of local tissues	Chemoattractants, autocrine motility factors, attachment receptors, degradative enzymes
Circulating tumor cell arrest and extravasation	Tumor cell aggregation
Adherence to endothelium	Tumor cell interaction with fibrin, platelets, and RDG* type receptors
Retraction of endothelium	Platelet and tumor cell factors
Adhesion to basement membrane	Laminin and thrombospondin receptors
Dissolution of basement membrane	Type IV collagenase, other proteases
Locomotion	Autocrine motility factors, chemotaxis factors
Colony Formation at Secondary Site	Receptors for local tissue growth factors, angiogenesis factors
Evasion of Host Defenses and Resistance to Therapy	Tumor antigen modulation, amplification of drug resistance genes, production of immunosuppressive factor (e.g., TGFβ†)

* RDG = peptide recognition site for integrin binding (Arg-Gly-Asp).
† Transforming growth factor β.
Source: From Liotta,[1573] p 5, with permission.

cancer.[474] This suppressor gene also appears to be down-regulated in melanomas and human breast cancers with metastatic potential.

5. Alteration of calcium-mediated signal transduction. Recent evidence suggests that inhibiting stimulated calcium influx into tumor cells may suppress growth and dissemination of cancer cells.[478]
6. Expression of CD44R1 adhesion molecules appears to promote colon carcinoma metastasis[2058a,2549] while antibodies against the metastasis-specific domain prevent metastases.[2355]
7. Loss of angiogenesis inhibition perhaps related to loss or mutations of *p53*.[556a]

Within metastatic empowered tumors are clones with a predilection for particular organs of the body (see the following).

Vascularization

Metastasis depends on growth of the primary tumor. To grow beyond 1 to 2 mm^3, a tumor requires an adequate blood supply. Neoplasms ensure themselves of this blood supply by promoting new vessel formation facilitated by "tumor angiogenesis factors."[2773b] Tumor angiogenesis is important for growth of both the primary tumor and its metastases. Folkman and colleagues[808,809] have shown that tumors implanted in the anterior chamber of the eye grow only to 1 mm^3 unless they contact the cornea, ciliary body, or other tissue from which they can grow a capillary bed. Tumors grow slowly at a linear rate before neovascularization but switch to exponential growth after vascularization.

The development of a new capillary bed is

particularly important in the CNS because, as metastases grow within the substance of the brain or spinal cord, they vascularize themselves with capillaries that differ from normal brain vessels. These neovessels have a fenestrated rather than continuous endothelial surface; the cells also lack tight junctions. Thus, newly vascularized metastases have an absent or deficient blood–brain barrier (see Chapter 3).

Angiogenesis is not only required for tumor growth but also permits the newly formed vessels to shed tumor cells into the bloodstream, promoting additional metastasis (Fig. 2–1). The degree of angiogenesis in a tumor, as measured by vessel count and density, correlates with the likelihood of metastasis.[1632] Tumor angiogenesis requires several chemical factors, including tumor angiogenesis factor,[809] fibroblast growth factors (FGFs), or transforming growth factors (TGFs) derived from either normal or neoplastic cells, and perhaps heparin because tumor angiogenesis is inhibited by protamine.[809] Angiogenic factors belonging to the FGF family are stored in the basement membrane of blood vessels. Metastatic tumor cells secrete heparinase that may serve to release FGF.[1058] The brain is enriched in FGF and other growth factors, but whether these factors play a role in CNS metastasis is unknown. A combination of high-dose corticosteroids and heparin is reported to inhibit angiogenesis and decrease metastasis.[808] Heparin also augments the antimetastatic activity of interferon and tumor necrosis fac-

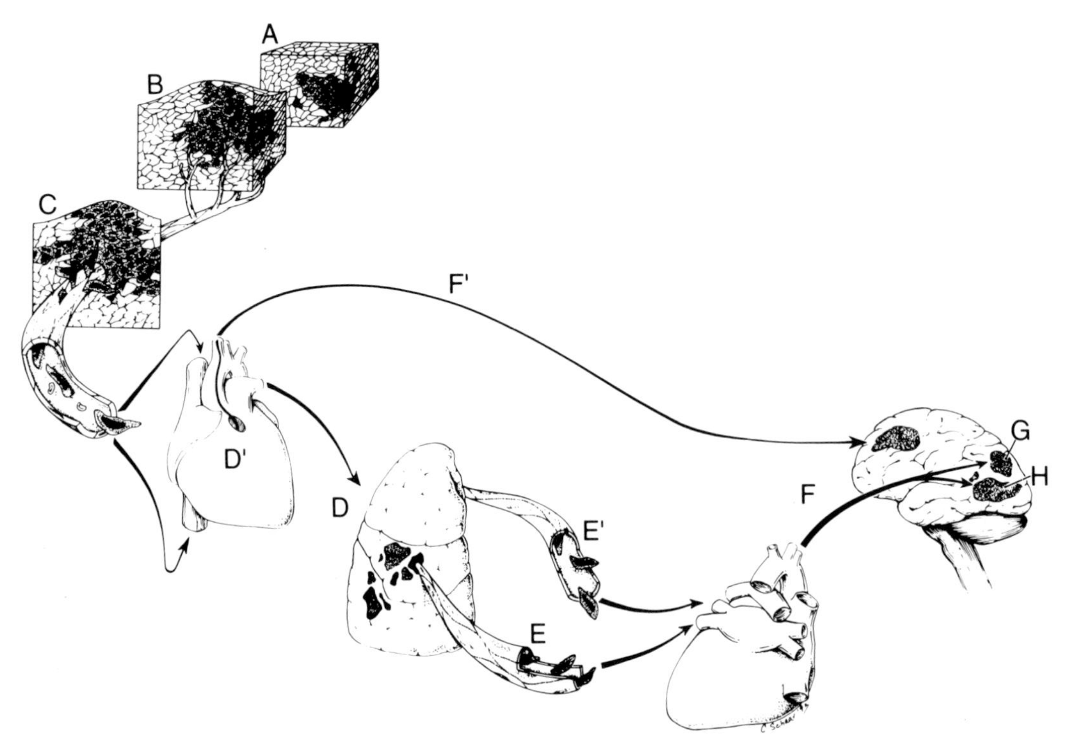

Figure 2–1. Pathophysiology of the metastatic process. Metastasis is a multistep process. In this schematic illustration, a malignant neoplasm arises in an organ distant from the central nervous system (CNS). (A) As it grows, it develops its own vascular supply. (B) Clones of malignant cells with metastatic potential enter blood or lymph channels and eventually reach the venous circulation. (C) The malignant cells enter the right heart with the venous circulation and either exit through the pulmonary artery to the lung (D) or cross a patent foramen ovale (D′) to enter the systemic circulation. Most tumors that enter the lung either arrest in the pulmonary capillary bed, grow as pulmonary metastases and subsequently seed the pulmonary venous circulation, or (E), alternately, traverse the pulmonary vascular bed without arresting (E′) to enter the pulmonary venous circulation. Malignant clones in the pulmonary venous circulation then enter the left heart and exit into the systemic circulation (F), along with those cells that may have crossed a patent foramen ovale (F′). Once in the systemic circulation, the likelihood of entering the cerebral circulation is high because, in the resting state, 15% to 20% of cardiac output supplies the CNS. (G, H) Tumor cells entering the cerebral circulation must then arrest in brain capillaries or venules, cross the vessel wall, and grow within the brain.

tor. Ingber and associates[1244] have reported synthesis of a family of angiogenesis inhibitors that are analogs of a naturally secreted fungal antibiotic, although their clinical role, if any, is as yet unknown.

Invasion

Before the vascularized primary tumor can spread, it must invade the host tissue in which it arose. Aznavoorian and colleagues[108] and Liotta and Kohn[1575] have described invasion as having three major steps: (1) tumor cell attachment to the matrix, promoted by specific attachment factors such as laminin, forming a bridge between the cell-surface laminin receptor and collagen of the host; (2) degradation of the matrix by tumor enzymes,[2491] and (3) locomotion, probably influenced by chemotactic factors.

Transport

Once the cells invade and detach, they must find a route to other tissues. Two important routes of metastatic spread are via the lymphatics and the vascular system. (Direct spread can occur via body fluids or along nerves; see Table 2–1.) The importance of vascular and lymphatic invasion to the development of metastases is emphasized by Freedman and coworkers,[834] whose work indicates that both vascular and lymphatic invasion are independently and significantly associated with risk of relapse. The lymphatic mode of spread is probably important in the peripheral nervous system (e.g., when the brachial plexus is involved by metastatic tumor from the lung or breast), but, because the CNS has no lymphatics, hematogenous spread is far more important in considering most metastatic neurologic complications of cancer. Separation of these two modes of spread is rather arbitrary because the blood and lymph systems are linked; lymphatic invasion can lead to the vascular system via venous-lymphatic anastomoses or via the thoracic duct. Batson's venous plexus probably is important in disseminating tumor cells to the vertebral bodies and skull (Fig. 2–2).[164,600]

Most tumor cells that reach the bloodstream die because physical (e.g., vascular turbulence), chemical, and immune factors kill them. Lethal deformation of large tumor cells in the microcirculation with surface membrane rupture also limits metastases.[2781] Probably fewer than 0.1% of cancer cells escaping into the circulation ever develop into metastases.[1574,2780] Studies of patients undergoing peritoneal-venous shunts to alleviate abdominal pain and distention from malignant ascites indicate that, although large numbers of malignant cells are introduced directly into the circulation, metastatic spread to other organs is uncommon, and, when metastasis does develop, it is often not in the first capillary network encountered.[2553] A similar situation occurs when cerebroventricular-peritoneal shunts are performed for the alleviation of hydrocephalus caused by either brain or leptomeningeal tumors. Seeding of the peritoneal cavity by the malignancy rarely occurs after ventriculoperitoneal shunting for leptomeningeal metastases and is almost never a clinical problem. Only rarely do clinically symptomatic metastases to the peritoneal cavity from medulloblastoma follow shunting when the CNS tumor is quiescent. Shunted tumor cells fail to seed the peritoneum because host-cell–to–tumor-cell recognition factors are lacking. Furthermore, the presence of tumor cells in the circulation does not indicate a poorer prognosis than the absence of tumor cells.

A few circulating tumor cells survive both physical destruction and identification and destruction by the host immune system,[501,762,894,2656a] in part because defective expression of MHC on their surface prevents their recognition by the immune system.[762] Tumors with metastatic potential are less likely to express class I MHC proteins than are nonmetastatic tumor cells. Likewise, metastases are usually MHC class I negative, whereas the primary tumor is usually positive.[501] Resistance to attack by natural killer cells also appears to aid survival of tumor cells in the circulation.[952]

Arrest

For a metastasis to develop, the tumor cells that survive the hazardous journey through

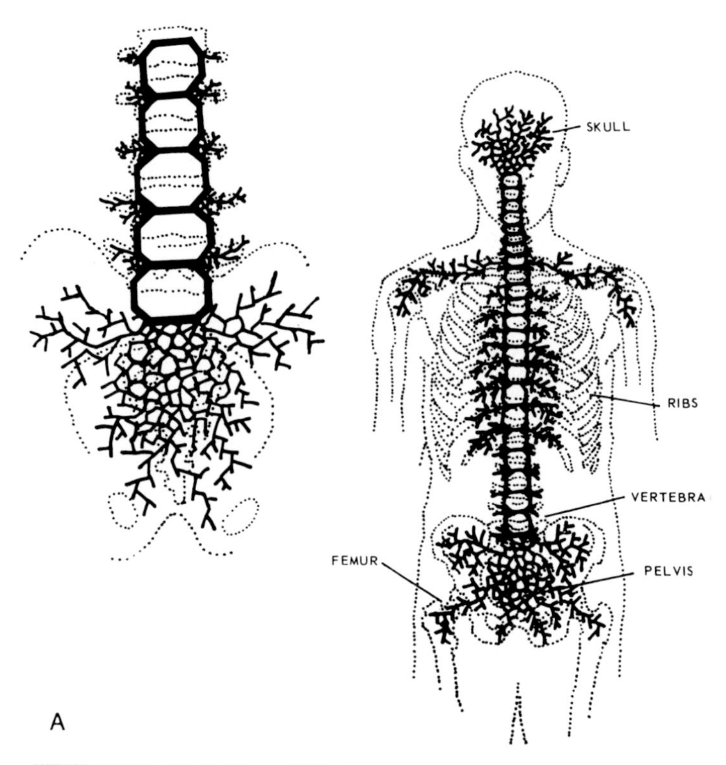

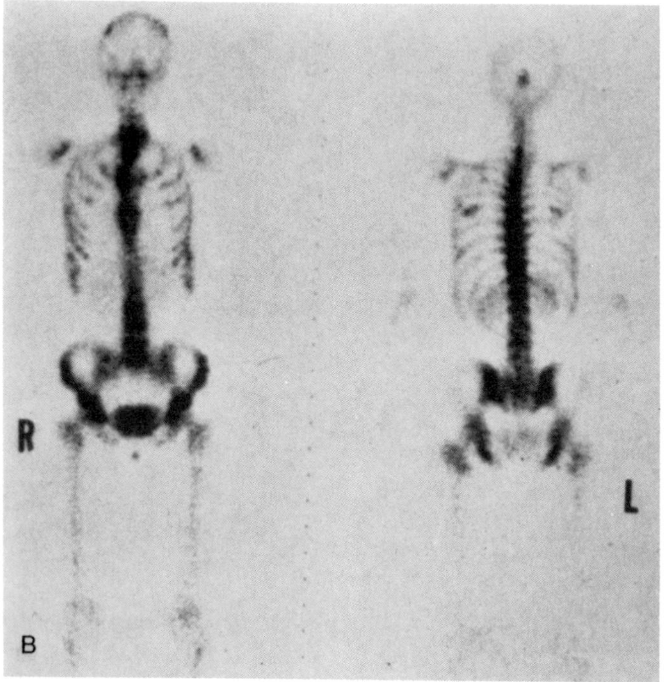

Figure 2–2. *A,* The vertebral venous system is a two-way thoroughfare frequently used by carcinoma of the prostate, breast, adrenal glands, and other types of cancer. (From del Regato,[600] p 36, with permission.) *B,* This bone scan of a patient with prostate carcinoma illustrates widespread metastases in vertebral bodies and other areas supplied by Batson's plexus. Virtually no metastases are observed in the axial skeleton and only a few in the skull. Parenchymal metastases were absent.

the vasculature must arrest on the vascular endothelium of the capillary bed of the organ in which they will eventually grow. They then must extravasate through the capillary and its basement membrane. Several factors influence the likelihood that a cancer cell will arrest in a capillary bed and adhere to the vascular endothelium.[2782] One important factor is thrombus formation. Arresting tumor cells secrete factors that cause platelet aggregation and intravascular thrombus formation. These factors activate platelets to secrete heparinase, widening endothelial gaps to enable invasion through the capillary wall.[1058] Platelets[1343] and fibrin both assist the cancer cell's adherence to the capillary wall. For a metastasis to be successful, a fibrin clot must protect it from circulation.[2747,2752] Experimental evidence indicates that anticoagulation with heparin or warfarin inhibits the formation of metastasis by injected tumor cells[484] and that glucocorticoids given as a single agent facilitate metastases[777] (but see reference 810). Prostacyclin may also inhibit metastases by anti-aggregatory effects on platelets.[2318] Anticoagulants appear to have little effect on human cancer metastases,[2883] however, and, although warfarin[416] and heparin[1489] may enhance survival in lung cancer, aspirin does not.[1488] Although the clinical implications of these findings are not entirely clear, many patients with cancer are known to be hypercoagulable (see Chapter 9); this state may enhance the tendency for a tumor to metastasize. Also, some reports indicate that tumors in patients with cancer who receive corticosteroids tend to metastasize to sites rarely selected in patients not receiving steroids.[1103,2382] It is not known whether the extensive use of glucocorticoids at the relatively high doses that are commonly used to treat patients with CNS metastases promotes further spread of the cancer.

Tumor Emboli

Most tumor emboli are small and do not obstruct vessels that are large enough to produce clinical symptoms. They distribute themselves much like small emboli and, in the brain, are likely to lodge in the watershed areas, that is, at the terminations of major end arteries (watersheds), and also in the gray-white junction where penetrating arterioles first separate into capillary beds (Fig. 2–3). An occasional tumor embolus to the brain is large enough to cause clinical symptoms that resemble a transient ischemic attack or, rarely, a full-blown stroke. If the symptoms clear and the tumor embolus invades the brain, the same symptoms may recur months later from the growing brain metastasis (see Chapter 5).

Extravasation and Growth

Experimental evidence indicates that adhesion of tumor cells to venular endothelium or the underlying basement membrane of specific organs plays a major role in site-specific tumor metastases. Tumor emboli can be trapped nonspecifically in capillaries of an organ, or the tumor cells may react with organ-specific receptors on endothelium and the underlying basement membrane.[1891] Tumors that attach specifically to capillary endothelium and venules are more likely to develop into metastases than those that lodge nonspecifically in capillaries. Furthermore, clumped tumor cells are more likely to become metastases than are single tumor cells because cells in the center of the embolus are protected from physical or immunologic destruction during the hazardous journey through the body's vasculature.

When a tumor clump causes a metastasis, that metastasis usually arises from a single cell within that clump.[778] Once the tumor cells have insinuated themselves between endothelial cells, they cross the basement membrane to reach the organ in which they choose to grow.[1347] A few hours or days after tumor cells are injected into the carotid artery, the cells form pseudopodia in regions facing the endothelial cells. The cytoplasm of the tumor cells and its projections completely breach the endothelial cells, resulting in exposure of the underlying basal lamina. The tumor cells then push the endothelial cells aside and attach directly to the basal lamina. They produce small pores into which the cytoplasmic projections are thrust, and the entire cell then streams into the extracellular space.

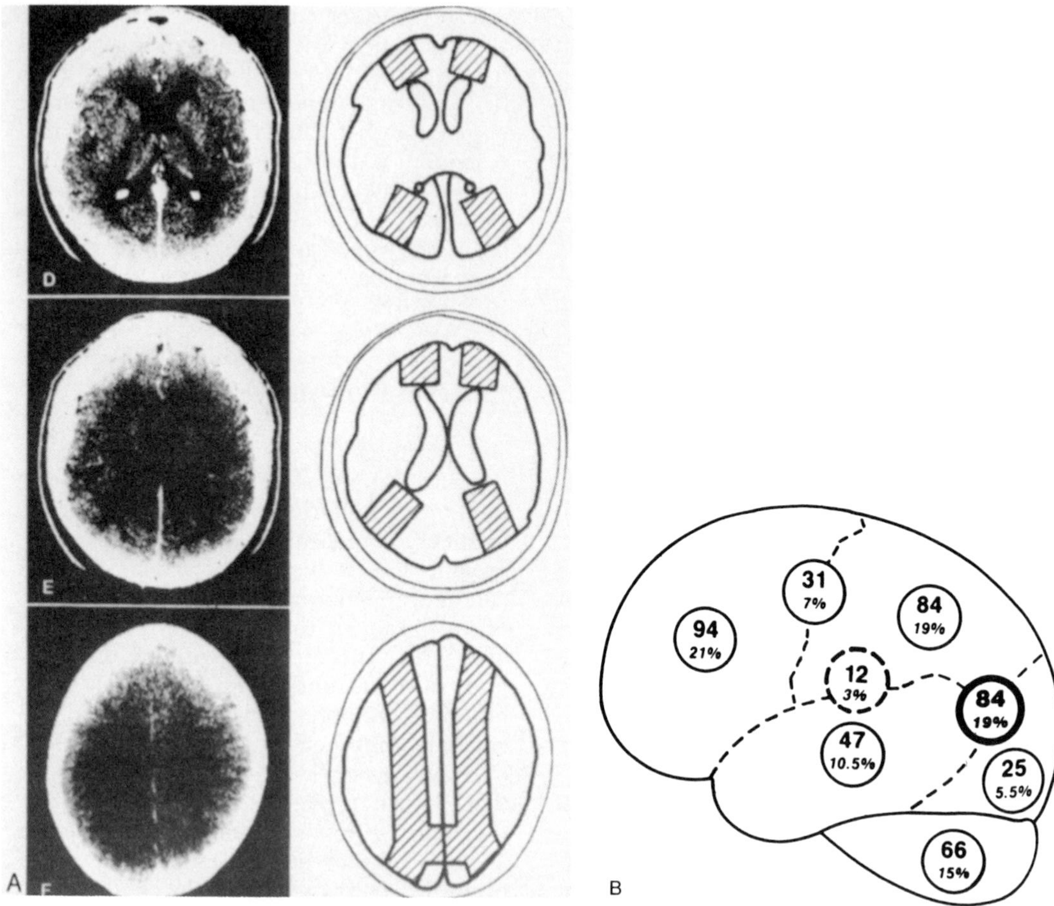

Figure 2–3. Distribution of brain metastases to watershed areas of brain. *A*, Lesions noted on computed tomographic (CT) scans were mapped and schematic representations were made of distal arterial fields in similar planes. Only three of six sections (D, E, and F) are shown. (From Toole,[2597] p 139, with permission.) *B*, Distribution of metastases noted on CT scan. There was a total of 443 metastases in 256 patients who each had fewer than five metastases. The *bold circle* indicates the overrepresentation of metastases in the watershed area between the middle and posterior cerebral arteries. There was also overrepresentation in the anterior border zone between the anterior and middle cerebral arteries. (From Delattre et al,[605] p 742, with permission.)

Despite the fact that the metastasis has a clonal origin, heterogeneity rapidly develops as the metastatic tumor grows, owing to mutations of the rapidly growing and genetically unstable tumor cells. Thus, in a patient with multiple metastases, each metastatic tumor may have arisen from a different clone within the primary tumor and may become even more heterogeneous as it grows, causing differential sensitivity to chemotherapeutic agents.[778]

Insinuation of tumor cells into the perivascular capillary space of an organ does not necessarily imply that a metastasis will develop; the number of cells that reach the pericapillary space of an organ far exceeds the actual number of metastases that eventually develop there.[932]

Organ-specific or tissue-specific growth or "repair" factors that are stimulated by tissue damage (e.g., trauma or ischemia) may promote tumor growth,[617] as may the normal organ-specific matrix,[1416] possibly explaining the observations that brain or spinal metastases are sometimes found at the site of prior CNS damage, considerably complicating the clinical diagnosis. Furthermore, organ-specific growth factors may promote the growth of individual tumor-cell clones that possess those specific growth factor receptors. The abundance of growth factors in brains may be one reason for the frequency of metastasis to that organ.

CLINICAL CONSIDERATIONS RELEVANT TO NERVOUS SYSTEM METASTASIS

Tumor Size

In general, the larger the primary tumor, the more likely it is to metastasize.[1414] Axillary metastases occur in fewer than 25% of women with breast tumors of 1 cm or less in diameter, but occur in 80% of those with tumors larger than 5 cm.[2091] Only 27% of patients with primary breast tumors less than 2.5 cm in diameter develop distant metastases at a median time of 42 months, whereas 92% of patients with primary tumors larger than 8.5 cm in diameter develop such metastases at a median time of 4 months.[2001b] The situation is similar in malignant melanoma. Only 4% of patients with tumors less than 1 mm in thickness develop distant metastases, compared with 72% of patients whose tumors are greater than 4 mm in thickness.[133] Furthermore, strong evidence indicates that local control of a tumor decreases the likelihood of distant metastasis if the local lymph nodes are negative, but local recurrence increases the likelihood, suggesting that the recurrent tumor cells that grow more rapidly and are genetically unstable develop the metastatic phenotype.[1515,1517,2867] Certain very small primary tumors, however (at times too small to be detected by clinical or laboratory tests), do metastasize, and some very large ones (even recurrent ones) do not.[133,2001b]

Properties of Metastases

The proliferative potential of a metastatic brain tumor, as measured by the 5-bromodeoxyuridine labeling index, is often greater than that of the primary tumor from which it arose,[448] accounting for a large brain metastasis from a small lung cancer. In addition, removal of the primary tumor may promote growth of the metastasis. The rate of accelerated growth is a function of the mass of the primary tumor.[247,2001b] Large primary tumors may synthesize more tumor-suppressive substances, which inhibit the growth of both the primary tumor and its metastases, than do smaller tumors.

The physician sometimes is confronted by a patient who has one or more brain metastases and who exhibits no clinical or laboratory evidence of a primary tumor.[2710] Even when patients die of brain metastases, the autopsy does not always disclose the primary site.

Differences Between a Primary Tumor and Its Metastasis

Whether the primary cancer is large or small, only certain cells within the tumor can metastasize to and grow within another organ. Because these cells may differ from the majority of cells in the primary tumor[1818] from which they arose, their biologic behavior, including their response to therapy, may differ from that of the primary tumor. Furthermore, two different metastases to the same or different organs may have different cellular characteristics, such as the presence or absence of estrogen receptors in breast cancer[1504] or the immunophenotype of melanoma metastases.[359] Factors in the host environment may also determine the response of metastases to therapy. Similar clones of tumor cells growing in different organs have different chemosensitivities. In one experiment,[778] a mouse fibrosarcoma implanted into skin or muscle responded to doxorubicin treatment, whereas the same clone of cells in the lung or liver did not,[779a] implying that radiation or chemotherapy that is effective for the primary tumor may not be similarly effective for a brain metastasis, or vice versa.[634]

Site of Metastases

Two major factors determine the site to which a tumor will metastasize: (1) the anatomic distribution of the blood and lymph drainage from the organ harboring the primary tumor (mechanical or hemodynamic hypothesis[744]), and (2) the receptivity of the organ receiving the metastasis (seed and soil hypothesis, or the molecular recognition hypothesis[1967]).

THE MECHANICAL OR HEMODYNAMIC HYPOTHESIS

The anatomy of the lymphatic and venous drainage explains some metastases.[2514] Some metastases arrest in the first capillary or lymph-node bed they encounter. Thus, the anatomy of the breast dictates that the first site of metastasis is often an axillary lymph node draining lymph channels from the breast, with potential compression of the brachial plexus. Another common site is the thoracic spine, reached via venous channels of Batson's plexus,[600] explaining the frequency of thoracic spinal cord compression from breast cancer. Cancer of the right side of the colon spreads via portal circulation to the liver first, but cancer of the left side spreads via systemic circulation to reach the lungs and, subsequently, at times, the brain (Fig. 2–4). Primary tumors of organs other than lung are likely to metastasize to lung first because, after reaching the systemic venous circulation and passing through the heart, the pulmonary capillary bed is the first encountered. Most patients with brain metastases that arise from a nonpulmonary primary cancer have lung metastases as well. Thus, in general, a patient with breast or colon cancer and no lung metastasis is less likely to have a brain metastasis.

Once tumor cells reach the systemic circulation, they are distributed in proportion to the blood supply to an organ. A primary tumor in the lung often causes brain metastasis because the brain receives about 20% of the resting body's cardiac output and, therefore, 20% of circulating tumor cells.

Hemodynamic factors, however, are not the sole determinant, as indicated by the observations that muscles, the largest organ of the body, and kidney, which also has a high blood flow, are rarely the site of metastasis (see the following), whereas the skull, with a low blood flow, is often a site for metastasis. Anatomic factors also do not explain the predilection for breast cancers to metastasize to endocrine organs.[2091] Why, for example, do cutaneous malignant melanoma and bladder cancer spread to the brain, or why are

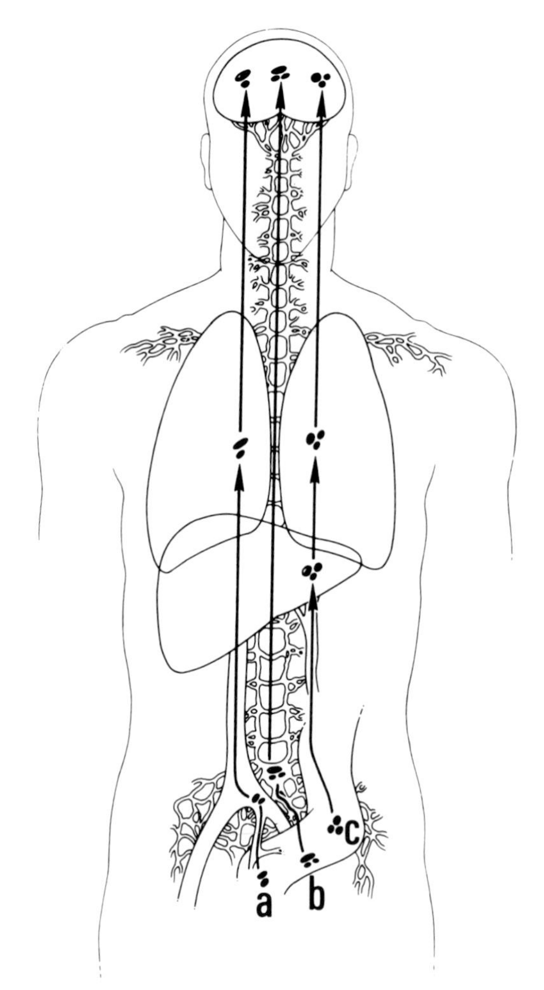

Figure 2–4. The cascade effect of possible routes of hematogenous metastasis of colonic cancer to the brain are (a) via the rectal plexus of veins into the inferior vena cava, bypassing the liver; (b) via Batson's vertebral plexus, bypassing the liver and lungs; (c) via the portal veins to the liver and lung and then the brain. (From Cascino et al,[397] p 207, with permission.)

more than 80% of bone metastases caused by breast, lung, and prostate cancers, which together account for only 42% of all cancers?[2310] The tendency for the axial skeleton, in particular the vertebral bodies, and the skull to be more involved than the appendicular skeleton may be explained by venous drainage through Batson's plexus.[600] The tendency of renal cancers to metastasize to the humerus,[2779] however, and the rarity of metastases to hand and foot bone cannot be explained by the vascular supply alone. In any event, the high frequency of vertebral metastases explains why epidural spinal cord compression (see Chapter 6) is such a common neurologic complication of cancer.

RECEPTIVITY OF THE RECEIVING ORGAN (THE SEED AND SOIL HYPOTHESIS)

The predilection of certain tumors to spread to certain organs involves interactions between the tumor cell itself (seed) and the organ receiving the metastasis (soil).[1891] The host organ may synthesize and secrete factors such as hormones or growth factors that attract certain clones of circulating tumor cells and promote their growth. Clones of tumor cells themselves may have factors on their surface that react with the endothelium of particular organs and allow preferential growth in a particular organ environment.[1892] For example, B16 melanoma will spread to an implanted artificial "organ" that releases lung extract (the organ of preference for that tumor) but not liver extract.[2475]

Subtypes

Specific cancer subtypes tend to spread to different organs.[1891] For example, infiltrating ductal carcinoma of the breast has a predilection to cause parenchymal brain metastasis, whereas infiltrating lobular carcinoma is more likely to affect the leptomeninges.[2445] Metastatic non-Hodgkin's lymphoma has a predilection to spread to the leptomeninges,[2135] but primary lymphomas of the CNS usually cause mass lesions within the brain.[587] Breast cancer often metastasizes either to bone (vertebral bodies) or to the brain, but usually not to both.[2692]

Even within the brain itself, selectivity is evident. Delattre and colleagues[605] found that, although most primary tumors distribute themselves within the brain in a fashion that relates to cerebral vasculature, certain pelvic tumors prefer to metastasize to the cerebellum rather than to supratentorial structures (Fig. 2–5). Most brain metastases are in white matter, but melanoma chooses gray matter. Also, mouse melanoma cell lines have been developed that have specific predilection either for brain parenchyma or leptomeninges.[1894]

Clinical and experimental evidence supports the concept that both the hemodynamic and the seed-and-soil hypotheses are important in the development and distribution of metastases in general and CNS metastases in particular. Molecular recognition (seed and soil) is probably the more important of the two. Intravenously injected tumor cells usually lodge in the lung, although many are found in other organs, indicating that cells can pass through the pulmonary capillary bed.[2078,2891] Intra-arterially injected tumor cells are distributed in many organs, primarily in proportion to their blood supply. Despite the fact that many such cells lodge in the brain, only a few metastatic lesions can be found there; multiple and diffuse metastases are uncommon.[1311,1894] Tumor clones can be developed that, even after intravenous injection, locate and grow in the brain.[1894] These experimental data are consistent with the clinical data indicated previously that certain tumor types preferentially metastasize to the brain whereas other tumor types rarely do so. Thus, the brain is a likely site of spread for many tumors partly because it receives a large portion of the cardiac output and partly because many common tumors have a propensity to grow in the brain.

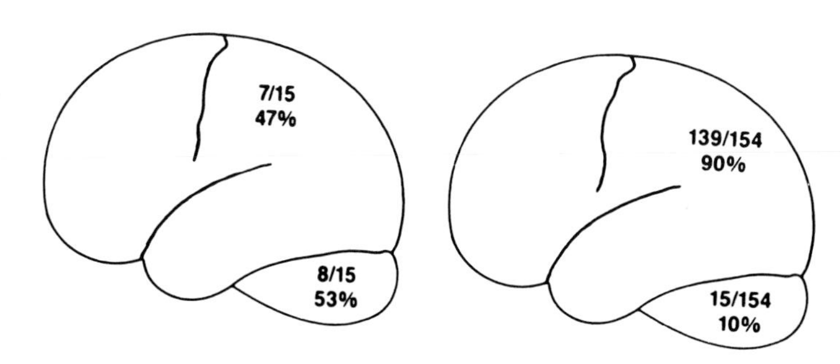

Figure 2–5. This schematic drawing shows the distribution of single metastases to the brain. The posterior fossa is significantly overrepresented in patients with pelvic (prostate or uterus) tumors and gastrointestinal primary tumors (*left*), compared with patients with other primary tumors (*right*) ($p < .001$). (From Delattre et al,[605] p 743, with permission.)

Time of Metastasis

Primary cancers differ not only in their likelihood of spreading to the brain, but also in the time at which a metastasis will occur. Lung cancer often, but not always, metastasizes early, so that a significant percentage (10% to 20%) of patients with lung cancer develop symptoms of brain metastasis before the pulmonary lesion is identified. Carcinomas of the breast and malignant melanoma are other tumors that commonly metastasize to the brain, but they rarely cause neurologic symptoms before the cancer has been identified (only 1 in 137 patients with brain metastases from breast cancer[267]); they may not cause neurologic symptoms for many years after the primary cancer has been discovered and effectively treated.

The Cascade Process

Although experimental evidence indicates that tumor cells can pass through the pulmonary capillary bed to reach organs such as the brain,[2891] clinical evidence suggests that this process occurs in only a minority of patients with CNS metastases. In animal experiments, only pulmonary metastases were encountered after foot-pad implantation of tumor, but widespread metastatic lesions developed after the lungs were bypassed by intra-arterial injection.[73] In most patients (about 70% in one series[605]), the CNS appears to be reached by tumor cells that have entered the arterial circulation from the lung, either because the primary tumor originated in the lung or because the primary tumor has metastasized to the lung via the systemic venous or lymphatic circulation. Thus, when the primary tumor arises outside the lung and metastasizes to the nervous system, it usually does so via a secondary metastasis from a metastatic lung tumor, the so-called cascade process.[318,487] Bross'[318] cascade hypothesis posits that certain metastatic patterns enable particular tumors to spread to particular organs, depending on their venous drainage. Only after metastases grow in a primary receptor organ and metastasize themselves to a secondary receptor organ will widespread dissemination of tumor occur (see Fig. 2–3).

Clinical and experimental evidence supports the cascade hypothesis. In the laboratory,[487] a tumor was developed for its brain-homing properties and then implanted into the hind limb and allowed to grow. The leg was amputated, curing the primary tumor. At autopsy, all animals had pulmonary metastases. In addition, 80% had metastases in the brain, suggesting that the tumor had metastasized first to the lungs and then to its preferential site, the brain. A transplantable colon carcinoma in mice, first grown in the liver and then injected into the arterial, portal venous, or systemic venous circulation, yields different patterns of metastatic spread and degrees of colonization from the same tumor grown in the lung, suggesting that cancerous growth in different anatomic sites can modify the subsequent arterial metastatic patterns, thus supporting the cascade hypothesis.[2783]

Other experimental evidence questions the cascade hypothesis, however. In nude mice, implantation of human tumor cells into the organ from which the human tumor cells arose often leads to rapid growth and metastases. By contrast, the same human cancer cells implanted at ectopic sites (usually subcutaneously or intramuscularly) result in slow growth and only rarely in metastases. These data imply that metastatic tumors have less potential to metastasize than do primary tumors. In addition, brain-derived melanoma cells from both mice and humans are not more malignant than those from lymph nodes, as would be expected by the cascade hypothesis.[2896] The issue of whether the cascade hypothesis is valid is clinically important because, if secondary spread of a lung metastasis goes to the brain rather than a primary spread to both organs, more aggressive treatment of the lung metastasis is warranted.

For the neuro-oncologist, another important question is whether CNS metastases can themselves metastasize outside the nervous system. If so, earlier treatment might be required. Because experimental evidence demonstrates that glucocorticoids enhance metastatic spread, probably by increasing the arrest of tumor emboli in capillaries, this phenomenon is particularly important in the management of brain metastases.[777]

The Bross hypothesis leads to the conclusion that brain metastasis can originate either from a primary cancer in the lung or from a pulmonary metastasis. An exception occurs when a skull metastasis from Batson's plexus causes direct growth of tumor into the brain. In most instances, the cascade hypothesis seems to hold. The most common tumor causing brain metastasis is lung carcinoma (see Table 1–2). Furthermore, in most instances, when a brain metastasis is discovered from a nonpulmonary primary cancer, careful chest x-ray or CT examination usually reveals evidence of a pulmonary metastasis.

CNS metastases do occur, however, in the absence of obvious pulmonary metastases. These exceptions to Bross' cascade theory must be explained. Several possible explanations have been adduced, although the clinical evidence for each is limited:

(1) *Paradoxic embolization.* Because most cancer cells travel by entering the systemic venous circulation and returning to the right heart, the first capillary bed they encounter after they have traversed the pulmonary artery is in the lungs. In some instances, a patent or potentially patent foramen ovale may allow tumor cells to shift from the right to the left heart without passing through the pulmonary circulation. Increasing evidence indicates that this is an important mechanism for cerebral emboli.[2347] One recent study suggests that about 40% of patients with cryptogenic stroke have contrast echocardiographic evidence of a patent foramen ovale.[650] Large paradoxic emboli from tumors sometimes occlude brain vessels. In one patient,[2588] the middle cerebral artery was occluded by tumor cells from a testicular carcinoma; a second tumor embolus was seen at autopsy lying astride a patent foramen ovale. It is unknown how often paradoxic embolization causes brain metastasis.

(2) *Batson's plexus.* Batson's plexus, previously mentioned, is a valvular system of veins lying in the epidural space. It drains vertebral bodies, the skull, and parts of the pelvis. Increases in intra-abdominal or intrathoracic pressure, such as coughing or straining, usually shift blood from the systemic venous system into this vertebral venous system. Batson[164] originally proposed that this system was a potential source of metastases to the CNS, including the brain. It is clearly a source of metastases to vertebral bodies and skull, according to the clinical studies of del Regato[600] and the experimental studies of Coman and DeLong[486] and Harada and associates.[1085] In both studies, tumor cells were injected into the tail vein of rodents with or without abdominal compression. Those animals without abdominal compression developed liver and lung metastases, while those with abdominal compression developed vertebral metastases. The unanswered question is whether tumor cells traveling via Batson's plexus can seed the parenchyma of the brain or spinal cord. Veins of Batson's plexus do communicate with the cerebral venous sinus system and through that system with veins draining the brain, so that a potential communication with the brain exists. Such a system may account for the small number of patients who have only solitary brain metastases in whom, even at autopsy, no metastases are found in the lungs. Delattre and associates,[605] however, found no patient with a brain metastasis who did not, after a careful search at autopsy, have metastatic disease in the lungs. Therefore, if this system plays any role in generating brain metastases, it must be a rare one; its importance in spinal metastasis is unequivocal[600] (see Fig. 2–2B).

(3) *Passage through pulmonary vessels.* It is well established that tumor cells can pass through capillary beds and, thus, can pass through the lungs to reach the systemic circulation. Because the brain receives a large blood supply, the likelihood of a brain metastasis occurring is high simply because of blood flow. Much clinical data, however, indicate that the vascular distribution of tumor cells after injection, which relates to the blood flow to an organ, plays virtually no role in the likelihood that a metastasis actually will develop.[775] Thus, in experimental studies, injected B16 melanoma cells metastasize to and grow in fragments of pulmonary or ovarian tissue implanted in the quadriceps femoris muscle but not in the quadriceps femoris muscle tissue itself, despite the fact that the number of cells that lodged in both muscle and implanted fragments was approximately the same. The reason that muscles, a major recipient of the cardiac output, are rarely the site of metastatic tumors is unclear.

(4) *Microlung metastases.* Occasionally, a large metastatic brain tumor is encountered in a patient and only later is it found that the patient has a very small pulmonary tumor. The micrometastasis in the lung was probably the source of the metastasis to the brain. This situation is different from the usual one in which the pulmonary metastasis is larger than the brain metastasis, although the brain metastasis may have been observed first symptomatically. As previously mentioned, growth of metastatic brain tumors may be rapid when compared to the primary tumor.[448]

(5) *Other factors.* Once tumor cells reach the nervous system, what determines whether or not they will grow? The nervous system itself may play a role in metastatic spread. Recent evidence suggests that destruction of the sympathetic nervous system by chemical axotomy increases the number of metastases without affecting normal cell activity or the immune reaction to prior tumor exposure.[305] Cell adhesion molecules probably play an important role.[1102] The expression of MHC class 1 antigens on the tumor cell surface allows an immune reaction that may protect against metastases. In some human tumors, human lymphocyte antigen expression is lost on metastatic but not nonmetastatic cells.[501]

Damage to an organ is also influential. Systemic cancers have a predilection to metastasize to vertebral bodies that have been the site of previous injury or of Paget's disease.[2083] This situation can cause considerable diagnostic confusion, both clinically, because the patient may have had back pain for a long time, and radiographically, because the vertebral collapse could be due to either the old trauma or the more recent metastatic lesion. Similarly, in the CNS, tumor cells occasionally may seed an ischemic area caused by cerebral vascular disease but spare normal brain.[1896]

DIRECT SPREAD

Direct spread of tumor cells from a primary cancer can compress or invade structures of both the central and peripheral nervous systems in one (or more) of several ways (see Table 2–1):

(1) The tumor or a metastasis from the tumor, such as in the lymph node, is in direct contact with a portion of the nervous system. An example is a lung cancer arising in the superior sulcus of the lung (Pancoast tumor). As the tumor grows, it encounters the inferior portion of the brachial plexus, compressing but usually not invading it. The nerves damaged by the compressing tumor first cause pain and the loss of neurologic function (see Chapter 8). Similarly, if the compressing tumor or other tumors (e.g., neuroblastoma or lymphoma) grow in the paravertebral area, portions of the tumor may grow through the intervertebral foramina to compress the spinal cord (see Chapter 6). Tumors of the skull, such as osteogenic sarcomas, or those growing near the base of the skull, such as nasopharyngeal carcinomas, may grow through the bone to compress or invade the brain or the cranial nerves exiting at the base of the brain. The presenting symptoms of nasopharyngeal carcinoma are neurologic in 15% to 35% of patients.[2582]

(2) Microscopic growth of tumor occurs along perineural sheaths (see Chapter 8). Certain tumors have a propensity for invading nerves in the primary organ affected by the cancer. The tumor cells then grow along the nerve sheath to reach the CNS, resulting in either microscopic or macroscopic CNS tumor. Neurologic symptoms often begin long after the primary tumor has been removed and presumably cured. At times, the growth is microscopic in the peripheral or cranial nerve but becomes macroscopic once it reaches the CNS. Particular examples include squamous cell carcinomas of the face, which may slowly grow along the trigeminal nerve to first cause numbness in the face and subsequently involve other cranial nerves as the tumor enters the cavernous sinus. Such tumors track along cranial nerves as far as the brainstem and may cause mass lesions in the posterior fossa of the brain. So-called neurotropic melanomas have a similar propensity. A similar mechanism has been imputed to prostate cancer as a cause for the lumbar vertebral metastases that frequently occur with that cancer. Microscopic evidence suggests that if perineural invasion can be found within the prostate, metastatic disease in the vertebral bodies is more likely to develop than if no such perineural invasion can be found. Microscopic invasion by tumor, destroying nerves and causing symptoms but

not causing apparent mass lesions by either inspection or imaging, represents a particular challenge for the neuro-oncologist (see Chapter 8).

(3) When, by either bulk growth or perineural invasion, tumor cells reach the CSF, they may spread throughout the neuraxis along the CSF pathways. This phenomenon, perhaps analogous to ovarian cancer seeding the peritoneal cavity and some tumors seeding the pleural cavity, usually occurs in the absence of metastatic spread to the brain or spinal cord. The clinical symptoms are usually those of widespread leptomeningeal metastasis (see Chapter 7).

PATHOPHYSIOLOGIC FACTORS RELEVANT TO SPREAD AND GROWTH OF CANCER TO SPECIFIC NEURAL STRUCTURES

Brain

Most metastatic brain tumors arise by embolization of tumor cells to the brain (see Fig. 2–1). Emboli of any kind in the brain arrest in the white matter at the gray/white matter junction.[605] As already mentioned, brain metastases generally lodge in the terminal ends of the arterial supply, the so-called watershed areas[605] (see Fig. 2–3A). Most tumors distribute themselves between the supratentorial and infratentorial compartments in proportion to the weight and the blood supply of those structures, that is, 85% hemispheres, 15% posterior fossa (see Fig. 2–3B). Certain tumors, however, particularly those arising in the pelvis (prostate or uterus) or gastrointestinal tract,[397,605] have a predilection to metastasize to the cerebellum. Thus, about 50% of single brain metastases from these organs are found in the cerebellum, whereas only 10% of single brain metastases from other organs evolve to the cerebellum (see Fig. 2–5). The reason for the cerebellar predilection of some tumors is unknown. It does not apply to all pelvic or abdominal tumors; renal-cell cancer, for instance, does not appear to select the cerebellum.[893] Experimental evidence is currently unavailable to support the Batson's plexus hypothesis of how these tumors spread, but evidence is available for skull and intracranial dural metastases.

Although edema of the white matter, wet-appearing and somewhat grayish, surrounds all metastatic brain tumors, its amount varies. Some small tumors are surrounded by massive amounts of edema and other large tumors by lesser amounts. Some investigators believe that adenocarcinomas, particularly from the lung, are associated with more brain edema than other metastatic tumors, but we have not been able to confirm such observations.

Most metastases in the brain grow as spherical masses, displacing rather than destroying brain tissue and creating edema in the surrounding white matter. Other intracranial metastases are more irregular (see Chapter 5). Brain metastases have a granular, fleshy appearance and are soft to the touch. They are usually well demarcated from surrounding brain, both grossly and microscopically, and, thus, often can be completely excised surgically. Certain cancers, particularly poorly differentiated lymphomas, renal carcinoma, and melanoma, may invade surrounding brain tissue microscopically although they appear grossly to be well demarcated. Brain metastases are usually solid but, because they grow rapidly, they often undergo central necrosis. Cystic lesions occasionally occur, particularly from primary breast cancer. Metastatic brain tumors are usually highly vascular, despite the fact that they appear avascular on arteriographic study. Metastases from melanomas, choriocarcinomas, and testicular carcinomas may be hemorrhagic, because these tumors either invade the walls of blood vessels[1407,2104] or promote extensive neovascularization.[2306] Those from melanomas and lymphomas tend to invade gray matter. Occasionally, widespread miliary metastases invade the cerebral cortex as small or microscopic foci of tumor, which may or may not be identifiable on CT or MR scan, giving rise to the clinical syndrome of "carcinomatous encephalitis."[802,1645,1770]

The microscopic appearance of a brain metastasis resembles the primary tumor from which it arises. Therefore, in patients with an unknown primary cancer, extirpation of the cerebral metastasis with microscopic examination often provides a significant clue as to the original site of the primary tumor, although a metastatic brain tumor may have a different appearance (and growth rate) from the primary. In mixed epidermoid and adenocarcinomas of the lung, it is the adenocarcinoma component that is more likely to metastasize to the brain; in mixed testicular tumors, choriocarcinoma elements are more likely to metastasize than the other portions.[2544]

Spinal Cord

Unlike the brain, in which most metastases are parenchymal, metastases affecting the spinal cord usually act by compressing the cord from the epidural space. Metastatic tumor reaches the epidural space in one of three ways (Fig. 2–6): (1) extension from a vertebral metastasis, (2) invasion through the intervertebral foramina by a paravertebral mass, or (3) direct hematogenous spread to the epidural space.

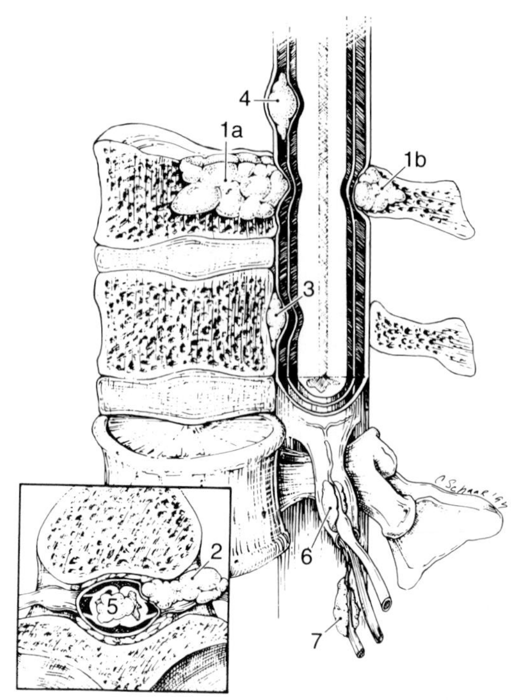

Figure 2–6. Most spinal cord dysfunction is caused by a metastasis to a vertebral body that invades the epidural space and compresses the anterior portion of the spinal cord. (1a) The vertebral body may also collapse, causing bone to herniate into the epidural space. Less common are metastases to the spinous process (1b) or vertebral lamina that compress the posterior or lateral portion of the spinal cord. Somewhat less common than vertebral metastases are those that compress the lateral portion of the cord by growing from the paravertebral space through the intervertebral foramen (2). The vertebral body may or may not be involved. Even less common are hematogenous metastases directly to the epidural space (3), intradural or leptomeningeal metastases (4), or parenchymal metastases (5). Metastatic lesions may rarely cause symptoms by compressing a radicular artery (6) or cause radicular symptoms, but not spinal cord symptoms, by invading or compressing the nerve root as it exits the intervertebral foramen (7).

VERTEBRAL METASTASES

Metastases to bone are much more common than might be predicted from bone's low overall blood flow (11 mg/kg per minute) or from the fact that skeletal blood flow accounts for only 4% to 10% of cardiac output.[1094] The high incidence of bone metastases results from:

1. The large capacity of the bone marrow's capillary bed, six to eight times that of the arterial system, allows the circulation to come to a virtual standstill at times.
2. The walls of sinusoids have discontinuities that allow tumor cells to escape blood vessels.
3. The intersinusoidal cords of hematopoietic tissue form culs-de-sac in which tumor cells can lodge and proliferate.
4. Production by the tumor of prostaglandin E_2, osteoblast-activating factor(s), parathormonelike substances and TGFα, serves to stimulate osteoblastic activity. Products of bone resorption[1674] stimulate tumor growth and monocytes that produce interleukin-1 may promote bone resorption.

The most common mechanism for spinal cord compression is hematogenous metastasis to the vertebral body or, less commonly, the vertebral lamina, pedicle, or spinous process. These posterior vertebral elements are involved about 15% as often as the vertebral body. Metastatic clones appear to have a predilection to invade bone already damaged by trauma or Paget's disease,[2083] complicating the diagnosis. Tumor invasion of the vertebral body often leads to collapse followed by progressive kyphosis. The tumor, collapsed bone, and occasionally intervertebral disc herniate posteriorly into the spinal canal to compress the cord. The posterior longitudinal ligament, which separates the vertebral bodies from the epidural space, may be buckled backward by the tumor or actually may be invaded and breached by the tumor to promote direct entry of tumor into the anterior or anterolateral portion of the epidural space (see Fig. 2–6). If the posterior elements are also destroyed by tumor or by prior laminectomy[783,1093,1094] (see Chapter 6), a forward-flexion deformity results. Less commonly but especially in children, the pedicles, lamina, or posterior spinous process may compress the posterior or posterolateral portion of the cord.

Vertebral invasion is the mechanism of epidural spinal compression in 85% to 90% of patients; as a result, most patients with spinal cord compression have identifiable abnormalities of the vertebral body at the compression site by plain x-ray, radionuclide bone scan, or CT or MR scan.

The tumor may reach the vertebral body or the epidural space hematogenously, either arterially[72] or by venous dissemination via Batson's plexus.[164] Other modes include spread along the lymphatics[790] and direct extension from retroperitoneal or posterior mediastinal tumor.[2106] Individual tumors drain differently into Batson's plexus and thus reach different portions of the vertebral column. The breast drains principally by the azygos vein into the thoracic level of the plexus. Cervical cancers metastasize to lumbar spine and sacrum,[790] usually to the left side, probably representing direct drainage from tumor-bearing lymph nodes. The prostate drains through the pelvic venous plexus, reaching Batson's plexus in the pelvis and lower spine. Some tumors, by contrast, drain principally via the pulmonary vein into the left heart and, thus, reach the vertebral body via the arterial circulation. In humans, particularly those with carcinomas of the breast and prostate, bony metastases are often distributed in a pattern outlining Batson's plexus; that is, they involve the axial skeleton and spare the appendicular skeleton (see Fig. 2–2B). Such patients are likely to have multiple vertebral metastases and often skull metastases without involvement of long bones.

The anatomy of Batson's plexus is not the whole explanation for the very high incidence of vertebral body and epidural metastases, however. The sinusoidal pattern of the vasculature of vertebral bone marrow makes that structure particularly vulnerable to metastases. Furthermore, certain tumors have a predilection to invade and grow in bone, probably because they produce osteoclastic substances, including osteoclast-activating factor and prostaglandins, that allow them to grow more easily within vertebral structures. Bone marrow stromal cells and hematopoietic growth factors in vertebral bodies also promote growth of the metastatic cancer. Conversely, many tumors promote bone growth and cause blastic rather than lytic lesions. Anecdotal evidence suggests that vertebral metastases are more likely to occur at the site of a previous injury to a vertebral body. A single vertebral metastasis may affect a previously documented traumatic compression fracture, considerably complicating early diagnosis.

Arguello and colleagues[72] constructed an experimental model of arterial spread to the epidural space. This model, produced by injection of tumor into the heart, led to invasion of the vertebral bodies near the cartilaginous plate at the site where end arterioles terminate as tortuous loops. The growing tumor then compressed and thrombosed vertebral veins and entered the spinal canal where the thrombosed veins traversed the intervertebral foramina. In the spinal canal, the tumor either can grow as an anterior mass compressing the spinal cord or can work its way around the cord, causing a more posterior mass. In this experimental model, the site of the mass depended on the nature of the tumor.

FORAMINAL INVASION

Less common than vertebral metastasis is invasion (10% to 15%) of the epidural space through the intervertebral foramen by paravertebral tumor. Lymphomas[730] and neuroblastomas[1184,2106] are particular offenders. The tumor usually remains in the extradural space and compresses the lateral portion of the spinal cord. The clinical implication is that spinal cord compression can occur in the absence of involvement of the vertebral bodies, so that the results of x-rays and nuclide scans of the vertebral bodies may be normal. A CT or MR scan (see Chapter 6) usually identifies both the paravertebral mass and the intraspinal extension.

EPIDURAL METASTASES

Direct hematogenous spread of tumor to the epidural space is uncommon. Most such exclusively epidural tumors are leukemias or lymphomas.[673,1622] About 5% of spinal lymphomas originate in the epidural space rather than metastasize there from elsewhere.[1627] The same phenomenon occasionally is encountered in leukemia[2845] and isolated cases of primary epidural Ewing's sarcoma[1344] and osteosarcoma.[2314] In this situation, x-rays of neither the vertebral bodies nor the paravertebral space provide a clue that the epidural space has been invaded. Furthermore, even CT or MR scan may fail to distinguish this epidural tumor from other epidural masses such as herniated disk[947] or extramedullary hematopoiesis.[156]

CONSEQUENCES OF SPINAL CORD COMPRESSION

Whatever the mode of spread, once the tumor reaches the epidural space, it not only compresses the cord at its entry site (anterior for vertebral metastases, lateral for those that enter through the intervertebral foramen), but also may spread in a circumferential fashion around the cord to compress it from all sides.[1918] The clinical implication of this anatomic fact is that the time-honored surgical operation for spinal cord compression, simple decompressive laminectomy, which removes the spinous processes and lamina, only temporarily decompresses the cord and may, in fact, promote instability, thus worsening rather than alleviating the situation.[783,1093]

Leptomeninges

Malignant cells can reach the CSF by several routes[1402,2544] (Fig. 2–7):

(1) *Direct extension.* Tumor metastases to brain or spinal cord that abut either the subarachnoid or ventricular surface can directly seed cells into the CSF.[1779,1780] Cerebellar lesions are particularly likely to cause meningeal metastases because of the large subarachnoid surface of the cisterna magna. About one-third of our patients whose cerebellar metastases have been surgically resected subsequently develop leptomeningeal metastases.[1992] Direct spread from brain or spinal cord is not a frequent mode of CSF entry for two reasons: First, metastatic tumor of the brain tends to originate in white matter (at the gray/white matter junction); the lesions grow largely below the subarachnoid surface but do not reach the ventricular surface. Second, even when tumor grows through the cortex to the subarachnoid surface, a reactive response develops in the leptomeninges that often seals off that tumor, leading to a focal leptomeningeal deposit but not the diffuse or the widespread multifocal leptomeningeal process encountered with tumor disseminated throughout the CSF. Because tumors rarely metastasize to the spinal cord parenchyma (see Chapter 6), this is a rare source of leptomeningeal tumor. Primary CNS lymphomas in the brain usually grow periventricularly and, thus, frequently seed the ventricles and leptomeninges.[580]

(2) *Hematogenous.* Tumor spread via the arterial circulation to the choroid plexus and from the choroid plexus into the cerebral ventricles is probably also uncommon. When leptomeningeal tumors develop from a choroid plexus metastasis, the cells are carried by CSF flow into the subarachnoid space.[1789,2398] Because the ventricles have a smooth ependymal surface without areas of stasis, tumor cells generally do not adhere to the ventricular wall (although exceptions have been observed), but instead find their way into the subarachnoid space, in which regions of stasis permit growth. Choroid plexus metastases are, in my experience, a rare source of leptomeningeal tumor.

(3) *Venous access.* Tumor cells may metastasize directly to the subarachnoid space, entering through leptomeningeal veins.[110,2095] This probably represents a common site of entry of leukemia cells.

(4) *Venous drainage from bone marrow.* Tumor cells involving the bone marrow of vertebrae or skull may grow along veins exiting the marrow to reach the dura and then along perivenous adventitial tissue connecting the dura mater with the subarachnoid space. A high incidence of bone marrow infiltration in patients who develop leptomeningeal metastases and a high incidence of leptomeningeal metastases in those tumors that either arise in or commonly affect the marrow indicates that this is a common source of spread

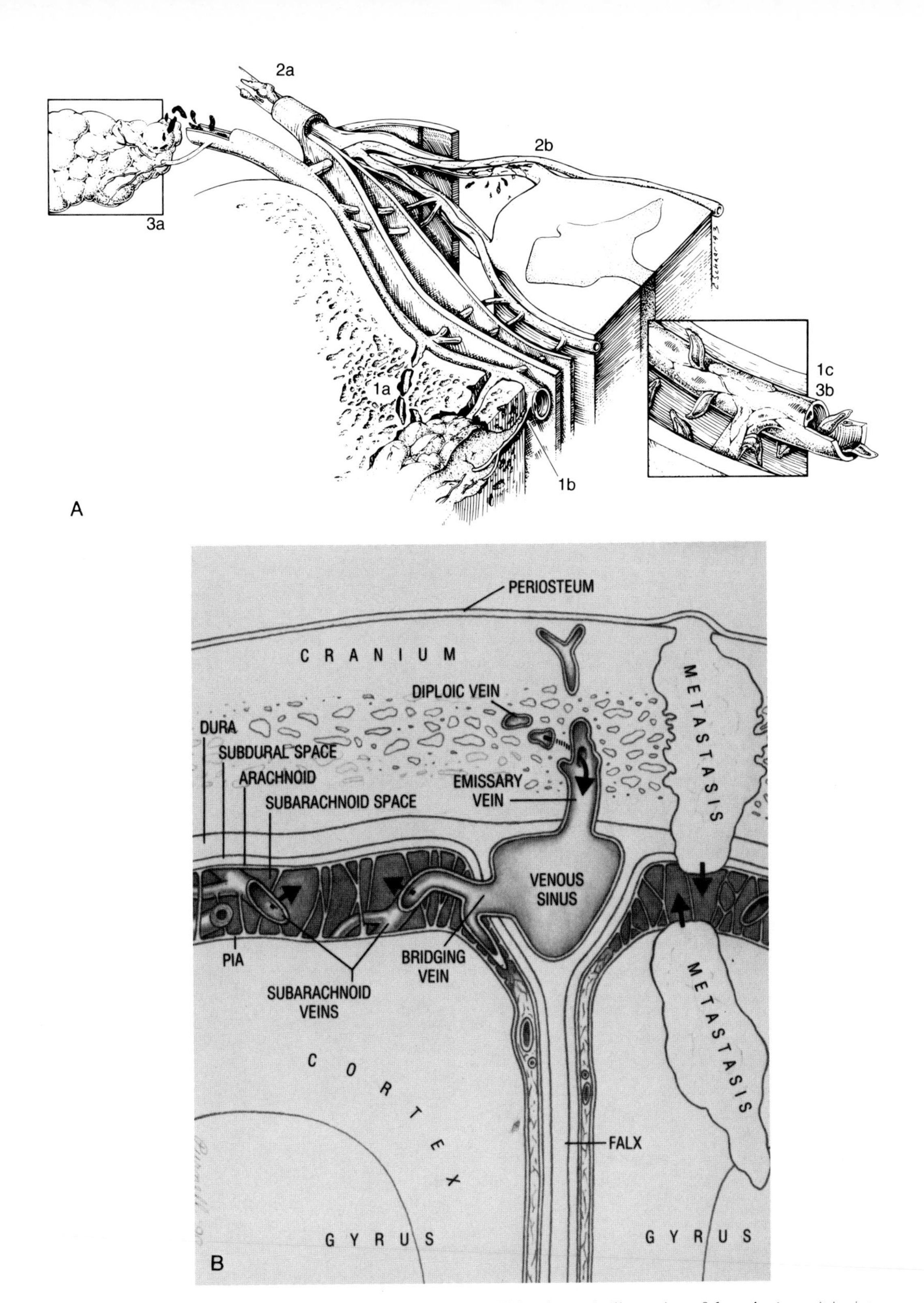

Figure 2–7. Pathophysiology of leptomeningeal metastases: *A,* This schematic illustration of the spinal canal depicts the mechanisms of tumor cell entry into the spinal subarachnoid space. The tumor may invade the vertebral body (1a) and grow along vertebral veins (1b) into the subarachnoid space (1c). The tumor may invade peripheral nerves or nerve roots outside the vertebral canal (2a) and grow along the nerve sheath into the spinal canal to seed the leptomeninges (2b). The tumor can invade blood vessels outside the CNS (3a) and traverse subarachnoid veins into the subarachnoid space (3b). *B,* This schematic drawing of the skull illustrates the possible mechanisms of tumor entry into the cerebral subarachnoid space. Tumor may enter the cranial subarachnoid space via metastases either to the skull or brain, diploic veins of the skull, or directly from subarachnoid veins. The choroid plexus (not shown) is also an occasional site for the formation of leptomeningeal tumor. (*B* is from Henson and Posner,[1141] p 2274, with permission.)

to the subarachnoid space.[112] A recent study contrasting the different histology of breast cancers metastatic to brain with those metastasizing to the leptomeninges also supports this mode of spread. Parenchymal cerebral metastases were associated almost exclusively with infiltrating ductal carcinoma and meningeal infiltration with infiltrating lobular carcinoma, the histologic variety that tends to metastasize to bone marrow.[2445]

(5) *Cranial and peripheral nerves.* Tumor may grow along cranial or peripheral nerves to enter the subarachnoid space with those nerves and then spread cells into the CSF.[1402,2140] The high frequency of paravertebral metastases in patients with leptomeningeal metastases, as well as pathologic evidence of growth along spinal and cranial nerves that lead to the subarachnoid space, supports this mode of spread as a common one.[1402]

To summarize, the two common sites of entry of tumor cells into the subarachnoid space are along vascular structures from the bone marrow of skull or vertebral body or along spinal or cranial nerves innervating extracranial structures containing the tumor.

Once the tumor has reached the CSF, it can seed any portion of the nervous system that contacts the CSF. The seeding, usually widespread with a particular predilection for the base of the brain and the cauda equina, includes the depths of the sulci (rather than the surface of the gyri); the lateral surface of the hemispheres; and the quadrigeminal, ambient, and peduncular cisterns surrounding the brainstem.[1942,2641] Tumor tissue is often found in the lateral recesses of the fourth ventricle and in the Sylvian fissure between the frontal and temporal lobes. In the cauda equina, it tends to be concentrated over the dorsal portions of that structure rather than the ventral surface. The dorsal surface of the brain usually is seeded more sparsely than the ventral surface, and the ependyma usually is spared. At times, tumor cells are found in the arachnoid villi. Because the villi are the site of CSF resorption, plugging of the arachnoid villi is one potential cause of hydrocephalus.

In many instances, even with extensive seeding of the leptomeninges, no abnormalities are apparent to the naked eye. Sometimes, the arachnoid membrane has a slight milky appearance that may indicate to the pathologist that leptomeningeal metastases are present, particularly in younger patients whose arachnoid membranes usually are transparent. Sometimes the tumor forms macroscopic masses, particularly along nerve roots of the cauda equina, making it evident in life to the radiologist on myelogram or gadolinium-enhanced MR scans and to the inspection of the pathologist at autopsy.

Microscopically, the metastatic tumor grows in sheets along the surface of the brain, spinal cord, cranial nerves, and spinal roots. Several different patterns of meningeal reaction commonly are seen but do not appear to characterize individual tumors:

1. Dense infiltration of the leptomeninges by tumor entirely obliterates normal meningeal structures but with little inflammatory or fibrotic reaction.
2. More sparse infiltration with tumor cells is organized in a linear fashion following the outline of the pia arachnoid and interconnecting trabeculae; the subarachnoid space may be relatively preserved with little evidence of reactive fibrosis.
3. Focally dense reactions of the leptomeninges result when a few tumor cells cause meningeal fibrosis with a moderate number of reactive meningothelial cells.
4. A thick exudative reaction is caused by a large number of tumor cells accompanied by a marked inflammatory reaction; many inflammatory and cancer cells infiltrate the leptomeninges and seed into the CSF, producing an inflammatory picture on lumbar puncture and giving rise to the commonly used term "carcinomatous meningitis."

Leptomeningeal metastases may remain restricted to the subarachnoid space or may infiltrate the parenchyma of the brain and spinal cord by growing down the Virchow-Robin spaces. These potential spaces are a tunnellike extension of the subarachnoid space formed by blood vessels that penetrate from the surface of the brain into its depths. Virchow-Robin spaces, strictly speaking, lie outside the brain, separated from it by pia and astrocytic foot processes. As the tumor grows in this space, however, it may penetrate the space to invade brain or spinal cord parenchyma itself. This tendency for tumor to settle deep in the sulci of brains and to invade the Virchow-Robin spaces has led some investigators to believe that intrathecally injected drugs would not reach all tumor and that more penetrating agents, such as radiation therapy, are required for adequate prophylaxis or treatment.

Leptomeningeal metastases also invade cranial and peripheral nerves as they pass through the subarachnoid space, a more common invasion than those to the brain or spinal cord. The first pathologic change appears to be interruption of the myelin sheath with relative preservation of axis cylinders, but if the tumor continues to grow, the nerve is entirely disrupted.

Cranial and Peripheral Nerves

Metastatic cancers affect peripheral nerves either by compression or direct invasion. Nerves can be compressed by the growing primary tumor or by metastases to bone or lymph nodes. Compression by primary tumors includes Pancoast tumors that compress the brachial plexus, nasopharyngeal tumors that compress cranial nerves exiting the base of the skull, and pelvic tumors, including colonic and cervical carcinomas that compress the sacral plexus with direct posterior growth. In addition, lung and breast cancers often metastasize to the bones of the skull base, compressing cranial nerves; tumors metastasizing to pelvic bones can compress the sciatic nerve; lymph node metastases compress brachial plexus in some patients with metastatic breast cancer and the lumbar or sacral plexus in patients with metastatic spread of colon, prostate, or bladder cancer. Rarely, peripheral nerves, such as the ulnar nerve, may be compressed by enlargement of nearby lymph nodes because of metastatic tumor.

An infrequent cause of peripheral nerve dysfunction is direct invasion of the nerve by the tumor either from hematogenous spread of tumor to peripheral nerve or dorsal root ganglion[640] or, more commonly, by direct extension to the nerve from a surrounding structure. An example of the latter is nerve invasion in the subarachnoid space in a patient with leptomeningeal metastases (see Chapter 7). The epineurium and perineurium generally form an effective barrier against tumor penetration. Often metastases entirely encompass the nerve and sometimes grow down its perineural septa, causing severe compressive damage but not actually invading the nerve.

Whether neurologic dysfunction is caused by compression or invasion of the nerve is clinically important. Nerve compression lesions tend to be more painful but associated with less neurologic dysfunction than nerve invasion. Compressive lesions of the nerve usually cause radicular pain accompanied by severe local aching. Invasive lesions are more likely to cause dysesthetic, tingling or burning pain, or, occasionally, even neuralgialike pains (sharp, shooting, short-lived, lightning-like pains resembling trigeminal neuralgia or the lightning pains of tabes dorsalis). Invasive lesions of mixed sensory-motor nerves often cause selective motor weakness, sometimes without pain and with relative sparing of sensory fibers. A similar situation is seen in the vascular disorder of nerves that causes diabetic amyotrophy.[1086]

Because compressive lesions of the nerve come either from tumor in bone or from enlarging lymph nodes or organs, they are more easily detected by imaging techniques than are invasive lesions, which are usually microscopic.

Although the mechanism by which tumor compression causes nerve dysfunction is not entirely known, direct pressure and ischemia probably both participate. The first pathologic change in compressive lesions appears to be demyelination with relative preservation of the axon. Later, axon loss occurs as well, suggesting ischemia of the nerve. How invasive lesions of the nerve cause their symptoms also is not known entirely. At some point in the invasion of a nerve by tumor, the entire nerve is destroyed, but before that, changes may be produced by interference with vascular supply or by competition for essential metabolites. Early destruction of myelin sheaths often appears with relative preservation of axons, similar to the effects of compressive lesions.

The CNS and peripheral nervous systems differ from each other in several respects that influence their response to treatment of metastases. Peripheral-nerve myelin sheaths are formed and nourished by Schwann cells rather than by oligodendroglial cells as in the CNS. Peripheral nerves have a better regenerative capacity and, thus, treatment is likely to be more effective if the primary process can be relieved. If the peripheral-nerve lesion arises near the cell body, however, there may be enough dying back to destroy the cell body, thus eliminating the possibility of regeneration.

The CNS and peripheral nervous systems are similar in two important and relevant aspects: (1) A blood–nerve barrier similar to the blood–brain barrier (see Chapter 3) serves to exclude water-soluble chemotherapeutic agents providing a sanctuary for cells.[1943,2137] (2) The peripheral nerve is encased in a relatively unyielding perineural sheath and, like the CNS, is susceptible to edema, which may, in and of itself, produce neurologic disability. These physiologic aspects of the peripheral nervous system have not been studied as carefully as they have in the CNS, however; thus, their exact relevance to the pathophysiology of neural dysfunction and its treatment has not been established.

Once a tumor invades a peripheral nerve, it can grow along the nerve, sometimes for a considerable distance, actually entering the CNS via that route.[463] The opposite situation, in which leptomeningeal tumor invades nerve roots and follows them outside the CNS, has been shown in experimental animals.[2641]

CHAPTER 3

BLOOD–NERVOUS SYSTEM BARRIER DYSFUNCTION: PATHOPHYSIOLOGY AND TREATMENT

Three aspects of the anatomy and physiology of the nervous system make it particularly vulnerable to the effects of metastases:

1. The CNS is enclosed by bone. The skull protectively encloses the brain, and the vertebral column surrounds the spinal cord. The result is that when tumors grow, they not only distort and compress normal tissue nearby, but they also raise tissue pressure both in the immediate area and at a distance (i.e., overall intracranial pressure), thus interfering with functions of neural tissue that is not directly invaded or compressed by the tumor (see Fig. 1–3). Once peripheral and cranial nerves leave the skull and/or spinal canal, they are not encased in bone but in an unyielding connective tissue sheath, the perineurium. The clinical consequence is the same as in the CNS; that is, compression and distortion increase tissue pressure, often causing serious interference with neural function before the tumor causes significant direct destruction.
2. Physiologic barriers termed the blood–brain barrier, blood–spinal fluid bar-

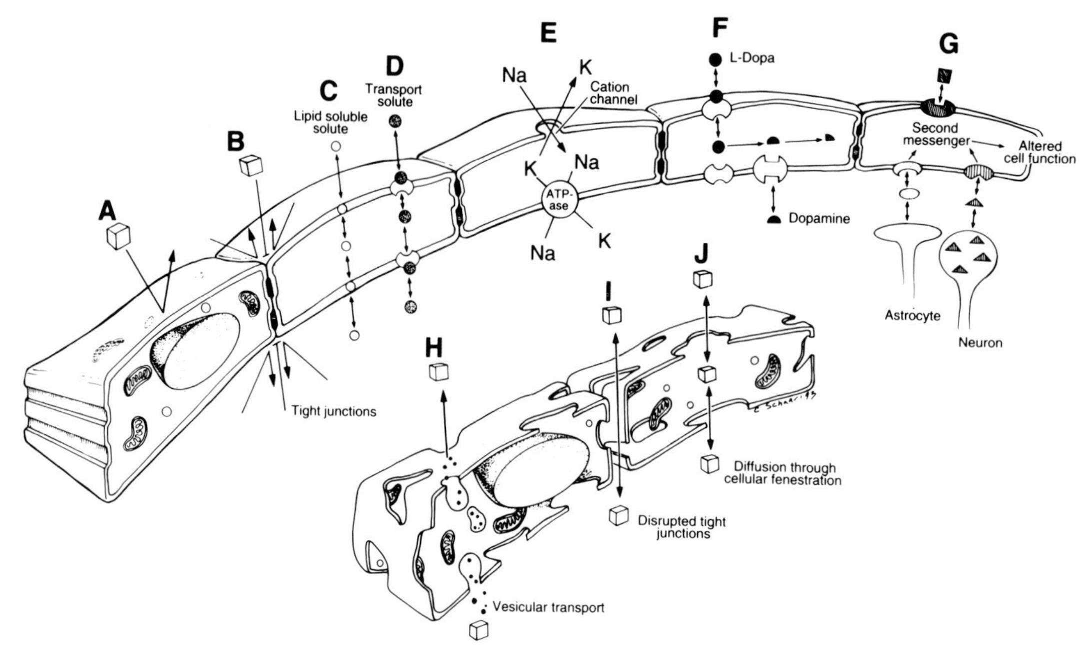

Figure 3–1. A schematic representation of the normal (*top*) and disrupted (*bottom*) blood–brain barrier. The endothelial cell lipid membrane (A) and tight junctions connecting endothelial cells (B) prevent the movement of polar solids between the blood and the brain. Lipid-soluble solids (C) and solutes for which the endothelial cell had transporters, such as glucose, some amino acids, and some micronutrients such as thiamine (D), cross from blood to brain by two-way transport systems. Other substances, such as potassium and sodium, are transported asymmetrically from either the blood to the brain or the brain to the blood (E). Some molecules that cross the luminal endothelial membrane, such as L-dopa (F), are metabolized within the endothelial cell so that a metabolic product such as dopamine reaches the brain. Receptors on the endothelial surface, including selectrins and integrins, react with circulating messengers that affect the brain via a second messenger system (G). In patients with brain tumors or other lesions, the blood–brain barrier is disrupted. This occurs in part via increased vesicular transport (H), in part because the tight junctions are disrupted, allowing polar solutes to cross from the blood to the brain (I), and, in part, because fenestrations in the endothelial cell allow increased diffusion of polar solutes through the cell (J). (Adapted from Betz,[209] pp 56, 57, 62, 65, 67.)

rier, and blood–nerve barrier separate the systemic circulation from the neuraxis* (Fig. 3–1). These barriers reside largely in the endothelium of the vessels feeding the nervous system, supported by perivascular astrocytes, but they also exist in choroid plexus and pia mater[1292] (Fig. 3–2). They retard entry of most water-soluble substances into the nervous system. One clinical consequence of these barriers is that many chemotherapeutic agents do not have access to tumor cells sequestered behind them,[767] perhaps causing the increased incidence of brain metastases from certain primary tumors that have been controlled by systemic chemotherapy (see Chapter 1). Once the tumors reach a size beyond a few millimeters, they promote angiogenesis with capillaries that lack tight junctions and other qualities of normal brain capillaries (see Fig. 3–1).[808,1927,2895] The process at least partially disrupts the blood–brain barrier.[2895] Water-soluble agents can gain access to tumor cells behind the disrupted barrier, although often not in concentrations equal to that achieved in systemic organs. Disruption of the blood–brain barrier in and immediately around metastatic tumors exposes the tumor and, by dif-

* References 209, 288, 350, 606, 767, 830, 941, 1233, 1875-1877, 1925, 2275.

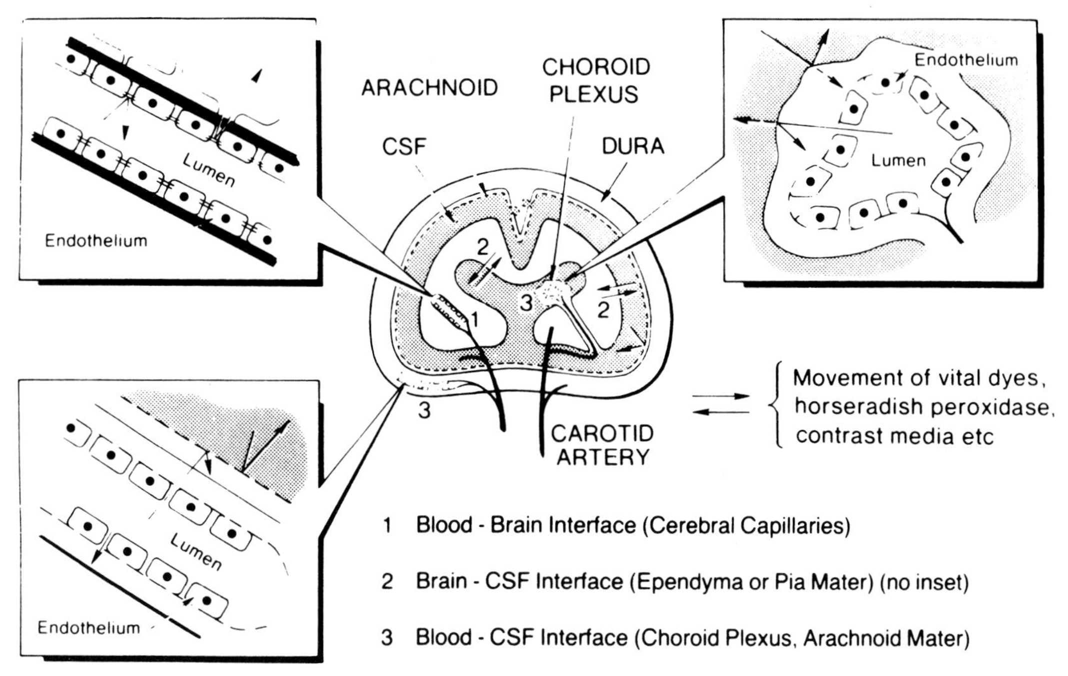

Figure 3–2. Major compartments of the CNS and interfaces between blood, CSF, and brain tissue. Relatively free passage (*straight arrows*) of vital dyes, horseradish peroxidase, and contrast media occurs between CSF and brain tissue and between vessels and tissue of the choroid plexus. However, such substances are prevented (*deflected arrows*) from passing freely between cerebral blood vessels and tissues by tight junctions, between dural vessels and CSF by arachnoid mater, and between tissues of choroid plexus and CSF by ependyma. (From Sage,[2266] p 128, with permission.)

fusion, exposes the normal brain surrounding the tumor to potentially neurotoxic chemotherapeutic agents. The disruption also allows the entry of many normal substances, including electrolytes and proteins, that usually do not have access to the brain. In addition to their own potential toxicity, these osmolar particles bring water with them and cause edema, thus adding mass to the already-expanding tumor (see Fig. 1–3).

3. The brain lacks lymphatics. Lymph channels that are positioned along cranial nerves, especially the olfactory nerve, and spinal roots may absorb some CSF and its macromolecules[532,533] (Fig. 3–3). The amount, however, is not sufficient to prevent brain edema and increased intracranial pressure. When disruption of the blood–brain barrier leads to accumulation of fluids, proteins, and other substances, absorption occurs by a long, tortuous route of convection or bulk flow through the brain substance to the ventricular system or subarachnoid space, where it is eventually absorbed with spinal fluid.[1687a] The tumor and its resulting increased intracranial pressure often disrupt the normal CSF absorptive pathways, compounding the problem of brain edema.[2654]

The ultimate result of these three anatomic-physiologic factors is that, when the blood–brain barrier is disrupted, plasma-derived fluid enters the brain and increases brain mass,[599] further raising already-increased tissue pressure in the tumor,[646] first locally, and then at a distance from the tumor (see Fig. 1–3). The increasing mass distorts surrounding normal tissue and interferes with its blood flow,[646,1010] often leading to ischemia, more edema, and more neurologic dysfunction. Furthermore, substances in the edema fluid (e.g., potassium and glutamate) may be neurotoxic, adding to the dysfunction. Distant neural structures physiologically linked to the area of tumor and edema also

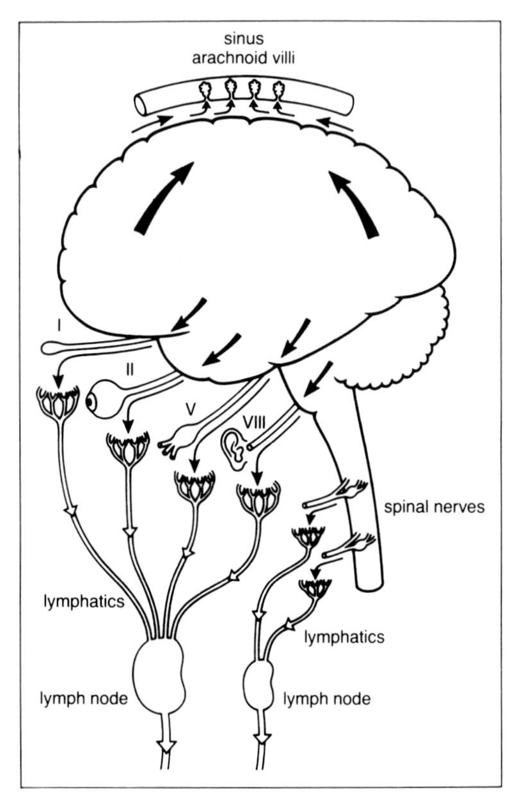

Figure 3–3. This schematic diagram illustrates outflow pathways from the cranial and spinal subarachnoid space across the arachnoid villi to dural sinus blood or along certain cranial nerves and spinal nerve roots to lymphatics: olfactory nerve (I), optic nerve (II), trigeminal nerve (V), and acoustic nerve (VIII). (From Cserr and Knopf,[533] p 509, with permission.)

fail to function normally, presumably because of remote transsynaptic impairment (diaschisis), and may contribute to neurologic dysfunction.[2231] The sum of these physiologic abnormalities often causes more symptoms than does the tumor itself, a principle proved by the rapid clinical response to corticosteroids, which restore the integrity of the blood–brain barrier and with time decrease edema.[31,2147]

ANATOMY AND PHYSIOLOGY

Normal brain capillaries of the blood–brain barrier differ from most of those elsewhere in the body (see Fig. 3–1) (Table 3–1). Exceptions are testis and skin, which have similar barriers.

Blood–Brain Barrier

As shown on Figure 3–1, five anatomic features of the blood–brain barrier retard the entry of most water-soluble but not lipid-soluble agents: (1) Capillary endothelial cells are connected by tight rather than gap junctions[311,2145,2209] that are perforated by aqueous channels with diameters no larger than 0.6 to 0.8 nm, restricting free diffusion of most substances. Even water does not move as freely across the blood–brain barrier as into other organs.[2117] (2) Large molecules, including proteins, find their way into the interstitial space of most organs through capillary fenestrations. Brain capillaries lack these fenestrations.[311] This lack in the CNS substantially retards movement of these molecules. (3) Pinocytotic vesicles transport plasma or interstitial fluid contents bidirectionally across the endothelium. The density of pinocytotic vesicles in the brain is about 5% of that in other organs, substantially diminishing the opportunity for this kind of transport. (4) Mitochondria that supply the energy for active transport across the endothelium are as much as 10 times more abundant in brain endothelial cells as in those of other organs.[1934] Increased density of mitochondria in the brain fuels several pumps

Table 3–1. **PHYSICAL CHARACTERISTICS OF THE BLOOD–BRAIN BARRIER AS A MODIFIED TIGHT EPITHELIUM**

- It is a sheet of cells on a basement membrane.
- The cells are connected by tight junctions.
- Permeability to hydrophilic nonelectrolytes is very low in the absence of a membrane carrier.
- Transport of certain organic solutes is facilitated with saturation kinetics, as well as stereospecificity and competitive interactions between related compounds.
- It has features of a tight epithelium, including low hydraulic conductance, low ionic permeability, and high electrical resistance.
- These characteristics hold for endothelial cells (blood–brain barrier) and the choroidal epithelium (blood–CSF barrier).

Source: Adapted from Fishman,[795] p 44.

that permit the entry of water-soluble substances that would not otherwise cross the blood–brain barrier. These pumps also promote the exit of potentially toxic substances that might accumulate as a result of brain activity (e.g., potassium).[1934,1978] (5) P-glycoprotein, a unique membrane glycoprotein with a molecular weight of 170 to 180 kd, is encoded by a multidrug resistance gene. Increased expression of P-glycoprotein has been associated with resistance of tumors to several chemotherapeutic agents including doxorubicin, etoposide, and vincristine. P-glycoprotein is expressed in the endothelial cells of blood–tissue barriers, including brain, skin, and testis. It is not expressed in those parts of the brain without a blood–brain barrier, except the pineal gland. P-glycoprotein appears to play a role in the blood–brain barrier and in keeping water-soluble chemotherapeutic agents out of the brain.[502,1139,2315a] Primary and metastatic tumors of the brain express little or no P-glycoprotein, although other normal capillary markers such as Factor VIII are present.[1139] Other unique proteins are expressed in brain endothelial cells.[2487]

Many water-soluble agents not synthesized by the brain, including proteins and amino acids, are necessary for brain function and must be conveyed either by active or carrier-facilitated transport across the blood–brain barrier (see Fig. 3–1). The brain is an obligate user of glucose, and the density of the glucose transporter moiety in its capillaries is 10 to 20 times higher than in the membranes of other endothelial tissues.[1090,1321,1977] Transporters exist for neutral, acidic, and basic amino acids[767,1089]; monocarboxylic acids such as lactic acid[1116] (primarily for efflux of lactic acid produced by the brain); ketones; and electrolytes. A sodium-potassium adenosine triphosphatase pump regulates the concentration of potassium in extracellular space of the brain at about 2.8 mEq/L, compared with the concentration of 3 to 5 mEq/L in the plasma. Higher levels of potassium that follow blood–brain barrier breakdown may lead to seizures and other abnormalities of neurologic function.

The capillary endothelium of the brain is surrounded by a basement membrane in which pericytes are embedded that help determine capillary diameter and, thus, control cerebral blood flow. In addition, cerebral capillaries are ensheathed by astrocytic foot processes that apparently are not vital to ongoing function of the blood–brain barrier, but they, and perhaps neurons,[2596] are essential to maintaining the structure of the blood–brain barrier.[512,2421,2497] Cerebral capillaries in vitro maintain tight junctions when cocultured with astrocytes or astrocytic-conditioned media, but, if cultured alone, lose their tight junctions.[2421] Astrocytic damage caused by primary and metastatic tumors may contribute to blood–brain barrier disruption.

Both the brain and peripheral nerves have anatomic areas that lack barrier function. In the brain, these areas are the area postrema, the median eminence, the preoptic recess (collectively referred to as the circumventricular organs), and the pineal gland. The area postrema is particularly interesting because it contains an emetic chemoreceptor trigger zone that may explain, in part, the nausea and vomiting that occur when patients are given chemotherapeutic agents that do not normally cross the blood–brain barrier.

Blood–Peripheral Nerve Barrier

Less is known about the blood–peripheral nerve barrier.* Like the blood–brain barrier, it restricts movement of water, proteins, ions, and certain other water-soluble agents between the blood and peripheral nerve, although it is somewhat less restrictive than the blood–brain barrier. The barrier site appears to be at endoneurial capillaries; epineurial vessel permeability does not differ from that of vessels elsewhere in the body. Endoneurial capillaries, like brain capillaries, possess tight junctions, no fenestrations, and few pinocytotic vessels.[168] The blood–peripheral nerve barrier is absent both at the dorsal root ganglion[350] (the cell body of sensory nerves) and in the terminal branches of both sensory and motor nerves. The absence of a blood–nerve barrier at the dorsal root ganglion may explain in part the sensory neuronopathy that sometimes follows *cis*-platinum chemo-

* References 1943, 2022, 2051, 2136, 2137.

therapy (see Chapter 12). The absence of a barrier in terminal branches of the nerve may permit ingress and retrograde transport of chemotherapeutic agents such as vincristine, which are likewise neurotoxic. Tumor cells, particularly leukemia and lymphoma cells that traverse the endoneurium, appear to be protected from most systemic chemotherapeutic agents. This resistance may explain some episodes of peripheral neuropathy from tumor invasion in patients after apparently successful systemic treatment for leukemia or lymphoma (see Chapter 8).

Blood–Cerebrospinal Fluid Barrier

The blood–CSF barrier differs from the blood–brain barrier in several respects.[1292] It has a substantially smaller surface area than that of the brain (5000-fold less). The major sites of transport across the blood–CSF barrier are at the choroid plexi (where a substantial portion of the spinal fluid is secreted and the composition of newly formed CSF is determined) and at the arachnoid villi (and probably, to a lesser extent, along nerve root sheaths), where spinal fluid is reabsorbed by bulk flow. Certain trace elements essential for brain nutrition, such as folic acid and vitamin B_{12}, which do not cross the blood–brain barrier, may be transported into the nervous system via the choroid plexus and reach the brain by diffusion.[2469] Certain acidic substances such as penicillin and methotrexate are transported from the CSF to the blood by the choroid plexus, particularly that of the fourth ventricle.[248,1292]

The CSF is reabsorbed by bulk flow through the arachnoid villi. The rate of spinal fluid formation and absorption is about 0.35 mL/min. The CSF volume in the adult is approximately 150 mL, which is achieved by children at about 4 years of age. Thus, the intrathecal dose of methotrexate or other drugs should be about the same in children older than 4 years as in adults.[235] The total CSF volume turns over approximately four times a day. A barrier does not exist between the CSF and the brain because the ependyma lining the ventricles and the pia-arachnoid surrounding the brain and spinal cord allow free diffusion of substances, including proteins such as albumin. However, the diffusion rate into and through brain parenchyma is considerably slower than that of bulk flow. Furthermore, many substances are reabsorbed by the brain capillary bed once they have diffused a short distance into the parenchyma. Thus, most substances introduced into the CSF do not penetrate very far into the brain or spinal cord. The result is that drugs injected intrathecally, while exposing leptomeningeal tumor to high concentrations, usually fail to reach parenchymal lesions in significant concentration. Consequently, the method is unreliable for treating intraparenchymal lesions.[1018] In experimental animals, appreciable concentrations of methotrexate have been shown to reach about 40% of the brain within an hour after intraventricular administration, but this cannot be achieved in humans. In both experimental animals and humans, white matter adjacent to CSF contains the highest drug concentration, possibly explaining the tendency for drug-induced leukoencephalopathy to be periventricular.

The CSF also serves as the brain's lymphatic system. Substances that either cross the blood–brain barrier to enter brain interstitial space or are secreted or excreted by neurons and glia leave the nervous system by diffusing into the CSF and then are absorbed by bulk flow. In addition to diffusion, hydrostatic pressure may drive substances either toward or away from the spinal fluid. Thus, in the presence of a brain tumor, the tumor and the surrounding plasma-derived edema cause increased tissue pressure; the pressure drives substances from the tumor through the normal brain toward the subarachnoid space. Conversely, when subarachnoid pathways are blocked, pressure may drive substances from the CSF into the brain. Intrathecal methotrexate appears to be more toxic in patients with leptomeningeal tumor (with partial blockage of subarachnoid absorptive pathways) than when given prophylactically to individuals with normal subarachnoid pathways. Toxicity may be severe with intraventricular injection in patients with obstructive hydrocephalus.[2365]

Most lipid-soluble substances enter the brain with little difficulty. Some examples common in neuro-oncologic practice are phenytoin, codeine, methadone, and 1,3-bis-chloro(2-chloroethyl)-1-nitrosourea (BCNU)

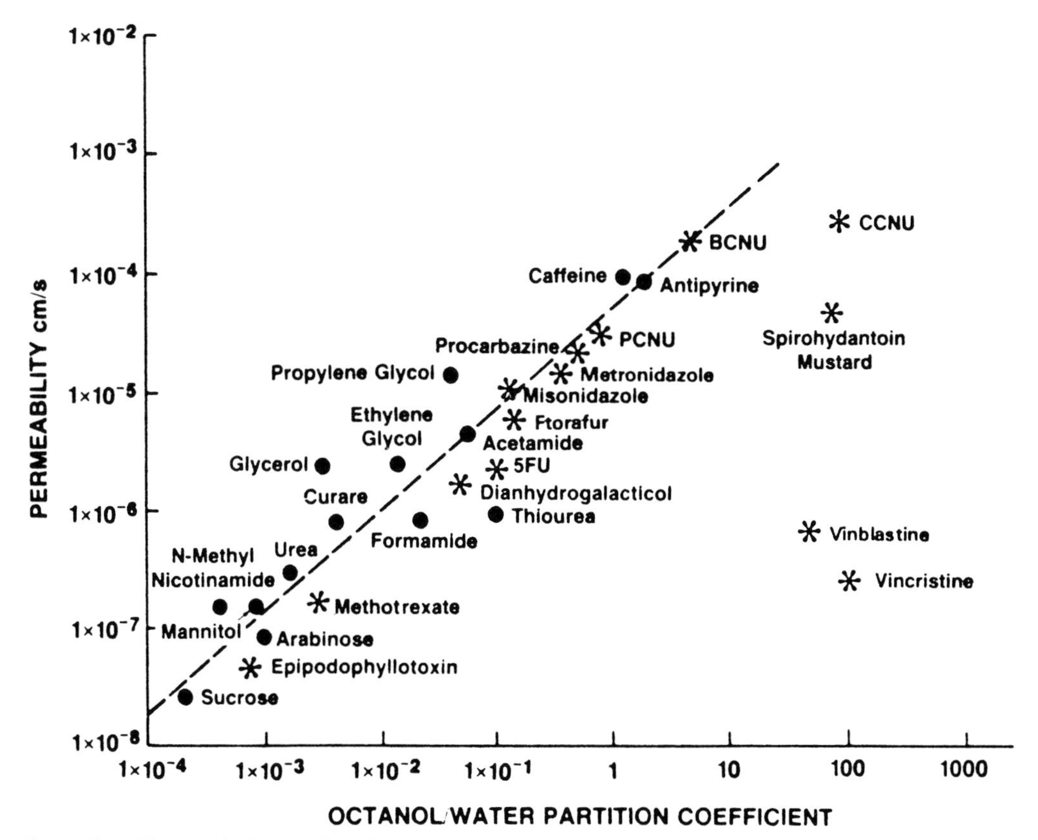

Figure 3–4. This graph depicts the relationship between octanol-water partition coefficient and cerebrovascular permeability. *Asterisks* indicate anticancer drugs. BCNU = 1,3-Bis-chloro(2-chloroethyl)-1-nitrosourea; CCNU = 1-(2-Chloroethyl)-3-cyclohexyl-1-nitrosourea; PCNU = 1-(2-Chloroethyl)-3-(2,6-dioxo-3-piperidyl)-nitrosourea; 5FU = 5-fluorouracil. (From Greig,[993] p 313, with permission.)

(Fig. 3–4). Morphine and aspirin enter the brain poorly. Most water-soluble chemotherapeutic agents, such as cytarabine and methotrexate, also enter the brain poorly, although the physician can substantially increase the concentration of these substances in the brain by raising the parenteral dose. Figure 3–4 shows several drugs and the degree to which they cross blood–CNS barriers.

DISRUPTION OF BLOOD–CENTRAL NERVOUS SYSTEM BARRIERS

Because metastatic tumors within the nervous system can grow to 1 to 2 mm without acquiring their own blood supply,[808,2895] these small tumors find sanctuary from many chemotherapeutic agents behind the blood–brain barrier. Most water-soluble chemotherapeutic agents do not reach them in adequate concentrations, giving the tumors an opportunity to grow even if they are sensitive to the parenteral drugs received by the patient. As noted previously, this activity may explain the increasing frequency of brain tumors in patients whose systemic tumor is well controlled with chemotherapeutic treatment (see Chapter 1).

As tumors enlarge, they produce angiogenic factors[808] that promote the emergence of new capillaries to supply the growing tumors.[1245] As mentioned earlier, newly formed capillaries in metastatic brain tumors are fenestrated, lack tight junctions, and have an increased number of pinocytotic vesicles and an irregular basal lamina.[1165,1599,2385] As a result, they do not possess a normal blood–CNS barrier, so that they are more accessible to water-soluble chemotherapeutic agents than normal cells. Even with an altered blood–brain barrier, experimental studies indicate that a water-soluble chemotherapeutic agent is less likely to reach a metastatic brain tumor than the same tumor found in other sites in the body.[2368] Furthermore, blood vessels surrounding primary brain tumors probably also do not have a normal blood–brain barrier.[1926,1927,2496] In some instances, this is due to an invasion of tumor cells into the parenchyma beyond the bulk of the tumor, a phenomenon uncommon in brain metastases except for renal-cell carcinomas and lymphomas. However, the disruption of the barrier does not depend on direct contact with tumor cells.[1926] The degree of macrophage infiltration seen on immunoperoxidase staining is correlated with the amount of peritumoral edema. Macrophagic infiltration is particularly prominent in metastatic brain tumors, perhaps partially explaining the marked edema that even small metastatic tumors often cause.[2393] In addition, tumor disruption of the barrier is rarely complete; it varies from tumor to tumor and within different regions of a single tumor. Substantial variability is found in the degree of breakdown of the blood–brain barrier in primary brain tumors implanted into rats. For instance, the nitrosourea-induced oligodendroglioma has an almost-normal blood–brain barrier, whereas the avian sarcoma virus–induced tumor is substantially leaky.[230,1798]

The clinical counterpart of this experimental observation is the difference in contrast enhancement when using iodinated dyes for CT scan or gadolinium for MR scan in various brain tumors. Low-grade gliomas, for example, often enhance poorly, if at all, whereas glioblastomas generally enhance intensely. Most metastatic tumors show substantial contrast enhancement. The commonly found enhancing rim and nonenhancing center does not indicate intact blood–brain barrier within the tumor center but represents low blood flow to the poorly vascularized tumor center. Delayed scans, after an injection of contrast, usually yield enhancement in the tumor center. If invaded by tumor, the leptomeninges, peripheral nerves, and nerve roots can also enhance on gadolinium MR scan.

Paradoxically, chemotherapy of established brain tumors that have broken down the blood–brain barrier is easier than such treatment of microscopic tumors that reside behind the barrier. Interesting experiments by Ushio and colleagues[2642,2646] have demonstrated in laboratory animals with brain or leptomeningeal tumors that the tumors are less susceptible to systemically administered chemotherapeutic agents early in their growth, when the blood–brain barrier is relatively intact, than they are later, when the barrier has been disrupted.

Brain Edema

As previously mentioned, when the blood–brain barrier is focally disrupted, water-soluble substances and large molecules such as proteins can enter the brain more easily. Because the brain has no lymphatics, these substances are not easily eliminated but are often driven into surrounding normal brain by increased hydrostatic pressure within the tumor, eventually to be eliminated by filtering through the white matter and then into the cerebral ventricles to be reabsorbed by bulk flow. Experimental evidence suggests that some protein can be reabsorbed by reverse vesicular transport across endothelial cells in the edematous brain,[2711] but few data are available to determine whether this mechanism is clinically significant.

The edema caused by brain tumors develops primarily in white matter rather than the more closely packed gray matter. It is extracellular and tends to follow white matter fiber tracts rather than to diffuse in a spherical pattern. Thus, a small occipital tumor may cause edema infiltrating along fiber tracts all the way to the tip of the temporal lobe, leading to a characteristic MR scan with the hyperintense edema fluid extending like fingers into the white matter outlining the cerebral cortex.

Brain tumors cause vasogenic edema (Table 3–2). The edema fluid has an elevated protein content including albumin, and the fluid volume of the extracellular space is increased. Most studies suggest that vasogenic edema, no matter how it is produced, is similar in content. One study of human tumors suggested, however, that the mean serum protein content in tissues adjacent to

Table 3–2. **CLASSIFICATION OF BRAIN EDEMA**

	Vasogenic	Cellular (Cytotoxic)	Hydrocephalic (Interstitial)
		CHARACTERISTICS	
Pathogenesis	Increased capillary permeability	Cellular swelling: glial, neuronal, endothelial	Increased brain fluid from blockage of CSF absorption
Location of edema	Chiefly white matter	Gray and white matter	Chiefly periventricular white matter, hydrocephalus
Edema fluid composition	Plasma filtrate including plasma proteins	Increased intracellular water and sodium levels	CSF
Extracellular fluid volume	Increased	Decreased	Increased
Capillary permeability to large molecules (RIHSA, inulin)	Increased	Normal	Normal
		CLINICAL DISORDERS	
Syndromes	Brain tumor, abscess, infarction, trauma, hemorrhage, lead encephalopathy Ischemia Purulent meningitis (granulocytic edema)	Hypoxia, hypo-osmolality (e.g., water intoxication) Dysequilibrium syndromes Ischemia Purulent meningitis (granulocytic edema) Reye's syndrome	Obstructive hydrocephalus Pseudotumor Purulent meningitis (granulocytic edema)
EEG changes	Focal slowing common	Generalized slowing	EEG often normal
		THERAPEUTIC EFFECTS	
Steroids	Beneficial in brain tumor, abscess	Not effective (possibly Reye's syndrome)	Uncertain effectiveness (possibly pseudotumor or meningitis)
Osmotherapy	Reduces volume of normal brain tissue only, *acutely*	Reduces brain volume *acutely* in hypo-osmolality	Rarely useful Improves compliance
Acetazolamide	Uncertain effect	No direct effect	Minor usefulness
Furosemide	Uncertain effect	No direct effect	Minor usefulness

After Klatzo, I: Neuropathological aspects of brain edema. J Neuropathol Exp Neurol 26:1–14, 1967; Manz, HJ: The pathology of cerebral edema. Hum Pathol 5:291–313, 1974; Fishman, RA: Brain edema. N Engl J Med 273:706–711, 1975.

CSF = cerebrospinal fluid; EEG = electroencephalogram; RIHSA = radioiodinated human serum albumin.

Source: Adapted from Fishman,[795] p 122.

the tumor varied considerably, depending on the nature of the tumor; it was high in glioblastomas and low in peritumoral edema surrounding metastases.[249] Dexamethasone has similar salutary effects on water content in either malignant gliomas or metastases.[249] Because the edema fluid has more water and is less dense than normal brain, it is relatively easily imaged by MR or CT scans. Characteristically, edema fluid is hypodense on CT scan and hyperintense on the T_2-weighted MR scan. Edema fluid does not enhance with contrast, making it easy to differentiate from tumor (Fig. 3–5).

The mechanism by which tumors cause vasogenic CNS edema is complex and multifactorial. Increased vascular permeability to plasma constituents, including albumin, results in the following: (1) Conductance of osmotically active solutes increases and their reflection coefficients decrease across the capillary wall; (2) a decrease in the concentration gradient of osmotically active solutes between plasma and brain extracellular fluid (ECF) (plasma > ECF) creates an imbalance between osmotic and hydrostatic pressures across brain and tumor capillaries, favoring fluid movement from blood to brain; (3) an increase in hydraulic conductivity of tumor vessels augments the transcapillary movement of plasma-derived fluid from blood to brain; (4) within the tissue, hydrostatic pressure gradients drive fluid movement from areas of blood–brain barrier breakdown into surrounding normal brain. The tissue hydrostatic pressure gradients and movement of edema fluid through the brain depend on arterial blood pressure and the hydraulic conductivity of the tissue (white matter > gray matter).

The formation within the tumors of new vessels that do not have a blood–brain barrier is certainly important to the pathogenesis of brain edema, but new vessel formation (i.e., angiogenesis) may not be the only way that edema is formed in brain tumors. Substantial

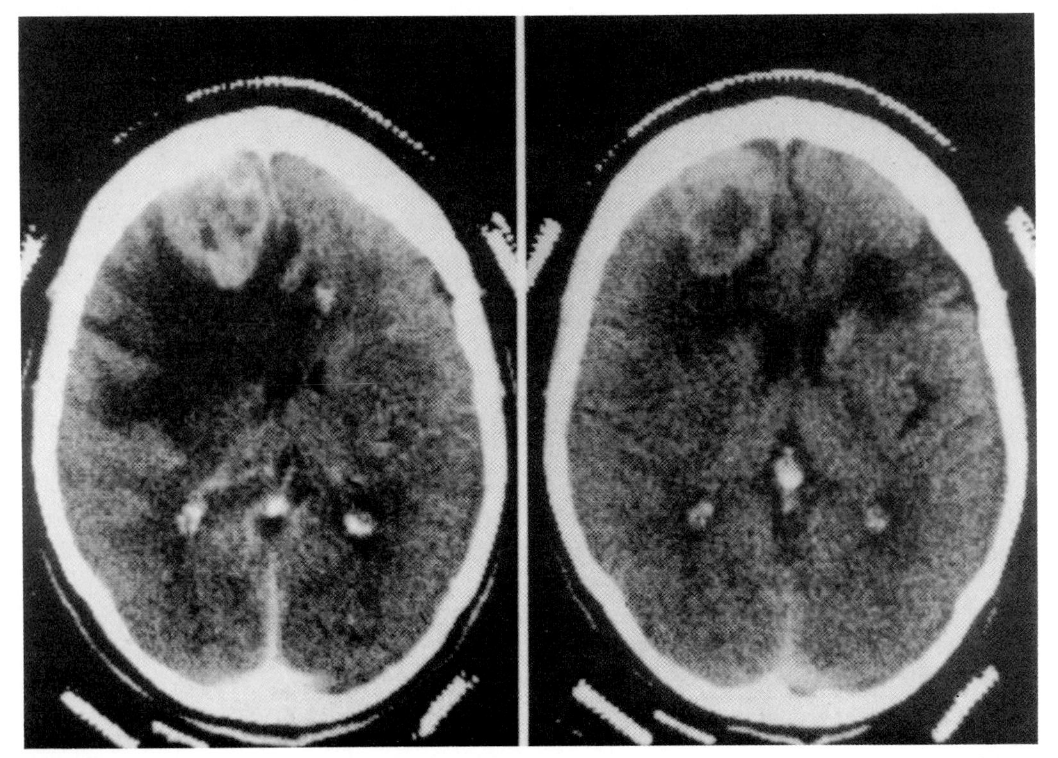

Figure 3–5. A contrast-enhanced CT showing the response of a frontal-lobe metastatic brain tumor to dexamethasone. *Left,* Massive edema with deformity and compression of lateral ventricles as well as herniation across the midline was present before dexamethasone treatment (see also Fig. 1–3); *right,* remarkable decrease in edema volume at the end of the follow-up period after the administration of dexamethasone. Note the decreased enhancement of the tumor without a change in size. (From Hatam et al,[1108] p 591, with permission.)

evidence indicates that, in addition to angiogenic substances, tumors secrete substances that not only promote angiogenesis of new vessels lacking a blood–brain barrier but also promote leakiness of normal brain capillaries in the area of brain immediately surrounding the tumor.[525,1926,1927,2512a] Interleukin-1, for example, injected into the brain, stimulates angiogenesis.[927] The nature of all of those substances that cause normal brain capillaries to leak has not been defined completely, but some investigators believe that arachidonic acid and its metabolites and cytokines (e.g., interleukin-1) may play an important role.* Ohnishi and his colleagues[1926] have found two different substances, poorly characterized at present, that, when injected into normal brain, disrupt the blood–brain barrier. The interference of glucocorticoids with arachidonic acid metabolism by inhibition of cyclo-oxygenase may partially explain why steroids restore a disrupted blood–brain barrier. Lipoxygenase inhibitors may also contribute to blood–brain barrier disruption.[113,875] Other substances implicated as possible mediators of vasogenic edema include bradykinin,[1241a] histamine, leukotriene, free radicals and serotonin,[2719] and, experimentally, the mucopolysaccharide, carrageenan.[875,876]

Other Sources of Disruption

Tumor growth is not the only mechanism that can disrupt the barrier. An increase in hydrostatic pressure, such as that caused by severe arterial hypertension, can disrupt the barrier[2528] and lead to brain edema. Compression of nervous system tissue can also disrupt the barrier, probably by interfering with venous drainage and increasing capillary hydrostatic pressure; this is possibly the mechanism of tissue edema caused by tumors compressing the brain or spinal cord but not directly invading them.[2644] Thus, mechanisms of edema formation in metastatic brain tumors and epidural spinal cord compression appear different. In metastatic brain tumors, leaky neovessels within the substance of the tumor and altered normal vessels in the brain surrounding the tumor lead to the formation of brain edema. Whether increased tissue pressure disrupts the blood–brain barrier in the brain surrounding a tumor is not entirely clear. In the patient with epidural spinal cord compression, on the other hand, the tumor is not in direct contact with the spinal cord, and neovascularity is absent; the edema is a result of normal vessels leaking within the spinal cord. It is not fully established whether hydrostatic pressure disrupts the blood–spinal cord barrier or whether some other damaging effect of spinal cord compression occurs. Edema caused by either intrinsic or extrinsic tumors responds to treatment with glucocorticoids (see the following). Other forms of edema are less amenable to steroid therapy (see Table 3–2).

Whether edema fluid in and of itself is toxic to the brain or whether all of its symptoms are a consequence of mass effect distorting normal tissue is not clear. No clinical or experimental evidence has defined whether or not symptoms are caused by the edema fluid itself. Edema fluid has a higher potassium concentration than does normal brain extracellular fluid, possibly promoting depolarization of neurons, which could lead to seizures. The pragmatic issue is that cerebral edema unquestionably is instrumental in causing symptoms in patients with metastatic tumors; amelioration of the edema with steroids or other substances (see the following) often substantially improves the symptoms even before the tumor itself is treated.

Other Substances Causing Blood–Brain Barrier Breakdown

In experimental animals, the intracarotid infusion of the chemotherapeutic agent etoposide has been shown to exert a dose-dependent effect on the blood–brain barrier, leading to its breakdown,[1190,2471,2472] as do intracarotid protamine sulfate[2509] and leukotreine C_4.[225,2635] Seizures can lead to breakdown of the blood–brain barrier[1901]; the subsequent formation of brain edema is probably related to seizure-induced arterial hypertension.[2528] The sudden accumulation of brain edema following a seizure may

* References 36, 224, 423, 445, 1835, 1925, 1927.

worsen neurologic symptoms in patients with metastatic brain tumors and is one reason to try to control seizures in such patients. Therapeutic irradiation also increases permeability across the blood–CNS barrier. Levin and associates[1538] observed a significantly increased permeability of blood–brain barrier during the first 24 hours after cranial radiation with 200 to 400 rad. Permeability was reduced after 2000 rad in 10 fractions. Experimental studies conducted at Memorial Sloan-Kettering Cancer Center (MSKCC) have shown increased permeability for the blood–brain barrier after application of radiation doses equivalent to those applied to humans therapeutically. The disruption of the blood–brain barrier may explain acute radiation reactions sometimes encountered clinically.[607,609,2032] Delattre and colleagues[609] report that, in an experimental brain tumor animal model, a single dose of 3000 rad and a total dose of 3000 rad delivered in 10 fractions increased the blood-to-brain transport of small molecules and partially disrupted the blood–brain barrier. No change was seen in the already partially disrupted barrier in the brain tumor. The clinical implication is that concurrent radiation and chemotherapy may promote the entry of additional chemotherapeutic agent into the brain without promoting entry into the tumor. Magnetic resonance scanning has been reported to temporarily alter the blood–brain barrier in the rat.[2394]

Chemotherapeutic substances may also alter the blood–brain barrier. Phillips and coworkers[2033] demonstrated that high-dose intravenous (IV) methotrexate impaired blood–brain barrier function, thus enhancing its own penetration into the CNS. Intracarotid administration of *cis*-platinum and etoposide appear to open the blood–brain barrier in the infused hemisphere for up to 96 hours. Interleukin-2 may have a similar effect[1925] because, when conjugated to a monoclonal antibody, it selectively promotes entry of the antibody into the tumor.[1490] One report[1592] suggests an increase in blood–CSF permeability following combined intrathecal methotrexate and CNS radiation. Corticosteroids often used to treat brain edema (see the following) tend to stabilize the blood–brain barrier and could decrease the entry of water-soluble chemotherapeutic agents into a tumor and surrounding brain. The clinical importance of this phenomenon is not established.

Transient "opening" of the blood–brain barrier by the intracarotid infusion of hyperosmolar agents (blood–brain barrier disruption) has been used therapeutically to treat patients with brain or leptomeningeal metastases[1874,2124] and some primary brain tumors, including lymphomas. The barrier remains open for only a few minutes, at least in baboons, and then returns to normal.[2907] The increase in barrier permeability is both greater and longer lasting in normal brain than in the brain tumor.[392] The hyperosmolar agent must be introduced intra-arterially and must exceed 1.4 mol/L. An intra-arterial infusion of 25% mannitol opens the blood–brain barrier in experimental animals and humans. During the time the barrier is open, water-soluble agents administered systemically or intra-arterially can enter the brain at a substantially greater rate. The procedure is usually but not always without complication[1471]; whether it is efficacious is controversial.[794] The mechanism by which hyperosmolar agents open the blood–brain barrier is also controversial. The best evidence indicates that shrinkage of endothelial cells widens interendothelial cell junctions, allowing substances to cross capillaries.[2125] Other studies suggest increased transendothelial vesicular transport.[510,756,1014] Experimentally, several studies have shown that modification of the blood–brain barrier has a far greater effect on drug entry into normal brain than into the tumor, thus exposing normal brain to greater concentrations of potentially neurotoxic drugs.[2368] The role of blood–brain barrier disruption combined with the delivery of potentially therapeutic monoclonal antibodies is currently under investigation.[2125] Friden and colleagues[838] have developed a novel method of circumventing an intact blood–brain barrier by conjugating the therapeutic molecule to an antibody against the transferrin receptor.

Measurement of Blood–Brain Barrier Function

The entry of substances from the bloodstream into the nervous system can be quantified in experimental animals by quantitative autoradiography (QAR) and in human beings by positron emission tomography (PET) scanning. Both techniques involve the injection of a radioactive tracer dose of the substances of interest and a comparison of radioactivity in the brain with that measured in the blood over time. The calculations yield a term called the plasma clearance constant (K_1), which reflects permeability of the capillaries to the substance of interest as well as the capillary surface area.

A variety of radioactive substances have been used to measure blood–nervous system barrier function in experimental animals by using QAR. The favorite substance is an artificial amino acid called "alpha amino isobutyric acid." C14 methotrexate and C14-labeled 1-(2-Chlorethyl)-3-(2,6-dioxo-3-piperidyl)-nitrosourea (PCNU) have also been used, as well as several other substances. In the human, blood–brain barrier function has been measured using rubidium (an element similar to potassium).

In general, normal brain has an exceedingly low transfer coefficient. In most brain tumors, the transfer coefficient is 4 to 20 times higher than in normal brain, although it varies from area to area. In the edematous brain immediately surrounding a tumor, the transfer coefficient may be two to four times that in normal brain. These findings apply to experimental animals with brain tumors. In the human, increased transfer constants are found within the brain tumor, but the resolution of PET is not sufficient to define the transfer constant in the edematous tissue immediately surrounding the tumor. As indicated previously, substantial alterations can be induced in the blood–brain barrier by such manipulations as the intracarotid injection of hyperosmolar agents.

CONSEQUENCES OF BLOOD–BRAIN BARRIER DISRUPTION: INCREASED INTRACRANIAL PRESSURE, PLATEAU WAVES, AND CEREBRAL HERNIATION

In patients with mass lesions involving or compressing nervous system structures, the breakdown of blood–nervous system barriers and the production of brain edema often lead to increased intracranial pressure. The pressure may be distributed evenly throughout the brain, such as when obstruction of the superior vena cava or sagittal sinus obstruction raises the pressure diffusely, or it may be distributed unevenly, as exemplified in patients with focal mass lesions.[2762] Evenly distributed increased intracranial pressure probably causes no symptoms until the intracranial pressure approaches the arterial blood pressure, resulting in cerebral ischemia. Focally increased tissue pressure causes herniation of portions of normal brain into areas of lower pressure. The most common sites of herniation, as illustrated in Figure 1–3, include herniation of the medial frontal lobe under the falx cerebri, herniation of the medial temporal lobe through the tentorium cerebelli, and herniation of the cerebellar tonsils through the foramen magnum. The clinical consequences of these herniations are described in Chapter 5. Focally increased tissue pressure can also cause symptoms by interfering with the local blood supply. Both mechanisms are probably responsible for many of the symptoms caused by brain and spinal cord tumors.

Some patients with normal or slightly elevated intracranial pressure at rest, or with chronically elevated intracranial pressure from mass lesions or compensated hydrocephalus from leptomeningeal tumors, suffer from intermittent episodes of neurologic dysfunction that result from sudden rises in intracranial pressure called *plateau waves*.[1119,1616,2225] These episodes last 5 to 20 minutes and then cease (Table 3–3). The waves, first described by Lundberg[1616] in 1960 (Fig. 3–6), appear to result from an increase in cerebral blood volume that is due to a sudden decrease in cerebral vascular resistance[1120,1703]; blood flow may actually decrease as the blood volume rises. Patients in whom the intracranial mass and elevated pressure have caused diminished CSF absorption are more likely to develop plateau waves than those with normal CSF absorption.[1121] Conversely, patients who have plateau waves develop signs of cerebral herniation at a higher pressure than do those who do not. One suggestion is that CSF pooling resulting from decreased CSF absorption forms a buffer to protect against herniation.[1121]

Plateau waves either can occur spontaneously or be precipitated in patients with

Table 3–3. CHARACTERISTICS OF PLATEAU WAVES

- Usually associated with intracranial hypertension
- May occur without any appreciable increase in blood pressure
- Usually not observed in hydrocephalic infants with an open fontanelle
- Often preceded by hypercarbia, painful stimuli, activity, increase in blood pressure, or change in body position
- Temporarily controlled by ventricular drainage, administration of hypertonic solution, hyperventilation
- Wider vessels in the arterial phase than in the interval between waves shown by angiograms during spontaneous plateau waves, but venous phase unaffected
- Increased cerebral blood volume and reduced cerebral blood flow reported during plateau waves

Source: Adapted from Fishman,[795] p 76.

increased intracranial pressure or with hydrocephalus. Common precipitating causes include tracheal suctioning, coughing or sneezing, and, particularly, rising from a lying or sitting position,[1646] especially in the early morning after a night's sleep. Plateau waves are often asymptomatic even when they cause a dramatic increase in intracranial pressure. The symptoms can be several and varied (Table 3–4), the most common of which are headache, restlessness and altered consciousness, and sudden weakness of both lower extremities with collapse but preservation of consciousness. Plateau waves respond dramatically to relief of raised intracranial pressure either by steroids or other mechanisms. Because of their dramatic symptomatology, plateau waves can be mistaken for seizures, transient attacks of cerebral ischemia (which may cause the symptoms of plateau waves), hemorrhage into a metastatic tumor, or migraine equivalents. A correct diagnosis of plateau waves depends on the physician's suspecting that plateau waves are responsible for the patient's symptoms. Intracranial pressure monitoring may also establish the diagnosis but is not always feasible or necessary. The diagnosis is often established on the basis of a therapeutic trial with corticosteroids. Plateau waves can lead to cerebral herniation, respiratory arrest, and death.[1121]

Treatment of Cerebral Herniation

Immediate treatment of increased intracranial pressure is required to reverse or

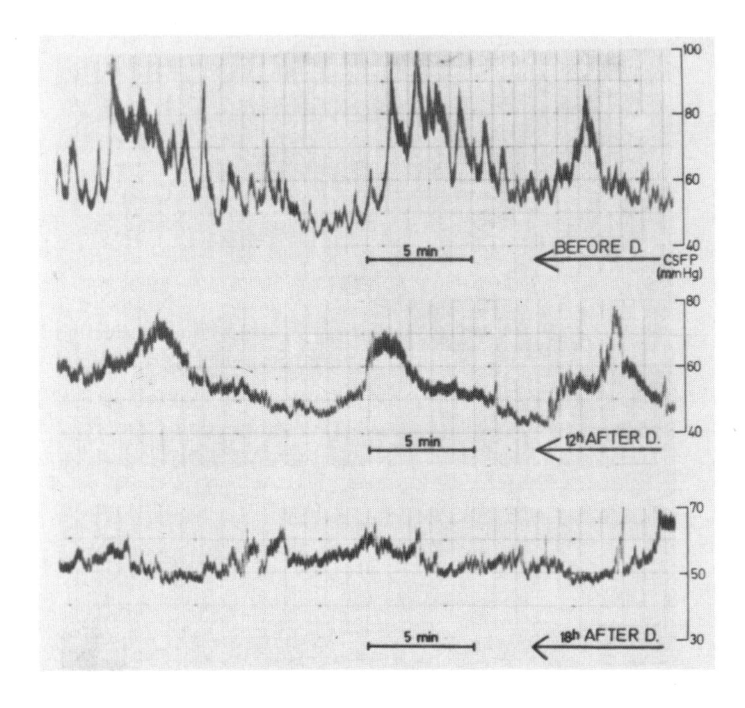

Figure 3–6. Continuous registration of the cerebrospinal fluid pressure (CSFP) in a patient with increased intracranial pressure before and after being treated with dexamethasone (D). The curves read from right to left. The amplitude and frequency of the plateau waves diminish rapidly; the overall intracranial pressure diminishes more slowly (see scales). (From Alberti et al,[31] p 177, with permission.)

Table 3–4. **PAROXYSMAL SYMPTOMS FROM PLATEAU WAVES IN PATIENTS WITH INTRACRANIAL SPACE-OCCUPYING LESIONS**

Impairment of consciousness
Trancelike state
Unreality/warmth
Confusion, disorientation
Restlessness, agitation
Disorganized motor activity, carphologia
Sense of suffocation, air hunger
Cardiovascular/respiratory disturbances
Headache
Pain in the neck and shoulders
Nasal itch
Blurring of vision, amaurosis
Mydriasis, pupillary areflexia
Nystagmus
Oculomotor/abducens paresis
Conjugate deviation of the eyes
External ophthalmoplegia
Dysphagia, dysarthria
Nuchal rigidity
Retroflexion of the neck
Opisthotonus, trismus
Rigidity and tonic extension/flexion of the arms and legs
Bilateral extensor plantar responses
Sluggish/absent deep tendon reflexes
Generalized muscular weakness
Facial twitching
Clonic movements of the arms and legs
Facial/limb paresthesias
Rise in temperature
Nausea, vomiting
Facial flushing
Pallor, cyanosis
Sweating
Shivering and "goose flesh"
Thirst
Salivation
Yawning, hiccoughing
Urinary and fecal urgency/incontinence

Source: Adapted from Lundberg,[1616] p 69.

prevent cerebral herniation and prevent death. The treatment of increased intracranial pressure and cerebral herniation is discussed extensively elsewhere[218,2132,2201,2224] and includes hyperventilation, hyperosmolar agents, and adrenocorticosteroids (Table 3–5).

Hyperventilation is the most rapid technique for lowering intracranial pressure and reversing herniation. Hyperventilation lowers pCO_2, causing cerebral vasoconstriction and decreasing cerebral blood volume. If the patient is unconscious, an endotracheal tube should be inserted and the patient ventilated to a pCO_2 level between 25 and 30 mm Hg, which lowers intracranial pressure rapidly in most patients but only transiently. Many patients with cerebral herniation spontaneously hyperventilate to these levels and require no additional respiratory intervention from the physician. However, intubation is advisable to protect the airway. Respiratory function must be monitored carefully because brain herniation can cause respiratory failure. Mechanical ventilation can raise as well as lower intracranial pressure. Patients who have brain lesions and require ventilation are at risk.[480]

Hyperosmolar agents decrease the water content of the brain by creating an osmolar gradient between the blood and that portion of the brain with an intact blood–brain barrier (Table 3–6). The agent of choice is mannitol given IV over 10 to 20 minutes as a

Table 3–5. **EMERGENCY TREATMENT OF IMPENDING HERNIATION IN ACUTELY DECOMPENSATING PATIENTS**

Therapy	Dosage or Procedure	Onset (Duration) of Action
Hyperventilation	Lower pCO_2 to 25 to 30 mm Hg	Seconds (minutes)
Osmotherapy	Mannitol, 0.5 to 2.0 g/kg (IV) over 15 minutes, followed by 25 g (IV "boosters") as needed	Minutes (hours)
Corticosteroids	Dexamethasone, 100 mg IV push, followed by 40–100 mg/24 hr, depending on symptoms	Hours (days)

Table 3–6. **PRINCIPLES OF OSMOTHERAPY**

1. Brain volume and elastance decrease in the presence of an osmotic gradient.
2. Osmotic gradients are short-lived; solutes reach equilibrium in the brain after a delay of a few hours.
3. With vasogenic edema, the normal brain areas "shrink"; edematous regions do not.
4. Osmotherapy is most effective in reducing intracranial pressure in normal subjects and least effective when the blood–brain barrier is impaired.
5. Rebound may follow the administration of any hypertonic solutions.
6. Brain adapts to sustained hyperosmolality with the equilibration of the administered solute and the appearance of "idiogenic" osmoles.

Source: From Fishman,[795] p 95, with permission.

20% solution at a dose of 0.5 to 2 g/kg.[2132] This drug also may decrease CSF formation and volume.[666] In a few patients with severe and sustained increased intracranial pressure, pressure can be monitored and the dose tailored to maintain decreased pressure.[2132] In patients with normal intracranial pressure, mannitol actually may increase the pressure briefly, probably because of a transient increase in cerebral blood flow and volume. This does not appear to occur in patients with increased intracranial pressure.[795,2132] The mannitol effects are rapid and last several hours. Mannitol injections may be repeated in smaller doses if the patient responds and subsequently relapses. Glycerol and urea are less widely used. Urea eventually finds its way across the blood–brain barrier and may produce a late reverse osmolar effect.[2224] Glycerol can be taken orally and was once used for more long-term management,[2721] but it is rapidly metabolized in the liver and also may cause a reverse osmotic effect. Repeated doses of mannitol also can cause a reverse osmotic effect. The addition of a diuretic (furosemide) enhances and prolongs the mannitol effect.[2055]

Dexamethasone (100 mg IV) is given immediately, followed by doses of 40 to 100 mg/24 hr, depending on the patient's response to treatment. Some physicians add furosemide (40 to 120 mg IV) to the steroids and believe that the combination is better than steroids alone.[2224]

Barbiturate anesthesia proved successful in one patient with intractable increased intracranial pressure from choriocarcinoma metastases.[2837] She subsequently responded to chemotherapy. The drug is rarely used to treat herniation from brain tumors because other methods are so effective.

With such vigorous treatment, most patients who herniate from brain metastasis can be stabilized and many have complete amelioration of their symptoms within a few days.

TRANSPORT OF CHEMOTHERAPEUTIC DRUGS ACROSS THE BLOOD–BRAIN BARRIER

Lipid-soluble drugs penetrate the blood–brain barrier with ease and are carried to the brain and tumors in direct proportion to blood flow. Blood flow is heterogeneous in most primary and metastatic tumors, and, in many areas, the flow may be quite low.[1010] Thus, in general, when lipid-soluble chemotherapeutic agents are used, the normal brain receives greater exposure than does the tumor. A few substances, such as melphalan, are transported across capillary endothelium by facilitated diffusion.[1011]

Several factors determine how much chemotherapeutic agent, lipid- or water-soluble, will enter the brain[767,830]: (1) One factor is the concentration of free drug in the plasma unbound to plasma proteins. Binding of a drug to a plasma protein usually limits its entry into the brain, but some plasma protein bound substances may become more available for transport through the barrier because of specific interactions between plasma proteins and the endothelial surface, interactions called *endothelial-enhanced absorption* of ligand-protein. The degree to which a given ligand is transported through the blood–brain barrier depends on which site the ligand binds. Albumin has at least six different endothelial binding sites. (2) Another factor determining entry of a drug into the brain is the drug's ionization. An ionized drug crosses the blood–brain barrier with much more difficulty (10,000 times) than the non-ionized form. (3) Both plasma concentration level and the drug's duration in the circulation are also important. The area under a concentration-versus-time curve expresses the total exposure of tissue to a chemotherapeutic agent. (4) For water-soluble drugs, the permeability of the capillaries and their total surface area is the most important factor. The increased capillary permeability in tumors leads to the entry of a greater amount of water-soluble chemotherapeutic agents into the tumor than into the normal brain. (5) The route of administration is also important. Intra-arterial injection generally leads to a greater entry of drug into both tumor and normal brain than does IV injection.[1154] The result affects both the flow in the injected artery relative to cardiac output and the rapidity of drug clearance from the circulation. The technique allows one to expose the tumor to more chemotherapeutic agent than the bone marrow at a given dose. The distribution of intra-arterially injected drugs is variable and not entirely predictable because streaming within the arterial lumen affects drug distribution.

Chemotherapeutic agents can be cleared from the brain by efflux, metabolism, or transport into other tissue regions via the CSF. Each factor may be important in determining the exposure of tumor cells to the drug. Experimental studies indicate how to measure the transfer constant and predict the exposure of a given tumor to a specific chemotherapeutic agent (Table 3–7).

Table 3–7. **CENTRAL NERVOUS SYSTEM PENETRATION BY ANTILEUKEMIC DRUGS**

Drug	CSF/Plasma (%)
Methotrexate	3
6-Mercaptopurine	26
Cytarabine	10–25
Daunomycin	ND
Vincristine	5
Teniposide	1–3
Prednisone	8 (dose dependent)
L-asparaginase	ND
Cyclophosphamide	
Parent drug	ND
Active metabolite	17

ND = not detectable in CSF.

RESTORATION OF BLOOD–CENTRAL NERVOUS SYSTEM BARRIERS

Lowering Intracranial Pressure

The breakdown of blood–CNS barriers leads to the formation of edema. Several agents and methods are used to decrease nervous system edema and to lower tissue pressure. Physical methods include hyperventilation (lowering the arterial pCO_2 causes cerebral vasoconstriction with decreased cerebral blood flow and volume, acutely lowering intracranial pressure but not directly affecting brain edema) and IV injection of hyperosmolar agents such as mannitol. The exact mechanism of mannitol's effect is controversial,[1104,2055] but the conventional belief is that it does not cross a normal blood–brain barrier and, therefore, increases the osmotic pressure of blood relative to brain. This, in turn, causes a shift of water from the brain to the blood and decreases brain water content. At sites in which the blood–brain barrier is no longer functional, mannitol can cross into the brain. Under such circumstances, the agent will not remove water as effectively from brain tumor or the surrounding edematous tissue as it does from the normal brain. In experimental animals given mannitol, maximal intracranial pressure reduction occurs within 20 minutes, whereas white matter water content in the normal hemisphere begins to decrease later, reaching a minimum at 60 minutes. The water content in the white matter of the edematous hemisphere does not change.[1104] Other effects on blood flow and volume also have been imputed as potential causes of lowering intracranial pressure but not affecting edema.

A wide variety of drugs, including glutamate inhibitors, nonsteroidal anti-inflammatory agents (indomethacin), and lazeroids have also been proposed for the treatment of edema of the brain and spinal cord,[9,1376,2147,2414] but their clinical efficacy is unproved. Corticotropin-releasing factor (CRF) has proved effective in ameliorating tumor-induced brain edema in experimental animals. The mechanism of action is not known. The edema-ameliorating effects are not a result of CRF-induced cortisol release because CRF is effective in adrenalectomized brain-tumor–bearing animals.[2592a] Clinical trials are now under way.

Steroids

The most widely used drugs in neuro-oncology are the synthetic glucocorticoids, commonly referred to simply as steroids.[711,2784] They are the mainstay of treatment for nervous system edema and increased pressure. Kofman and colleagues[1401] first demonstrated in 1957 the effectiveness of steroids in relieving symptoms of breast cancer metastatic to the brain (an effect that may have, in part, been oncolytic); Galicich and French[870] subsequently demonstrated amelioration of symptoms of primary brain tumors by dexamethasone (see the following). Since that time, these drugs have been used in virtually all patients suffering from metastatic brain and spinal cord tumors. Steroids have an oncolytic effect on a few tumors such as lymphomas and breast carcinoma but are used by the neuro-oncologist primarily to relieve the symptoms of edema affecting the brain, spinal cord, and, possibly, nerves and nerve roots. They are also frequently used to treat symptomatic leptomeningeal and peripheral nerve metastases as well as CNS edema that occurs as a side effect of chemotherapy or radiation therapy. Steroids probably exert their major effect by partially reversing the disruption of the blood–brain barrier, blood–spinal cord barrier, or blood–nerve barrier caused by metastases to those organs.[50,2864] A 1-day prevalence study in 1986 indicated that 33% (13 of 40) of patients on the General Neurology Service at The New York Hospital and 69% (22 of 32) of the patients on the Neuro-oncology Service at MSKCC were receiving corticosteroids. Overall, about 15% of all patients hospitalized at MSKCC receive corticosteroids at some time.

The optimal dose and best preparation of corticosteroids are not established.[1931] The dosage probably should differ with both the nature of the problem and its severity.[2155] Equivalent doses of the steroids commonly used by neuro-oncologists are indicated in Table 3–8.

The steroid most widely used remains dexamethasone, largely because it was the drug established by Galicich and French[870] to treat brain tumors. Dexamethasone may be preferred to other synthetic glucocorticoids for several theoretical reasons. First, because it has no mineralocorticoid effect, it is the least likely steroid to cause salt retention and systemic edema formation. Some investigators believe it is also less likely than other synthetic steroids to cause cognitive and behavioral dysfunction[795] (see Chapter 4). Dexamethasone also inhibits leukocyte

Table 3–8. **RELATIVE POTENCY OF STEROIDS**

Steroid	Glucocorticoid Activity*	Mineralocorticoid Activity*	Equivalent Dose (mg)
Short-acting (8–12 hr†)			
Cortisol (hydrocortisone)	1.0	1.0	20.0
Cortisone	0.8	1.0	25.0
Intermediate (12–36 hr†)			
Prednisolone	4.0	0.8	5.0
Prednisone	4.0	0.8	5.0
Methylprednisolone	5.0	0.5	4.0
Long-acting (>36 hr†)			
Dexamethasone	25.0	0.0	0.75

*Relative to cortisol.
†Biologic half-life.

migration to a lesser extent than other synthetic glucocorticoids, perhaps decreasing the risk of infection.[2016] On the other hand, experimental evidence indicates that dexamethasone and other fluorinated steroids are more likely to cause steroid myopathy. For many disorders, prednisone often is given every other day to minimize side effects; however, every-other-day prednisone is ineffective in controlling brain edema and its symptoms. Because dexamethasone has a long half-life, an every-other-day dosage does not lessen side effects. On balance, dexamethasone appears to be the best drug to treat metastatic CNS tumors.

Only a few experiments address a dose-response curve for CNS effects of corticosteroids. One such experiment in an animal model of spinal cord compression suggests that doses equivalent to 100 mg/24 hr of dexamethasone may be superior to lesser doses both in decreasing edema and in ameliorating clinical symptomatology.[603] Because reports thus far give no indication that these higher doses given for a few days are deleterious, our practice is to use high doses in seriously symptomatic or deteriorating patients, tapering the dose after a few days to the lowest dose consistent with symptomatic control.

Steroid treatment begins with the physician's selecting a dose appropriate for the neurologic disorder and its severity[2784] (see the following). Because of its long half-life, dexamethasone can be given twice daily, although most physicians give four divided doses. The drug is well absorbed from the gastrointestinal tract, but first-pass hepatic metabolism may decrease the effectiveness of an oral dose, especially in patients taking phenytoin (see Chapter 4). Because side effects are numerous and often serious, patients should be maintained on the lowest dose of steroids that affords relief of symptoms. Thus, once symptomatic control is established and more definitive therapy (e.g., surgery, radiation, and chemotherapy) is under way, the steroid should be tapered to the lowest possible dose (see the following). Other agents that might control brain edema (e.g., 21-aminosteroids) are being tested, but none have yet proved to be clinically effective.[1194,1726] The following paragraphs describe the use of steroids to relieve symptoms caused by metastatic and some nonmetastatic effects of cancer on the nervous system.

BRAIN METASTASES

Symptomatic but stable patients can begin on 16 mg of dexamethasone daily (one report suggests that 4 mg or 8 mg is as effective as 16 mg).[2682] About 70% to 80% of patients with brain metastases achieve symptomatic improvement. The improvement is more dramatic in patients with symptoms and signs of "generalized brain dysfunction," that is, headache, lethargy, and papilledema, caused by distortion of the intracranial contents by tumor and edema, and in patients with signs of cerebral herniation. The drug is slightly less effective in patients who have only focal signs, that is, hemiparesis without headache or lethargy, aphasia, and visual field defects. If the standard dose fails to produce a clinical response within 48 hours, the dose should be doubled each 48 hours until this response is achieved. Up to 100 mg/24 hr of dexamethasone may be required.[1564,2155] For patients with signs of increased intracranial pressure, cerebral herniation, or plateau waves, an IV bolus of 40 to 100 mg may be given, followed by a daily dose equal to the size of the effective bolus. It was recently proposed that controlled-release polymers could deliver dexamethasone to the brain by direct implantation, effectively treating peritumoral edema without the use of the systemic drug.[2547]

SPINAL CORD COMPRESSION

Steroid effects seem to be less dramatic in epidural spinal cord compression than in metastatic brain tumor. This difference may be because most patients with spinal cord compression receive other therapy (i.e., surgical decompression, radiation therapy, or cytotoxic drugs) almost immediately, without an opportunity for the physician to assess steroid effects. By contrast, in patients with metastatic brain tumors, other therapy is often deferred 2 or 3 days until the full effects of steroids have occurred. Also, spinal cord edema arises from a mechanism different from that of brain metastases. The edema results from compression of the spinal cord vasculature rather than from direct contact of tumor with the CNS. Nevertheless, animal experiments demonstrate the presence of vasogenic edema when the spinal cord is compressed by epidural tumor, and have shown that the edema can be reversed (and neurologic symptoms improved) by steroids[2644]; higher doses are more effective than lower ones.[603]

Steroids alone have a salutary effect on the neurologic signs and symptoms of epidural cord compression in some patients and are effective in relieving the pain in most.[378,984,2654,2681] For patients with clinical or MR-scan evidence of cord compression but without neurologic symptoms except for moderate pain, one can begin with the standard dose (16 mg/24 hr of dexamethasone), increasing the dose if pain persists or new symptoms develop. For patients with severe pain, or evidence of myelopathy, an IV bolus of 100 mg of dexamethasone should be administered, followed by 100 mg/24 hr in divided doses orally. The drug should be tapered as the patient is treated with more definitive modalities (see Chapter 6). IV dexamethasone is infused slowly over a period of 5 to 10 minutes; some patients complain of severe genital burning as the drug is infused, but this lasts only a few minutes and is easily tolerated by the patient, particularly if he or she is forewarned.[542] One study suggests that no additional benefit is obtained from these higher doses,[2681] but animal experiments[603] along with a great deal of anecdotal human experience suggest an advantage. A recent randomized trial of high-dose steroids versus no steroids indicated improved function in the steroid group at 6 months after radiation.[2464]

STEROIDS FOR OTHER NEUROLOGIC COMPLICATIONS OF CANCER

The indications for steroids in the treatment of leptomeningeal metastases involving nerve roots, or of tumor involving peripheral nerves or nerve plexuses, are not established. Many patients are relieved of pain at standard or somewhat higher doses; some appear to have improved neurologic function. The drugs are worth trying in the initial treatment of patients with these conditions but should be abandoned if a clinical response is not achieved.

Steroids may also help treat chemotherapy-induced leukoencephalopathy (see Chapter 12) and some of the delayed effects of radiation on the nervous system (see Chapter 13). Although the dosage for these effects is not established, it is probably best to start with large doses and either taper rapidly or abandon the treatment if a response is not observed in a few days.

Patients with metastatic tumors of the brain, and sometimes the spinal cord, begin to improve within an hour after an IV injection of dexamethasone. Maximal clinical improvement on continued treatment occurs within 24 to 72 hours. In patients with spinal cord compression, pain may improve within an hour. Patients with brain tumor headache, lethargy, and sometimes weakness are demonstrably better within a few hours. Alberti and colleagues[31] have shown that the first change is a decrease in plateau waves (see Fig. 3–6), followed by gradual decline of the initially increased intracranial pressure over a period of 48 to 72 hours. The CT and MR scans often fail to show a substantial amelioration of edema in patients who have shown dramatic clinical improvement, but many scans do show decreased contrast enhancement within the tumor, suggesting partial restoration of the integrity of the blood–brain barrier. On rare occasions, the tumor, as defined by contrast enhancement, disappears after the corticosteroid treatment. The brain tumor that responds most dramatically to steroids is lymphoma. About 40% of contrast-enhancing masses that are due to lymphoma in the brain disappear with steroid treatment, probably reflecting a direct oncolytic effect. With gliomas and metastatic brain tumors, dramatic changes in the size or intensity of contrast areas occur only rarely, usually with small metastases. Thus, in most patients suspected of harboring neoplasms in the CNS, scans should be performed before steroids are administered unless the drugs are necessary to control serious symptoms.

Experimental evidence in animals with epidural tumor–induced spinal cord compression suggests that within 1 hour after steroids are injected, the transfer constant of water-soluble substances from blood to spinal cord has decreased; this effect is greater at 12 hours after a single large dose of steroids.[2366]

The PET scans of humans with brain tumors show an effect on the blood–brain barrier as early as 6 hours after a 100 mg IV bolus of dexamethasone. The transfer constant of rubidium, a water-soluble substance resembling potassium, is the marker used.[1278] The apparent blood and tissue volumes in and around the tumor also decrease at a later time.

STEROID TAPER

Because of deleterious effects of corticosteroids (see Chapter 4), patients should be treated with the smallest effective dose for the shortest time possible. Virtually all patients begun on corticosteroid therapy for brain metastases or spinal cord compression are treated subsequently with either radiation therapy or chemotherapy. During or after this more definitive treatment, the patient should be weaned from the steroids entirely, if possible. The steroid taper begins 3 to 4 days after surgery or during week 2 of radiation therapy and should be tapered gradually enough to prevent the development of steroid withdrawal symptoms but rapidly enough so that the patient is not taking the drugs for an extended period. For patients receiving 16 mg of dexamethasone, the drug should be tapered by 2 to 4 mg every fifth day. If at any time during the tapering the patient develops symptoms of either brain tumor or steroid withdrawal, the drug is increased to the next dose for 4 to 8 days before tapering again. If, after drug withdrawal, the patient develops brain tumor symptoms, it is probably wise to start the full regimen of 16 mg/24 hr of dexamethasone.

For patients who have been on steroids for many months and fail the usual taper schedule or have large amounts of residual tumor, the drug is tapered more slowly (e.g., 1-2 mg/wk) to the lowest dose tolerable. For patients taking large doses of steroids (e.g., 100 mg/24 hr dexamethasone) who have stabilized and are receiving more definitive treatment, the dose can be halved every 4 to 5 days, depending on the patient's clinical state. The dose should be raised again if the clinical state deteriorates.

Weissman and colleagues[2786] propose a more rapid taper schedule beginning at 16 mg/day (8 mg bid) for 4 days followed by 8 mg/24 hr for 4 days and 4 mg/24 hr until completion of radiation therapy. This procedure was well tolerated by their patients.

MECHANISMS OF STEROID ACTION

The mechanisms by which steroids stabilize blood–brain barriers, blood–spinal cord barriers, and probably blood–CSF barriers are not entirely known, although several have been proposed. Glucocorticoids inhibit the production or release of a number of biochemical substances shown to increase vascular permeability and to induce vasodilatation (an effect that, by increased hydrostatic pressure, also increases permeability). Glucocorticoids induce formation of lipocortins, which inhibit phosphorylase A2, thus preventing the release of arachidonic acid.[423] Arachidonic acid and its metabolites increase vascular permeability; thus, the reduction of arachidonic acid by steroids may reduce brain edema. Nonetheless, other inhibitors of this pathway, such as indomethacin, do not stabilize the blood–brain barrier or ameliorate the symptoms of brain tumors as effectively as do corticosteroids. Also, steroids inhibit the release of interleukin-1; whether the interleukins play a role in blood–brain barrier breakdown is not known. Steroids also appear to have a direct effect on endothelial cells in several organisms, inhibiting the increased permeability that results from their interaction with a number of chemical agents.[2788] Experimental evidence suggests that steroids can induce the synthesis of a protein that inhibits microvascular permeability, a direct action on the endothelial cell. The inhibitory protein appears to be distinct from lipocortin, and, thus, the effect is independent from the inhibition of phosphorylase A2. Whatever the mechanism, steroids appear to be unique in their ability to ameliorate clinical symptoms and stabilize the blood–brain barrier.

In addition to restoring capillary impermeability,[2818] dexamethasone also decreases cerebral blood flow and volume[1278,2543] and increases the fractional extraction of oxygen throughout the brain without affecting oxygen utilization. Reports suggest that the drug probably has a direct vasoconstrictive effect on cerebral blood vessels.[1508] Dexamethasone treatment reduces or eliminates the filtration of plasma-derived fluid across tumor capillaries and also reduces the movement of albumin through the extracellular space by solvent drag. These effects may be mediated by reducing the size of the extracellular space or decreasing the pore size of tumor capillaries, probably representing an important mechanism for corticosteroid control of tumor in peritumoral brain edema.[1851] Although most studies have not demonstrated an effect of dexamethasone on the blood–brain barrier of normal brain, at least one study[1127] suggests that dexamethasone may decrease the permeability to macromolecules of even normal cerebral vasculature, possibly by interfering with vesicular transport.[1127]

CHAPTER 4

SUPPORTIVE CARE AGENTS AND THEIR COMPLICATIONS

Patients with neuro-oncologic disorders often suffer pain and other symptoms that are not strictly neurologic but either mimic neurologic complications of cancer or occur more commonly in patients who have neurologic complications or who are being treated for them. Some of these nonneurologic abnormalities, such as cachexia,[1736] generalized weakness[733,1217] and fatigue,[2444] gastrointestinal (GI) ulcerations, deep vein thromboses, and side effects of the many drugs used for supportive care, are particularly common in patients with neuro-oncologic disorders. Effectively managing these disorders and their attendant symptoms can improve the quality of the patient's life and promote survival.[1550,2071,2563] Supportive care and symptom management is a vast field. Only a few problems of particular relevance to neuro-oncology can be addressed here. These include the side effects of several drugs used for supportive care of patients with cancer (Table 4–1).

GLUCOCORTICOID HORMONES

Glucocorticoids are among the most frequently used drugs in oncology. In one survey of patients with cancer admitted to hospice, one-third were receiving glucocorticoids.[1865] More than two-thirds of the patients on the inpatient Neuro-oncology Ward at Memorial Sloan-Kettering Cancer Center (MSKCC) are receiving corticosteroids. The major use of glucocorticoid hormones is to control brain and spinal cord edema (see Chapter 3). They are also useful as chemotherapeutic agents for several cancers, such as breast cancer and lymphoma, and have other important salutary effects: They improve appetite, elevate mood, decrease pain, and restore the integrity of the blood–brain barrier.

Salutary Effects

In controlled trials, steroids increased the quality of life in patients with preterminal or

Table 4–1. **COMMON AGENTS USED FOR SUPPORTIVE CARE OF THE NEURO-ONCOLOGY PATIENT**

Glucocorticoids	Analgesics
Gastroprotectors	Psychotropics
Laxatives	Anti-emetics
Anticonvulsants	Antibiotics
Anticoagulants	

terminal cancer.[332,610,2059,2551] They improve appetite,[328] decrease nausea and vomiting,[403] enhance the feeling of well-being in many patients, and appear to have substantial pain-relieving qualities.[2551] The exact mechanism of pain relief is unclear, although several steroid properties, including their anti-inflammatory and anti-edema effects, their ability to reduce ectopic firing of damaged peripheral nerves,[630] and their inhibition of nociceptive cytokine release, may play a role. In patients with spinal cord compression, pain relief is often dramatic and is clinically independent of its effect on other spinal cord dysfunction. Many patients with severe pain can decrease their intake of opioids when they begin taking steroids, and, in some, the pain relief from steroids is more complete than that from opioids.

Steroids are also useful to manage nausea and vomiting caused by either the cancer or its chemotherapy.[1686] A number of trials have documented the usefulness of corticosteroids either alone or in conjunction with other anti-emetic agents in the control of chemotherapy-induced nausea and vomiting. In at least one of these studies, the steroids also improved mood and reduced the sense of fatigue.[403] The mechanism by which steroids reduce nausea and vomiting is unknown but may be a direct effect of steroids on the vomiting center of the brainstem.[534]

Corticosteroids increase appetite and redistribute fat, undesirable side effects in most instances but beneficial in cachectic patients with terminal cancer.[332] The increase in appetite and the weight gain, however, are usually offset by the catabolic effects of steroids, which decrease muscle mass (see the following). Other drugs that may increase appetite without the side effects of steroids include cryohepatidine,[1341] a serotonin antagonist, dronabinol,[167a] and megestrol.[2564]

The specific corticosteroid that achieves the best effect, the dose, and the timing of divided doses has not been established. Prednisolone, methylprednisolone, and dexamethasone have all been used in various studies and have yielded approximately comparable results. Relative potencies of individual preparations can be found in Table 3–8 and in the references.[1132] Relatively low doses of the drug (e.g., 32 mg/24 hr of methylprednisolone[332]) appear to suffice for most indications, but our experience at MSKCC suggests that in spinal cord compression, higher doses are necessary to control pain (see Chapter 3). The side effects of high-dose steroids (e.g., 100 mg/24 hr of dexamethasone) appear to be no greater than those from lower doses (16 mg/24 hr dexamethasone) if given for only a short period.[1691] At least one study, however, suggests a higher frequency of serious side effects with high-dose steroids.[1131] Dexamethasone is the steroid preparation most used by neurologists, partially for historical reasons but partially because its lack of mineralocorticoid effect obviates the salt retention sometimes induced by other corticosteroids. The absence of mineralocorticoid effect is so complete that the physician must remember that in patients with adrenal failure associated with cancer, such as adrenal metastases or adrenalectomy, dexamethasone cannot be substituted for hydrocortisone without risking volume depletion and vascular collapse (adrenal crisis).[1262]

Protein binding of prednisone and dexamethasone differs. At standard doses, less dexamethasone is bound, so that relatively more dexamethasone than prednisone can be found in the brain and CSF after systemic administration. This difference is probably the reason that patients with acute leukemia receiving dexamethasone have only half as many meningeal relapses as those receiving prednisone.[137]

One report suggests that dexamethasone is less inhibiting to the migration of white cells into injured tissue, and thus it may be less immunosuppressive than other steroids.[2016] On the other hand, some investigators believe that the fluorinated steroids are more likely to produce steroid myopathy than nonfluorinated glucocorticoids.[1466]

Increasing evidence indicates that corticosteroids with antibiotics are useful in treating bacterial meningitis as well as certain other infections such as pneumonia resulting from *Pneumocystis carinii* in the immunosuppressed patient (see Chapter 10). Whether these considerations apply in the patient with cancer who suffers a CNS infection is unclear. Corticosteroids may also suppress the aseptic meningitis (probably caused by blood in the subarachnoid space) that sometimes follows neurosurgical procedures for primary or metastatic brain or spinal tumors[384] (see Chapter 14).

Unwanted Effects

Table 4–2 summarizes the common side effects of steroids. Details of these and other effects may be found in a number of reviews and most textbooks of pharmacology.[106,1691,1928,2785] In one study[2785] of patients treated with steroids for spinal cord compression, 50% developed at least one side effect; 20% required hospital admission. The side effects included hyperglycemia (19%), infections (22%), GI disturbances (14%), myopathy (19%), and psychiatric problems (3%). Side effects were most widespread in patients with a low serum albumin level. These developments and other important, relevant effects are discussed in the following paragraphs.

MYOPATHY

Most patients receiving conventional doses (16 mg/24 hr of dexamethasone or equivalent) of steroids for more than 2 or 3 weeks develop at least mild steroid myopathy,[285,2560] characterized histologically by bland atrophy of type 2 (fast twitch) fibers. The disorder begins with proximal muscle weakness in the hip girdle, with wasting of thigh muscles.[94,1200] Affected patients have difficulty rising from the toilet seat or a low chair without pushing off with their hands. When the disorder is more severe, it affects the ability to climb stairs. Weakness may spread to the proximal arm muscles (Fig. 4–1), preventing the lifting of heavy objects above the head.[1362,2560] At its most florid, severe weakness is noted in the shoulder and pelvic girdles and in the neck muscles, particularly the flexors. The onset is usually slow but may be sudden with accompanying myalgia. In some instances, respiratory function is compromised.[583,2560] Rarely, high-dose intravenous steroids (e.g., 1 g/24 hr methylprednisolone), especially when combined with nondepolarizing, muscle-blocking agents,[150a,2904] cause quadriplegic myopathy within 2 weeks.[1167,1455] Distal weakness is

Table 4–2. **SIDE EFFECTS OF STEROIDS**

Common But Usually Mild	Nonneurologic But Serious	Neurologic (Common)	Neurologic (Uncommon)
Insomnia	Gastrointestinal bleeding	Myopathy	Psychosis
Sensation of abdominal bloating	Bowel perforation	Behavioral alterations	Paraparesis
Increased appetite	Osteoporosis	Hallucinations (high dose)	Seizures
Visual blurring	Avascular osteonecrosis (usually hip)	Hiccoughs	
Urinary frequency and nocturia	Glaucoma	Tremor	
Acne	Opportunistic infections	Visual blurring	
Edema	Hyperglycemia		
Lipomatosis	Kaposi's sarcoma		
Genital burning (IV push)	Pancreatitis		
Oral candidiasis			

IV = intravenous.

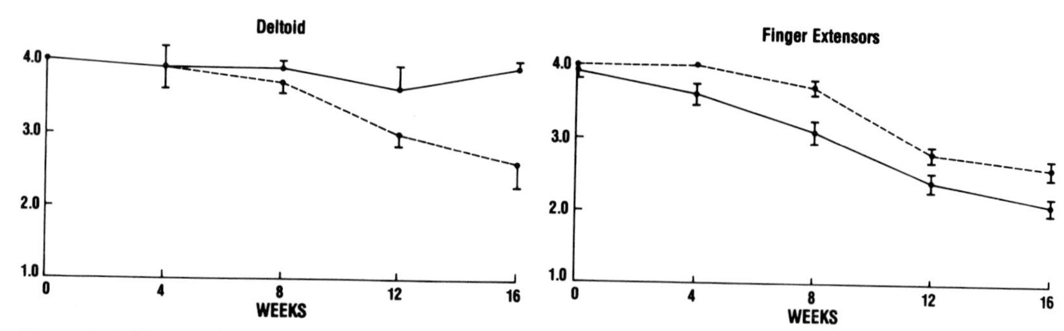

Figure 4–1. This graph illustrates muscle strength (ordinate) over time (abscissa) in patients receiving steroids for systemic lymphoma. *Vertical bars* indicate the standard deviation. The low-dose dexamethasone group (*solid line*) received 25 mg 3 times a week and the high-dose group (*broken line*) 50 mg 3 times a week. Proximal weakness in the deltoids was evident by week 12 and more pronounced by week 16 in all patients receiving high-dose corticosteroids. Distal muscles most affected by vincristine, such as the finger extensors, were not affected by the corticosteroid dose; patients receiving the higher dose of dexamethasone had less weakness in distal muscles than those patients receiving the lower dose. An identical pattern of weakness was seen in the leg muscles (not shown). (From DeAngelis et al,[583] p 2244, with permission.)

rare. Sensation remains normal, and deep tendon reflexes are preserved.

The differential diagnosis of proximal muscle weakness in patients with cancer who are taking steroids includes metabolic and nutritional myopathies, leptomeningeal tumor, spinal cord compression causing predominantly proximal weakness, the Lambert-Eaton myasthenic syndrome, and polymyositis (see Chapter 15). It is particularly important to consider polymyositis because that disorder is treated with steroids. Laboratory abnormalities in polymyositis include electromyographic changes of increased insertional activity of muscle, elevated muscle enzyme concentrations in serum, and histologic findings of muscle necrosis or inflammation. These laboratory findings are absent in patients with steroid myopathy. Progressive spinal cord compression in patients being treated with steroids may cause increasing proximal leg weakness that should be distinguished from steroid myopathy because the compression may require an increase in the steroid dose.

Steroid myopathy is treated by discontinuing the drug, if possible, after which the myopathy usually resolves over time.[492] Anabolic steroids, B-complex vitamins, and a high-protein diet have been reported to hasten the resolution of steroid myopathy in experimental animals[2270] but do not appear to be effective in humans.[492] Some evidence indicates that exercise attenuates the disorder.[453] One report suggests that patients with brain tumors treated with phenytoin are at lower risk (8%) for developing steroid myopathy than those not taking the anticonvulsant (16%).[686]

STEROID PSYCHOSIS

Psychotic changes[2498] caused by steroids were common when adrenocorticotropic hormone and naturally occurring glucocorticoids were more widely used. With synthetic steroids, psychosis is less common, and with dexamethasone, florid steroid psychosis is rare. Divided doses of enteric-coated steroid preparations may increase the incidence of steroid-induced psychosis. The Boston Collaborative Group reports the dose-related incidence of acute psychotic reaction as 3% of patients treated with prednisone.[278] Psychosis does not appear to be correlated with duration of treatment, however; psychiatric symptoms can follow a single dose. A double-blind prospective trial of prednisone, 80 mg/24 hr, given to normal volunteers for 5 days revealed that 11 of 12 subjects developed at least mild psychiatric reactions during treatment or withdrawal.[2842] Symptoms included irritability, anxiety, insomnia, trouble concentrating, euphoria, or depression.[302]

More severe psychiatric reactions are of three general types: affective, schizoid, and delirious.[1553] A reversible dementia unassociated with psychotic symptoms has also been reported.[2676]

Affective disorders cannot be distinguished from non–steroid-associated psychiatric illness. Mania is more common with exogenous steroid therapy; depression is more common with Cushing's syndrome. The disorder usually begins early in the course of therapy, is more likely to affect women, and may be dose-related. It resolves when the steroids are withdrawn and can be treated with neuroleptic drugs, although tricyclic agents are not effective and may worsen symptoms. Clonazepam has been used to treat steroid-induced mania.[2699] Affective disorders occasionally begin during the tapering of steroids but resolve once the steroids are discontinued entirely. Three patients taking alternate-day steroids have been reported to cycle with mood elevation on the on-days and depression on the off-days[2370]; the phenomenon appeared to be dose-related. A single report[752] suggests that lithium used prophylactically may prevent the affective form of steroid psychosis. A history of steroid psychosis does not predict recurrent psychosis with a second course of steroids.

Schizophrenia may be mimicked by steroids. The disorder usually begins acutely. The patient becomes withdrawn, paranoid, or both, and may experience auditory or visual hallucinations. The disorder cannot be distinguished from the primary psychiatric illness but always responds to either steroid withdrawal or neuroleptic treatment.

Delirium may be caused by steroids. Affected patients become distractible, confused, and unable to attend appropriately to environmental stimuli; visual hallucinations are common. Mild delirium often is not reported because patients attribute hallucinations to the drug and are neither surprised nor concerned about them.

The affective and schizoid steroid psychoses occurring in a patient under the stress of cancer treatment must be differentiated from a psychiatric disorder. Steroid-induced delirium must be distinguished from similar symptoms that are due to other metabolic disorders that may complicate the cancer or its treatment (see Chapter 11).

INSOMNIA

Insomnia and other sleep disturbances are common in patients with cancer and are particularly prominent if the patients are on steroids as well.[1221] The insomnia, often exacerbated by steroid-induced nocturia, should be treated with hypnotics.

BONE DISORDERS

Osteoporosis, a common side effect of prolonged steroid use,[1614] sometimes causes vertebral fractures. The back pain from the fracture may lead the physician to suspect a vertebral tumor. Steroid-induced osteoporosis reverses itself, at least in young persons, when the drug is discontinued.[2050] One study suggests that a second-generation biphosphonate with calcium can prevent the disorder.[2148]

Avascular osteonecrosis of the hips[727,757] or occasionally of the shoulders, wrist, clavicle, or vertebral body[1862] may be confused with spinal cord compression or peripheral neuropathy. Affected patients have usually been on steroids for months, although occasional patients develop osteonecrosis after only a few weeks of treatment.[757,1909] Dose and risk appear to be correlated.[766] The hip disorder is characterized by pain, often radiating down the anterior aspect of the thigh to the knee and resembling, in some respects, a femoral neuropathy or lumbar radiculopathy. Sometimes the pain may be localized to the buttock or groin, hindering the diagnosis. The pain is exacerbated by walking. The diagnosis is suggested by reproducing the pain on rotation of the hip. In some patients, a click can be heard as the hip is passively flexed and extended. The results of plain x-rays, nuclide bone scans, and CT scans may be normal early in the course of the disorder, but eventually they will reveal the necrosis. The most sensitive diagnostic test is MRI.[1113,2183,2787]

LIPOMATOSIS

Steroids cause redistribution of fat to the face, causing the characteristic moon facies; to the abdomen, causing a "pot belly"; and to the posterior lower neck, causing the characteristic "buffalo hump." Many patients suffer a sensation of chronic abdominal bloating. Additionally, fat redistributes to the retro-orbital space (causing exophthalmos),[2436] to the mediastinum, and to the epidural space. Excess fat in the epidural space can cause spinal cord compression.[1046,1332,2253] In some instances, surgical decompression of the cord has been necessary to relieve neurologic symptoms. Both MR and CT scans easily differentiate the typical fat density of the steroid-induced lesions in the epidural and mediastinal spaces from other lesions such as metastases.

VISUAL PROBLEMS

The visual system can be affected by steroids in several ways. Many patients receiving corticosteroids complain of visual blurring, which appears to be due to a change in refraction associated with the corticosteroids. The symptoms may be precipitated by either an increase or decrease in steroid dose but generally disappear when the agents are discontinued. Cataracts are common in patients on long-term steroids and have been reported to be caused by intermittent dexamethasone used as an anti-emetic.[244] Steroids have also been reported to induce mydriasis and ptosis in experimental animals[1881] and may increase intraocular pressure, leading to glaucoma.[24]

GASTROINTESTINAL DYSFUNCTION

GI bleeding and bowel perforation are two well-recognized complications of steroid therapy.[1752,2295] Although GI ulceration and bleeding are generally more common, GI perforation is the more serious complication in neurologic patients receiving steroids.

Gastrointestinal Ulceration. Upper GI bleeding is rare in patients taking steroids who do not have a history of GI bleeding; only 2.8 cases per 10,000 patients have been reported.[391] The incidence of GI bleeding is much higher if patients receive anticoagulant treatment or have a history of GI bleeding. A major question is whether prophylaxis prevents ulceration and bleeding. One study in experimental animals[656] suggests that cimetidine can prevent the development of gastric ulcers induced by steroids. A small, double-blind, controlled study in humans suggests that GI symptoms and antacid consumption were lower in the group treated with cimetidine and steroids than in the group treated with a placebo and steroids.[372] A study of patients with spinal cord trauma treated with either high-dose steroids (1 g/24 hr of methylprednisolone) or low-dose steroids (160 mg/24 hr of methylprednisolone) and protected either by antacids alone or by antacids and cimetidine showed no difference in GI bleeding. Unfortunately, the study had no group that did not receive GI prophylaxis.

The issue would be trivial were it not for the fact that GI prophylaxis carries its own side effects.[2611] The histamine (H_2) blockers have been associated with encephalopathy and occasionally coma in the elderly. Whether H_2 blockers react synergistically with other drugs to promote sedation needs clarification. They often cause thrombocytopenia and interact with chemotherapeutic agents.[1542] Cimetidine decreases the clearance of some drugs eliminated by hepatic metabolism, including phenytoin and 1-3-bis-chloro(2-chloroethyl)-1-nitrosourea (BCNU).[1542] Carbamazepine is not affected. In the absence of firm evidence that H_2 blockers are helpful, they are probably best avoided. Alkalinization with antacids leads to a significant increase in colonization of Gram-negative bacteria in the stomach, with a possible increase in aspiration pneumonia.[2611] Sucralfate is not absorbed and thus should be safe, but it binds a number of drugs in the stomach, preventing adequate absorption. Thus, if it is used, it should be given either 2 hours before or after other oral agents that require absorption to be efficacious. It is my policy not to use GI prophylaxis of any sort in patients on steroids unless a history of peptic ulceration has been noted.[391] In that case, I prefer sucralfate, taking care that it is not given at the same time as other oral agents. At least one other neuro-oncologist agrees.[2694]

Bowel Perforation. Bowel perforation generally affects the sigmoid colon.[749,2153,2772] The affected patients are usually constipated because of bowel dysfunction that is due to spinal cord compression, drugs, or inactivity. Clinical symptoms usually begin with moderate-to-severe pain in the abdomen, but the physician is often misled because bowel sounds persist and the rebound tenderness characteristic of peritonitis is often not present, being masked by the steroids or abdominal muscle weakness resulting from spinal cord compression. The diagnosis can be confirmed by finding free air under the diaphragm on upright abdominal or lateral decubitus radiographs. The patient usually must be treated surgically, although a few bowel perforations apparently heal spontaneously. The risk is particularly high in patients with spinal cord compression because they are more prone to constipation and they receive corticosteroids. Prevention or early treatment of constipation might avert this serious complication.

Pneumatosis Cystoides Intestinalis. Pneumatosis cystoides intestinalis is a benign syndrome related to steroid therapy. Within the intestinal wall, air appears as cysts or linear streaks.[862] The cysts may rupture, but they heal spontaneously and do not require surgical repair.

Colonic Ileus. Colonic ileus, or pseudo-obstruction of the colon (Ogilvie's syndrome), is a disorder of bowel motility that affects severely ill patients, including those with spinal cord compression. The cecum may enlarge enough to cause colonic rupture.[1057,1289]

Laxatives are particularly important drugs for patients with neurologic complications of cancer, particularly for those taking glucocorticoids. Strong efforts should be made to maintain bowel function in any patient taking corticosteroids. Virtually all patients on opioids, and those who are not but who are constipated, should take a stool softener; laxatives should be administered, as needed, to maintain normal bowel function. Patients should be encouraged to increase bulk in their diet and to drink adequate liquids to maintain stool softening. In some patients in whom opioids have produced severe constipation, oral naloxone[536,2537] appears to relieve constipation without altering the analgesic effect of the opioids.

MISCELLANEOUS SIDE EFFECTS

Several other side effects of steroids are occasionally encountered in neuro-oncologic practice. A particularly unpleasant one is hiccough,[123,1554] a dose-related but idiosyncratic corticosteroid effect that afflicts a few patients. Treatment of steroid hiccough is often difficult unless the dose is decreased. Phenothiazines, nifedipine, valproate, and carbamazepine sometimes suppress the symptom.

Hypersensitivity and even anaphylaxis to corticosteroids have been reported.[485,835] Occasional patients develop psychological dependence.[797] A peculiar side effect of IV bolus injection of dexamethasone is a severe anogenital itching or tingling that is extremely distressing but generally subsides within a few minutes. The patient who is warned of the possibility in advance finds it tolerable.[126,542] Steroid-enhanced free-water clearance may cause nocturia and sometimes may awaken the patient hourly. Corticosteroids diminish the senses of taste and smell and occasionally cause anorexia. Intrathecal administration of corticosteroids can cause a severe pachymeningitis.[197,1867]

Because of their known immune-suppressing capacities, steroids, whether exogenous or endogenous, can lead to opportunistic infections[961,1140] (see Chapter 10). In the neuro-oncologic setting, a common problem is *P. carinii* in patients who have been on steroids and are being tapered to lower doses.[1140,2358,2440] Some physicians recommend prophylaxis with trimethoprim-sulfamethoxazole given as one double-strength tablet twice a day for 3 consecutive days each week.[1229] The drug is generally given to patients who will be on prolonged treatment with steroids, and it is discontinued a month after steroids are stopped.

Steroid Interactions with Other Drugs

Because patients with neuro-oncologic problems treated with steroids often also take other drugs, it is important to be aware of untoward drug interactions, especially interactions with drugs that induce hepatic microsomal enzymes (cytochrome P-450 system). Drugs such as phenytoin, phenobarbital,[317] and perhaps carbamazepine increase the metabolic clearance of steroids and may decrease their therapeutic effect. In one study, an oral dose of dexamethasone was decreased to 20% of its previous bioavailability after the addition of phenytoin.[419] As a result, some patients who have brain metastases and are on stable doses of steroids develop increased symptoms when they are started on anticonvulsants. Conversely, one report[1484] suggests that administration of dexamethasone may increase phenytoin levels, but my own experience has been the opposite. I have found that some patients on stable doses of phenytoin develop toxicity as the steroid dose is decreased, or they develop seizures because phenytoin levels become subtherapeutic when the steroid dose is increased.[1453]

Steroid Withdrawal Syndrome

Withdrawal of patients from steroids also causes neurologic disability (Table 4–3).[42]

"Steroid pseudorheumatism"[651,2221] is the most common withdrawal symptom. Patients develop acute myalgias, arthralgias, or both, sometimes severe. One such patient was admitted to MSKCC with a presumptive diagnosis of spinal cord compression because severe pain in his legs prevented him from walking. In others the disorder is milder and can be ameliorated by increasing the dose of steroids for a few days and then tapering more slowly. Steroid pseudorheumatism usually follows a rapid taper of steroids but occasionally occurs when the drug is decreased by as little as 2 mg of dexamethasone a week. In affected patients, each reduction seems to produce an exacerbation of the arthralgia, which then disappears over a period of 36 to 48 hours.

Headache, lethargy, and sometimes low-grade fever are also common symptoms of steroid withdrawal. The steroid withdrawal syndrome was first described by Amatruda and colleagues[42] in patients who had no underlying neurologic disease. When it occurs in patients with CNS disease, the physician may believe that the symptoms are due to recurrent brain tumor rather than to steroid withdrawal.

In children, pseudotumor cerebri can complicate withdrawal from prolonged steroid treatment.[2722] This finding may be caused by decreased CSF absorption associated with steroid withdrawal.[1299]

Adrenal insufficiency may result when steroids are tapered too rapidly; the disease often clinically manifests when the patient suffers the stress of a medical or surgical illness.

Table 4–3. **STEROID WITHDRAWAL SYNDROME**

Myalgia, arthralgia (steroid pseudorheumatism)
Headache
Lethargy
Fever
Nausea, vomiting, anorexia
Postural hypotension
Papilledema
Pneumocystis pneumonia

Source: Adapted from Amatruda et al,[42] p 1209.

OTHER SUPPORTIVE CARE AGENTS

Table 4–4 lists other supportive care agents that are considered in the following pages.

Anticonvulsants

Seizures are a presenting complaint in about 20% of patients with brain metastases. They probably occur in 30% to 40% of patients at some time during their clinical course.[470] They also occur in patients with leptomeningeal metastases or CNS infections, after bone marrow transplantation, and with several other neurologic complications of cancer[1973,2482] (Table 4–5).

Generalized seizures can be lethal if they induce status epilepticus. Seizures both exhaust brain metabolic reserves and raise cerebral blood flow, blood volume, and intracranial pressure, potentially causing cerebral herniation (see Chapter 3). Focal seizures, if repetitive, can also cause permanent neurologic damage in patients with brain metastases. Repetitive seizures should be stopped first with IV diazepam (5 to 10 mg over 1 to 2 minutes) or lorazepam (0.5 to 2 mg over 1 to 2 minutes) followed by 1000 mg phenytoin by slow IV injection (no more than 50 mg/min) (Table 4–6). A discussion of maintenance therapy follows.

When a patient has a seizure, it is treated by most physicians with anticonvulsants. To my knowledge, however, no published studies

Table 4–4. OTHER SUPPORTIVE CARE AGENTS

Analgesics	*Antibiotics*	*Anticoagulants*	*Anticonvulsants*
NSAIDs	Amphotericin B	Heparin	Phenytoin
Aspirin	Aminoglycosides	Warfarin (Coumadin)	Carbamazepine
Acetaminophen	Acyclovir		Phenobarbital
Opioids			Valproic acid
Meperidine (Demerol)			
Others			
Anti-emetics	*Gastroprotectors*	*Hormones*	
Metoclopramide	Antacids	Megestrol	
Ondansetron	Cimetidine		
Prochlorperazine	Ranitidine		
Lorazepam	Sucralfate		

NSAIDs = nonsteroidal anti-inflammatory drugs.

Table 4–5. CAUSES OF SEIZURES IN THE PATIENT WITH CANCER

Metastatic Central Nervous System Neoplasms	*Treatment-Related Causes*
Parenchymal metastases	Radiation therapy
Dural-based metastases	Acute
Leptomeningeal metastases	Delayed
	Early
Metabolic Conditions	Late
Hyponatremia	Chemotherapy
Hypoglycemia	Antimetabolites
Hypoxia	Methotrexate
Hypocalcemia	L-asparaginase
Hypomagnesemia	Ara-C
Cerebral Infarction	*Vinca* alkaloids
	Topoisomerase inhibitors
Cerebral Hemorrhage	Alkylators
Infections	Ifosfamide
Bacterial	Nitrosoureas
Listeria monocytogenes	*Cis*-platinum
Viral	Biologic response modifiers
Cytomegalovirus	Interferon
Herpes simplex	Interleukin-2
Fungal	Opioids
Cryptococcus neoformans	Meperidine
Aspergillus fumigatus	Anti-emetics
Candida species	Phenothiazines
Parasites	Butyrophenones
Toxoplasma gondii	Antibiotics
	Penicillins
	Imipenem-cilastatin

CNS = central nervous system.

Source: Adapted from Stein and Chamberlain,[2482] p 34.

Table 4–6. **MANAGEMENT OF CONVULSIVE STATUS EPILEPTICUS**

Treatment	*Time*
Restore homeostasis	0–15 min
Airway, blood pressure, nasal O_2, record ECG, intubate only if necessary	
Administer 50 mL of 50% glucose and 100 mg of thiamine IV	
Start isotonic saline slow drip IV	
Send blood for laboratory analysis	
Stop convulsive seizures	
Diazepam 0.25 mg/kg IV up to 20 mg (<5 mg/min) followed immediately by phenytoin 18 mg/kg IV (<50 mg/min)	
Monitor blood pressure and ECG; repeat phenytoin 7 mg/kg × 1 if necessary	
or	
Lorazepam 0.1 mg/kg IV (<2 mg/min) with subsequent medication determined by serum drug levels or, if necessary, phenytoin IV as above	15–60 min
If seizures persist:	
Intubate; EEG should be used at this point	60–120 min
Phenobarbital 20 mg/kg IV (<100 mg/min)	
or	
Midazolam 200 μ/kg IV bolus followed by 0.75–11 μg/kg per min[1979a]	
If seizures persist:	
General anesthesia with short-acting barbiturates (e.g., pentobarbital 5 mg/kg, then 1–3 mg/kg per hour); adjust dose to obtain burst suppression pattern on EEG without depressing blood pressure severely and titrate to keep patient seizure-free	
Use additional anticonvulsants as necessary	

ECG = electrocardiogram; EEG = electroencephalogram; IV = intravenous.

Source: Adapted from Engel,[728] p 267. See also Dodson et al,[657] p 857.

address whether anticonvulsant agents prevent further seizures in patients with brain metastases or other neurologic complications of cancer even when blood levels of the agents are kept within accepted therapeutic ranges. Some evidence suggests a poor correlation between "therapeutic" serum phenytoin levels and partial seizures despite a correlation between such concentrations and generalized seizures.[2622] Nonetheless, even in the absence of proof, the use of anticonvulsant agents to prevent further seizures seems warranted.

PROPHYLACTIC ANTICONVULSANTS

The use of prophylactic anticonvulsants for patients who have not had seizures but who are at increased risk is more controversial. Two retrospective studies failed to show a decrease in the incidence of seizures when patients with known brain metastases were treated with prophylactic anticonvulsants,[470,1230] but another study suggests that seizures were prevented in patients with cerebral gliomas.[245] In a study of patients operated on for other brain lesions, prophylactic anticonvulsants did not prevent seizures.[826]

A recent double-blind randomized placebo-controlled trial of anticonvulsant prophylaxis in adults with newly diagnosed brain metastases indicates that anticonvulsant prophylaxis does not decrease seizures.[927a] Although this study was small, the results are supported by an ongoing prospective analysis of prophylactic anticonvulsant therapy in brain metastases at MSKCC (unpublished data).

One problem with anticonvulsant treatment is the difficulty of maintaining a therapeutic blood level, especially in patients with metastatic cancer, at least in part because anticonvulsants interact with anticancer agents. For example, several studies show that during a course of BCNU, *cis*-platinum, carboplatin, and other drugs, the serum concentration of anticonvulsants decreases, presumably because of microsomal enzyme induction[255,658,913,1019,1866] or decreased absorption.[255] Conversely, anticonvulsants such as phenytoin and phenobarbital may lower the serum concentration of antineoplastic agents,[913,2748] decreasing their effectiveness.

In occasional patients, a decrease in anticonvulsant serum concentration is clinically significant and leads to seizures. To compensate for the lower anticonvulsant levels, the physician may decide to increase the dose, only to have the level overshoot to toxic ranges. To compound the problem, elevated levels of several anticonvulsant drugs cause toxicity that may mimic the symptoms of brain tumor or may even increase seizure activity.[368,2502] Thus, my policy is not to use prophylactic anticonvulsants in patients with brain metastases, except in patients with metastatic melanoma, in whom the incidence of seizures may be as high as 50% because of the predilection to involve gray matter.[357] Nevertheless, many physicians do give prophylactic anticonvulsants after craniotomy and sometimes before CT scans because iodinated contrast provokes a seizure within minutes of its administration in some patients with asymptomatic brain metastases. An oral prophylactic dose of a benzodiazepine (e.g., 5 to 10 mg of diazepam given 30 minutes before contrast injection) substantially decreases the likelihood of seizures.[1964] IV gadolinium, the contrast agent for MR scan, is not associated with seizures.

CHOICE OF DRUGS

For chronic treatment of focal or generalized convulsions associated with systemic cancer, four major agents are available: phenytoin, carbamazepine, phenobarbital, and valproate. Other less commonly used agents include primidone and clonazepam. Little evidence supports the superiority of one drug over another in the prevention of further seizures,[1707,2325] although evidence indicates that monotherapy (using maximal tolerated doses of a single agent) is superior to polytherapy (multiple agents) to manage epileptic patients.

All anticonvulsant agents have side effects (Table 4–7). Lethargy and cognitive dysfunction can be caused by any of the agents listed in Table 4–7, even when blood levels are within the "therapeutic" range.[691] Recent evidence[2889] suggests that all anticonvulsant agents produce about the same degree of drowsiness and cognitive dysfunction, although individual patients may tolerate one anticonvulsant better than another. Carbamazepine and primidone, if given initially at full doses, cause profound drowsiness and may not be tolerated. These drugs must be started at low dose and gradually increased to reach appropriate levels. Both phenytoin and, less frequently, carbamazepine have been reported to cause the Stevens-Johnson syndrome, particularly in patients who receive whole-brain radiation while on a decreasing dose of steroids.[608] If the patient has taken the anticonvulsant drug for more than a month without toxicity, radiation treatment to the brain while steroids are being tapered appears to be safe. Phenytoin has been reported to cause granulomatous vasculitis[859] and has, on occasion, caused pulmonary failure; it has also been associated with osteomalacia.[59] The levels of alkaline phosphatase and other liver enzymes in the serum may increase in patients receiving phenytoin.[34] Involuntary movements, particularly choreoathetosis, may be a sign of phenytoin intoxi-

Table 4–7. **SIDE EFFECTS OF ANTICONVULSANTS**

Idiosyncratic
Stevens-Johnson syndrome (phenytoin, carbamazepine)
Vasculitis (phenytoin)
Arthritis, shoulder–hand syndrome (phenobarbital)
Stupor (valproate)
Meningitis (carbamazepine)
Agranulocytosis (carbamazepine)
Pseudolymphoma (phenytoin)
Dose-related
Seizures (phenytoin, carbamazepine)
Cognitive dysfunction (all)
Diplopia (carbamazepine, phenytoin)
Ataxia-nystagmus (phenytoin)
Asterixis (all)
Metabolic
Microsomal enzyme inducer (phenytoin, carbamazepine)
Osteomalacia (phenytoin)
Increased liver enzymes (phenytoin, valproate)

cation, substituting for the more common and recognized toxic signs of ataxia and nystagmus.[18] A severe but reversible myopathy has been related to phenytoin therapy[147] despite its reported protective effect on steroid myopathy. Myelotoxicity from phenytoin is rare[2133] but serious, particularly in the patient with cancer who might receive other myelosuppressive agents. Phenytoin clearance may be increased by chemotherapy.[1279] Additionally, this drug has been reported to increase the cytotoxicity of vincristine in either wild or multiresistant-type tumor cells.[878] Its advantage is that it is available in IV and oral preparations and is amenable to loading by high-dose oral or IV treatment.

Many patients taking carbamazepine complain of intermittent diplopia as well as drowsiness even at "therapeutic" doses. Carbamazepine lowers the white cell count, which may cause concern in patients being treated with myelosuppressive chemotherapeutic agents, but it very seldom leads to true agranulocytosis, and it is not clear that it potentiates the myelosuppression from chemotherapeutic agents. The syndrome of inappropriate antidiuretic hormone secretion with resultant hyponatremia occurs rarely as a carbamazepine side effect.[1456,2651] The drug has been reported to cause aseptic meningitis.[1162] Prolonged "absence status epilepticus" mimicking stupor has been reported to be caused by carbamazepine in one patient.[368] A parenteral preparation is not available, but the drug can be given rectally.[2504]

About 20% of patients with brain tumor who take phenobarbital as a therapeutic agent develop pain and dysfunction in the shoulder, and sometimes in the entire upper extremity (shoulder–hand syndrome).[2561] This syndrome is usually contralateral to the tumor site and may occur even in patients without motor deficit.

Valproate, which occasionally causes hepatic dysfunction in young children receiving multiple anticonvulsant agents,[965] also occasionally causes thrombocytopenia[917a] and interferes with the synthesis of coagulation factors such as fibrinogen. Because so many patients with neurologic complications of cancer take multiple drugs, I have been reluctant to use valproate, although some clinicians have reported the drug to be safe and effective. Patients taking valproate sometimes develop stupor or coma that clears when the valproate is discontinued.[965,2259] This syndrome may be a result of valproate-induced hyperammonemia, although the pathogenesis is not entirely understood. Reversible extrapyramidal signs resembling Parkinson's disease may complicate valproate therapy.[2293a]

If anticonvulsants are used, the physician should probably measure blood levels frequently, certainly when untoward effects relate to them. So-called therapeutic levels are only guidelines, however; many patients achieve seizure control at lower levels, and others with blood levels substantially above the therapeutic range have no signs of toxicity. Thus physicians should treat patients, not blood levels. Because of the long half-life and nonlinear kinetics of drugs such as phenytoin, attempts to adjust levels within the therapeutic range often lead to toxicity without altering the patient's susceptibility to seizures.

Obviously it is difficult to propose an ideal anticonvulsant agent. The drug of choice is probably phenytoin, followed in order by carbamazepine, phenobarbital, and valproate. The failure of one of these agents does not predict the failure of the others. If seizures persist, switching to another drug may be effective. The role of newly available chemotherapeutic agents (e.g., felbamate and gabapentin) is not yet known.

Anticoagulants

Most patients with cancer have coagulation disorders (see Chapter 9); circulating fibrinogen degradation products may be found in as many as 90%. Thrombophlebitis, with or without pulmonary embolism, is a major problem in patients with both primary and metastatic brain tumors, particularly in those who undergo surgical treatment.[2085,2244,2312] In addition to these general risk factors for thrombophlebitis, patients with brain lesions often suffer immobility of the extremities, predisposing to stagnation of venous blood and clotting. Even in patients without motor deficits, when thrombophlebitis develops, it is twice as likely to occur in the extremity contralateral to a primary metastatic brain tumor than in the ipsilateral limb.[2244]

Precautions may help decrease the frequency of thrombophlebitis in patients with cancer, particularly in the postoperative period. External pneumatic calf compression boots applied in the operating and recovery room and continued until the patient is fully ambulatory appear to substantially decrease the incidence of thrombophlebitis and pulmonary embolism.[226,2625] The venous compression does not alter intracranial pressure even in brain-injured patients.[568] The role of low-dose heparin in postoperative treatment is not clear[1319]; many surgeons are reluctant to use the agent because of the possibility of intracranial bleeding, although it does not appear to cause GI bleeding.[732] Low–molecular-weight heparin may prove to be safer and as effective as low-dose heparin.[981]

When thrombophlebitis develops in postoperative patients or in those with an unoperated brain tumor, many physicians hesitate to use therapeutic anticoagulation because of their fear of brain hemorrhage.[1422,2532] Their apprehension appears to be poorly founded. In patients with both primary and metastatic brain tumors, the incidence of intratumoral hemorrhage is no greater in anticoagulated patients than in those not treated with anticoagulants.[1936,2244] Thus, for patients who are more than 4 or 5 days into the postoperative period or patients who are harboring brain tumors and have not had surgery, thrombophlebitis should be treated as vigorously as it would be in a patient without a brain tumor. Prophylactic low-dose heparin (5000 U twice daily), beginning the day after craniotomy, appears to be both safe and effective.[841] The use of anticoagulants in patients with or without cancer is not without other risks, however. Heparin can induce thrombocytopenia and thrombosis,[99] and warfarin occasionally can induce necrosis of the skin and sometimes of the breast, penis, or toe.[1723]

Because of the risk of bleeding and these other anticoagulant complications, many physicians place inferior vena cava filters to prevent pulmonary emboli in patients with cancer and lower extremity thrombophlebitis.[171,2732] Although these filters are usually effective, a significant percentage of patients still suffer pulmonary embolism (12%)[1535]; progressive vena caval, leg, or pelvic thrombosis[2312]; or massive edema of the lower extremities, which interferes with function. I prefer, when possible, to use anticoagulation with heparin followed by warfarin, reserving the filters for those patients in whom anticoagulation is clearly contraindicated.[2732] In occasional patients, anticoagulation with warfarin is not effective; such patients are maintained on subcutaneous heparin to prevent further thrombosis (see Chapter 9).

Analgesic Agents

Most patients with end-stage cancer experience pain; it is a particular problem in those patients with epidural spinal cord compression or peripheral nerve invasion or compression. A vast literature addresses the problem of pain relief in patients with cancer[6,441,1077,2001,2061]; only a few principles can be mentioned here. The major problem in providing adequate analgesia to patients with neurologic complications of cancer is that the best analgesic drugs, the opioids, often add to the existing neurologic dysfunction. The side effects of morphine, including sedation, may augment or mask the symptoms caused by a growing mass lesion in the brain. Furthermore, opioid overdose can decrease respiration, thus increasing pCO_2 and causing a rise in intracranial pressure that may exacerbate brain tumor symptoms.[477] Multifocal myoclonus[115] and seizures[991,2807] may complicate the use of any opioid, especially meperidine (see Chapter 11). Despite these potential shortcomings, pain in patients with cancer who suffer neurologic complications must be treated vigorously.

In general, this pain may be divided into the broad categories of nociceptive (systemic) and neuropathic pain.[2001,2061,2819] The importance of distinguishing between the two is that nociceptive pain probably responds better to opioids and neural blockade than does neuropathic pain, which may respond to the tricyclic antidepressants. For mild nociceptive pain, such as pain caused by bony metastases, the clinician should begin with a peripherally acting analgesic such as acetaminophen, aspirin, or a nonsteroidal anti-inflammatory drug (NSAID). It is probably unwise to use aspirin or NSAIDs in patients on glucocorticoids because the drugs may augment GI bleeding. (Choline magnesium trisalicylate may have less GI toxicity.) Most cancer pain will not respond to these drugs, however; one should quickly begin opioids, starting with codeine or oxycodone in conjunction with acetaminophen or aspirin and, if ineffective, escalating promptly to morphine or morphinelike agents. Large doses of opioid drugs are sometimes required to control pain and should be used if they do not produce substantial side effects. If the pain is relieved by other means, however, such as treatment directly to the tumor, the same dose of opioid that was previously well tolerated may now cause excessive sedation and even respiratory insufficiency. Also, if the pain is relieved by other means, the patient may cease taking the opioids abruptly and, if physically dependent, may suffer withdrawal unless instructed to taper the drugs even in the absence of pain.

Neuropathic pain (e.g., that produced by tumor invading nerves such as the brachial plexus) may be exceedingly difficult to treat and often responds poorly to opioids. Tricyclic antidepressants, sometimes at surprisingly low doses such as 10 to 25 mg at bedtime, may be more effective agents in some patients.[373] These drugs, or other adjuvant analgesics often used for neuropathic pain, including anticonvulsants, baclofen, corticosteroids, oral local anesthetics, and clonidine, are usually combined with opioids. The effect of tricyclic antidepressant agents on neuropathic pain is independent of their effect on mood.

Corticosteroids have been advocated for treating bone pain and nerve compression pain as well. In one controlled trial, corticosteroids produced a significant reduction in both pain and analgesic consumption when compared with a placebo.[332] The response to high-dose IV corticosteroids in patients with epidural spinal cord compression is particularly dramatic.[984]

Although aspirin and the NSAIDs can cause GI bleeding, they rarely cause neurotoxicity. Sometimes NSAIDs cause acute aseptic meningitis with headache, fever, stiff neck, and pleocytosis.[2112] As CSF eosinophilia is common in this drug-induced aseptic meningitis, it should prompt one to suspect a drug side effect before considering infectious meningitis or meningeal metastases.

Psychotropic Drugs

Anxiety and depression frequently are significant complications of cancer, particularly in patients with neurologic complications.[373,380,1185,1186] Many physicians are reluctant to use antidepressants to treat psychological distress in patients with cancer, falsely believing that the anxiety or depression, which the physician feels is appropriate for the patient's situation, will not respond to drug therapy. In fact, antidepressant drugs quite effectively treat depression associated with cancer, just as anxiolytic drugs appear effective in treating anxiety.[380] Many patients with cancer not only are anxious and depressed but also suffer insomnia and anorexia. Tricyclic antidepressants with sedative properties, such as amitriptyline, are often extremely effective in such patients. The patient receives both the sedative and the antidepressant effects of the drug, administered as a single dose at night, gradually increased from 10–25 to 150 mg or more. The sedative effects take hold immediately, and patients often feel substantially better after their first good night's sleep. Antidepressant effects take somewhat longer. The role of newer anxiolytic antidepressant agents, such as alprazolam and fluoxetine, remains to be elucidated. At low doses, most of these drugs appear to have minimal side effects in the cancer population, but neurotoxic reactions do occasionally occur.[1552] Tricyclic antidepressants have been reported to stimulate tumor growth in experimental animals, but no evidence supports such an effect in humans.[295] Psychotropic drugs can also cause psychiatric symptoms.[6a] An extensive list of these, as well as other drugs that cause psychiatric symptoms, has recently been published.[62]

Anti-emetic Agents

Anti-emetic agents such as metoclopramide, prochlorperazine, and haloperidol have dopamine-blocking activity that can cause acute extrapyramidal reactions[1275] or respiratory dyskinesias.[1191] Extrapyramidal signs generally occur in the young and are characterized by dystonic posturing associated with akathisia and often severe agitation, much greater than that appropriate for any fright caused by the physical symptoms. One patient experienced dystonic sensations in an amputated limb during metoclopramide treatment.[1275] The disorder can usually be reversed by IV diphenhydramine (Benadryl). In rare instances, however, diphenhydramine itself causes dystonia.[1481] Extrapyramidal reactions usually begin while the patient is taking the drug but occasionally may begin as long as 48 hours after the offending agent has been discontinued. The reaction may follow a single dose. The diagnosis may be difficult, particularly if the physician is unaware that the patient has received an anti-emetic. Ondansetron, a serotonergic receptor antagonist, also can cause an extrapyramidal reaction.[1068] Classic parkinsonian syndromes may occur but are much less common than are acute dyskinesias. Metoclopramide sometimes causes multifocal myoclonus[1236] as well as extrapyramidal reactions. The disorders are always reversible. Marijuana is still advocated as an anti-emetic by some oncologists.[654]

Antibiotic Drugs

Penicillinlike agents, as well as other antibiotics, can cause multifocal myoclonus and seizures, especially in patients with renal failure in whom the blood–brain barrier has been disrupted.[1008] Seizures usually occur in patients receiving high-dose IV therapy and are often preceded by multifocal myoclonus. When seizures or myoclonus develops, the dose should be decreased; anticonvulsants are unnecessary. A single patient developed a chronic granulomatous pachymeningitis associated with penicillin therapy. Headache, deafness, vertigo, and tinnitus associated with increased intracranial pressure and CSF pleocytosis were the findings.[754] Penicillin can also cause aseptic meningitis.[2177a]

Aminoglycosides such as gentamicin can cause ototoxicity and vestibulotoxicity. Patients develop tinnitus and hearing loss as the first symptom. The vestibulotoxicity may be more insidious. An ill, bedridden patient may complain only of mild dizziness while receiving the medication. After the course of the antibiotic has been completed, when the patient begins to ambulate, he or she discovers striking gait ataxia, which impairs walking. A characteristic complaint is oscillopsia; that is, when the patient attempts to walk, the environment does not appear to be stationary but instead bounces. Examination reveals absent vestibular responses to caloric stimulation and sometimes high-frequency hearing loss. Patients receiving aminoglycoside antibiotics should be monitored carefully and questioned about dizziness or vertigo; the dose should be decreased or the drug discontinued if these occur. The toxicity is usually associated with a prolonged antibiotic course, high serum levels of the drug, and renal failure. The aminoglycosides also cause synergistic ototoxicity with *cis*-platinum even if the drugs are not given simultaneously. The vestibular failure rarely reverses, but younger patients can compensate. Physical therapy, sometimes with the use of a neck collar to stabilize the head, helps with walking.

Amphotericin B occasionally causes brain white matter damage.[626,2728] The disorder occurs after bone marrow transplantation, when the amphotericin has been given to treat an opportunistic fungal infection. The disorder is characterized by encephalopathy with confusion and disorientation progressing to akinetic mutism or coma. Corticospinal tract signs include hyperactive reflexes, upgoing toes, and sometimes diffuse extensor rigidity. Stupor may begin abruptly sometime after the course of therapy is completed, even after the patient has fully recovered from the marrow transplant and returned home. The illness may be irreversible[2828]; patients who lapse into coma usually die. White matter changes are identified on the MR scan as nonenhancing lesions best seen on T_2 images. Pathologic changes are typical of leukoencephalopathy and are indistinguishable from encephalopathy caused by methotrexate (see Chapter 12) or radiation (see Chapter 13).

Trimethoprim-sulfamethoxazole has been reported to be responsible for aseptic meningitis[383,1291,2177a] as well as a painful sensory and autonomic neuropathy.[522] A case of acute but reversible psychosis following the use of ciprofloxacin and trimethoprim-sulfamethoxazole has been reported.[1720]

Sulfadiazine and pyrimethamine used together to treat toxoplasmosis have been reported to cause carnitine deficiency, leading to hyperammonemia and hepatic encephalopathy.[2356]

Pentamidine used to treat *P. carinii* pneumonia may cause severe hypoglycemia with stupor or coma.[2749] The hypoglycemia usually is caused by systemically administered pentamidine but occasionally has been associated with aerosolized drugs. When hypoglycemic coma occurs in a patient with a known lesion, the diagnosis may not be apparent.

Antiviral agents, including vidarabine (ara-A) and ganciclovir used for the treatment of herpes infection, are usually not neurotoxic. Occasionally, acute encephalopathy, reversible after discontinuation of the drugs, occurs.[535,569]

Acyclovir can be neurotoxic, causing tremor or myoclonus and delirium.[1048,2127] Occasionally, focal symptoms are also present. The neurotoxicity may occur at peak serum levels 24 to 48 hours after the drug is initially administered.[1048]

PART 2

Metastases

CHAPTER 5

INTRACRANIAL METASTASES

Metastases to the cranium and the intracranial contents are the most common metastatic neurologic complication of cancer. Although metastases to the skull are more common than parenchymal brain metas–tases, the latter are more likely to be symptomatic (Fig. 5–1). Symptoms of brain metastases are often the presenting complaint in patients not known to have cancer. In one series from a general hospital, 42% of patients with autopsy-confirmed lung cancer presented with symptoms of a brain metastasis[2594]; in my experience, the first symptom is neurologic in about 10% of patients with lung cancer. Before CT and MR scans were available, such patients were often misdiagnosed as suffering from strokes.[2774] Mistakes are still made, especially if the diagnostic procedure is a CT scan without contrast enhancement. Cerebral symptoms such as seizures, dementia, hemiparesis, aphasia, and headache make brain metastases the most feared by patients and often lead physicians to abandon treatment. With early diagnosis and vigorous treatment, however, the symptoms can usually be reversed, often returning the patient to a useful life, at least for a time. About 15% of patients with intracranial metastases from breast cancer survive more than 1 year, and because prognosis is not easy to predict,[261,267,1324,2462] all patients deserve treatment. Good pretreatment performance status is a favorable prognostic sign.[591] Several monographs and reviews address various aspects of incidence, symptoms, and therapy of brain metastases.*

CLASSIFICATION

A bewildering variety of metastatic lesions to the cranial vault or its contents may cause neurologic symptoms. Even metastases to brain parenchyma vary widely in number and pathology (Fig. 5–2). Table 5–1 classifies intracranial metastases by their anatomic sites. Metastases to the skull are particularly common in patients with carcinoma of the breast and prostate. Skull metastases can be subdivided into those affecting the calvaria and those affecting the base of the skull. Calvarial

*References 1991, 2544, 2626, 2777, 2851.

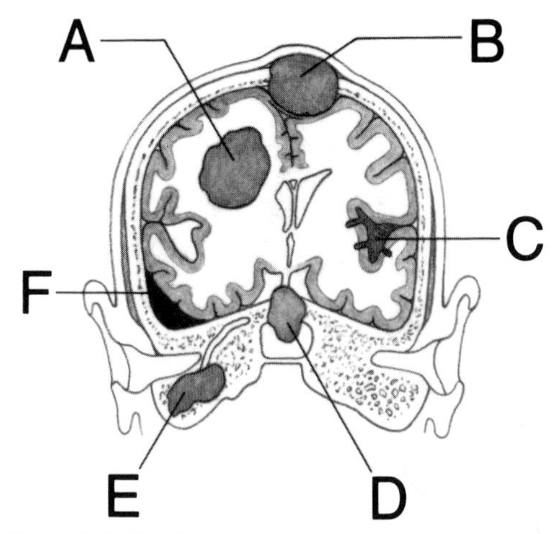

Figure 5–1. Cranial metastases. Most metastases affect the brain directly by hematogenous spread to the white matter of the cerebral hemispheres (A) (see also Fig. 1–3). The brain may be affected secondarily by a skull metastasis that invades the epidural space and compresses the brain. The skull metastasis may also compress the sagittal sinus (B) (see also Fig. 5–11). The tumor may involve the cranial leptomeninges and invade the brain by growing down the Virchow-Robin spaces (C) (see also Fig. 2–7B). A metastasis to the base of the skull may affect the pituitary gland (D) or cranial nerves (E) as they exit from the skull. Subdural metastasis may cause effusions (F) that compress the brain.

metastases are usually asymptomatic (symptomatic calvarial metastases are discussed on p. 108), whereas those to the base often cause pain and cranial nerve dysfunction (see Chapter 8). Pachymeningeal (dural) metastases include those to the epidural space, usually by direct extension from skull metastases, and those to the subdural space, either by direct extension from an epidural metastasis or by hematogenous spread. The extensive neovascularization of dural metastases may cause subdural hematomas or effusions that are larger and more symptomatic than the tumor itself.[1776,2623,2708] Leptomeningeal metastases are discussed in Chapter 7.

Several other intracranial sites are sometimes affected by metastatic spread. Pituitary metastases are common, particularly in patients with breast cancer; these usually involve the posterior lobe and are typically asymptomatic but may cause diabetes insipidus[516,1700,1711,2190] or cranial nerve abnormalities by extension to the leptomeninges or the cavernous sinus.[1715] The pineal[1951,2766] and choroid plexus are less common sites. Even rarer are metastases from a systemic primary cancer to an already extant intracranialbrain tumor[2546] such as a meningioma,[1593,1972] a glioma,[2546] an acoustic neurinoma,[1491] an ependymoma, a pituitary adenoma,[1795] or even to an arteriovenous malformation.[985] Brain metastases may arise in areas of cerebral damage from ischemic infarction[1896] or in chronic subdural hematoma membranes.[435]

FREQUENCY

Autopsy studies find intracranial metastases in about 25% of patients who die of cancer.* As shown in Table 5–2, the brain parenchyma is involved in about 15% of patients and is the exclusive site of intracranial metastases in about 10%. The term "solitary brain metastasis" implies the absence of other metastatic lesions either in the brain or elsewhere in the body. "Single brain metastasis" indicates one lesion in the brain but implies that extracranial tumor also is present.

Epidemiologic studies based on death certificates, hospital records,[2723] tumor registries,[805] or a combination of these,[1031,2005] substantially underestimate the frequency of even symptomatic intracranial metastases. Most such studies suggest an incidence of brain metastases similar to that of primary brain tumors, whereas the autopsy studies (see Tables 5–1 and 5–2) indicate that they are far more frequent.

Evidence demonstrates that the frequency of intracranial metastases increased in the years between 1959 and 1979, when the last large surveys were completed[2037,2073] (see Fig. 1–2). Although the cause of this increase is unknown, some investigators suggest that it may result from better control of the primary tumors and of systemic metastases, allowing time for cells sequestered behind the blood–brain barrier to grow and cause symptoms.

---

*References 2037, 2073, 2544, 2779, 2851.

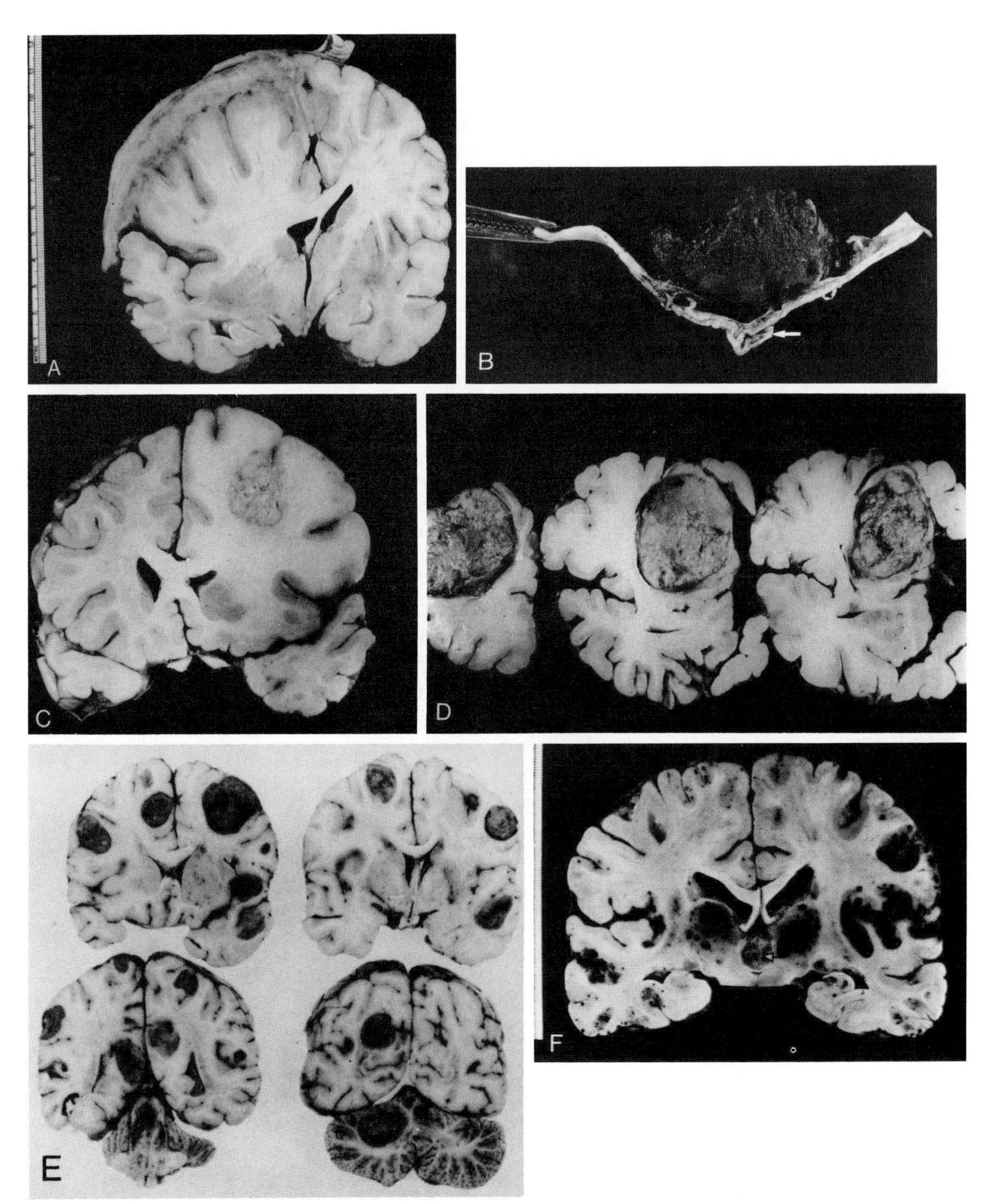

Figure 5–2. Various intracranial metastases are depicted. *A,* Skull metastasis from lung carcinoma growing into and through the epidural space to compress the sagittal sinus and invade the subdural space, leptomeninges, and cerebral cortex. Although the tumor itself is not very thick, massive edema of the hemisphere is shown with lateral shift and herniation. *B,* Metastasis from carcinoma of the breast to the skull, compressing yet not invading the dura but occluding the sagittal sinus *(arrow).* *C,* A single brain metastasis from lung carcinoma. Note the location of the fleshy-appearing tumor at the junction of the gray and white matter and its clear demarcation from surrounding brain. The white matter of the entire hemisphere shows massive edema with lateral shift. *D,* Single brain metastasis from carcinoma of the thyroid. Despite the massive size of the tumor and the resultant lateral shift, considerably less edema is noted than in *panel C. E,* Metastases from malignant melanoma. Most of the tumors are at the gray matter and white matter junction, with a few gray matter lesions. The lesions are mostly nonhemorrhagic. *F,* Malignant melanoma with an uncountable number of gray matter metastases. In this patient, the white matter is largely spared, although tumor has spread diffusely through the gray matter of the cerebral cortex and basal ganglia. The pineal gland is also involved *(arrow).*

Continued.

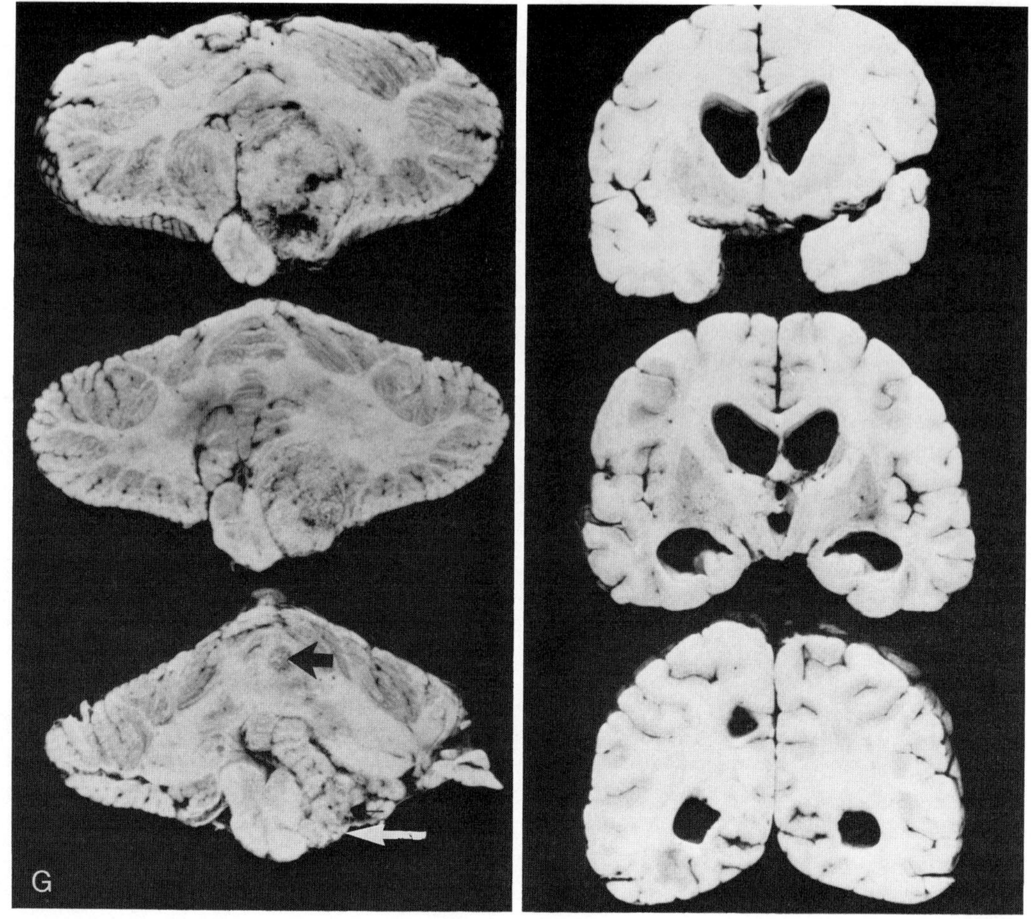

Figure 5–2. ***Continued.*** *G,* Cerebellar metastases *(left).* This patient had breast carcinoma. A large metastasis is visible in the cerebellar tonsil *(white arrow).* A smaller one is present superiorly *(black arrow).* The larger metastasis occludes the outflow foramina of the fourth ventricle, thus obstructing CSF flow *(right).* The cerebral hemispheres from the same patient show marked hydrocephalus. Both lateral ventricles, including the temporal horn and third ventricle, are enlarged.

BRAIN METASTASES

Relationship to Systemic Cancers

Table 5–3 lists the primary tumors from a group of 210 patients encountered at Memorial Sloan-Kettering Cancer Center (MSKCC) during the first 10 months of 1994. Brain metastases can arise from any primary systemic cancer,[2715] but certain tumors, such as melanoma[357,1745] and breast[261,267,1505,2693] and lung cancer,[874,2462] have a particular predilection to metastasize to the brain. Others, which include prostate[407,1438,2292] and ovarian cancer*, osteosarcomas,[144,1682] other sarcomas,[1551] and Hodgkin's disease,[2290] rarely result in metastasis to the brain. Furthermore, certain tumors such as melanoma are more likely to cause multiple metastases, whereas those such as breast cancer usually cause single lesions. Table 5–4 lists the likelihood of single or multiple (greater than one) metastases from different primary tumors, based on CT scans.[605] Because half

*References 565, 1529, 1713, 2483, 2897.

Table 5–1. **CLASSIFICATION OF INTRACRANIAL METASTASES BY ANATOMIC SITE**

- I. Skull
  - A. Calvarium
  - B. Base (see Chapter 8)
- II. Cerebral Meninges
  - A. Epidural
    - (1) Extension from skull metastases
    - (2) Hematogenous to dura
      - (a) Compressing brain
      - (b) Compressing venous sinus(es)
  - B. Subdural
    - (1) Causing mass lesion
    - (2) Causing effusion
  - C. Leptomeningeal (see Chapter 7)
    - (1) Focal
    - (2) Diffuse
- III. Brain
  - A. Cerebral hemisphere(s)
  - B. Brainstem
  - C. Cerebellum
- IV. Other Intracranial Sites
  - A. Pituitary
  - B. Pineal
  - C. Choroid plexus
  - D. Pre-existing brain lesion (e.g., tumor, infarct, vascular malformation)

of the patients have a single lesion and an additional 20% have only two, the clinical implication is that at least 70% of patients are potential candidates for focal therapy.[16,605,2068]

Most brain metastases originate from cancers of the lung, especially small-cell cancer[874] and adenocarcinoma,[780,2462] or cancer of the breast and of the skin (melanoma).[1745] Quite a few patients develop brain metastases from an unknown primary source.[700,703] In series reported from general neurologic or neurosurgical services, the percentage of unknown primary tumors is greater than in series reported from a cancer hospital because of referral patterns. The primary site of such lesions, if eventually discovered, is usually the lung, or, less often, other sites including the gastrointestinal tract or kidney.[1438,1497,2710,2779] Often the primary site is not found,[703,1485,1747,2710] even at autopsy.[700] A CT scan of the chest, abdomen, and pelvis will usually locate the primary site if it can be found. In the absence of organ-specific symptoms or signs, other laboratory tests are rarely helpful.[1747,2710]

Most brain metastases, particularly those that arise from primary neoplasms other than lung cancer, occur at a late stage in the dissemination of most cancers, when metastases are usually also present elsewhere in the body. The presence of more than one

Table 5–2. **INCIDENCE OF INTRACRANIAL METASTASES IN AUTOPSY STUDIES**

	Posner and Chernik[2073] (1978)	**Takakura and colleagues[2544] (1982)**	**Pickren and colleagues[2037] (1983)**
Total No. of Autopsies	2375	3359	10,916
Site of Metastases			
Intracranial	572 (24%)	860 (26%)	
Dural	467 (20%)	645 (19%)	
Leptomeningeal	184 (8%)	90 (3%)	
Brain	361 (15%)	555 (17%)	954 (8.7%)
Brain Only	225 (9%)	—	—
Single	106 (47%)*	—	378 (39%)
Solitary†			32 (0.3%)

*% of total brain metastases that are single.
†No other systemic metastases.

Table 5–3. **PRIMARY TUMORS IN 210 PATIENTS WITH BRAIN METASTASES**

Lung	85	
Non–small-cell		73
Small-cell		12
Breast	39	
Melanoma	20	
Genitourinary	15	
Renal		7
Testis		4
Bladder		2
Prostate		2
Gastrointestinal	14	
Colon		8
Esophagus		4
Gastric		1
Pancreas		1
Gynecologic	10	
Ovary		3
Choriocarcinoma		3
Cervix		3
Endometrium		1
Sarcoma	7	
Unknown Primary	5	
Head and Neck	4	
Thyroid	4	
Miscellaneous	7	
Lymphoma		2
Thymoma		1
Neuroendocrine		2
Adrenal		1
Mediastinal germ cell		1

brain metastasis also suggests a broad dissemination of the primary tumor. In 201 patients with brain metastases treated at MSKCC,[363] only 38 (19%) were without evidence of other metastatic disease, and several of these developed clinical evidence of systemic metastases within a few weeks after the initial negative evaluation. In a large autopsy study of patients who had lung cancer, brain metastases were present in 25% but were solitary in only 3%.[874] About 67% of patients with brain metastases from organs other than the lung also have pulmonary metastases; about 25% have bone metastases.[605]

At times, brain metastases may appear as isolated lesions years after "successful" treatment of the primary tumors. In patients with primary lung cancer, the brain is often the only site of metastasis.[780] Such lung lesions are likely to be peripheral or apical rather than central, and the brain lesion is more likely to be single[2594] than multiple, making both pulmonary and brain lesions more amenable to resection. Nevertheless, only 20 of 100 patients who died of lung cancer were found to have a solitary brain metastasis.[2594]

As a result of their late appearance, at a time when the systemic cancer has disseminated widely, brain metastases often are discovered only at autopsy, having been asymptomatic prior to the patient's death in as many as 25% to 30% of patients.[363] Occasionally, CT or MR screening scans will detect asymptomatic metastases in the brain. Jacobs and colleagues[1259] report a 6% incidence of asymptomatic metastases detected by CT scan in patients scheduled for surgery for lung cancer. Salbeck and associates[2274] found asymptomatic brain metastases on CT scans at the initial evaluation for lung cancer

Table 5–4. **NUMBER OF METASTASES AND PRIMARY SITE OF TUMORS IN 288 PATIENTS[605] WITH BRAIN METASTASES**

No. of Metastases	No. of Patients (%)	Primary Site	Single %	Multiple % (Two or More)
1	141 (49)	Lung	46	54
2	60 (21)	Melanoma	41	59
3	38 (13)	Unknown	32	68
4	17 (6)	Breast	56	44
5+	32 (11)	Pelvis-abdomen	69	31

in 11% of 232 patients. Most often, these patients had either limited small-cell lung cancer or stage III, but not stage I or II, non–small-cell lung cancer. Preoperative scans should be routine in patients at high risk for brain metastases in whom major surgery for the primary tumor is planned, because the presence of a silent brain metastasis may change the treatment; for example, the brain tumor may be treated first.

Pathophysiology of Symptoms and Signs

The pathophysiology of the metastatic process is discussed in Chapter 2. As illustrated in Figure 5–2, most brain metastases begin in the white matter of the watershed area of the brain at the junction of the gray and white matter. This section describes how brain metastases cause neurologic symptoms or signs (Table 5–5). Neurologic symptoms and signs can be classified as focal, generalized, or false-localizing. Focal signs may either identify the site of the brain metastasis or be false-localizing[1969,2066] (see the following). Generalized signs are the result of increases in intracranial pressure, either gradual or sudden, as in plateau waves, which are discussed in Chapter 3. Increased intracranial pressure in and of itself, as in the syndrome of idiopathic intracranial hypertension, can cause several confusing symptoms such as tinnitus, stiff neck, paresthesias in the legs, and back pain, all of which can be relieved by lowering intracranial pressure. False-localizing signs result from distortion or compression of structures distant from the actual tumor.[87,481,891,1284,1393]

Neurologic symptoms and signs have multiple causes:

1. *Destruction or replacement of brain tissue* by a metastatic tumor is probably unusual. The central necrosis often seen pathologically and on CT or MR scans is due to tumor necrosis, not to destruction of the underlying brain tissue. When a metastatic tumor is effectively treated by steroids, radiation, or surgical extirpation, neurologic signs usually improve substantially or disappear altogether. If a substantial portion of brain tissue has been destroyed by the tumor, neurologic signs should persist.
2. *Displacement of brain tissue by the rapidly growing metastatic tumor* is the common cause of focal neurologic symptoms. The growing mass compresses surrounding brain tissue, squeezes out blood and interstitial fluid, and distorts normal anatomy. In addition, hemorrhage, cyst formation, or necrosis within the tumor can suddenly increase its size, rapidly compressing normal brain and causing acute focal symptoms.
3. *"Irritation" by the tumor or the surrounding*

Table 5–5. **PATHOPHYSIOLOGY OF SIGNS AND SYMPTOMS OF BRAIN METASTASIS**

Signs/Symptoms	Examples	Causes
Focal	Hemiparesis (hemiplegia) Visual field defects Aphasia Focal seizures Ataxia	Direct effect of metastasis (plus hemorrhage or cyst) Secondary effect of edema Remote effect of cerebral herniation (false-localizing signs)
Generalized	Headache Confusion, memory loss Lethargy Vomiting Ataxia	Increased intracranial pressure Hydrocephalus
False-Localizing	Abducens nerve palsy Ipsilateral hemiparesis	Shifts of structure Cerebral herniation

edema of the overlying gray matter probably accounts for the high incidence of focal seizures. Although the exact mechanism is unknown, it is likely that changes in the extracellular fluid composition caused by blood–brain barrier disruption are important. In patients who have melanoma that has invaded the gray matter directly, seizures are more frequent than they are with metastases that are more likely to invade white matter.

4. *Cerebral edema* increases the size of the mass in the hemisphere, further compressing surrounding brain.
5. *Cerebral herniations* (i.e., the shifting of cerebral structures from one compartment to another) may result from increased tissue pressure caused by the metastasis and its surrounding cerebral edema. Common sites and effects of herniation caused by supratentorial tumors (Fig. 1-3) are:
   A. Herniation of the cingulate gyrus under the falx compresses both anterior frontal lobes and leads to urgency incontinence and bilateral extensor plantar responses. The ipsilateral anterior cerebral artery also may be compressed, causing frontal lobe ischemia.
   B. At the tentorium cerebelli, the uncus of the temporal lobe or the hippocampal gyrus, or both, herniate, displacing the brainstem toward the opposite side and compressing the opposite peduncle against the tentorium cerebelli (Kernohan's notch), leading to an ipsilateral hemiparesis. The herniated uncus may also compress the third nerve and the posterior cerebral artery. Compression of the third nerve leads initially to ipsilateral pupillary dilatation and subsequently to total third-nerve palsy. Compression of the posterior cerebral artery may cause ischemia or infarction of the ipsilateral occipital lobe, with a contralateral homonymous hemianopia. On rare occasions, both posterior cerebral arteries are compressed by massive herniation, causing bilateral occipital infarction and cortical blindness.
   C. The enlarging supratentorial mass also shifts the diencephalon both contralaterally and caudally, resulting in progressive loss of consciousness, beginning with drowsiness and proceeding to stupor and finally to coma. Whether lateral or caudal shifts are primarily responsible for coma is disputed.[764,1243,2146,2200] Lateral shifts also obstruct the third ventricle and Monro's foramen, leading to contralateral enlargement of the lateral ventricle(s) and further increasing tissue pressure in the supratentorial compartment. Rostral-caudal shifts compress the midbrain and pons, possibly causing brainstem hemorrhage (Duret's lesion).
   D. A large supratentorial mass causes herniation of the cerebellar tonsils through the foramen magnum in about one-third of cases; tonsillar herniation is particularly common in patients with posterior fossa masses.
   E. Herniation of brain substance through the tentorial notch interferes with cerebrospinal fluid (CSF) absorptive pathways, leading to hydrocephalus. The same is true of tonsillar herniation through the foramen magnum.

Infratentorial mass lesions also cause herniations, most commonly herniation of the cerebellar tonsils through the foramen magnum. The low brainstem is compressed; when the compression is acute, it can cause apnea as a first sign, followed by loss of consciousness. Cough syncope may be a symptom of a cerebellar metastasis.[1472] Tonsillar herniation probably causes the sudden death that sometimes follows lumbar puncture in patients with brain tumors or meningitis.[2047] A second form of herniation from posterior fossa tumors is that of the superior vermis of the cerebellum through the tentorial notch (upward herniation).[537] Upward herniation compresses the brainstem at the mesencephalic level, causing pupillary and eye-movement abnormalities; it may interfere with subarachnoid absorptive pathways either by aqueductal stenosis (causing obstructive hydrocephalus) or by obliteration of perimesencephalic cisterns (causing communicating hydrocephalus). Although not a herniation, enlarging cerebellar masses also push the brainstem forward, compressing it against the clivus anteriorly, sometimes obstructing the fourth ventricle.

6. *Compression of venous structures and increased resistance to CSF absorption* caused by the tumor mass elevate intracranial pressure.[2653,2655] The mass, with its attendant elevation of intracranial pressure, often causes intermittent vasoparalysis, leading to plateau waves[1109,1616] (see Chapter 3).

Clinical Findings

SYMPTOMS AND SIGNS

Presenting Symptoms

The presenting symptoms of brain metastases are summarized in Table 5–6. The percentages total more than 100% because many patients present with more than one symptom or sign.

Headache. This presenting complaint, which may be focal or generalized, occurs in about 50% or fewer patients with brain metastases.[716,822a,823,2251] When the headache is focal, it has localizing value. Simonescu[2428] reports that, in 72% of his patients, the headache was localized at the site of the metastasis, but in most brain tumor patients examined at MSKCC, the headache has been diffuse or bilateral in the frontal or occipital regions, and thus without localizing value. The classic "brain tumor headache," which occurs in only a minority of patients,[716] is mild at onset, begins when the patient awakens in the morning, disappears shortly after he or she arises, and recurs the following morning. The headaches gradually increase in frequency, duration, and severity until, in their later stages, they are almost constant and may be associated with other signs of increased intracranial pressure, including drowsiness, nausea, and vomiting. Headache as an isolated symptom is more common in patients with multiple metastases than in those with single lesions. It also is more common in patients with cerebellar metastases than in those with cerebral hemisphere metastases. Rarely, patients with large frontal lesions will report severe and recurrent headache without other signs or symptoms, but nearly all brain tumor patients with headache have other symptoms or signs. An otherwise occult brain tumor may occasionally present as a typical common or classic migraine.[2004]

Brain tumor headaches probably result when the mass lesion causes traction on pain-sensitive intracranial structures such as the dura at the base of the brain, the cranial nerves, and the large venous sinuses. The brain itself is pain-insensitive. Such headaches imply an increase in intracranial pressure, either focal or diffuse. The clinical implication is that many patients, particularly older patients with atrophic brains that can accommodate the tumor mass without increasing pressure, are less likely to suffer headache.

Table 5–6. **PRESENTING SYMPTOMS AND SIGNS OF BRAIN METASTASIS**

Symptoms	% of 363 Patients*	Signs	% of 363 Patients*
Headache	49	Impaired cognitive function	58
Focal weakness	30	Hemiparesis	59
Mental disturbances	32	Mild-moderate	27
Gait ataxia	21	Severe	31
Seizures	18	Hemisensory loss	21
Focal motor	4	Papilledema	20
Generalized	7	Gait ataxia	19
Other focal	7	Aphasia	18
Speech difficulty	12	Visual field cut	7
Visual disturbance	6	Limb ataxia	6
Sensory disturbance	6	Depressed level of consciousness	4
Limb ataxia	6		

*Patients may present with more than one symptom or sign.
Source: Data from Cairncross et al[363] and Young et al.[2871]

Because headaches caused by a metastasis are usually accompanied by increased intracranial pressure, one might expect a high frequency of papilledema in such patients. The contrary is true.[524] In the series reported by Young and colleagues,[2871] 53% of patients reported headaches but only 26% had papilledema. In patients with cerebellar tumors, headaches were present in 70% and papilledema in only 25%. In short, almost 50% of the patients with brain metastases do not have headache as a presenting complaint, and 75% of the patients do not have papilledema. The absence of these two textbook hallmarks of brain tumor does not exclude a symptomatic brain metastasis.

Focal Weakness. The second-ranking complaint reported in most patient series is focal weakness, which may range from a gradually developing mild monoparesis or hemiparesis to acute hemiplegia. Focal weakness was a presenting complaint in 18% of the Paillas and Pellet series[1969] but was present in 67% of patients by the time the diagnosis was confirmed. Focal weakness usually accurately localizes the tumor to the contralateral cerebral hemisphere, but because the effects of the tumor and its surrounding edema are so widespread, it does not accurately localize the lesion to the motor area of that hemisphere. If only one extremity is weak, the tumor is more likely to be located in the white matter directly below the cortical area subserving that function. Paillas and Pellet[1969] note that motor disturbances are found more often than sensory disturbances even though more metastatic tumors are in the postcentral than in the precentral gyrus.

Mental Disturbances. The initial complaint in about 30% of patients is mental disturbance; for example, a patient or family member reports a change in personality or memory. Mental and behavioral changes may be a result of either focal disturbances of brain function or more generalized cerebral abnormalities. Focal abnormalities of mental function include such disorders as aphasia, alexia, acalculia, agnosia, apraxia, amnesia,[2871] and sometimes affective changes,[1658] usually depression. When present in pure form, these disorders have localizing value. Dressing apraxia that results from a right parietal lesion is a surprisingly common presenting complaint.

Much more common are mental and behavioral changes that result either from multiple cerebral metastases or from strategically placed lesions that cause increased intracranial pressure. In the early stages, patients typically are awake and alert, although they may find that they sleep more than usual and take an unaccustomed afternoon nap. They complain of difficulty with memory and concentration, or the family reports increased apathy, withdrawal, irritability, and forgetfulness. Occasionally, business colleagues complain that the patient's judgment has become poor. Despite the patient's denial of being depressed, psychiatric consultation is often sought before a brain scan is procured.

Although mental changes may occur in the absence of any other neurologic symptom, headache is a commonly associated symptom because both symptoms are related to increased intracranial pressure. If a diagnosis is not made and the patient is not treated, symptoms usually progress and intensify, with loss of alertness, increasing drowsiness, increasing memory impairment, and, finally, loss of orientation (first, for time, and later, for place and person).

Seizures. Whether focal or generalized, seizures are most common in patients with multiple metastases and in patients with combined brain and leptomeningeal metastases.[1260] They also occur more frequently with melanoma metastases because these lesions are more likely to be multiple and to reside in the cortex rather than in the subcortical white matter. Cascino and colleagues[397] report that seizures affected 25% of the patients studied who had metastatic colon cancer (50% multiple lesions); Byrne and coworkers[357] note seizures in 56% of patients with melanoma metastases (60% multiple lesions). The seizures are usually focal in onset and have localizing value; rarely are they false-localizing.[87] In the Paillas and Pellet[1969] series, seizures were a presenting complaint in 19% of the patients studied, but by the time the diagnosis was confirmed, 39% suffered from seizures. Of the patients studied by Simonescu,[2428] 29% had seizures. Cohen and associates[470] report an 18% incidence of seizures as the presenting complaint, with a 10% incidence of late seizures whether or not prophylactic anticonvulsants were given. Although seizures are common, status epilepticus is rare, but it can be devastating in patients with brain metastases. The treatment of seizures and status epilepticus as well as the use of prophylactic anticonvulsants is discussed in Chapter 4.

The characteristic seizure is a focal motor seizure beginning with a clonic jerking of the face or of one extremity. The seizure may progress to involve the other extremity on the same side (Jacksonian march) or may generalize to a grand mal convulsion. Following the seizure, the patient often suffers Todd's paralysis of the extremities. The paralysis is usually transient, with recovery ranging from several minutes to hours, but, on occasion, single or repetitive seizures lead to permanent paralysis of the involved extremities. Todd's paralysis occurs more frequently in patients with brain metastases than in those with focal seizures without tumor; it probably results when seizures increase blood flow and blood volume, worsening previously elevated intracranial pressure and leading to focal ischemia and sometimes to infarction. Seizures sometimes cause transtentorial herniation.

Episodes of transient paralysis or other loss of neurologic function may mimic transient ischemic attacks or complicated migraine but probably represent either nonconvulsive seizures or plateau waves.[787]

Other Presenting Symptoms. Gait ataxia is a prominent presenting complaint when the tumor lies in the cerebellum or brainstem. Ataxia also occasionally occurs as a result of a large frontal lobe metastasis or hydrocephalus caused by obstruction of CSF pathways.[1708] Ataxia from hydrocephalus can be relieved by shunting of the ventricular system. Rarely, parietal lesions cause a particular form of unilateral ataxia called optic ataxia, in which visually guided limb movements are poorly performed.[556]

Aphasia was a prominent presenting complaint in about 10% of the patients in the series reported by Young and colleagues,[2871] was an isolated complaint in only 1% of Paillas and Pellet's[1969] patients, and was seen in 4% of Hildebrand's[1156] patients. Aphasia is an excellent localizing symptom when it occurs in the absence of other cognitive changes, but it may be confused with nonaphasic naming difficulties, a common result of more generalized brain dysfunction.

Sensory changes are an uncommon complaint in all series, despite the fact that the parietal lobe, the site of the sensory cortex, is involved in many patients. Visual abnormalities, usually a hemianopia, were a prominent presenting complaint in one surgical series.[877] Some patients with hemianopia are aware that they have visual difficulty, although they cannot exactly specify its nature. Other patients are totally unaware of any visual deficit until, for example, they are involved in an automobile accident because they failed to see a car or other object in their hemianopic field.

Presenting Signs

In most series, signs and symptoms are lumped together. Young and associates[2871] and Cairncross and colleagues,[363] however, separately describe the presenting signs and symptoms of brain metastases in 363 patients (Table 5–6). The major finding was that careful neurologic examination often revealed signs of which the patient was unaware. For example, although 30% (108) of the patients complained of focal weakness, examination revealed evidence of focal weakness in over 50% (214).

More striking was the high incidence of impaired cognitive or behavioral function in patients at the time of diagnosis. Young and associates[2871] found that 75% of the patients studied could not perform normally on the standard tests of mental status. This figure is higher than most reported in other literature but does suggest that careful testing of patients suspected of brain metastases often reveals subtle and unexpected changes in cognitive function. Paillas and Pellet[1969] report mental disturbances at the time of diagnosis in 24% of their patients, and generalized asthenia, including clouding of consciousness and torpor, in an additional 24%. Elkington[718] reports mental changes in 75% of patients. Part of the discrepancy among these series may be associated with unclear and inconsistent definitions of mental disturbances.

When usually safe doses of opioids or sedative agents provoke delirium or impaired cognition, the presence of previously asymptomatic brain metastases may be suspected. Early hydrocephalus from obstruction of the fourth ventricle may cause cognitive or behavioral changes mimicking depression.

Although neurologic findings on examination are often more prominent than those noted by the patient, ataxia in cerebellar tumors is an exception. Patient complaints of gait unsteadiness are often strikingly out of proportion to the little found on examination. Patients with a single metastasis in the cerebellum usually present with gait ataxia with or without limb ataxia. Headache, dizziness, diplopia, and vomiting are initial symptoms in fewer than 50% of the patients with cerebellar metastases, as are papilledema and nystagmus.[524,748] Vomiting with or without nausea is an occasional presentation of a posterior fossa metastasis. Particularly suggestive is vomiting on first awakening in the morning. If the patient is known to have disseminated cancer, especially in the liver or abdomen, the physician may fail to consider a brain lesion as a potential cause.

Unusual and perplexing focal signs are associated with tumors in unusual places. Examples are bilateral arm weakness sparing the legs ("man-in-a-barrel" syndrome) associated with symmetric tumors of the arm area of the motor strip,[1802] hemichorea associated with basal ganglia tumors,[2242] symptoms of a diffuse encephalopathy associated with miliary metastases to the brain,[802,1645] and the syndrome of pseudobulbar palsy from bilateral, symmetric lesions of the frontal operculum. Brainstem metastases can also cause perplexing symptoms including gaze and cranial nerve palsies, ptosis, and ataxia.[588,616,2492] Other unusual signs of posterior fossa tumors include hypertension,[742] orthostatic hypotension,[1220] hiccoughs,[2506] achalasia,[4] night terrors,[1746] inability to sneeze,[1695] and neurogenic hyperventilation.[1267] Because such brainstem metastases may be quite small, they may not be detected on CT scan but are invariably detected by MR scan.

Onset of Neurologic Dysfunction

The signs and symptoms of a brain metastasis usually begin insidiously and evolve over a period of days or a few weeks or, more rarely, over a period of weeks or months. Sometimes the onset of the neurologic symptoms is sudden, occasionally because of hemorrhage into a tumor,[1407,1673] although the acute worsening of pre-existing, slowly evolving symptoms is the more common presentation of intratumoral hemorrhage. Paillas and Pellet[1969] report an acute onset of symptoms in 47% (83) of 178 cases: 19% (34) had seizures, 18% (32) had an acute strokelike syndrome with hemiplegia, and the rest had other acutely developing neurologic signs such as sensory loss, aphasia, and dementia. Van Eck and associates[2665] indicate that 30 of their 104 patients with brain metastases had a "more or less acute onset of symptoms" but do not specify further. Our own experience has been that if seizures are excluded (15%), acute or apoplectic onset of neurologic symptoms occurs in fewer than 10% of patients. Metastatic tumor can mimic transient ischemic attacks, stroke-in-evolution, completed stroke, or multi-infarct dementia.[2774]

Paillas and Pellet[1969] report a three-stage course beginning with an acute onset of neurologic symptoms, which they believe represents a tumor embolus occluding a blood vessel.[1569] Next is a phase of improvement that may last several weeks to months, followed by recurrent and progressive neurologic symptoms. The phase of improvement reflects the return of function in an ischemic but not infarcted area; the secondary increase in neurologic symptoms represents the growth of tumor from the tumor embolus. We have encountered such events only rarely in patients at MSKCC.

Metastases that present with apoplectic onset, the three-stage course, or transient attacks have all been grouped together under the term "pseudovascular syndromes."[578] The clinical importance of these unusual modes of onset is that they may be mistaken for stroke rather than tumor.

The pathogenesis of gradually developing symptoms is that of a slowly increasing, space-occupying mass with surrounding edema. The pathogenesis of the acutely developing symptoms other than seizures is more perplexing. In some instances, acute onset heralds a hemorrhage into a previously silent metastatic tumor. This mode of onset is particularly common with uterine or testicular choriocarcinomas and with malignant melanomas, but hemorrhage into a brain metastasis can occur with any primary tumor and is most common in lung metastases[1673] because of their large numbers (see Table 1–2). Hemorrhage is suggested clinically by the acute onset of symptoms and can be confirmed by CT scan. In many instances, however, patients with brain metastasis suffer the apoplectic onset of hemiplegia or other neurologic signs without clinical or pathologic evidence of hemorrhage. In these cases, the pathogenesis is not certain. In some instances tumor may compromise arterial circulation, causing a cerebral infarct.

More perplexing are patients with brain metastases who suffer episodic neurologic symptoms often lasting a few hours, after which the symptoms clear.[737,787,1247] These symptoms are usually not motor but, instead, are behavioral abnormalities, vaguely described episodes of dizziness, or difficulties in comprehending a situation or the environment. Several explanations are possible. (1) They may represent partial seizures originating in the limbic system. Although partial seizures (nonconvulsive status epilepticus) can last for a long period, they are usually shorter than the 30- to 90-minute episodes seen in patients with brain tumors. (2) The episodes may result from transient ischemia, although they last longer than the few minutes of most transient ischemic attacks. Furthermore, most transient ischemic attacks cause motor or sensory abnormalities rather than behavioral disturbances. (3) The episodic symptoms may result from plateau waves.[737,1247] I think most are probably seizures and should be so treated (see Chapter 3).

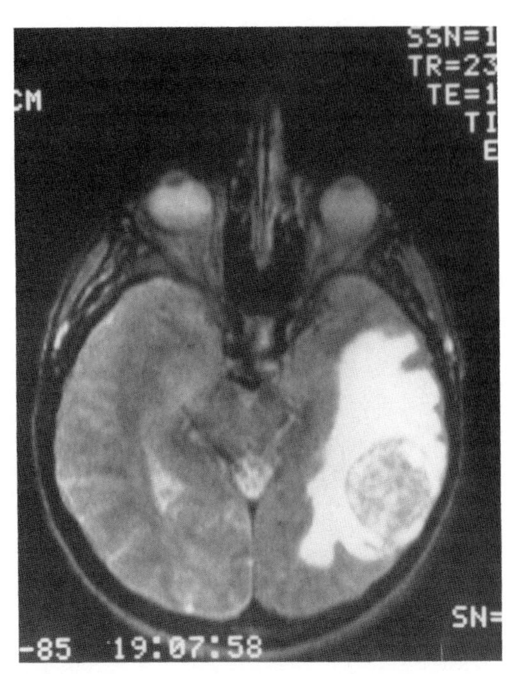

Figure 5–3. A T_2-weighted MR scan of a patient with metastatic malignant melanoma. The tumor is visible as a heterogeneous mass surrounded by hyperintense edema in the white matter. Notice how the fingerlike projections of the edema invade the white matter and spare the cortex of the temporal lobe.

Laboratory Findings

MAGNETIC RESONANCE

An MR scan is the best diagnostic test for brain metastases (Fig. 5–3). A carefully done, contrast-enhanced MR scan, if negative, effectively rules out brain metastasis, except for miliary cortical metastases (see Chapter 7), as a cause of neurologic symptomatology. MR with gadolinium enhancement is preferable to CT scanning because it is more sensitive, revealing small lesions not detected by CT, particularly in the brainstem or cerebellum,[573,748,2430,2881] thus potentially altering management. It also is preferable because the contrast material is safer. Because almost any single symptom or constellation of neurologic symptoms can be caused by metastatic brain tumors, including no symptoms, an MR scan should be performed on any patient with cancer who has an unexplained alteration in brain function, as well as in those patients who are at high risk for brain metastases and are about to undergo potentially curative systemic treatment. Examples include patients with lung cancer who are being considered for surgical resection of the primary tumor and patients with metastatic melanoma or small-cell lung cancer who are about to undergo systemic chemotherapy or immunotherapy.

If MR is selected, T_1- and T_2-weighted images should be performed before the injection of contrast material (Fig. 5–4). The unenhanced T_1-weighted image often fails to show a metastatic lesion unless it is hemorrhagic, in which case the intensity is increased. Calcified lesions may be associated with areas of absent signal. The T_2-weighted image is almost always positive, revealing an area or areas of increased intensity in the white matter, usually encompassing both the tumor and the surrounding edema. Occasionally, the intensity of the tumor is less than that of the surrounding edema, permitting easy identification and localization

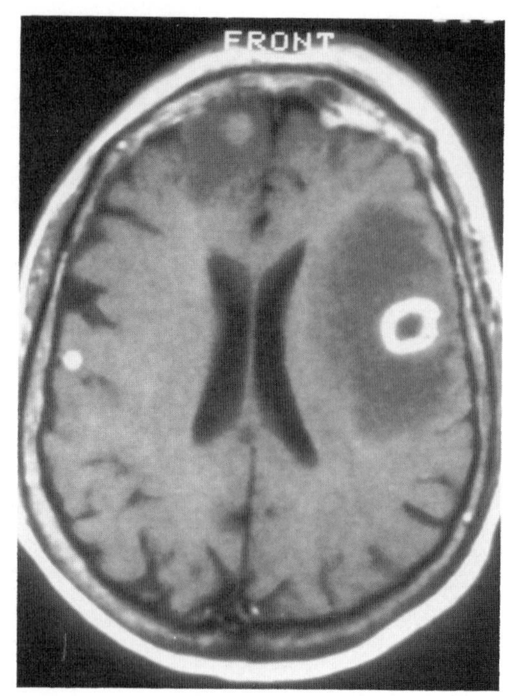

Figure 5–4. Enhanced T_1-weighted MR scan in patients with multiple metastases from lung adenocarcinoma. Notice the ringlike enhancement of the largest metastasis in the left frontal lobe *(right side of figure)*. A massive amount of edema appears as hypointensity surrounding the tumor. A moderate amount of edema surrounds the slightly contrast-enhancing smaller lesion in the right anterior frontal lobe. A small, uniformly contrast-enhancing lesion more posteriorly in the right frontal lobe is not surrounded by edema.

(see Fig. 5–3). Almost all metastatic tumors are hyperintense after the injection of contrast (gadolinium) on the T_1-weighted image, allowing for clear identification of the size, shape, and location of the metastasis. An enhanced brain metastasis usually is spherical and well demarcated from surrounding brain. The center is devoid of contrast but surrounded by a rim of enhancement. If the images are performed in more than one plane, the tumor can be exquisitely localized by the area of enhancement, which is especially useful if focal therapy is contemplated.[1427] High-dose gadolinium MR scans appear to increase the number of metastases detected and to improve the image quality.[2881]

OTHER LABORATORY TESTS

If an MR scan cannot be performed, a CT scan should take place both before and after the injection of contrast (iodine). If a brain metastasis is strongly suspected, 5 to 10 mg of diazepam should be given 30 minutes before the contrast injection to prevent seizure induced by the contrast material[1901] (see Chapter 4). Most metastatic lesions of the brain are hypodense or isodense on the precontrast CT except for melanoma, choriocarcinoma, colon cancers, and leukemia,[2794] which are often hyperdense. Virtually all metastatic tumors increase their density after the injection of contrast. A CT scan without contrast can identify those rare metastases that calcify.[2858]

If the diagnosis cannot be made with reasonable certainty by CT or MR scanning, no other test short of biopsy (or CSF evaluation for malignant cells when coexisting leptomeningeal tumor is present) can establish the diagnosis. Cerebral angiography is not helpful; neither is the obsolete (in this context) radionuclide brain scanning, electroencephalography, or plain skull radiographs. PET and single-photon emission computed tomography have not been shown to be useful in diagnosing metastatic tumors and are less sensitive than CT and MR scans. When fluorodeoxyglucose was used to image the metabolic rate of brain metastases, fewer than 70% of tumors were detected because either they were below the resolution of the PET scanner or they were not hypermetabolic.[999]

Radionuclide brain scanning after the cisterna magna injection of radioiodinated Indium (i.e., Indium cisternography) often demonstrates asymmetric obstruction of the flow of CSF through the subarachnoid space, which may help to explain elevated CSF pressure with supratentorial lesions, but RIHSA scans are not helpful diagnostically.[2653]

A few reports suggest that an elevated plasma carcinoembryonic antigen (CEA) level may be an early sign of brain metastasis from lung or breast cancer and that an increased CSF/serum ratio of beta human chorionic gonadotropin (βHCG) may be the first sign of brain metastasis from choriocarcinoma. Even with choriocarcinoma, however, MR scans are more sensitive than βHCG.[96] A caveat: One patient with a meningioma and a history of breast cancer developed an elevated plasma CEA caused by the meningioma, not by recurrent or metastatic breast cancer.[1605]

Differential Diagnosis

Usually, the clinical history, combined with the results of an MR scan, establishes the diagnosis of brain metastasis with reasonable certainty. A definitive diagnosis of metastatic brain tumor cannot be made on scan results alone; absolute certainty requires stereotactic needle biopsy.[840,1756] Even a typical scan only suggests, but does not prove, that the lesion is a brain metastasis rather than a primary brain tumor, a cerebral abscess,[515] or another lesion[1993] (Table 5–7). Multiple lesions increase the likelihood of brain metastasis, and a known systemic cancer makes the diagnosis even more likely. In one study, however, 6 of 54 patients with known cancer and single brain lesions did not have metastases on biopsy; 3 did not even have a neoplastic lesion.[1993] Stereotactic needle biopsy will settle the issue if doubt exists.[840,1756]

Table 5–7. **BRAIN METASTASIS: DIFFERENTIAL DIAGNOSIS**

- I. Primary brain tumors
  - A. Meningioma
  - B. Glioma
  - C. Pituitary adenoma
  - D. Acoustic neurinoma
- II. Vascular disease
  - A. Cerebral hemorrhage
    - 1. Intratumoral (metastasis or primary brain tumor)
    - 2. Vascular anomaly
  - B. Cerebral embolus
    - 1. Nonbacterial endocarditis
    - 2. Tumor
  - C. Cerebral thrombosis
    - 1. Arterial
    - 2. Venous
- III. Infections
  - A. Abscess—especially Hodgkin's disease and lymphoma
  - B. Viral infection—progressive multifocal leukoencephalopathy
- IV. Side effects of therapy
  - A. Methotrexate leukoencephalopathy
  - B. Radionecrosis
- V. Other disorders
  - A. Related to cancer—"paraneoplastic syndromes"
  - B. Not related to cancer (e.g., multiple sclerosis)

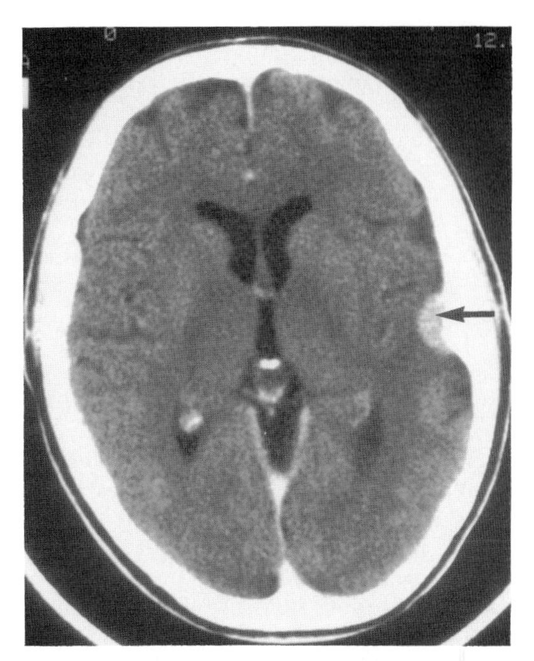

Figure 5–5. Meningioma in a patient with metastatic breast cancer *(arrow)*. The lesion presented with a seizure. CT scan shows the typical dural location and uniform contrast enhancement of the lesion, with thickening of the bone caused by the tumor. These abnormalities indicate meningioma rather than metastatic breast cancer.

Recognizing that the diagnosis by scan is never certain, particular clues suggest brain metastasis rather than another brain lesion. For example, whereas brain metastases tend to be spherical, primary gliomas often are irregular, with fingerlike extensions of contrast-enhancing tumor material running along white matter bundles and fiber tracts. Primary brain lymphomas are often multiple, periventricular in distribution, uniform rather than ring enhanced, and have irregular margins.[577] Meningiomas are distinguished from brain metastases because of their usual homogeneous contrast enhancement, relative lack of peritumoral edema, and their attachment to the dura of the calvarium, falx, or the base of the brain (Fig. 5–5). Metastatic breast, prostate, myeloma, and other cancers also arise from the calvarium or falx (dural metastasis), however, and can even be supplied by branches of the external carotid artery, at times making the distinction between metastatic brain tumors and meningiomas impossible except by biopsy.[1577,2364] Meningiomas, benign and potentially curable tumors, are reported to occur more frequently in women with breast carcinoma than in women without this malignancy[2239,2446] (other investigators have disputed that observation[1258]) and in men and women with other cancers.[179] Therefore, if the neurologic symptoms have developed very slowly or if the scan suggests a lesion abutting the falx or the inner table of the skull, serious consideration must be given to a meningioma. To further complicate the issue, breast cancer may metastasize to a meningioma.

Other primary brain tumors, such as acoustic neurinomas or pituitary adenomas, are at times impossible to distinguish from metastases in the same area. Cerebral infarction may be confused with a brain metastasis, but the problem does not arise if the patient is seen during the acute stage because the infarcts do not enhance; in fact, the scan may be entirely normal for 24 to 48 hours after an acute cerebral infarct. If the scan is delayed several days, however, contrast enhancement develops and may become intense between 10 days and 3 weeks after the ictus. Contrast enhancement of an infarct characteristically involves the pial surface of the overlying brain and has a serpiginous outline corresponding to the cortical gyri, unlike the usual spherical, ringlike contrast enhancement of a brain metastasis. After several weeks, the contrast enhancement in an infarct diminishes and finally disappears; the area of infarction changes to a low-density, fluid-filled cavity.

An acute cerebral hemorrhage is hyperdense on the noncontrast CT scan but may appear normal on the MR scan. If the hemorrhage ruptures into the ventricles, blood can be identified in the ventricular cavities or in the subarachnoid space. Contrast enhancement is not seen early but may appear 3 to 6 weeks after the hemorrhage, at which time the clot is isodense and a ring of contrast enhancement develops, resembling a metastasis or abscess. Early enhancement suggests that the hemorrhage has occurred in an underlying metastasis.

Cerebral abscess cannot be distinguished from brain metastasis by scan alone. Cerebral abscesses usually occur in immunosuppressed patients (see Chapter 10), particularly in those suffering from conditions in which brain metastases are uncommon, such as Hodgkin's disease and other lymphomas. In Hodgkin's disease, a toxoplasma abscess may mimic a brain tumor. Biopsy may be required for correct diagnosis.

Radiation necrosis of the brain produces a hypodense or isodense lesion surrounded by edema. The lesion often contrast enhances and the enhancement may be either ringlike (resembling a metastatic tumor or an abscess [see Chapter 13]) or homogeneous. Radiation necrosis may be difficult to differentiate from recurrent brain metastases in a patient previously irradiated for a brain metastasis.

Multiple sclerosis (MS) may be characterized by one or more contrast-enhancing lesions indistinguishable from a brain tumor.[1359,2020] With MS, however, the enhancement disappears in 6 to 8 weeks and other nonenhancing lesions may be present, findings unlikely with brain metastases.

Methotrexate leukoencephalopathy will cause hyperintensity of the white matter on T_2-weighted MR images (decreased density on CT scan), usually bilaterally and associated with ventricular enlargement. The lack of contrast enhancement distinguishes it from a metastatic brain tumor.

Progressive multifocal leukoencephalopathy (see Chapter 10) causes white matter lesions of diminished density on CT or hyperintensity on T_2-weighted MR images, which are irregular in outline and without contrast enhancement.

Meningeal hematopoiesis in a patient with myelofibrosis can appear as multiple enhancing masses mimicking dural-based neoplasms.

Transient changes in scans sometimes follow focal or generalized epilepsy in the absence of an underlying primary or metastatic brain tumor. The lesions may occasionally mimic brain tumors, but they are usually small, lack significant edema, and disappear within a few weeks after seizures are controlled.[1419]

THE ROLE OF MR SCANS IN PATIENT MANAGEMENT

Contrast-enhanced MR or CT scanning plays an important role in the surgical management of patients with brain metastases.

Preoperative localization of intracranial lesions by MR scan[1427] allows the surgeon to locate and remove even small lesions with minimal damage to overlying cortical structures. Similarly, scanning plays an important role in the postoperative period,[724] allowing the surgeon to determine how complete lesion removal has been. Although this is more of a problem with infiltrating primary tumors than with well-localized metastatic tumors, a postoperative, contrast-enhanced scan is useful after metastases have been extirpated. The scans should be performed within the first 72 hours after surgery; after that time, contrast enhancement resulting from neovascularization from surgical trauma may mimic residual tumor even when surgical removal has been complete. The operatively induced contrast enhancement may not disappear for several months.[364,724,2720] Scans performed after radiation therapy (RT) also must be interpreted with caution because tumor progression may be mimicked by radiation changes weeks to months after completion of cranial RT.[960]

STEREOTACTIC NEEDLE BIOPSY

This relatively simple diagnostic procedure has gained great popularity. It may be performed under local anesthesia with a small scalp incision and requires only 1 day of hospitalization, yet a definitive diagnosis can be made more than 95% of the time.[1823] A small sample size sometimes prevents an adequate diagnosis, although this usually is not a major issue when the question is one of metastasis versus nonmetastasis. More important, a small risk of hemorrhage attends worsening neurologic signs; neurologic worsening also may result from cerebral edema caused by trauma from the biopsy needle. Brain edema sometimes increases after the biopsy, leading to neurologic worsening even when corticosteroid doses are increased.

The major indication for stereotactic needle biopsy in patients with cancer is to distinguish among metastases, primary brain tumor, and non-neoplastic (usually inflammatory) lesions. Since most neoplastic lesions are better treated by surgical removal, however, stereotactic biopsy is indicated only when the physician suspects either a non-neoplastic lesion that would not benefit by direct surgical attack or a primary CNS lymphoma.[580]

Approach to Diagnosis in the Patient Not Known to Have Cancer

Figure 5–6 outlines an approach for use in diagnosing metastasis in patients with known cancer. Sometimes, however, patients in whom no systemic cancer has been found may exhibit neurologic symptoms and be suspected of harboring a brain metastasis. An approach to these patients is shown in Figure 5–7. The first and best diagnostic test, as indicated previously, is an MR scan. If a patient without known cancer presents with neurologic symptoms and the results of his or her MR scan show a contrast-enhancing lesion suggesting metastatic brain disease, one should search for a malignant primary tumor site before treating the brain metastasis.[2710] Because most such brain metastases originate from the lung, either because the tumor originated in the lung or because pulmonary metastases are present, careful attention should be directed to the chest. In one series[1156] of 19 brain metastases of unknown source, 11 were found to originate in the lung. In another series of 23 patients, the primary site could be identified at autopsy in only 14 (10 lung, 3 kidney, 1 colon).[2710] If a routine chest radiograph and sputum cytology test are not productive, a chest CT or MR scan may be fruitful. A suspicious lesion should lead to bronchoscopy, needle biopsy, or surgical exploration. A careful physical examination will usually detect tumors originating in the rectum, testicle, prostate gland, breast, or skin (melanoma). A radionuclide bone scan may detect bone metastases amenable to biopsy examination. A stool test for occult blood should be performed in all patients. An abdominal and pelvic CT scan to look for an occult renal or other cancer is also useful. Biochemical markers are only occasionally helpful. Upper and lower GI series are generally unrewarding and probably not warranted as part of the routine workup. If no lesion is found on this screening battery and if the lesion in the brain is single and surgically accessible, extirpation is indicated to establish the diagnosis and for therapy. If

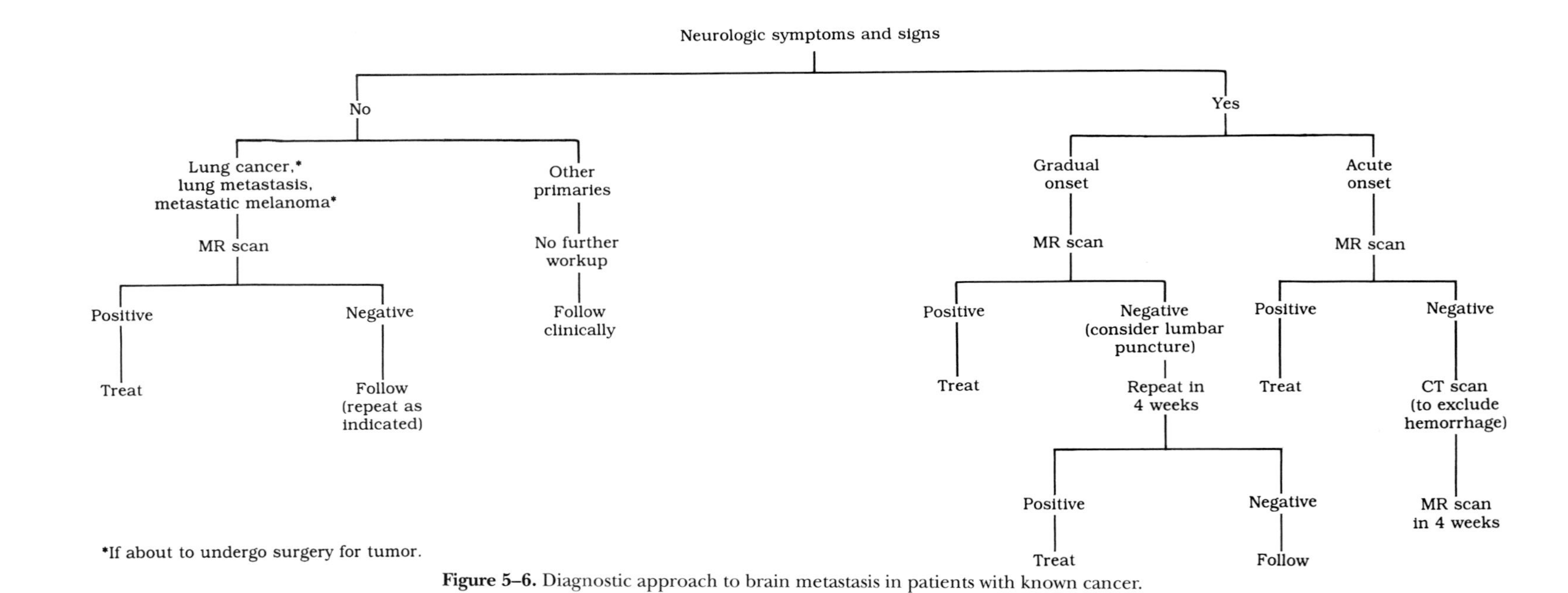

*If about to undergo surgery for tumor.

Figure 5–6. Diagnostic approach to brain metastasis in patients with known cancer.

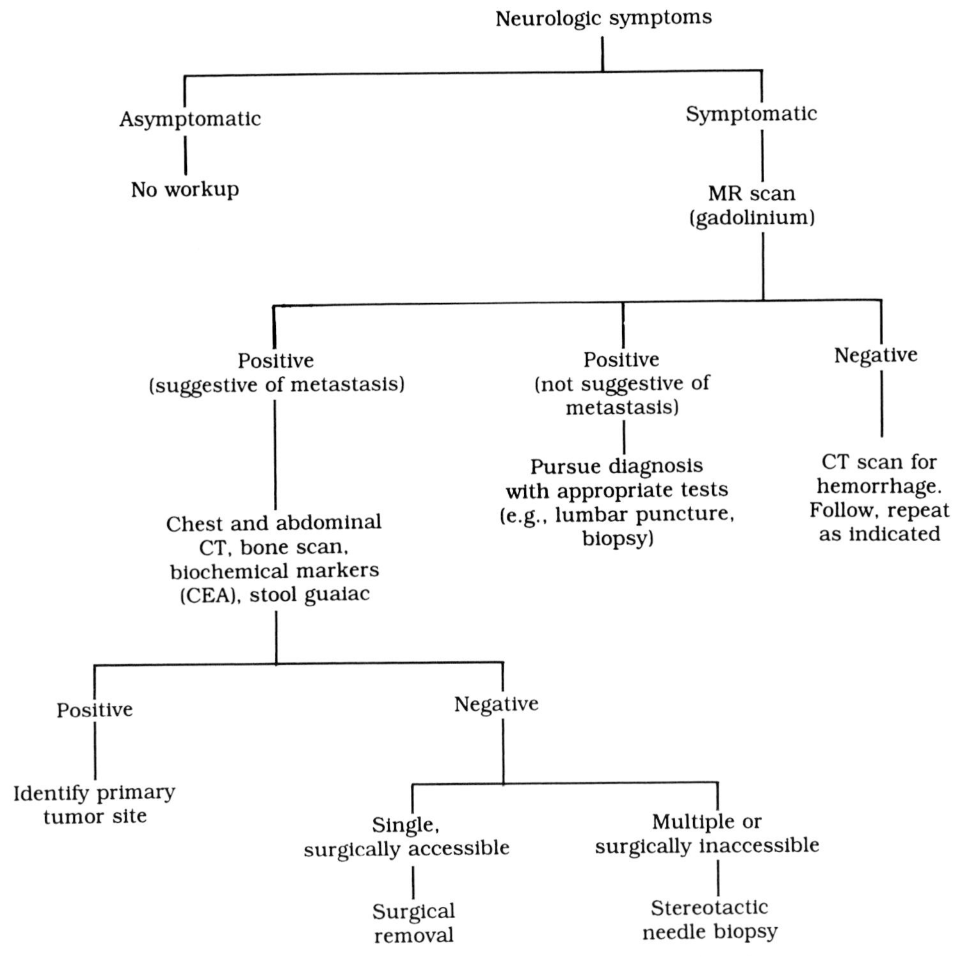

Figure 5–7. Diagnostic approach to brain metastasis in patients without known cancer.

the lesions are multiple or if a single lesion is not surgically accessible, stereotactic needle biopsy is indicated.

Treatment of Brain Metastases

The first step in treating brain metastases is stabilizing neurologically unstable patients,[157,218,2199] that is, those with either increased intracranial pressure threatening cerebral herniation or with repetitive seizures or status epilepticus. The treatment of increased intracranial pressure is considered in Chapter 3 and treatment of seizures is discussed in Chapter 4.

Once stabilized, the physician should classify the patient into one of two categories:

1. A. Multiple brain metastases
   B. A single brain metastasis in a critical location (e.g., brainstem)
   C. Brain metastases associated with widespread untreatable systemic disease likely to be fatal within the next several months
2. A. A single, surgically approachable brain metastasis (or occasionally two) and no known remaining systemic cancer
   B. Systemic cancer amenable to surgical treatment
   C. Systemic cancer believed controllable for at least 6 to 12 months by RT or chemotherapy.

In addition, one should consider the nature of the primary tumor site with respect to its sensitivity to RT and chemotherapy.[803,1425]

Treating stable patients who have widespread systemic disease or multiple brain metastases (more than two) is not particularly controversial because surgery is rarely an option. Treating patients who have a single metastasis has been controversial, but recent studies strongly suggest that surgical extirpation is the preferred therapy.[1852a,1903a,1993,2680]

SYMPTOMATIC THERAPY

To my knowledge, no controlled studies have compared the effects of managing metastatic brain tumors without treatment or with symptomatic therapy only. The available literature on the natural history of brain metastases suggests a median survival of fewer than 7 weeks if a symptomatic metastasis is not treated.[426,1125] Symptoms almost never remit spontaneously, and patients develop increasing intracranial pressure, obtundation, stupor, and coma. Death results from cerebral herniation and brainstem compression or from intercurrent infection (e.g., pneumonia) in neurologically crippled patients. Spontaneous regressions are extremely rare.[167,1944] All available evidence indicates that survival is longer and quality of life better if brain metastases are treated.

STEROIDS AND RADIATION THERAPY

All patients with metastatic brain tumors should receive steroids, approximately 16 mg/24 hr of dexamethasone (or equivalent) for 48 to 72 hours prior to starting RT (see Chapter 3). Few studies address the question of steroid therapy as the sole treatment for brain metastases, that is, without subsequent surgery or radiation. Evidence that steroids alone prolong life is sparse; the median duration of remission for patients treated with steroids alone is approximately 2 months.[1125] Horton and colleagues[1207] found that patients treated with prednisone alone had shorter remissions and shorter survival than patients treated with prednisone plus radiation. The data of Hazra and colleagues [1125] are similar. Nevertheless, as indicated in Chapter 3, steroids rapidly ameliorate many symptoms of brain metastasis and should be used at the onset of therapy for all symptomatic patients.

RADIATION THERAPY

RT is the appropriate treatment for all patients with multiple brain metastases or a single brain metastasis associated with widespread systemic disease.[363,430,476,1212] Present evidence suggests that RT is also indicated after total extirpation of a single metastatic focus,[584,1050] but there is disagreement[83a] that will be settled only by a controlled trial. Prophylactic RT decreases the incidence of brain metastases and may improve survival[2213] in patients with small-cell lung cancer and perhaps other neoplasms, but disagreement exists here also.[2372a]

The standard treatment (Table 5–8) is to deliver external-beam, megavoltage radiation to the whole brain in varying dose and fractionation schedules (see the following). A vast literature reports the outcome of whole-brain irradiation therapy for treating brain metastases. Several findings are worth emphasizing. The median survival of patients with brain metastases treated by RT is between 3 to 6 months, with a 10% to 15% 1-year survival rate. There are occasional long-term survivors[362] (Table 5–9). In general, patients with good performance on admission live longer.

Table 5–8. **RADIATION THERAPY OF BRAIN TUMOR: OPTIONS**

I. Whole-brain—external beam
 A. With focal boost
 B. High fraction—short course
 C. Low fraction—prolonged course
II. Focal radiation therapy
 A. External beam
 B. Brachytherapy
 C. Stereotactic
  1. Heavy particles
  2. Photons
III. Enhancers
 A. Chemotherapy
 B. Hypoxic enhancers
IV. Protectors

Table 5–9. **RADIATION THERAPY FOR BRAIN METASTASES**

Series	Year	No. of Patients	Radiation Therapy/ Protocol	Response (%)	Median Survival (Months)	1-Year Survival (%)
Young and colleagues[2871]	1974	83*	1500 rad/2 fr/3 days	57	2	—
		79	3000 rad/3 wk	62	4	—
Berry and colleagues[204]	1974	124*	Variable	63	4	10
Hendrickson[1136]	1977	1001	1000 rad/1 fr to 4000 rad/3 wk	52	4	15
Markesbery and colleagues[1684]	1978	129	3000 rad/3 wk	—	4	12
Cairncross and colleagues[363]	1980	183	3900 rad/17 days	78	3	8
Zimm and colleagues[2899]	1981	156	Variable	—	3	12
Patchell and colleagues[1993]	1990	23	3600 rad/12 fr/2 wk	—	4	10

*Includes patients who had surgery for the metastases.
fr = fractions.
Source: From Hoang-Xuan and Delattre,[1172] with permission.

Studies of the Radiation Therapy Oncology Group and others* who have used fractionation schedules varying from 1000 cGy × 1 fraction to 400 cGy × 4 weeks indicate that virtually all radiation doses and fractionation schedules yield similar results with respect to survival. The exception is ultra-rapid, high-dose schedules; for example, 1000 cGy as a single fraction[272,1136,1164] or 1500 cGy in 2 fractions over 3 days[1136,2871] yield shorter survival and earlier relapse. Multiple daily fractionation, either hyperfractionation or accelerated fractionation, has no advantage over conventional daily treatment. The equivalence of schedules holds even when patients with a more favorable prognosis are selected.[895] The data must be accepted with caution, however, because follow-up scans are not available in most studies, and survival was the measured outcome. Survival is not the best measure of RT's effect on brain metastasis because many patients die of systemic disease.[363] The only way of confidently evaluating treatment effectiveness is by neurologic evaluation coupled with follow-up scan.[2663,2897a] No studies carried out in this way have assessed the effects of different fractionation schedules of RT.

Dose and fractionation schedules do affect outcome in some patients. Although some investigators report few acute side effects from large fractions such as 600 cGy or more,[1054] we have noted that such fractions often lead to acute side effects, including headache, worsening of neurologic symptoms, and, in rare instances, cerebral herniation and death.[2871] Patients particularly at risk are those with grossly elevated intracranial pressure or hydrocephalus from posterior fossa tumors. Such patients should be started on a lower dose/fraction of 150 to 200 cGy. Furthermore, current evidence[582] suggests that at least 10% of patients who survive longer than a year after the conventional 300 cGy × 10 whole-brain radiation for metastases develop radiation-induced brain damage. As a result, for patients who have a good prognosis, we recommend lower daily fractions of 200 cGy and a more protracted course of radiation, such as 4 to 5 weeks.

In brain metastases from melanoma, no advantage to large fraction size is evident, as has been reported with cutaneous lesions.[1408,2130] Using high daily fractions, the palliative rate is 40%,[494,1408] but median sur-

*References 271, 272, 545, 1136, 1164, 2378.

vival is not prolonged,[2130] although some patients survive more than a year.[449]

Certain tumors are usually more sensitive to RT than others in individual patients. The clone of cells that have metastasized from that tumor to the brain may vary greatly in sensitivity. Most series have reported no statistically significant differences in survival among patients by tumor type after treatment of brain metastases. Studies from MSKCC indicate that patients harboring metastases from breast and lung carcinoma are likely to respond, both clinically and by CT scan, to radiation therapy and, if they respond, are unlikely to die of their metastatic brain tumor.[363] In patients who have single brain metastasis from lung cancer and whose systemic disease is otherwise under control, the most common cause of death after whole-brain RT is recurrence of the brain metastasis.[1993] Patients with melanoma,[357,1745,2130,2510] colon cancer,[397] and renal cancer[893,1677] are unlikely to have a CT response to steroids and RT therapy even when there is an apparent clinical response, and they are more likely to die of metastatic brain tumor than of systemic disease. Occasional responses by these patients to RT, documented by CT or MR scan,[397,2160] however, make treatment of all patients desirable.

RT is effective palliative therapy. Depending on the series, between 66% and 75% of patients improve clinically. Patients whose neurologic symptoms are mildest at the time treatment is undertaken improve most. Occasional patients who enter the hospital stuporous or comatose from herniation have a dramatic and very useful response to steroids combined with RT, and even a failure to respond to steroids does not indicate that RT will fail. By CT criteria, an objective response (50% or greater shrinkage) is seen in 50% to 60% of patients at 6 weeks after RT[363,2663] (Fig. 5–8). Smaller tumors respond better than larger tumors. The presence of more than three lesions is a poor prognostic sign for survival.[2535] In occasional patients, RT sterilizes the tumor, and if there is no other disease, the patient is cured.[362] A residual contrast-enhancing mass on CT scan may mark the site of necrosis in the sterilized tumor.[1562]

Several clinical issues remain unresolved (Table 5–10):

Focal Versus Whole-Brain Radiation Therapy. For initial treatment, whole-brain RT is preferred, partially because multiple metastases may be present even if some are too small to be detected on scanning; when they become apparent later, they are more difficult to treat. Focal RT with either external beam, stereotactic radiosurgery,[1594,1595,2820] or implantation of radioactive iodine sources[2086] (brachytherapy), however, is now a possible addition to whole-brain radiation to treat larger lesions. One study reports that focal boosts of 15 cGy in 8 fractions to the site of single metastases did not increase survival or tumor control.[1212]

Focal Radiation Techniques. Several recent reports recommend focal RT[801,1623,2031] if a single or, occasionally, two brain metastases are uncontrolled by conventional treatment or if brain metastases relapse after whole-brain RT. Such therapy has the advantage of sparing normal brain, thus preventing the side effects of dementia and brain necrosis. The treatment can be delivered by conformal three-dimensional RT,[1517] by a focused beam of photons (stereotactic radiosurgery),* or via the implantation of radioactive sources (interstitial irradiation or brachytherapy).[1516,2086] Stereotactic radiosurgery can be delivered as a single dose of radiation, 900 to 2500 cGy, via a linear accelerator or a gamma knife (a specially designed cobalt machine). Reports[1595] suggest excellent local control with minimal side effects. Most results have been achieved with metastatic adenocarcinoma, with lesser responses from melanoma,[566] renal cell carcinoma, and sarcoma. Most patients improved neurologically, although some developed either leptomeningeal tumor or metastatic lesions in the brain outside the radiation portal. Interstitial radiation requires a surgical procedure for the implantation of radioactive (usually ^{125}I) sources. Most reports involve high-activity iodine sources, which must be removed after 4 to 5 days. Responses and prolonged survival have been reported,[1516,2086] although the exact

*References 16, 387, 468, 800, 1594, 1595, 1729.

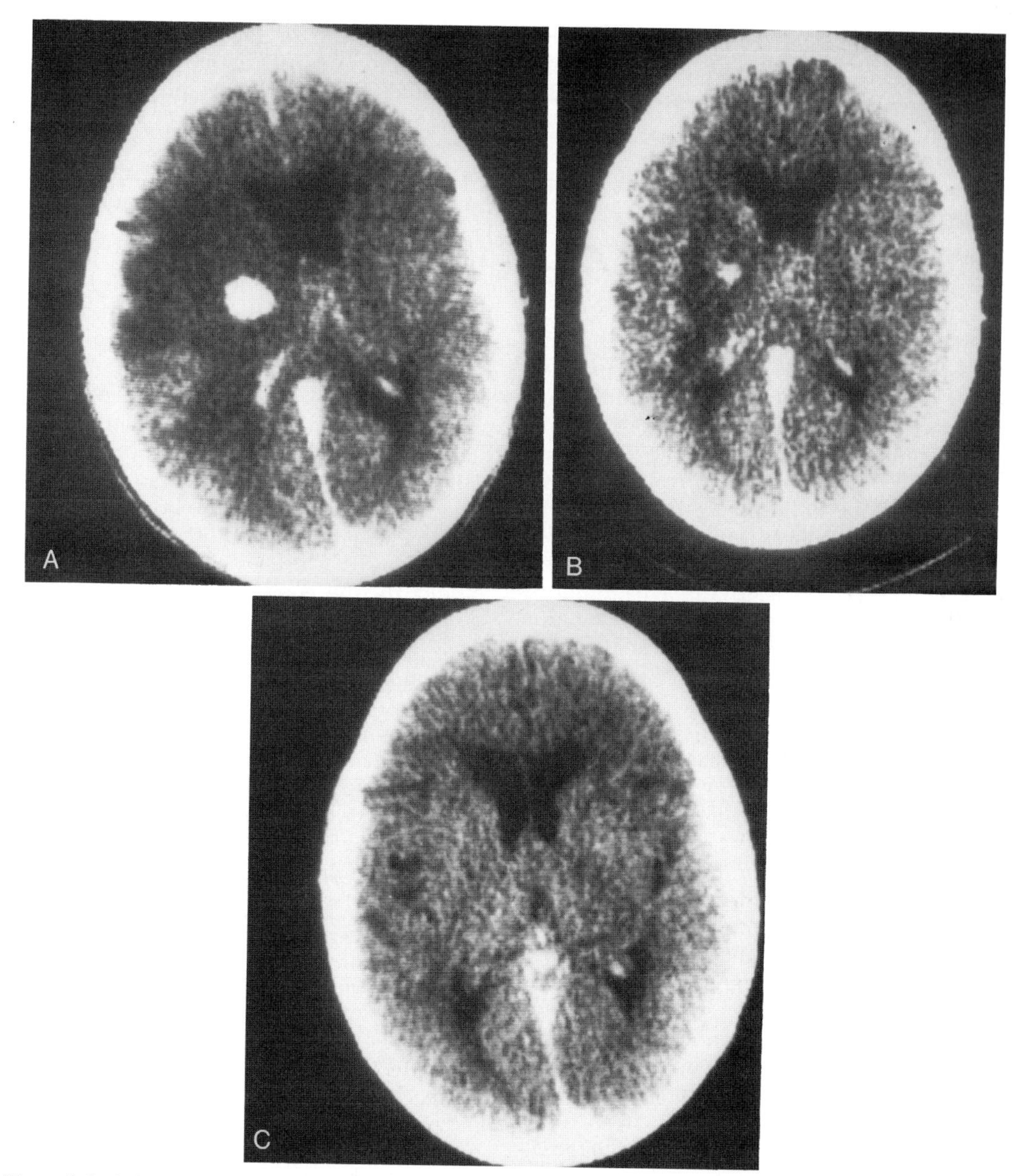

Figure 5–8. *A–C,* Serial CT scans of a patient with brain metastasis from uterine cancer. The large, homogeneously enhancing mass is found in the right hemisphere prior to RT. *B,* Two months later, the mass was still present but substantially smaller. *C,* Several months after RT, the mass had disappeared. It did not recur for the remaining 18 months of the patient's life.

role of these focused techniques in the treatment of metastatic brain tumors is still not established.

Prophylactic Radiation Therapy. Patients with acute lymphoblastic leukemia often receive prophylactic radiation therapy to the brain, as well as intrathecal chemotherapy, to eradicate sanctuaried cells and prevent the development of meningeal leukemia. A similar approach has been recommended for treating small-cell lung cancer to prevent the development of brain metastases. Clinical

Table 5–10. **UNRESOLVED ISSUES IN RADIATION THERAPY**

Focal versus whole-brain radiation
Brachytherapy, stereotactic radiosurgery
Prophylactic radiation
Re-irradiation after relapse
Radiosensitizers and radioprotectors

studies demonstrate that elective whole-brain RT significantly decreases the incidence of brain metastases.* Most small-cell lung cancer studies suggest little effect on overall survival, but others suggest survival improves with RT.[2213] A recent study from MSKCC supports the use of prophylactic radiation of the brain in small-cell lung cancer. When controlled for the confounding issue of thoracic failure, prophylactic cranial irradiation was associated with significant enhancement of survival (2-year survival 56% versus 14%; 5-year survival 3% versus 0%).[2213]

It has not been established whether prophylactic cranial irradiation decreases the frequency of brain metastases from non–small-cell lung cancer[518,1261] or delays the time to their development. Survival is not increased.

Some groups question the wisdom of prophylactic RT on the grounds that the few patients who develop symptomatic brain metastases can be treated effectively with RT and those who cannot are spared the side effects of brain radiation. Others support prophylactic RT on the grounds that once symptomatic brain metastasis develops, it is difficult to eradicate with RT. The issue is still undecided.

The timing of prophylactic cranial irradiation (PCI) is probably important. Lee and colleagues[1499] recommend early PCI, after two or three courses of chemotherapy, as opposed to late PCI, after five or six courses. A recent study by Laukkanen and associates[1479] addressed the question of long-term sequelae. They concluded that PCI, after intensive combination chemotherapy, did not induce gross dementia or neurologic dysfunction but that its risk-benefit ratio is not overwhelmingly favorable; it failed to prevent brain relapses in one of five patients and led to subtle, but detectable, motor findings and neuropsychologic impairment in the majority.

Reirradiation after Relapse. Patients who initially respond to RT and subsequently relapse are candidates for reirradiation.[495,680] Although the response rate (about 40%) is lower than after initial RT, some patients do respond after a second or even a third course. Delayed radiation necrosis (see Chapter 13) is more likely, but most patients do not survive long enough to develop this complication. Those patients who have had a good clinical and CT or MR scan response to RT and who survive longer than 6 months after the initial RT course are the best candidates for repeat irradiation. If the patient's systemic tumor is under control, he or she should also be considered a candidate for surgical extirpation or chemotherapy. Focal RT is playing an increasingly important role in treating recurrent metastases.[387,1516,1595]

Radiation Enhancers and Protectors. Several drugs that function as electron acceptors and appear to enhance the effect of RT on partially hypoxic tumor tissue are now being tested. These drugs should be ideal to help radiate brain tumors, including metastases, because the normal brain is fully oxygenated, whereas the tumor may be partially hypoxic. Thus, the radiation enhancers should enhance the effect of radiation only on the tumor, not on the normal brain. Despite this theoretic advantage, evidence is not available to suggest that radiation enhancers promote either clinical improvement or survival. Randomized studies using metronidazole[20,746,1404] or lonidamine[581] to treat metastatic tumors failed to yield a statistically significant difference between the control and radiation-enhancer–treated groups. Some chemotherapeutic agents also act as radiation enhancers, but little evidence supports the idea that chemotherapy synchronized with RT may prolong survival.

A new series of drugs called radiation protectors is also being developed. These drugs presumably protect normal tissue against the side effects of radiation, allowing increased doses of RT to be administered to eradicate tumor. They have not been tested in the CNS, so their efficacy is not known.[2333]

*References 1000, 1256, 1479, 1499, 2372a, 2702.

SURGICAL EXTIRPATION

Recent reviews describe in detail the technique and results of surgery.[1170,1993,2544,2851] Recently published randomized trials[1903a,1993,2680] support previous noncontrolled studies* that indicate that patients with a single brain metastasis live longer and have fewer brain recurrences and a better quality of life if treated by surgery followed by whole-brain irradiation than if they are treated by RT alone.[2003] In one recent series of selected brain metastases treated by surgery, 22% of patients survived more than 4 years, with a median survival of more than 2 years.[1823]

The rationale for surgically excising lesions includes the palliative rather than curative nature of RT (but see references 362, 1562); if one hopes to cure a solitary metastasis, the lesion must be surgically removed. Furthermore, the excellent pathologic demarcation of the metastatic tumor from surrounding brain usually allows complete removal with minimal operative morbidity and mortality. In one study[602] of 81 patients, however, complete resection (as judged by the surgeons) was possible in only 70% of patients. Mortality at 30 days was 7.4% and neurologic deficits worsened in 22%. At MSKCC, the rate of complete resection was 79%, the operative mortality 1%, and neurologic morbidity 5%. Careful preoperative[1427] or operative[2709] localization helps to lower morbidity. Computer-assisted stereotaxis may allow successful removal of deep-seated, previously inaccessible lesions.[1170,1354] Percutaneous cyst aspiration via an Ommaya reservoir system may help to control symptoms of cystic tumors not amenable to complete resection.[2192] A recent study of 207 consecutive craniotomies for brain tumors (74 metastatic) reports a mortality of 2.4% with major complications of 4.3%.[359a]

After successful removal of a single brain metastasis, steroids can usually be discontinued. It is much more difficult to discontinue steroids after RT because residual tumor often remains a nidus for continuing brain edema. The ability to discontinue steroids explains in part the better quality of life in patients whose tumor is removed surgically as opposed to those having RT alone.[1993]

*References 300, 347, 1076, 1631, 1992, 2899.

Surgical removal of a presumed metastatic brain tumor allows the diagnosis to be unequivocally established, which is particularly important in the patient not known to have cancer. Even with CT and MR scanning, mistakes will be made unless tissue samples can be microscopically examined. Because operative complications (in good hands) are almost as low after extirpation of the lesion as after stereotactic biopsy,[1076] surgical removal should be strongly considered if the diagnosis is questionable. Stereotactic biopsy is reserved for surgically inaccessible lesions or for the patient with numerous intracranial masses.

Although the study of Patchell and colleagues[1993] did not have any long-term survivors, other studies have shown long-term survivors among patients with solitary metastases from non–small-cell lung and other cancers. In one series, all of the 5-year survivors had limited pulmonary disease without nodal involvement and good performance status prior to treatment.[872] Another study[2002] suggests that extent of extracerebral disease, performance status (Karnofsky score better than 70), and histopathologic diagnosis were important prognostically. Adenocarcinoma of unknown primary and renal-cell carcinoma carried a better prognosis; melanoma, adenocarcinoma of the lung, and other tumors had worse prognoses. Occipital and parietal lobe tumors did better than cerebellar and temporal lobe tumors; also, patient's age greater than 55 was a minor prognostic variable.

Operative mortality in stable patients is almost nil. Operative morbidity in the form of increased neurologic disability affects about 10% of patients. In most, it is transient. The neurologic worsening may be present immediately after surgery or may begin 24 to 48 hours later. In most instances, this exacerbation of symptoms is due to brain swelling, and if steroids are continued or increased without anything further being done, the patient recovers in a few days. In other instances, however, the symptoms may be due to an accumulation of subdural or epidural blood, which must be evacuated by a second operation. Before CT scans were available, 5% to 15% of patients undergoing operative intervention for brain metastases developed sufficiently severe secondary symptoms to necessitate a re-exploration operation. Usually only brain swelling was found, and the patient recovered without incident. The advent of CT scanning, particularly useful for emergency situations, permits physicians to distinguish between hemorrhage and swelling, so that reoperation is done only for patients who hemorrhage.

Important advances in surgical technique have included preoperative localization,[1427] use of intraoperative ultrasound,[2709] CT-guided stereotactic removal of deep-lying tumors,[1354] and percutaneous cyst aspiration via an Ommaya reservoir system for control of symptoms in cystic tumors not amenable to complete resection.[2192] Late recurrence of brain metastases at the same site or a new site can be treated with a second resection if the patient is in good general neurologic and systemic condition.[67a,576,2522]

The surgical removal of solitary metastatic lesions in patients whose systemic disease is well controlled and whose performance status is good is now rarely debated. This applies to most tumors, but probably not to highly radiosensitive and chemosensitive lesions such as small-cell lung cancer and lymphomas and possibly not to breast cancer.[267] Metastases involving language areas can usually be successfully removed without rendering the patient worse; in fact, language is often improved. Some neurosurgeons now consider extirpation of two or three accessible, relatively radioresistant lesions in the brain, such as those from colon cancer, renal-cell cancer, or melanoma, to offer a longer and better-quality life. One report of 18 patients operated on for two or more metastases and treated with postoperative RT suggests that survival is poorer than with a single metastasis,[1126] but others suggest that if all metastases can be removed, the prognosis is the same.[219]

The number of patients who are candidates for surgical extirpation is limited. In the series reported by Cairncross and colleagues,[363] of 201 consecutive patients, only 18 were considered to be candidates for surgical extirpation. Of these, 4 had unknown primary tumors and the surgical extirpation was done in part for diagnosis. Half had no evidence of systemic disease, and in those who did, the disease was under good control.

Questions about Surgery. Some unresolved questions persist concerning surgical therapy of brain metastases. One concerns leptomeningeal tumor, which may develop in as many as 33% of patients after surgical extirpation of a cerebellar metastasis. These tumors occur in a much smaller percentage of patients with supratentorial lesions.[1779,1992] Tumor in the cerebellum likely spills into the cisterna magna, seeding the meninges. There is substantially less contact with the subarachnoid space when supratentorial lesions are operated on, unless the lateral ventricle is entered. Prophylactic intrathecal therapy with methotrexate might be considered in patients after successful extirpation of a single cerebellar metastasis.

A second unanswered question concerns postoperative RT, which has two purposes: (1) to eradicate residual tumor at the surgical site and (2) to treat micrometastases elsewhere in the brain. Although the evidence is skimpy and there are no controlled trials, most published evidence suggests that postoperative whole-brain radiation decreases relapse both at the site of the surgical removal and elsewhere in the brain.[584,675,2442,2443] Full therapeutic doses should probably be used because lower doses do not appear to prevent recurrence.[675] Current evidence supports postoperative RT even after the removal of relatively radioresistant metastatic melanomas.[1050] A recent study at MSKCC suggests marginal, if any, benefit from postoperative RT after resection of brain metastases from lung cancer.[83a] A randomized study by the Radiation Therapy Oncology Group was abandoned because of poor accrual, but no benefit was found in the small number of treated patients.

Indications for Surgery. I suggest the following indications for surgery (Table 5–11):

1. Uncertain diagnosis in patients not known to have systemic cancer but with a solitary, surgically accessible mass lesion in the brain. If a search for a primary tumor has been fruitless,[2710] surgical extirpation achieves both diagnosis and therapy. If the lesion is not surgically accessible, stereotactic needle biopsy is probably indicated.
2. A patient with cancer and one or two accessible lesions that cannot be controlled by RT or chemotherapy (i.e., not

Table 5–11. **INDICATIONS FOR SURGICAL REMOVAL OF BRAIN METASTASES**

1. Uncertain diagnosis
2. Established metastasis(es)
   A. Solitary metastasis—primary controlled or controllable
   B. Single metastasis—good systemic performance score
   C. Two (or rarely, three) metastases in some patients—radioresistant tumors, systemic disease controlled
3. Radiation therapy failure
4. Uncontrollable neurologic symptoms
5. Recurrence after successful surgery with or without radiation therapy

lymphoma, small-cell lung cancer, or germ-cell tumor). A few patients with one large and several small lesions are candidates for resection of the large lesion prior to RT of the smaller ones.

3. Failure of RT in a symptomatic patient. If a patient with a single brain metastasis undergoes RT and the therapy fails to improve neurologic symptoms or shrink the lesion, the patient should undergo surgical extirpation, provided systemic disease is under control.[1992] If the patient has no symptoms, or if the symptoms can be easily controlled by steroids (particularly in the presence of widespread systemic disease), surgical extirpation is probably not indicated. The point at which one should consider RT a failure is not clear, but if, 8 weeks following RT, the tumor has not shrunk and the patient remains symptomatic, radiation failure seems fairly certain. A patient who has been radiated successfully and then relapses 6 months to a year later should be carefully assessed concerning the advisability of surgical extirpation.[1992] The reinstitution of steroid hormones and a repeat course of RT are sometimes the best option.[680] In most instances, however, the lesion, if it is accessible, should be surgically excised.
4. Uncontrollable neurologic symptoms. In a few patients, symptoms of increased intracranial pressure that cannot be controlled by steroids or repetitive and intractable seizures that cannot be controlled with anticonvulsant drugs represent an indication for surgery even without the prior use of RT. If increased intracranial pressure cannot be controlled with steroids, RT may at least temporarily worsen the symptoms, so it may be wise, if the tumor is accessible, to remove it before RT is undertaken. This may be applicable even if the patient has multiple brain metastases, if one is the predominant cause of symptoms. For example, in addition to having numerous supratentorial metastases, such a patient may have a large lesion in the posterior fossa obstructing the fourth ventricle.
5. Recurrence after successful surgery. Relapse after surgical extirpation can be followed by reoperation in those patients who remain good surgical candidates.[67a] In one series, median survival following a second craniotomy was 9 months, and the actuarial 2-year survival was 25%.[2522] In another, it was 10 months.[67a]

CHEMOTHERAPY

Regimens. Increasing evidence shows that chemotherapy (Table 5–12), either alone or in combination with immunotherapy and

Table 5–12. **CHEMOTHERAPY OF BRAIN METASTASES**

1. Nonspecific
   A. Anticonvulsants
   B. Steroids
2. Specific
   A. Hormones
   B. Cytotoxic drugs
      (1) Oral or intravenous
      (2) Intra-arterial
      (3) Intravenous with osmotic opening of blood–brain barrier
      (4) As radiation therapy sensitizer
      (5) Intrathecal

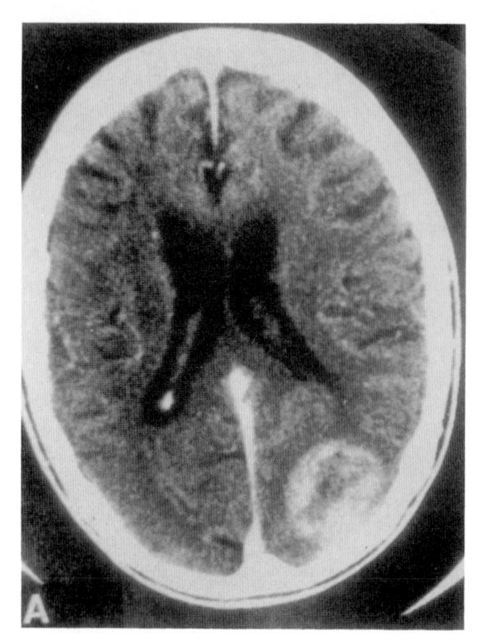

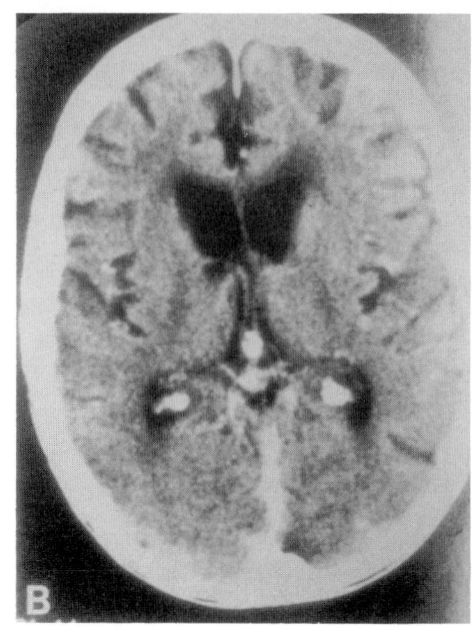

Figure 5–9. CT scan of the brain *(A)* before and *(B)* after three courses of chemotherapy with cyclophosphamide, adriamycin, and vincristine. The mass has entirely disappeared. The small-cell cancer of the lung also responded.

radiation, effectively treats some brain metastases* (Fig. 5–9).

Cytotoxic drugs can be administered orally or intravenously, into the carotid or vertebral artery supplying the brain metastases, or intrathecally, into the lumbar or ventricular CSF (see Chapter 7). The drugs can also be administered intravenously after opening the blood–brain barrier by intra-arterial hyperosmolar mannitol infusion.[1874]

Rosner and colleagues[2214] describe the results of systemic chemotherapy in 100 patients with brain metastases from breast cancer; 10 were complete responders and 40 were partial responders. Several combinations of chemotherapy appeared equally efficacious (Table 5–13). Similar responses were obtained in a smaller series by Cocconi and associates,[467] using a combination of platinum and etoposide. Hormonal therapy with tamoxifen[1082,2060] and bromocriptine[1006] proved efficacious in isolated cases of metastatic carcinoma of the breast. Adjuvant chemotherapy for breast cancer does not prevent brain metastases from developing later, however. In fact, it appears to increase the number of first recurrences in the brain.[267,1995] The same appears to be true with malignant melanoma[1009] and ovarian carcinoma.[338]

The series by Madajewicz and coworkers[1643,1644] and Cascino and associates[395] report responses to intra-arterial BCNU or etoposide and *cis*-platinum in various metastatic brain tumors, including lung cancer, breast cancer, and melanoma.[2770] Responses were usually partial and relatively short-lived. Jacquilliat and colleagues[1266] report a 25% response rate (9 of 36 partial responses) of brain metastasis from melanoma to the nitrosourea fotemustine. Lee's group[1498] treated 14 patients with brain metastases from small-cell lung cancer and found 1 complete response and 8 partial responses in 11 evaluable patients. Small-cell lung cancer in the brain usually responds to chemotherapy,[1425] and brain metastases from neuroblastoma respond to etoposide and ifosfamide.[2760] Melanoma has responded to interferon, dacarbazine,[1748] and fotemustine.[1266]

Factors Predicting Efficacy of Chemotherapy. Several factors must be considered when deciding to use chemotherapy:

*References 261, 337, 467, 992, 1082, 1390, 1395, 1425, 1468, 1540, 1643, 1644, 2188, 2214, 2255, 2468, 2595, 2640.

Table 5–13. **RESULTS OF CHEMOTHERAPY FOR BRAIN METASTASES**

Series	Year	Cancer	No. of Patients	Protocol	Response (%)	Median Survival (Months)	1-Year Survival (%)
Hildebrand	1975	Breast	11	CCNU,M,V	45	—	—
Rosner	1986	Breast	100	CFP ± MV MVP C,A	50	5.5	31
Cocconi	1990	Breast	22	CDDP,VP16	55	14*	55
Kleisbauer	1988	SCLC NSCLC	13	VP16	30	2.5	—
Postmus	1989	SCLC	23	VP16	43	—	—
Twelves	1990	SCLC	19	C,V,VP16	53	7*	20
Lee	1990	SCLC	11	C,A,V,VP16	82	8†	—
Kleisbauer	1990	SCLC NSCLC	24	CDDP	30	3.5*	12
Thomas	1990	SCLC NSCLC	60	VP16 CDDP	30	3	—
Robinet	1991	SCLC NSCLC	16	CDDP,F	50	9	30
Jacquillat	1990	Melanoma	39	Fotemustine	28	6.5	21

*Includes patients treated with radiotherapy while in remission or after failure of therapy.
†Chemotherapy associated with radiotherapy as primary treatment modality.
A = adriamycin; C = cyclophosphamide; CCNU = lomustine; CDDP = *cis*-platinum; F = 5-fluorouracil; M = methotrexate; NSCLC = non–small-cell lung cancer; P = prednisone; SCLC = small-cell lung cancer; V = vincristine; VP16 = etoposide.
Source: Adapted from Hoang-Xuan and Delattre,[1172] p 30.

1. An effective drug or combination of drugs must be available. Most patients develop brain metastases late in the course of their cancer, when few good therapeutic agents are available or when resistance to previously effective chemotherapy has developed. If the patient has a tumor likely to be responsive to a hormonal or chemotherapeutic agent, the presence of a brain metastasis should not prevent the physician from using the agent. If the brain metastasis is small but visible on a contrast-enhanced scan and relatively asymptomatic, it may be useful to try chemotherapy before delivering RT.
2. Even if the primary tumor is chemosensitive, it does not guarantee that all of the metastases will be. Metastatic tumors in general tend to be more resistant to chemotherapeutic agents than the primary tumor from which they arose. This may also be true in the brain. In clinical studies comparing brain metastases and simultaneous systemic lesions, however, the responses were the same[1425,2214] (Fig. 5–10).
3. The metastasis must be exposed to adequate concentrations of the drug. The blood–brain barrier excludes most water-soluble chemotherapeutic agents. At the time most metastatic brain tumors become symptomatic, the blood–brain barrier is partially or completely disrupted. (If it were not disrupted, enhancing agents would not show the metastasis on MR or CT scan.) The degree of disruption, however, varies both from tumor to tumor and in different areas of the same tumor.[842] Generally, less agent enters brain metastases than enters the primary tumor. When tumors are small and do not contrast enhance, the blood–brain barrier is intact. Lipid-soluble agents, such as the nitrosoureas, cross even an intact blood–brain barrier.
4. Attempts to circumvent the blood–brain barrier have included barrier opening with hyperosmolar agents and intrathecal administration. Intrathecal drugs are usually reabsorbed into the blood before they penetrate substantially into the brain, and they have not proved useful in treating metastatic tumors except those in the leptomeninges (see Chapter 7). Experimental evidence indicates that opening the blood–brain barrier increases the amount of drug that enters the normal brain surrounding the tumor more than it increases entry into the tumor. If the drugs are neurotoxic, toxicity may be enhanced with a limited increase in tumor destruction.[1406] Furthermore, although barrier opening appears to be safe, it is unclear that it does not have long-term toxicity of its own.[2271]

The preceding data suggest that chemotherapy should be attempted if appropriate agents are available. If the patient is asymptomatic or if the symptoms are minor enough not to require immediate radiation, the chemotherapy probably should be administered before RT, when the blood supply to the tumor is still optimal. The patient probably should not be on steroids, which decrease the transfer of water-soluble agents from blood to brain and may decrease the amount of water-soluble chemotherapeutic agents entering tumors. If the patient requires immediate RT and an effective chemotherapeutic agent is available, it can be given either concomitantly with the radiation, hoping for synergistic effects, or at the completion of RT. The combination, however, may increase myelotoxicity or perhaps even neurotoxicity.[1500]

Several questions remain unanswered. The first is how to predict drug resistance in brain metastases. In theory, if a brain metastasis develops after a patient has received chemotherapy, the metastasis is likely to be resistant to the previously used drugs and perhaps others as well.[628] This concept is supported by established evidence of better control by chemotherapy of CNS metastases occurring at the time of diagnosis of both lymphoma[2135] and small-cell lung cancer.[916,2666] Metastases developing late in the course are less responsive to treatment and often lead to the patient's demise. On the other hand, if microscopic tumor is sequestered behind the blood–brain barrier during the course of initial chemotherapy for the primary tumor, those cells may still be sensitive to the same drugs; also, because the blood–brain barrier breaks down as the tumor grows, it may respond to systemic therapy. Data suggest that chemotherapy prior to radiation is worth

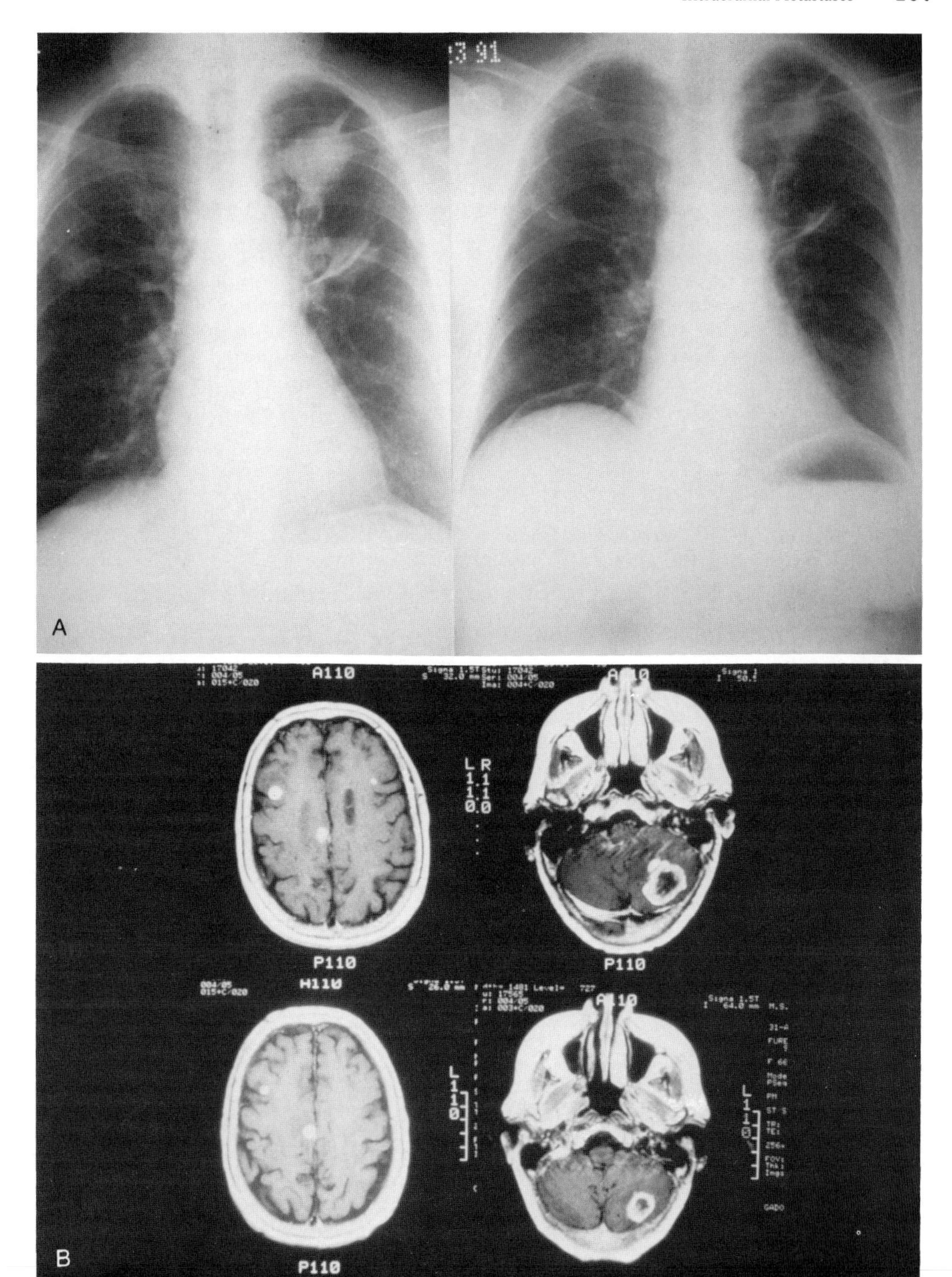

Figure 5–10. *A,* Chest film of a patient with breast carcinoma and pulmonary metastasis before *(left)* and after *(right)* chemotherapy. *B,* Contrast-enhanced T_1-weighted MR image of the brain in the same patient before *(top)* and after *(bottom)* chemotherapy. The brain metastases have decreased in size to about the same extent as the lung metastasis. The small lesion in the left frontal lobe has disappeared *(right side of figure)*. The patient subsequently underwent whole-brain RT with further shrinkage of the tumor but died a year later of systemic disease.

a try even in patients who have been treated previously with chemotherapy, but if chemotherapeutic treatment fails because of drug resistance, RT is indicated.

IMMUNOTHERAPY

Although immunotherapy dates to the turn of the century, immunotherapeutic agents and biologic response modifiers have had a resurgence in recent years[2206] (Table 5–14), although there is little or no evidence that they effectively treat metastatic brain tumors. Most protocols using biologic response modifiers specifically exclude patients with brain metastases because of the fear of increased blood–brain barrier leakage with interleukin-2 and of hemorrhagic necrosis with tumor necrosis factor. In addition, the steroids required by most brain tumor patients interfere with the efficacy of most immunotherapeutic agents. Whether these agents have a role in the treatment of brain metastases in the future is not established. Grooms and colleagues[1009] indicate that patients undergoing active immunotherapy with bacillus Calmette-Guérin for systemic melanoma have a higher incidence of brain metastases than those not being treated by immunotherapy.

In preliminary experiments, Neuwelt and colleagues[1873,1876] have used blood–brain barrier disruption to increase delivery of tumor-specific monoclonal antibodies to normal animals and patients with melanoma metastatic in the brain.[1876] One experimental study demonstrated that interleukin-2 alone or with lymphokine-activated killer cells reduces pulmonary metastasis but has no effect on brain metastases, suggesting organ-specific resistance, perhaps because of inadequate trafficking of lymphocytes or inadequate activation in situ.[1720a] The use of membranes of virally infected tumor cells (viral oncolysates) to treat systemic melanoma has been reported to increase inflammatory mononuclear cell infiltrates in subsequently developing brain metastases.[401]

Table 5–14. **IMMUNOTHERAPY OF BRAIN METASTASES**

I. Active
  A. Immune potentiators (e.g., bacillus Calmette-Guérin, bacterial toxins)
  B. Vaccines
    (1) Allogenic
    (2) Autologous
II. Passive
  A. Antibodies
    (1) Against tumor cells
    (2) Against growth factor receptors
III. Cytokines
  A. Interferon
  B. Interleukins
  C. Tumor necrosis factor

OTHER SITES OF INTRACRANIAL METASTASES

Calvarial Metastases

Metastases to the skull vault are usually asymptomatic and are discovered during routine radiographic evaluation of the patient with cancer. They probably reach the skull via Batson's plexus (see Chapter 2). Occasionally, expansion of the bones or involvement of the periosteum may cause pain or a palpable mass. Sometimes a painless mass becomes quite large and may be disfiguring.[2476] In some instances, a skull mass may be the first evidence that a known tumor has metastasized. A skull metastasis may reach sufficient size to cause brain compression. Symptoms result from direct compression of the brain by the tumor or from secondary edema.

If the calvarial mass is situated over the sagittal or lateral sinus, it may compress that structure and cause increased intracranial pressure, usually with papilledema and sometimes headaches (Fig. 5–11). The neurologic examination is otherwise normal. Papilledema is also associated with compression of a dominant jugular vein at the base of the skull.[978] RT should be delivered to the lesion to decompress the compressed venous structure. Hemorrhagic infarction of the brain involving one or both hemispheres and associated with severe headache and focal signs, including focal seizures, sometimes occurs with sagittal sinus obstruction caused

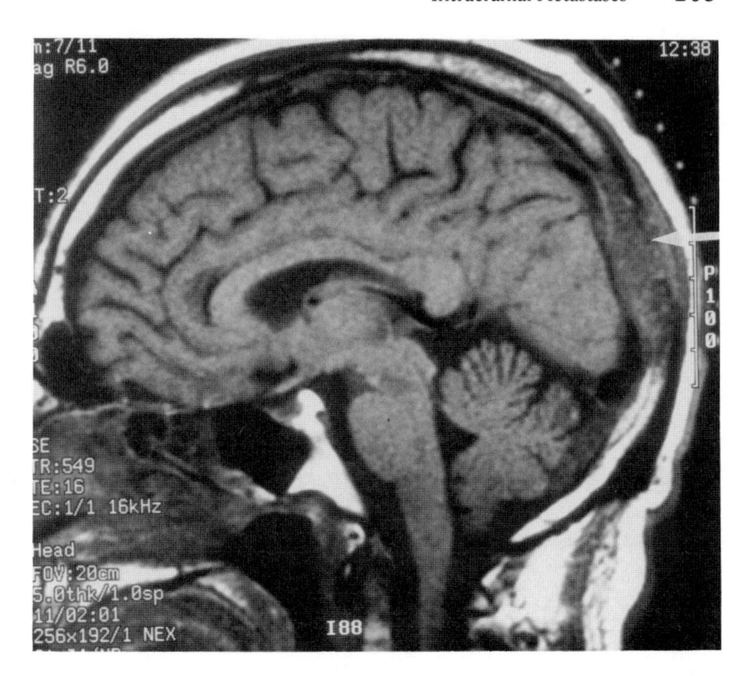

Figure 5–11. This MR scan shows metastasis of the skull compressing the sagittal sinus *(arrow)*. Metastatic breast tumor raised intracranial pressure and caused papilledema and headache. Other neurologic signs were absent.

by occlusion rather than compression (see Chapter 9), but it is rare with metastatic compression.

In general, the treatment of skull metastases is RT; surgical removal of a single large metastasis, particularly if it compresses the brain, may be indicated. Asymptomatic metastases do not require specific treatment.

A peculiar and unique phenomenon of skull metastasis occasionally occurs in children with neuroblastoma. The skull is widely seeded with metastatic tumor, the skull sutures split, and the skull expands as if the patient had hydrocephalus. The size of the brain and its ventricular system do not increase, however; the apparent hydrocephalus is a direct result of the tumor in both the skull and the underlying epidural space. CT scan easily establishes this diagnosis.

Dural Metastases

Metastases to the dura may arise either by extension from the skull or by direct hematogenous spread. Carcinomas of the lung, prostate, and breast have a predilection for this site. Other tumors, including Hodgkin's disease, pancreatic carcinoma, carcinoid,[1224] leukemia,[2853] and plasmacytoma,[102] have been reported as well.

Two clinicopathologic syndromes result. In the first, the tumor compresses or invades the underlying brain. The symptoms resemble those of a parenchymal brain metastasis, although focal seizures at onset may be somewhat more common. The location of the lesion is established in the symptomatic patient by CT or MR scanning. The bone may or may not be involved. It is often difficult to distinguish dural-based metastases from meningiomas by radiologic means. Surgical extirpation is the treatment of choice for a single large lesion. In patients who are not appropriate candidates for surgery, RT has salutary effects on most metastases and some meningiomas.

Alternatively, metastases to the subdural space may remain small and cause symptoms by exuding fluid into the subdural space, producing a subdural hematoma or effusion.[1322,1776] The fluid presumably represents a leakage of plasma and blood from blood vessels newly formed by the tumor. The neurologic signs and symptoms are similar to those of a subdural hematoma or hygroma. Patients complain of headache, lethargy, and sometimes contralateral weakness. On examination, changes in mental state are out of proportion to focal neurologic signs, and localized headache and skull tenderness may be present.

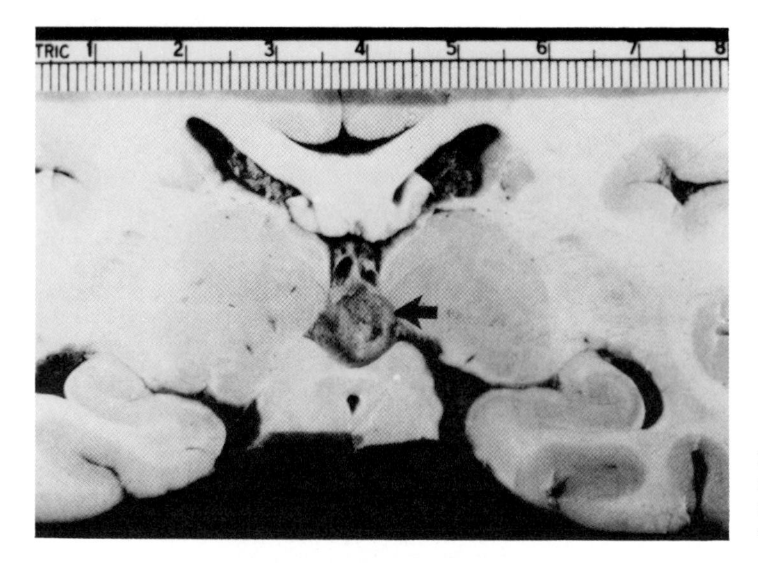

Figure 5–12. This figure shows a metastasis to the pineal gland *(arrow)*, compressing the tectum of the midbrain.

Additional Intracranial Metastases

Symptomatic metastases occasionally appear in the pineal body (Fig. 5–12), the choroid plexus, and the pituitary gland. Pineal metastases rarely cause symptoms unless they grow large enough to compress the cerebral aqueduct. A large pineal metastasis might cause symptoms similar to a primary pineal tumor, including hydrocephalus, large-fixed pupils, forced downward deviation of the eyes, and hearing loss. I have not encountered such a patient with a metastatic tumor. The diagnosis and treatment of pineal metastases resemble that of brain metastases.

Lesions of the choroid plexus rarely produce symptoms unless they either seed cells into the CSF, causing leptomeningeal metastasis (see Chapter 7), or obstruct outflow pathways of CSF at Monro's foramen, leading to hydrocephalus. The diagnosis and treatment resemble those of brain metastases.

Metastatic spread to the pituitary gland is more frequent than pineal or choroid metastases.* In one series of 100 autopsies, pituitary metastases were found in 1.8% of all cancer patients and in 9% with breast cancer.[7] In another study, metastases were found in about 10% of pituitary glands removed for treatment of breast carcinoma. Max and associates [1711] report findings from 16 patients with pituitary or parapituitary lesions, delineating both the endocrine and neurologic symptomatology of the group. It may be impossible clinically to distinguish a pituitary metastasis from the more common pituitary adenoma. If the tumor has grown into the suprasellar cistern, it may exude cells into the CSF; lumbar puncture may identify the malignant cells of a metastatic tumor. In one series from a general medical center, 20% of patients with diabetes insipidus had that symptom as a result of metastatic tumor.[1214] The tumor that metastasizes most frequently to the pituitary gland is breast carcinoma; others include melanoma; germ-cell tumors; leukemia; and colon, prostate, uterus, and larynx carcinomas.[1711] Metastasis rather than pituitary adenoma is indicated by the more rapid development of endocrine dysfunction; cranial nerve palsies, including visual field defects from optic chiasm compression and ocular muscle paralysis from cavernous sinus invasion; a larger size; and evidence that tumor has invaded the infundibulum or hypothalamus, as seen on MR scan.

*References 751, 1315, 1700, 1715, 2332, 2565.

CHAPTER 6

SPINAL METASTASES

As Chapter 5 indicates, most symptomatic intracranial metastases involve brain parenchyma. In the spinal canal, most symptomatic tumors compress the spinal cord or cauda equina from the epidural space and rarely directly involve the cord. In addition, several other complications of cancer can affect spinal cord function, mimicking metastatic disease (Table 6–1).

Epidural lesions are usually caused by a tumor that has metastasized to vertebral bodies; neurologic symptoms result from compression rather than invasion of the spinal cord (Fig. 6–1; see also Fig. 2–6). Epidural tumors rarely breach the dura; the dura compressed by tumor may be more than a millimeter thick and quite resistant to penetration.[1093] When the intradural space or the spinal cord is directly invaded, it is usually either by growth of the tumor along the spinal roots or by hematogenous spread directly to the spinal cord. Together, these invasions account for less than 5% of symptomatic spinal cord involvement.[513,708,2010,2077]

At autopsy, approximately 5% of patients who die from cancer exhibit spinal cord or cauda equina compression.[151] In patients with systemic cancer, Bansal and associates[143] report a 2% incidence of symptomatic spinal cord compression, which varied from 1% to 4% depending on tumor histology. Hildebrand[1156] reports that 1.3% of patients with cancer that he studied developed spinal cord compression. In one series, symptomatic spinal cord compression affected 5% of 2259 children with malignant solid tumors.[1386] The most likely offenders are cancers with a propensity to involve the vertebrae, including cancers of the breast, lung, myeloma, and prostate[246,921,984,1325,2847] (Table 6–2); spinal cord compression is less common with other tumors such as cervical cancer.[2288] Leukemia[1158,2845] and lymphoma[3] sometimes invade the epidural space without causing vertebral destruction.[1959,2014]

Symptoms and signs of spinal cord compression, other than pain, usually evolve rapidly. If untreated, weakness and ultimately paralysis invariably ensue.[921] When spinal cord compression is diagnosed and treated early, most patients either maintain or regain their ability to walk.[265,921,2142,2187] If diagnosis and treatment are delayed until the patient becomes paraplegic or quadriplegic, functional recovery is rare.[783,921] Therefore, early diagnosis of spinal cord compression is essential, and if the diagnosis is delayed until neurologic signs are rapidly worsening, treatment is urgent. The same considerations apply to compression of the nerve roots of the cauda equina, which occupy the spinal canal from vertebral body L-1 or L-2 to the sacrum. Because symptoms and prognosis are similar

Table 6–1. **SOME CAUSES OF SPINAL CORD DYSFUNCTION IN PATIENTS WITH CANCER**

I. Metastatic
  A. Epidural lesions
    1. From vertebral body
    2. From paravertebral structures
    3. Arising in epidural space
  B. Intradural metastases
    1. Single mass
    2. Leptomeningeal metastases
  C. Intramedullary metastases
II. Nonmetastatic
  A. Infections
    1. Epidural abscess
  B. Vascular disorders
    1. Hemorrhage
    2. Infarct
  C. Side effects of therapy
    1. Radiation
    2. Chemotherapy
  D. "Remote effects"

when either the cauda equina or the spinal cord is involved, they are discussed together in this chapter and are included under the general topic of spinal cord compression or invasion. Several recent reviews consider various aspects of diagnosis and treatment of spinal metastases* and spinal cord disease in general.[358,2848] Other reports consider specific tumors.†

EPIDURAL METASTASES

Frequency

The vertebral bodies, a common site of metastasis, are involved in 25% to 70% of patients with metastatic cancer.[820,865,1094,1525,2844] Fortunately, most vertebral metastases are either asymptomatic or cause pain only; a small percentage initiate significant spinal cord or cauda equina compression (Fig. 6–2). The spine is the most common site of bone metastasis irrespective of the responsible primary tumor[865,1093] (Table 6–3). So common are vertebral metastases that even a solitary vertebral tumor is more likely to be a metastasis than a primary bone tumor.[358] The pathophysiology and management of bone metastasis in general has been recently reviewed.[1895]

The exact incidence of spinal cord compression is not well established for several reasons: (1) Epidural spinal cord compression usually occurs late during the course of metastatic cancer, often during its terminal stages. Prior to CT and MR imaging, the diagnosis of spinal cord compression required a myelogram; many patients and their physicians chose not to pursue spinal cord signs with that invasive procedure, particularly if a patient was very ill. (2) Most pathologists do not routinely examine the spinal cord at autopsy, thus underestimating the incidence of spinal cord pathology. (3) Even when the spinal cord is examined at autopsy, pathologic changes may be minimal and not indicative that symptomatic spinal cord compression was present during life.[1918]

Epidural spinal cord compression, particularly from vertebral metastasis, is a relatively common neurologic complication of cancer. At Memorial Sloan-Kettering Cancer Center (MSKCC) in 1994, a diagnosis of epidural metastasis was made in 136 patients, a little over half the frequency of brain metastasis. In one 6-month period at MSKCC, neurologists evaluated these 136 patients with cancer and neck or back pain. Epidural tumor was present in 33% (44).[461] Back pain is the most common reason for neurologic consultation at MSKCC.[461] Of those referred, about 33% have epidural metastases and another 33% have vertebral metastases without epidural invasion. The remainder suffered degenerative spine disease or paravertebral or meningeal metastases. Overall, about 20,000 people—5% of 400,000 dying of cancer—develop spinal cord compression each year.[356]

Spinal cord compression may be the first sign of cancer. In a 10-year clinical study[2477] at the London Hospital, 131 patients with

*References 47, 117, 251, 356, 451, 969, 1016, 2129, 2778.

†References 475a, 702, 790, 1100, 1146, 1184, 1560, 1585, 1627, 2184, 2263, 2314.

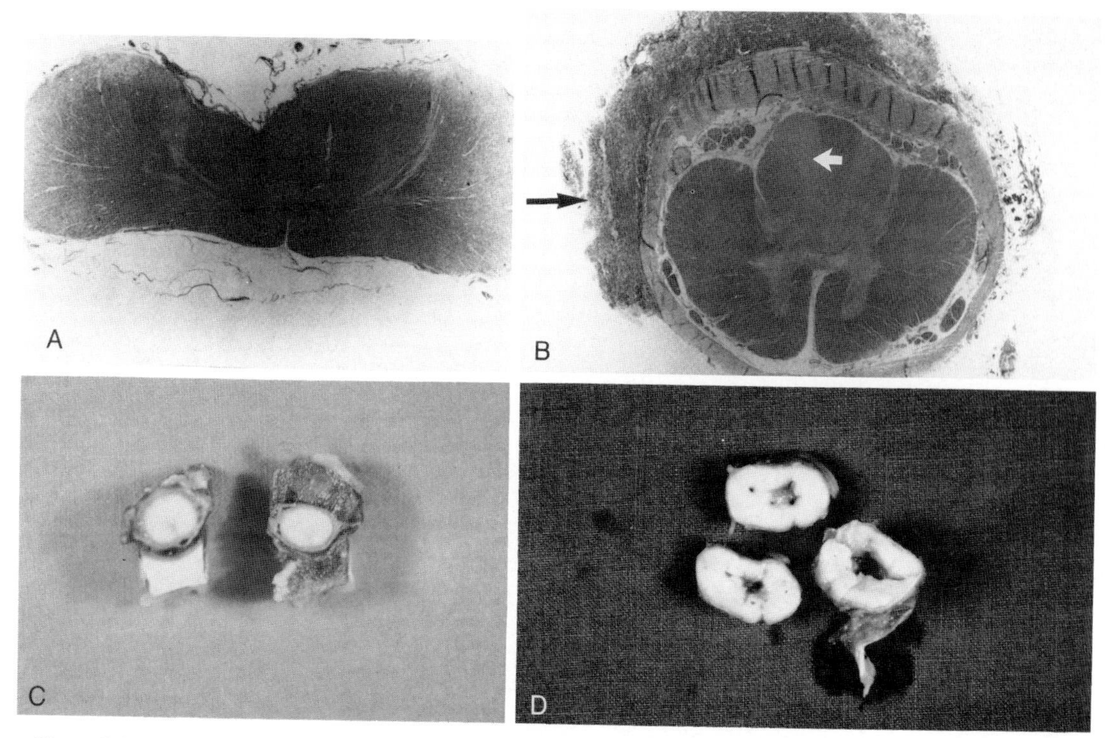

Figure 6–1. Anatomy and pathology of spinal cord dysfunction. *A,* Severe flattening of the spinal cord compressed by an anteriorly located epidural tumor. The lateral columns are demyelinated, but the anterior and posterior columns and the central gray area are relatively well preserved. *B,* An epidural tumor originating from a metastasis to the spinous process causing compression of the spinal cord posteriorly. Notice, in addition, that the tumor has partially surrounded the spinal cord on its lateral aspect (*black arrow*) and has caused demyelination in the dorsal columns (*white arrow*). *C,* A pathologic specimen at two levels from a patient suffering with spinal compression by malignant neuroblastoma. Although the tumor originated in the vertebral body, once it entered the epidural space it grew circumferentially around the cord, compressing the spinal cord anteriorly and posteriorly. Shrinkage artifact because of fixation makes the compression less apparent than it actually was. *D,* Central necrosis of a compressed spinal cord at the cervical level caused by epidural tumor metastatic to the C-5 vertebral body. Evidence of vascular occlusion was absent, although all of the radicular arteries were not carefully examined.

Continued.

cancers other than hematologic malignancies were found to have neurologic signs that were due to spinal cord or cauda equina compression; almost 50% were not known to have cancer when they presented with spinal symptoms. In 18 patients, the primary site was never discovered. In a similar study collected over 15 years by Paris and Naples,[511] of 600 patients with spinal metastases and neurologic signs, carcinomas of the breast (25%), lung (15%), and reproductive system (12%) were the common primary sites; in 12%, the primary site was unknown, fourth in the order of frequency. Hematologic tumors represented only 6%, perhaps because the report comes from a neurosurgical service; most patients with spinal cord compression from hematologic tumors are treated medically.

Table 6–4 lists the particular types of tumor and sites of spinal cord compression found in 265 patients with cancer at MSKCC. The thoracic spine is the most common location of epidural compression, followed by the lumbosacral and cervical spine in a ratio of about 4:2:1. Breast and lung cancer are distributed about equally through vertebral bodies, whereas prostate, renal, and GI tumors are more likely to affect the lower thoracic or lumbar vertebrae.

RT directed at the primary tumor also affects the incidence of metastases. Spinal

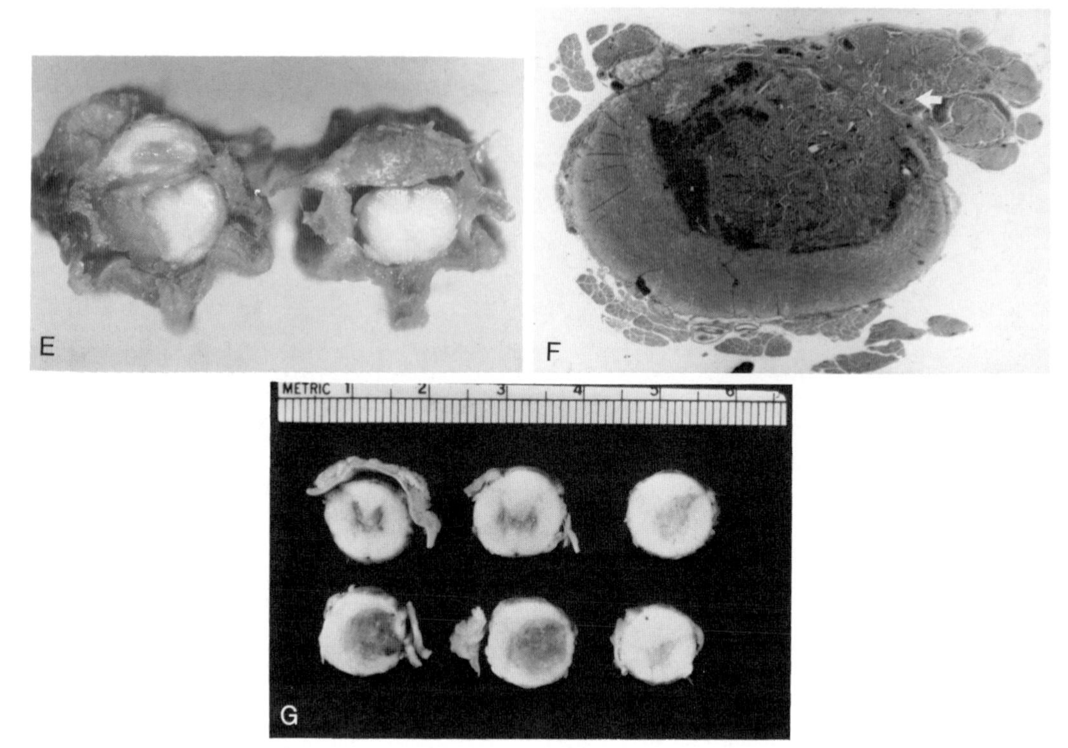

Figure 6–1. ***Continued.*** *E,* Spinal cord compression in a rat. The section on the right is taken from a normal animal. The section on the left demonstrates cord compression from a tumor that grew through the intravertebral foramen to compress the cord laterally. The bones of the vertebra are not affected. *F,* Intramedullary metastasis caused by small-cell lung cancer that invaded the spinal cord via the posterior root (*arrow*). Notice the infiltration of the posterior root and the apparent direct growth from the root into the spinal cord. *G,* Hematogenously spread intramedullary metastasis from malignant melanoma. The leptomeninges and the roots are not involved.

cord compression from malignant lymphoma has decreased at MSKCC over the years, probably because of RT delivered to the spinal column during the initial treatment of the lymphoma. A similar decrease in midthoracic spine metastases has been reported for patients with breast cancer who have received parasternal RT.[1146] Irradiation of these areas has not decreased the incidence of leptomeningeal tumor (see Chapter 7), probably because the tumor enters the CSF at sites outside the irradiated area. Irradiation of the lumbar vertebrae during primary therapy of prostate cancer also decreases the incidence of lumbar spinal metastases. It is not clear whether the vertebral irradiation has its effect by treating already-present micrometastases or by preventing development of future metastases by altering the vertebral environment.

Biology of Spinal Metastases

PATHOPHYSIOLOGY OF SIGNS AND SYMPTOMS

The mechanism(s) by which neurologic signs and symptoms are caused by epidural spinal cord compression is only partially understood. Direct compression, ischemia, and edema are probably all important. (1) In experimental animals, compression of the spinal cord by epidural tumor[1345] or abscess[761] causes weakness associated with white matter edema and axonal swelling at a time when spinal cord blood flow remains normal[1345] and blood vessels are patent. The edema appears to be a result of either direct compression of the cord or venous congestion from compression of the epidural venous plexus,[761] or both. At this stage, removal of the compression usually leads to full

Table 6–2. **PRIMARY CANCERS CAUSING SYMPTOMATIC SPINAL CORD COMPRESSION IN 583 PATIENTS AT MSKCC**

Primary Tumor	Number of Patients	(%)
Breast	127	(22)
Lung	90	(15)
Prostate	58	(10)
Lymphoreticular system	56	(10)
Sarcomas	52	(9)
Kidney	39	(7)
Gastrointestinal tract	29	(5)
Melanoma	23	(4)
Unknown primary	21	(4)
Head and neck	19	(3)
Miscellaneous	69	(12)
Total	**583**	**(100)**

MSKCC = Memorial Sloan-Kettering Cancer Center.

functional recovery. (2) With progressive compression, spinal cord blood flow decreases. The normal dilatation of spinal cord vessels in response to carbon dioxide inhalation (autoregulation) fails at the site of compression and caudally even before blood flow itself begins to decrease.[1345] Tumors located either posteriorly or anteriorly to the cord occlude the vasculature to the center of the cord, whereas lateral masses of larger size do not.[668] At this stage, if untreated, the cord eventually infarcts, causing irreversible neurologic damage. (3) The spinal cord edema caused by tumor compression is vasogenic[174,2645] and can be partially ameliorated by adrenocorticosteroids[603,2645] (Fig. 6–3), improving clinical symptoms.

The biochemical processes associated with spinal cord compression and edema are not fully understood. Pharmacologic evidence implicates an increase in the synthesis or release of prostaglandin E_2 and 6–ketoprostaglandin F-1α.[2412] Serotonin 5-hydroxytryptamine (5HT) metabolism may be altered as well; 5-hydroxyindoleacetic acid (5-HIAA)/ 5-HT ratios are elevated in the compressed cord, suggesting that 5HT utilization is increased; the type-2 serotonin receptor antagonists cyproheptadine or ketanserin reportedly delay the onset of paraplegia in experimental animals.[2406,2407] Release of the excitatory transmitter, glutamate, may also play a role because the glutamate receptor antagonists ketamine and MK-801 appear to decrease the edema induced by experimental cord compression.[2409] The role these substances play in clinical cord compression in humans is unknown.

The rate of spinal cord compression is important. Tarlov and Klinger,[2554] using inflated epidural balloons in dogs, have shown that the more rapidly spinal cord compression develops, the less likely recovery is after decompression, and, conversely, the more slowly compression develops, the longer the

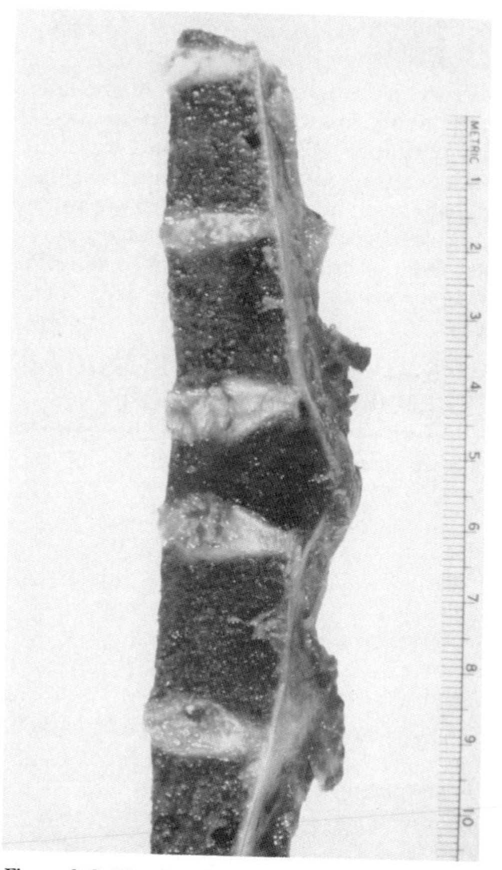

Figure 6–2. The thoracic spinal cord of a patient with a metastasis to a vertebral body. The vertebral body is collapsed anteriorly. Tumor and posterior protruding bone compromise the spinal canal but do not breach the posterior longitudinal ligament.

Table 6—3. **VERTEBRAL METASTASES IN PATIENTS WITH CANCER**

Primary Tumor	No. of Patients	% Metastases at Autopsy	% with Vertebral Metastases but Negative Radiograph (False-Negatives)	% Vertebral Collapse on Radiograph but No Metastases Pathologically (False-Positives)
Total	832	36	26(78/300)	22(34/155)
Breast	113	74	25	8
Lung	138	45	24	3
GI	115	25	38	4
Lymphoma	107	29	64	3
Female GU	78	20	25	3
Head and neck	35	20	40	3
Kidney	24	29	0	8
Prostate	21	90	10	5

GI = gastrointestinal tract; GU = genitourinary tract.
Source: Adapted from Wong et al,[2844] p 1.

animal can be paralyzed and still recover. Experiments in cats give similar results.[933] Data in humans[921,2449] suggest that metastatic tumors causing neurologic dysfunction that develops over hours to days carry a worse prognosis even after treatment than do those that evolve more slowly. For example, Smith[2449] found that fewer than 10% of patients with symptoms progressing over 2 months benefited from surgical decompression, whereas 33% of patients whose symptoms developed more slowly benefited. It is widely recognized that even paraplegic patients with slowly developing symptoms, such

Table 6—4. **SITE OF COMPRESSION IN 265 PATIENTS WITH EPIDURAL SPINAL CORD COMPRESSION**

Primary Tumor	No. of Patients	%	Cervical	T-1 to T-6	T-7 to T-12	Lumbosacral
Breast	58	21.9	7	25	26	11†
Lung	49	18.5	3	28	13	7
Prostate	25	9.4	1	7	10	9
Kidney	19	7.2	1	5	11	5
Lymphoreticular system	18	6.8	1	7	8	4
Melanoma	10	3.8	1	4	4	2
Gastrointestinal tract	14	5.3	3	1	5	6
Soft-tissue sarcoma	19	7.2	2	4	12	2
Unknown primary tumor	14	5.3	1	7	7	2
Miscellaneous*	39	14.7	3	17	15	8
Total	**265**	**100**	**22**	**105**	**111**	**56**

*Thyroid, bladder, Ewing's sarcoma, germ-cell tumors, neuroblastoma, and others.
†Some patients had more than one site of compression.

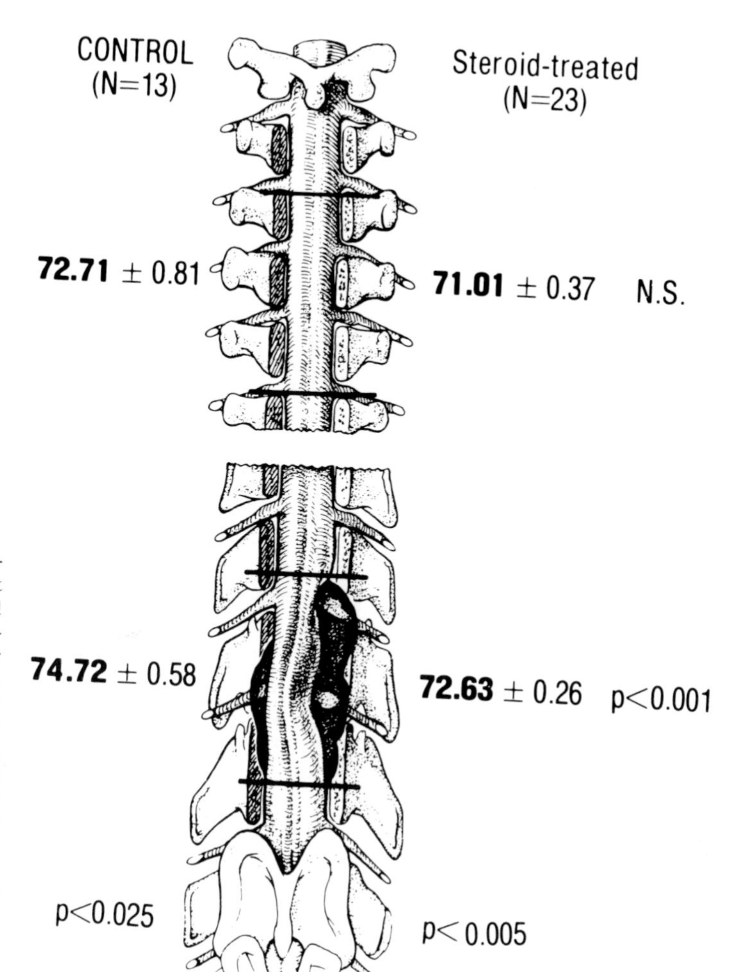

Figure 6–3. The effect of corticosteroids on the water content of the rat spinal cord. In this experimental model, the epidural tumor compressed the spinal cord anteriorly and laterally after growing through the intervertebral foramina at several levels (see Fig. 6–1*E*). A significantly higher ($p<.025$) water content is found in the compressed spinal cord than in the cord distant from the tumor. After steroid treatment, the water content of the compressed spinal cord drops significantly ($p<.001$) but is still greater than that of the normal cord. The animals improve symptomatically as well. (From Ushio et al,[2645] p 427, with permission.)

as caused by a meningioma, may regain neurologic function, a phenomenon much rarer with metastatic tumors.

In most patients with epidural spinal cord compression, neurologic symptoms other than pain evolve rapidly to paraplegia over several days to a few weeks. In some patients, with or without preceding pain, paraplegia begins suddenly, suggesting infarction of the cord. This sequence occurred in 28% of the patients reported by Costans and colleagues,[511] but much less frequently in our experience at MSKCC. Because the evolution of neurologic symptoms is usually rapid and because one cannot predict when slowly evolving symptoms will suddenly accelerate, early diagnosis and prompt treatment are essential.

PATHOLOGY

Displacement and distortion of the spinal cord may be present on gross inspection of a fixed pathologic specimen (see Fig. 6–1A) but more often are absent (see Fig. 6–1C). When present, the degree and extent of gross distortion do not correlate with the degree of abnormalities noted microscopically.[1717,1918] Almost all symptomatic patients with spinal cord compression exhibit pathologic changes identified microscopically, although the changes are often minor and consist of only white matter edema and axonal swelling. Demyelination may not be present, infarction may not have occurred, and the axon cylinders may remain intact. The extent of spinal cord or nerve root pathology does not reflect the degree of neurologic impairment. The absence of major pathologic changes strongly suggests that physiologic changes predominate early in cord compression, and it is only later that the anatomic changes participate in the pathogenesis of symptoms.

Despite the usually anterior or anterolateral location of the epidural metastasis, microscopic changes at the level of compression are most common and most severe in the dorsal and lateral funiculi, with relative sparing of the anterior funiculi and the central gray matter.[1320,1717] The earliest change in experimental cord compression appears to be extravasation of IV contrast into gray matter and small hemorrhagic areas in the dorsal columns.[761,1345] Microscopic abnormalities in the white matter may be limited to tract demyelination, or tissue necrosis may be diffuse and extensive. Even with severe white matter damage, the central gray matter is often fairly well preserved; the most common changes are degeneration of anterior horn cells and diffuse gliosis. Vacuolization of white matter indicating edema is most common at the cord periphery. Other changes include scattered small focal infarcts in white and gray matter, secondary tract degeneration away from the compression, and nerve root demyelination.

Pencil-shaped, longitudinal softening of the ventral portion of the posterior columns or posterior horns that extends over several segments is a relatively common complication of spinal cord compression,[1106] either from vascular compression (arterial circulation or venous drainage) or directly from mechanical compression. This disorder tends to occur in the upper thoracic cord and, in one series, was present in 6 of 15 patients with epidural spinal cord compression[1106] (see Fig. 6–1D). The lesion is always associated with either transverse or patchy necrosis or with status spongiosis of the cord. Filled with necrotic debris and macrophages, the cavity can actually form a mass lesion compressing the surrounding cord. Rarely, epidural metastases may cause a visible syrinx on MR scan that resolves after treatment.[1202] Infarction may occur as a result of vascular occlusion from compression of radicular arteries by tumor in the intervertebral foramen.

Clinical Findings

PAIN

Pain is the earliest and most frequent presenting symptom of spinal cord compression (Table 6–5). Pain from spinal metastasis is usually mild at first, but unless the diagnosis is established and treatment started, it becomes progressively more severe, often incapacitating the patient. Other signs and symptoms of spinal cord or cauda equina compression, including weakness, sensory loss, and autonomic dysfunction, develop later. The bone marrow is insensitive to pain so that vertebral metastases cause pain only when the enlarg-

Table 6–5. **SIGNS AND SYMPTOMS OF SPINAL CORD COMPRESSION IN 211 PATIENTS AT MSKCC**

	FIRST SYMPTOM		PRESENT AT DIAGNOSIS	
	No. of Patients	**% of Patients**	**No. of Patients**	**% of Patients**
Pain	201	94	207	97
Weakness	7	3	157	74
Autonomic dysfunction	0	0	111	52
Sensory loss	1	0.5	112	53
Ataxia	2	0.9	8	4

MSKCC = Memorial Sloan-Kettering Cancer Center.

ing mass breaks through the bony cortex to involve the periosteum, paravertebral soft tissues, or other pain-sensitive structures such as dural nerves. Pain and other symptoms are also caused by compression or invasion of nerve roots, by pathologic fractures of vertebrae, by spinal instability[863,864] that occurs when posterior vertebral elements are destroyed, and by spinal cord compression itself. The tumor often secretes osteoclast-activating factor as well as prostaglandins E_1 and E_2, substances that assist the tumor in invading the bone and also cause hyperalgesic effects.[1709] The clinical implication is that prostaglandin inhibitors may relieve pain and retard metastatic development. Other pain-producing substances, including acetylcholine, histamine, serotonin, bradykinin, and substance P, probably also play a role in producing pain by stimulating nociceptors.

The absence of pain does not mean an absence of cord compression. In one study, only 60% of patients with CT evidence of cord compression complained of back pain; neurologic signs also were absent.[1916] Even a "complete block" to myelographic contrast material may be painless.[1600] In most series, however, in more than 90% of patients,[921] pain is the first symptom; it may begin from hours to months (median = 7 weeks) before other neurologic symptoms or signs develop. The duration of pain before the development of other symptoms is shorter for lung cancer metastases than for breast cancer metastases.[2477] Treatment is most effective when pain is the only symptom. The physician must be prepared to pursue vigorously the workup of patients with cancer and spinal pain, and he or she must caution patients, many of whom have widespread cancer with multiple aches and pains, that pain in the neck or back or radicular pain should be reported immediately and not ignored.[1134a]

Failure to evaluate the patient when pain is the only symptom may result in missed opportunities for effective therapy that preserves function. For example, Gilbert and associates[921] report that, although 125 of 130 adults with spinal cord compression had pain as the first symptom, by the time the diagnosis was eventually made, 99 (76%) complained of weakness, 74 (57%) of autonomic dysfunction, and 66 (51%) of sensory loss. Only five patients presented with painless weakness of the lower extremities. Other series of adults give a somewhat lower incidence of pain: Costans and colleagues,[511] 61%; Stark and coworkers,[2477] 69%. But Bernat and associates[196] report pain in 99% of patients. Of these, 43% had only local pain; 13%, radicular pain; and 43%, both. Although pain is absent in only about 5% of adults with myelopathy from metastatic spinal cord compression, as many as 20% of children may be pain-free.

Local Pain. Back pain caused by cancer may be of several types. In most patients, the initial pain is local and perceived as steady and aching at the site of the involved vertebral body. The pain is often exacerbated by coughing, by straining (i.e., the Valsalva maneuver), and sometimes by movement, especially if the spine is unstable. Characteristically, it is more severe when the patient is supine.[452] The reason may relate to increased filling of the veins of Batson's plexus in this position. Nocturnal spine pain that is relieved by arising and walking suggests a spinal cord tumor and helps to differentiate this pain from herniated disk pain, which is usually relieved by lying down.[655] At times, the positional pain requires the patient to sleep sitting up; some physicians have found this sign unreliable.[1606] Local pain is usually associated with tenderness to percussion over the vertebral body, although some physicians question the usefulness of this sign. O'Rourke and associates[1916] found it in only 43% of patients with CT-positive vertebral metastases and in only 65% with epidural disease. When present, however, the sign helps localize the metastasis. At times the pain is exacerbated by neck flexion if the involved vertebral body is cervical or upper or midthoracic. Straight-leg raising often exacerbates the pain of lower thoracic or lumbar spinal metastases. Both signs suggest spinal cord compression rather than just vertebral metastasis.

Much local pain from spinal cord compression is probably not simply the result of vertebral body involvement but originates from compression of neural structures because it is usually dramatically relieved by administering corticosteroids (see the following), whereas other bone pain (such as hip metastasis) is not. The site of the local pain may help distinguish vertebral metastasis from the more common degenerative back lesion. Most degenerative back disease is either cervical or lumbar, causing neck or low back pain, whereas most epidural spinal cord compression is thoracic, yielding local thoracic pain.

Radicular Pain. Compression of nerve roots within the spinal canal or on exit through the intervertebral foramen generates radicular pain; although it usually follows local pain, it sometimes precedes or is independent of it. Radicular pain is present in 80% of patients with cervical lesions. It generally radiates down one arm or sometimes both arms. Of patients with thoracic compression, 55% characteristically have radiating pain in a tight band around the chest or abdomen, almost always bilaterally; 90% of patients with lumbar spine involvement have pain radiating down one or both legs.[921] While most of these patients have local pain as well, radicular pain may be the only pain, and it may be felt in only one portion of the dermatome remote from the cord compression site.[452] One of our patients underwent extensive workup for isolated knee pain before careful examination revealed that the pain could be reproduced by straight-leg raising; an epidural metastasis was found.

Referred and Funicular Pain. Referred pain applies to pain perceived at a distance from the lesion but not dermatomal (radicular) in distribution. For example, L-1 vertebral metastases can cause pain over the sacroiliac joint. In such cases, the physician may undertake a fruitless search for a lesion at the site of referred pain. Funicular pain is caused by compression of ascending spinal cord tracts; its presence can also mislead. For instance, cervical cord compression can cause funicular pain in the lower extremities, simulating sciatica,[2345,2679] and can also cause pain and paresthesias in a bandlike distribution around the thorax or abdomen. Pseudoclaudication in the legs may be the only symptom of lumbar nerve root compression.[750]

WEAKNESS

Weakness is the second most common finding.[921,984] It usually results from corticospinal tract dysfunction and therefore is associated with spasticity, hyperactive deep tendon reflexes, and extensor plantar responses (Babinski's sign).

Upper Motor Neuron Weakness. Spinal cord compression usually causes weakness that begins in the legs, regardless of the spinal compression site, and is more marked proximally than distally early in the course. Thus, the patient usually complains of difficulty walking and especially climbing stairs or rising from low chairs or toilet seats. The patient may notice that the knees buckle even when he or she walks on level ground. As the illness progresses, the weakness becomes more profound, both proximally and distally, leading to increased difficulty in walking. With an upper thoracic or cervical cord lesion, the patient may next notice a weak cough or difficulty in sitting up from a recumbent position because of weak abdominal muscles. Only late in the development of cervical cord compression do the arms become substantially weak.

Although weakness is usually bilateral and symmetric, at times it may predominate in one leg or arm. Examination during the early stages of upper motor neuron weakness may fail to reveal spasticity or hyperactive reflexes; only modest weakness of iliopsoas and hamstring muscles may be observed, with apparently normal strength in distal muscles. Even at this time, the patellar and achilles reflexes are usually slightly more active than the upper extremity reflexes; extensor plantar responses may also be elicited. As the illness progresses and the weakness becomes more profound, spasticity, hyperactive reflexes, and unequivocal extensor plantar responses develop. These signs are usually bilateral and symmetric, although one side may be more affected than the other. If the onset is sudden and leads to complete paraplegia, most patients are flaccid with areflexia, reflecting distal spinal reflex inhibition.

The distribution of the weakness and reflex changes do not identify the site of cord compression in the horizontal plane; that is, laterally placed lesions do not necessarily cause Brown-Séquard's syndrome[1399]: ipsilateral weakness and proprioceptive loss with contralateral temperature and pain loss resulting from hemicord dysfunction. Such lesions may cause more contralateral than ipsilateral weakness, probably because of torsion and ischemia of the cord. No clinical findings differentiate between anteriorly and posteriorly placed lesions.[1717] Slowly growing tumors are more likely to cause the anatomically expected localizing signs.

Lower Motor Neuron Weakness. When the cauda equina rather than the spinal cord is involved, the weakness reflects lower motor neuron dysfunction. Characterized by hypotonia, atrophy, fasciculations, and areflexia, lower motor neuron weakness can also occur with spinal cord compression as a result of dysfunction of anterior horn cells. This dysfunction is probably vascular rather than compressive. Lower motor neuron hand weakness, for example, may be an early and isolated sign of lower cervical cord compression. With cauda equina compression, the weakness is usually more marked distally than proximally, although buttock and hamstring muscles are usually affected as well. The distal weakness begins with foot-drop and proceeds to flail weakness below the knees. Initially, such patients may have more difficulty descending than climbing stairs; later, they catch their foot as they walk on an uneven surface or climb a curb. Achilles reflexes disappear early and the patellar reflexes follow. Plantar responses are absent or flexor. Fasciculations occasionally appear in the lower extremities, but severe atrophy is uncommon, probably because the disease evolves rapidly. In rare instances, fasciculations in the lower extremities have been reported with cervical cord compression[1375] or injury.[21] I have seen one patient in whom fasciculations in leg muscles disappeared after a C-7 epidural metastasis was treated successfully.

With lower motor neuron dysfunction from spinal cord compression, the segmental reflex disappears at the compression site, although reflexes below this site are hyperactive. For example, with C-5 cord compression, the biceps reflex disappears and unilateral selective weakness may develop in the deltoid and biceps muscles. The triceps and finger-stretch reflexes are hyperactive, with better strength in those muscles. With T-1 compression, pain in the upper back, radiating down the medial aspects of one or both arms or localized to the elbow(s), is accompanied by weakness of the small muscles of the hands and absent finger-stretch reflexes. The finger-stretch reflex (Hoffmann's sign) may be absent in normal individuals but is present in most patients stimulated by the anxiety, tension, and pain associated with the spinal metastases. Its unilateral absence is strongly suggestive of a T-1 spinal lesion. Some of our patients have further developed severe weakness and atrophy of the small hand muscles without long tract signs. This pattern is particularly important to recognize because plain radiographs of the cervical and thoracic spine rarely show the T-1 vertebra clearly because it is covered by the shoulder and other bony structures. One caveat: Atrophy of the small hand muscles, usually without much weakness, may accompany upper cervical cord compression as a false-localizing sign, possibly from compression of descending arteries.[1166]

SENSORY LOSS

Usually concurrent with the development of weakness or shortly afterward, patients notice paresthesias, loss of sensation and numbness, or both, in the lower extremities. Sensory complaints without pain are rare with spinal cord or cauda equina compression. Only 1 of 83 patients reported by Greenberg and colleagues[984] presented with sensory symptoms without pain, weakness, or ataxia. Sensory abnormalities usually begin in the toes and ascend in a stockinglike fashion, eventually reaching the level of the lesion. The patient may complain of either numbness ("as if I am wearing thick stockings") or paresthesias ("pins and needles" tingling of the lower extremities). They say, "My feet feel as if they are asleep." Although sensory changes evolve rapidly, the earliest sign appears to be a slight decrease of vibration and position sense, with pain and temperature loss ensuing. By the time most such patients present for diagnosis, sensory loss for both touch and pinprick are found to be one to five levels below the site of actual spinal cord compression. On occasion, the level of sensory loss is one or two segments *above* the site of spinal cord compression, presumably because of ischemia to the cord from compression of ascending vessels.

Sacral Sparing. Loss of sensation to pinprick in the legs and trunk with preservation in the perianal region and buttocks was originally believed to be characteristic of intramedullary disease but actually commonly occurs with epidural spinal cord compression. About 20% of our patients with extramedullary compression have exhibited some degree of sacral sparing. Usually limited to the buttocks, it may extend down the posterior aspect of the thighs (S2 dermatome) and, on rare occasions, down the posterior or even lateral aspect of the leg and foot (S1–L5 dermatome). Preserved sensation in the sacral area may explain why autonomic dysfunction is a late occurrence with spinal cord compression.

With cauda equina compression, the sensory loss is dermatomal and usually bilateral, involving the perianal area, the posterior thigh, and the lateral aspect of the leg. Substantial sensory loss is almost always associated with significant motor loss but sometimes occurs independently of motor change; therefore, a careful examination for a sensory level should be performed in all patients complaining of back pain.

Sensory loss is rarely as profound as weakness. Even in patients who are paraplegic, some appreciation of gross touch is usually present; that is, the patient perceives something happening when his or her leg is lightly squeezed. In some patients, however, loss of position sense may preclude independent walking even when strength is sufficient.

Lhermitte's Sign.[2687] Originally believed to be a pathognomonic symptom of multiple sclerosis, Lhermitte's sign is an electric shock-like sensation radiating into the back or legs when the neck is flexed. Unpleasant but not painful, it sometimes complicates cervical or thoracic spinal cord compression. The sign is more common in patients with radiation myelopathy (see Chapter 13) and *cis*-platinum neuropathy (see Chapter 12).

AUTONOMIC DYSFUNCTION

None of the patients whom we have studied at MSKCC have had autonomic dysfunction as the sole presenting complaint. Even when other neurologic signs are absent, the patient complains of back pain. Costans and coworkers[511] report isolated sphincter disturbances in 2% of patients studied. We have found bladder and bowel dysfunction in more than 50% of patients by the time the diagnosis of spinal cord or cauda equina compression is made. Most men are impotent. It is difficult to say whether impotence results from the cord compression or from pain and systemic illness. Constipation is usually present, but it may be a result of opioids taken to relieve pain. Occasional patients have observed that enemas or laxatives induce fecal incontinence.

The most characteristic autonomic abnormality is bladder dysfunction. Urinary urgency with incontinence is an occasional complaint if the motor symptoms are evolving slowly. More commonly, patients simply develop painless urinary retention, usually associated with severe weakness and sensory loss of the lower extremities. Patients may or may not be aware that they have not voided recently, and the bladder may grow to enormous size. As the bladder rises above the pelvic brim, some will suffer from diffuse abdominal pain, probably from peritoneal irritation, but many have no pain even when the bladder reaches the umbilicus. The physician suspecting cord compression is obligated to percuss the abdomen frequently and to ask the patient, if not hospitalized, to keep records of frequency and quantity of urinary output. If the bladder cannot be percussed because of a patient's obesity, one must measure residual urine. One woman referred because of weakness in the lower extremities was told that cancer was rapidly progressing because of an enlarging abdominal mass; the mass disappeared when 2000 mL of urine were gradually drained from her painless bladder.

Other autonomic changes of lesser importance but occasional clinical usefulness include a definable sweat level (i.e., the absence of sweating below the level of a spinal block) and Horner's syndrome. A sweat level usually develops only when weakness is profound, but sometimes, in patients unable to cooperate for sensory examination, the level of the lesion can be discerned by running one's hand or a dry tuning fork or a spoon up the back or abdomen. The tuning fork begins to stick or the finger perceives moisture at the level where sweating begins. In patients who are profoundly paraplegic, increased sweating above the level of the lesion is a normal mechanism for heat dissipation. Horner's syndrome is more common in patients with paravertebral tumors than with cord compression, but when cord compression is at C-8 to T-1, Horner's syndrome, either unilateral or bilateral, occasionally occurs.

An unusual autonomic presentation takes place when the cord is compressed at the T-10 to T-12 vertebral bodies at or just above the conus medullaris. Many patients, after experiencing pain for several days to weeks, suddenly develop urinary retention and severe constipation without weakness or sensory loss. The neurologic examination is usually normal save for a lax anal sphincter and an enlarged bladder. Vertebral tenderness is present over the lower thoracic and upper lumbar area.

Examination of all patients with suspected spinal cord compression should include a rectal examination to assess sphincter tone, the patient's ability to contract the sphincter voluntarily, and the reflex contraction of the sphincter when the skin around the anus is scratched (anal wink). If any one of the above findings is abnormal, cauda equina or conus medullaris compression should be suspected.

ATAXIA

Gait ataxia is common, but "cerebellar signs" are usually obscured by motor weakness and sensory loss. In occasional patients, isolated ataxia, either with or without pain, can be a major complaint.[921,1026,1060] Ataxia without pain is probably the most confusing sign of cord compression that the clinician encounters. An initial clinical diagnosis of either paraneoplastic cerebellar disease or hysteria has delayed proper diagnosis in several of our patients. One patient with pain and ataxia but no other neurologic signs was locked in a psychiatric ward after punching a house officer who told the patient he was "drunk and hysterical." The alcohol the patient drank was an attempt to control the severe thoracic pain resulting from an esophageal carcinoma metastatic to the T-4 vertebral body. A woman with painless cord compression from Hodgkin's disease was treated for several days for anxiety and "conversion symptoms" before a consultant suggested the correct diagnosis. Lack of dysarthria and upper extremity ataxia in the presence of severe gait and lower extremity ataxia should lead to a suspicion of spinal disease, although the same signs occur with lesions of the cerebellar vermis. The ataxia of spinal cord compression probably results from compression of the spinocerebellar tracts. Why these tracts should be selectively and symmetrically involved is not clear. Ataxia may persist after restoration of strength and sensation following treatment of spinal cord compression, making it impossible for the patient to walk. Sometimes gait training helps.

UNUSUAL FINDINGS

Unusual signs of spinal cord compression (Table 6–6) can lead to an incorrect diagnosis. Physiologically unexplained, rare signs include papilledema, hydrocephalus,[1785,1890] and nystagmus in patients with thoracic cord compression, as well as facial weakness, diplopia, and lower extremity fasciculations in patients with cervical or upper thoracic cord compression. Explainable physiologically are Brown-Séquard's syndrome,[1399] herpes zoster, pseudoclaudication, pain in the neck and numbness of the tongue on head turning (the neck-tongue syndrome),[1465] myoclonic contractions of abdomen and leg muscles, and the syndrome of painful legs and moving toes. Brown-Séquard's syndrome is more often encountered in radiation myelopathy (see Chapter 13). Its presence with cord compression does not necessarily indicate that the tumor is positioned ipsilaterally. Herpes

Table 6–6. UNUSUAL SIGNS AND SYMPTOMS IN PATIENTS WITH SPINAL CORD COMPRESSION

"Painful legs and moving toes"
Lhermitte's sign with cervical or thoracic tumor
Lower extremity fasciculations with cervical tumor
Sciatica with cervical tumor
Facial paresis with cervical tumor
Nystagmus with thoracic tumor
Pseudoclaudication
Hydrocephalus (papilledema)
Spinal myoclonus
Tongue numbness
Inverted knee jerk

zoster at the cord compression site has been noted by several authors[921]; it is believed to be due to activation of the latent virus from tumor compression of the dorsal root ganglion.

Facial pain and numbness sometimes may delay accurate diagnosis of upper cervical cord compression. The upper cervical sensory fibers, particularly from the C-2 and C-3 roots, supply the back of the head and also a variable portion of the face. The extent of sensory loss on the face caused by a cervical lesion can vary with physiologic manipulation of the spinal cord.[613] Some patients with compression of C-2 and C-3 roots complain of pain, often ticlike, and numbness involving the lateral portion of the cheek and jaw. The pain and numbness never reach the medial portion of the face but can mislead a physician into thinking that the symptoms originate with the trigeminal nerve rather than the upper cervical cord.

Laboratory Examination

APPROACH TO THE PATIENT

The most sensitive and specific diagnostic test for spinal lesions caused by cancer is an MR scan[2021a] (Fig. 6–4). If the entire spine is

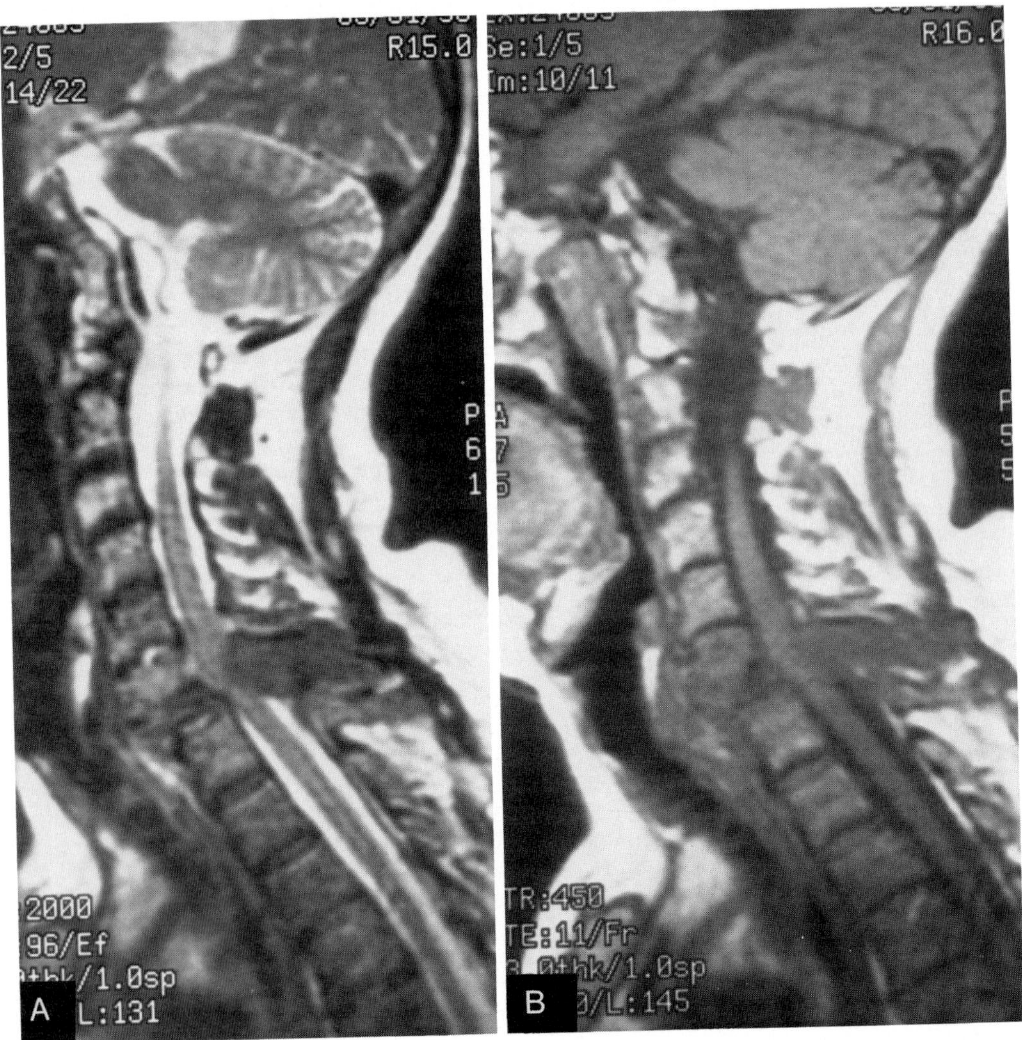

Figure 6–4. An MR scan in a patient with breast carcinoma reveals anterior and posterior epidural spinal cord compression. The posterior spinous process and the vertebral body were invaded by the tumor. Cord compression is more apparent in the T_2-weighted image (*A*) than the T_1-weighted image (*B*).

imaged both before and after contrast enhancement, a normal study effectively rules out vertebral and paravertebral metastases, epidural spinal cord compression, intramedullary spinal metastases, and many leptomeningeal tumors. Those rare occasions when epidural mass lesions are missed by MR scans, even after contrast enhancement, appear to be due to failure to examine the spine in its most lateral aspects and to obtain appropriate transverse as well as sagittal images. MR scans also distinguish malignant lesions from benign ones such as disk herniation. A complete MR study is expensive and arduous for a patient in pain. Less expensive and time-consuming diagnostic tests often suffice, but all too often, failure to begin with an MR scan results in the patient's undergoing a series of increasingly sophisticated images (e.g., plain radiographs to bone scan to CT), only to finally have the diagnosis established by MR after a significant delay and increased exposure. Particularly in patients with severe pain, pain localized to the thoracic area (where disk disease is uncommon), or pain of recent onset, MR scan may be the place to start. Because multiple lesions may be present, the entire spine should be imaged.

Noncontiguous metastatic lesions occur with high frequency, either near each other or at a distance.[2062,2243,2661] The presence of these other lesions may alter both the patient's symptoms and the physician's treatment plan. Thus, in most instances, it is important to image the entire spine. It is also important to try to determine if spinal cord compression associated with vertebral collapse is a result of tumor, bone in the epidural space, or (as is usual) both. If bone alone is the culprit, RT and chemotherapy will not work. Figure 6–5 is a modified algorithm initially devised by Portenoy and colleagues [2063] for the diagnosis and management of patients with back pain and cancer. The specific use of imaging techniques is detailed in the paragraphs that follow.[2067]

RADIOGRAPHS

Depending on the series, in 85% to 95%[1328,2062] of patients with spinal cord compression, plain radiographs identify the responsible vertebral lesion[921,1328,2062,2187] (Table 6–7). In a few others, radiographs will identify a paravertebral mass when vertebral bodies are normal. Vertebral body abnormalities include radiolucencies or radiodensities from direct involvement by tumor, erosion of pedicles, collapse, and sometimes subluxation of vertebral bodies. In one recent prospective study,[2187] 42 of 45 patients with spinal blocks identified by myelography had abnormalities on spine radiographs. Plain radiographs are also both highly sensitive (91%) and highly specific (86%) for predicting epidural disease. Particularly useful predictive features of epidural spinal cord compression are greater than 50% vertebral collapse and pedicle erosion (see Table 6–7). Fewer than 10% of patients with radiologic evidence of vertebral metastases without vertebral collapse suffer epidural spinal cord compression.[2062] Plain radiographs are not entirely reliable, however, for several reasons: (1) Certain vertebral bodies, such as T-1, may be obscured behind other bony shadows and not easily detected by routine spine radiographs. (2) Even when the vertebral body is seen, the tumor may not have destroyed enough bone to be identifiable. The estimate is that 30% to 50% of the vertebral body must be destroyed before noticeable changes are seen on radiographs. (3) If multiple vertebral bodies are involved by metastatic tumor, the radiographs will not identify which area is causing cord compression. (4) All too often, the oncologist or neurologist refers the patient to the radiologist with a note saying "suspected cord compression; please do cervical, lumbar, and thoracic spine films." In these instances, even a careful radiologist

Table 6–7. **PLAIN RADIOGRAPH FINDINGS AT THE SITE OF EPIDURAL SPINAL CORD COMPRESSION FROM METASTASES**

Finding	%
Vertebral collapse > 50%	87
Pedicle destroyed	66
Vertebral metastases without collapse	23
Normal radiograph	6

Source: Data from Graus et al.[973]

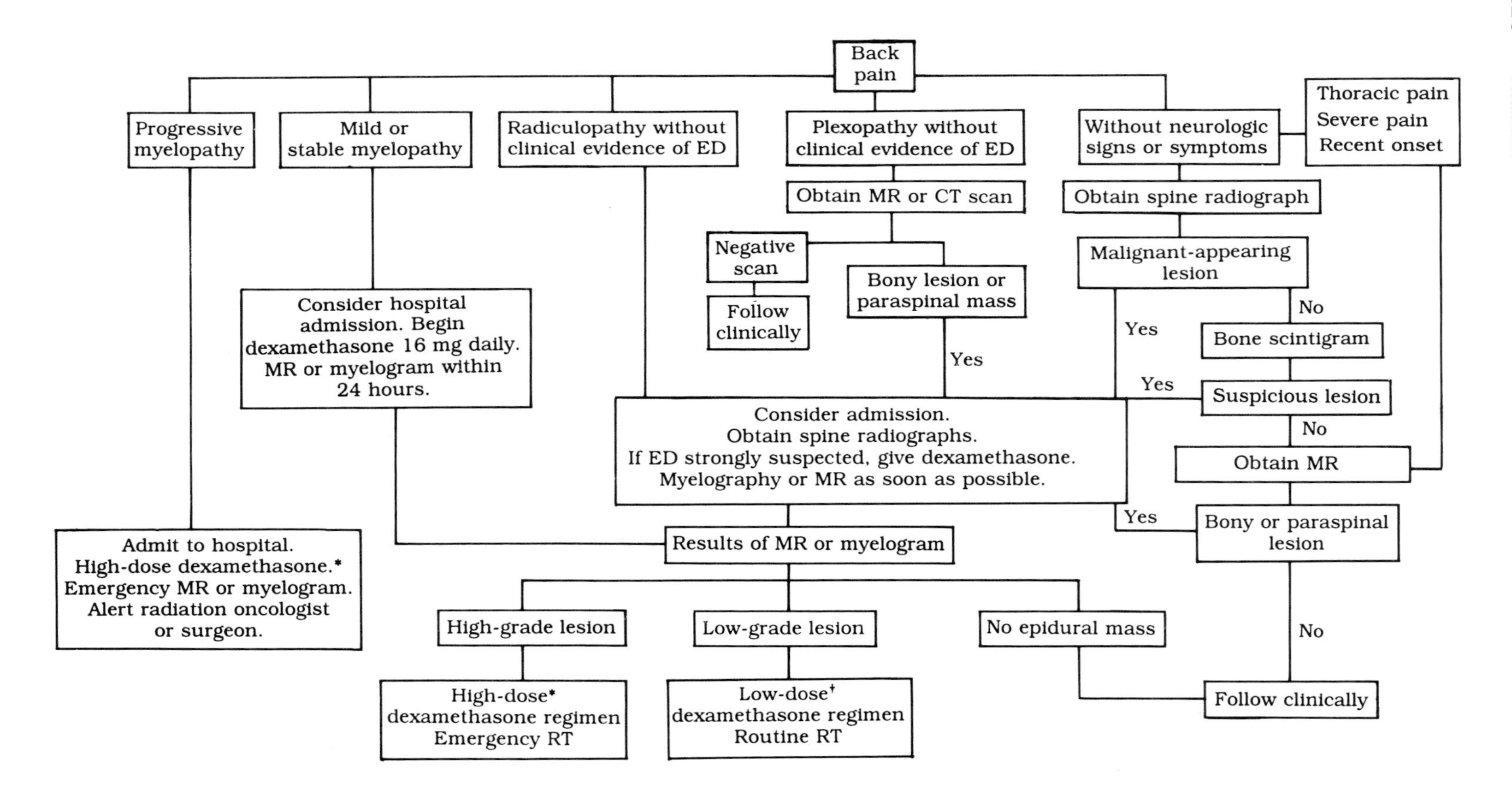

ED=Epidural disease
MR=Magnetic resonance imaging
CT=Computed tomography
RT=Radiation therapy

*High-dose=100 mg intravenous bolus followed by 100 mg po daily.
†Low-dose=16 mg po daily.

Figure 6–5. Management of back pain in the patient with cancer.

may miss a subtle lesion unless a localizing clue is available.

Recent autopsy studies suggest that about 25% of spinal lesions are not identifiable by plain radiographs[2844] (see Table 6–3). The incidence is highest in lymphomas (63%), testicular tumors (50%), and nasopharyngeal tumors (40%). By contrast, a collapsed vertebral body in a patient with cancer is not absolute evidence of metastatic disease. In one study, 34 of 155 patients with vertebral collapse did not have bony metastases, a false-positive rate of over 20%.[2844] Vertebral compression fractures with back and leg pain but without epidural disease may be a presenting symptom of acute lymphoblastic leukemia.[2163]

RADIONUCLIDE BONE SCAN

Bone scans are as sensitive as radiographs (91%) but less specific in predicting the site of spinal cord compression.[2062] They are more sensitive in identifying vertebral metastases that, even in asymptomatic patients, may be associated with a partial block.[1600] Bone scans, however, are often abnormal at sites in which vertebral bodies are diseased by processes other than cancer. In one prospective series, bone scans predicted with only 66% accuracy the presence and location of epidural metastases.[2187] In the few cases in which spinal abnormalities were visualized on bone scan but not on plain radiography, the myelogram was normal. As with radiographs, bone scans may reveal multiple uptake areas in the vertebral bodies but may fail to identify the block site.

Increased radionuclide uptake, the usual abnormal finding on bone scan, is due in part to increased blood flow and in part to sequestration of the technetium isotope at sites of new bone formation. When a destructive tumor neither substantially increases blood flow nor allows new bone formation, the scan may be negative despite extensive destruction. This occurs often with myeloma and occasionally with metastatic solid tumors and at the site of previous RT. In addition, the metastatic disease is sometimes so diffuse that the uptake by bone scan is uniform throughout, and the bone scan is interpreted as normal because there are no normal areas against which to compare those involved by metastatic tumor. Immunoscintigraphy, using a monoclonal antibody directed against the tumor, promises to be a more sensitive technique than standard radionuclide scanning for identifying spinal metastases.[2159]

COMPUTED TOMOGRAPHY SCAN

CT scans often identify metastatic lesions in vertebral bodies when plain radiographs and bone scans are negative,[1328] a particularly important point when a prior myelogram has identified a lesion that may be a herniated disk. CT scans can determine if a vertebral body metastasis has caused the disk to herniate.[2330] Furthermore, CT scans can identify paravertebral lesions that have grown into the spinal canal without bone destruction. Disruption of the bone cortex adjacent to the spinal cord on CT scan provides strong evidence that the spinal cord is compressed.[2062] CT scanning is limited, however, because only a few vertebral bodies can be examined, whereas the entire spine can be examined easily by plain radiographs, myelography, or MRI. Thus, to get the maximum information from CT scanning, the physician must direct the radiologist to a specific area as indicated by clinical examination or other radiographic study.

MAGNETIC RESONANCE SCAN

Because MR imaging is the procedure of choice to evaluate the vertebral column and the spinal cord, it usually eliminates the need for myelography (see the following), CT scans, and probably even bone scans and plain radiographs[2540] (Fig. 6–6). Although a few comparative studies still show that epidural cord compression is better identified by myelogram than by MR scanning,[1049,1052] refinements in MR technique have overcome this questionable advantage.* MR scans also are more sensitive in identifying metastatic disease in vertebral bodies than are plain radiographs and CT scans.[1612] Thus, although expensive, the MR scan has major clinical advantages both as a screening tool

*References 1135, 1328, 1557, 1560, 2451, 2540, 2541.

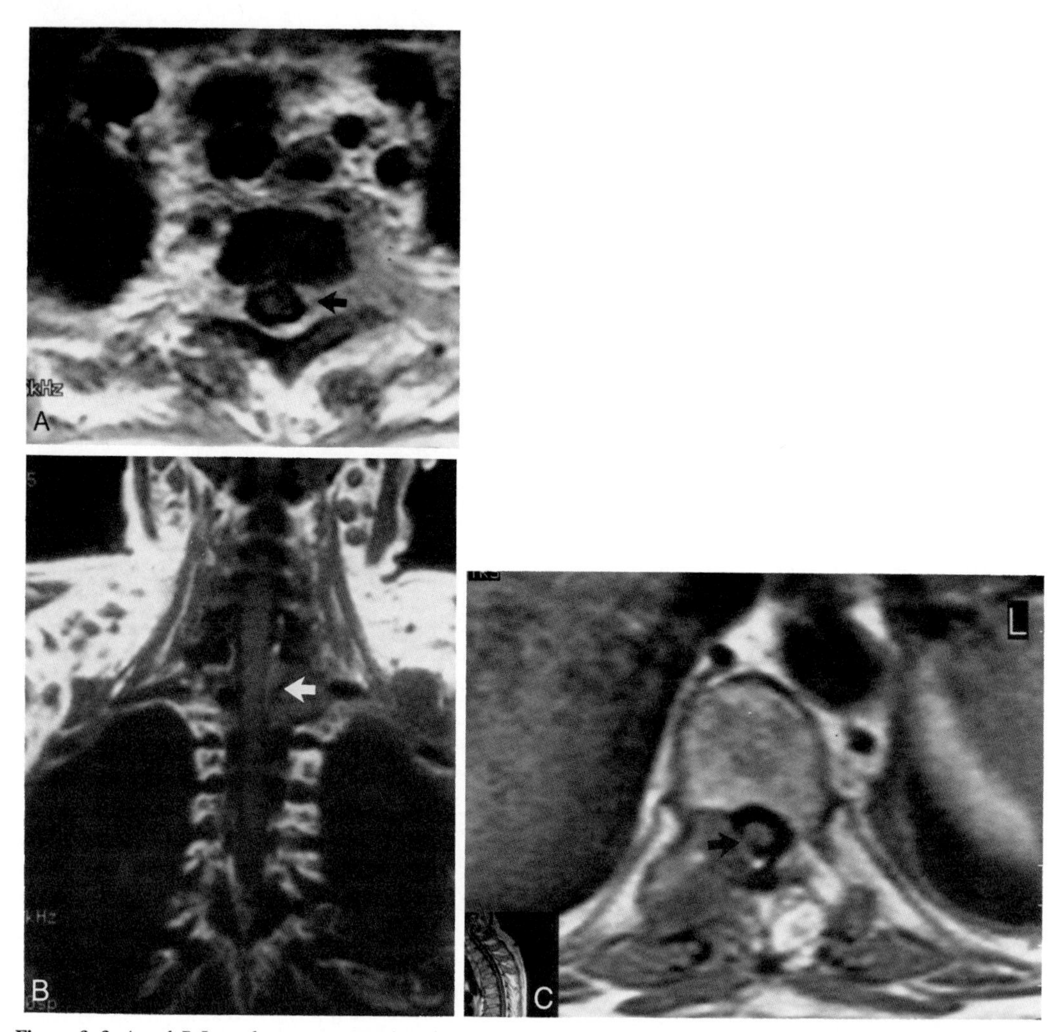

Figure 6–6. *A* and *B,* Lymphoma compressing the spinal cord. The tumor arose in the paravertebral space and grew through the intervertebral foramen to compress the spinal cord laterally (*arrow*). The bones are entirely normal. The tumor is distinguished from normal fat, as seen on the opposite side, by the difference in the signal and by the fact that the spinal cord is compressed (*arrow*). *C,* Metastases growing through the intervertebral foramen from a thyroid carcinoma. The spinal cord is compressed (*arrow*). Both anterior and posterior elements are partially destroyed by the primary growth, but the major growth is through the intervertebral foramen. The patient's clinical symptoms responded to radioactive iodine.

and as the ultimate diagnostic test to evaluate spinal cord compression.[1428] The disadvantages of MR scans are that they take more than 1 hour and that movement substantially degrades the MR image; many patients with severe back pain cannot lie quietly for that long. Faster MR scanning under development promises to shorten this time considerably. Steroids often give enough pain relief to allow the patient to lie still. Because myelography is faster, it may be chosen over MR in some instances.

MYELOGRAPHY

At MSKCC, improvements in MR scans, including faster imaging, have rendered myelography nearly obsolete. In those rare instances in which MR has not established the diagnosis in a patient strongly suspected of epidural spinal cord compression, the clinician should proceed to myelography. A complete myelogram is essential for two reasons: (1) to define the length of the block and (2) to determine whether additional lesions exist above the block encountered by the lumbar myelogram, which should be done first. About 10% of patients with epidural lesions have more than one lesion.

In a patient suspected of having a block, 3 mL of myelographic contrast material are inserted in the lumbar area under fluoroscopic observation to screen the subarachnoid space. If a complete block is encountered, contrast material is inserted via lateral C-1 to C-2 puncture into the cervical spinal canal, and the upper end of the block is discerned, completing the myelogram. The lipid-soluble contrast agents formerly used had the advantage of remaining in the spinal canal, so the myelogram could be repeated during follow-up examinations without the physician's requesting another lumbar puncture. In some patients, however, refluoroscopic myelography after treatment suggested a block even when none was present, probably because of asymptomatic arachnoiditis caused by irritation from the lipid-soluble agent exacerbated by either surgical trauma or RT. The water-soluble agents now universally used disappear rapidly, and if a repeat myelogram is required, another lumbar puncture is necessary. The newer agents often get past blocks that were impassable to lipid-soluble agents, and they are less irritating to the subarachnoid space. They also allow a postmyelographic CT scan to be performed to further delineate the site and nature of the lesion.

Lee and colleagues[1507] report that, in patients with apparently complete blocks to the passage of myelographic contrast material, an injection of up to 15 to 20 mL of air into the lumbar sac forced the contrast material past the block and allowed outlining of the upper end. They report "no apparent severe complications" in 240 patients; 39 of them had complete block, and in all, the "squeezing" maneuver was successful. I have had no experience with this approach but am concerned that forcing additional material into the spinal canal may be deleterious to spinal cord function.

The characteristic myelographic abnormality of epidural spinal cord compression is a complete or almost-complete block to the passage of myelographic dye at the site of a vertebral bony lesion or paravertebral mass, extending one to two segments. Longer blocks sometimes occur but are unusual. More commonly, when the myelographer encounters what appears to be a much longer block, such as a block at T-10 on lumbar myelogram and C-7 on cisternal myelogram, there are actually two separate lesions. The clinician can initiate steroid therapy (see the following), begin RT directed at the C-7 and T-12 vertebral bodies, and repeat the myelogram in 12 hours, hoping that some contrast material will move beyond the block to determine whether one or two lesions are present. If two lesions exist, then two RT portals can be drawn, decreasing the amount of bone marrow irradiated.

Like an MR scan, myelography can screen the entire spine to reveal additional lesions, including intradural metastatic nodules on cauda equina roots (see Chapter 7). Intramedullary metastases are not usually identified by myelography[708] but by MR scan. CSF obtained by myelography can be evaluated for malignant cells.

The major disadvantage of myelography is that the lumbar puncture can alter CSF dynamics in such a way that patients with a complete block may clinically worsen (see Chapter 14). One series reports a 15% incidence of increased clinical symptoms following lumbar myelograms in patients with spinal cord tumors.[1189] My experience suggests that this is a rare problem. Nonetheless, clinical worsening is an occasional risk. Some investigators believe that lateral cervical puncture alters the CSF dynamic less and is thus safer. Empiric evidence that supports this view is unavailable, although one report[1309] describes patients who developed spinal symptoms after undergoing ventricular decompression for hydrocephalus. If a complete block is suspected, steroids should be given immediately before the myelogram. The rapid onset of steroidal action may help prevent complications.

Differential Diagnosis

Many causes of myelopathy that may be confused clinically with epidural spinal cord compression (Table 6–8) are ruled out by MR scan or myelogram. The MR and myelographic pictures of intramedullary or extramedullary-intradural tumors, lepto-

Table 6–8. **DIFFERENTIAL DIAGNOSIS OF EPIDURAL SPINAL CORD COMPRESSION**

Diagnosis	Example(s)	Diagnostic Test
Intramedullary tumor	Glioma Metastasis	MR with gadolinium
Extramedullary-intradural tumor	Meningioma Neurofibroma Drop metastasis from primary brain tumor	MR with gadolinium
Leptomeningeal tumor	Primary lymphoma	MR with gadolinium, CSF cytology
Radiation myelopathy	Previous RT to spine	MR with gadolinium
Arteriovenous malformation		MR with gadolinium, myelogram, arteriogram
Transverse myelopathy	Postinfectious myelopathy	MR with gadolinium
Epidural hematoma	Thrombocytopenia (history of LP)	MR
Epidural abscess	Sepsis	Culture/MR
Herniated disk		CT or MR
Osteoporosis	Vertebral collapse	MR/Biopsy

CSF = cerebrospinal fluid; CT = computed tomography; LP = lumbar puncture; MR = magnetic resonance scan; RT = radiation therapy.

meningeal metastasis, radiation myelopathy, arteriovenous malformations, and subacute transverse myelopathy, all of which cause spinal cord dysfunction, are not easily confused with those of epidural spinal cord compression. Even epidural lipomatosis (see page 63) is easily distinguished from tumor by its density on CT or MR scan. Those illnesses that can be confused both clinically and radiographically with epidural spinal cord compression from systemic tumor include herniated disks, epidural hematoma or abscess, and, rarely, extradural hematopoiesis.

EPIDURAL HEMORRHAGE

On a few occasions, epidural hematomas are mistaken for spinal cord compression from a tumor and so treated. Epidural spinal hematomas associated with cancer usually occur in thrombocytopenic patients; are usually acute, without preceding pain; and are generally (although not invariably) painful at onset. The signs and symptoms usually evolve rapidly over minutes to hours rather than days to weeks. On scan, there is no evidence of vertebral involvement by tumor, and the epidural block usually covers several segments rather than the one or two segments characteristic of epidural spinal cord compression. Furthermore, the density characteristics of hemorrhage on the MR scan are different from those of tumor, except for a hemorrhagic tumor.[2845] When these clinical and radiographic factors are considered, epidural hematomas can usually be distinguished from epidural metastases, although at times the differential diagnosis cannot be made without biopsy. Unfortunately, most patients with epidural hematomas are profoundly thrombocytopenic and cannot undergo operative removal of the hematoma, which would confirm the diagnosis and treat the illness. Epidural hemorrhages from systemic vasculitis, as in polyarteritis nodosa, also occasionally cause spinal cord compression.[2186]

EPIDURAL ABSCESS

Epidural abscesses are rare in patients with cancer, but they can represent a problem in differential diagnosis. In these patients, an epidural abscess usually arises from either osteomyelitis of the vertebral body itself, a result of hematogenous spread of bacteremia, or from direct extension of an open wound of the head, neck, or back. The clinical picture of epidural abscess resembles epidural spinal cord compression. Pain, probably from vertebral body involvement, is the first symptom and is usually present for days or weeks before other neurologic signs appear, evolving either slowly or rapidly. Radiographs of the spine may be normal at onset but eventually almost always become abnormal; characteristically, two vertebral bodies across a disk space are destroyed. This is a hallmark of infection because it is rare for metastatic tumor to cross the disk space and involve two contiguous vertebral bodies, although two adjacent vertebral bodies may be involved independently with an intact disk between. Another characteristic is that the inflammatory response in the epidural space initiates a CSF pleocytosis; the CSF culture is negative. Most, but not all, patients with epidural abscess are febrile. To further complicate the diagnosis, epidural abscess may form at the site of a metastatic epidural tumor, but this is rare. If the diagnosis is in doubt, needle biopsy of the involved vertebral body will establish the diagnosis. Often, the patient can be treated by needle drainage of an abscess.

HERNIATED DISK

Herniation of lumbar or cervical disks (rarely thoracic disks) can mimic epidural spinal cord or cauda equina compression, leading to inappropriate treatment.[947] The signs, usually not those of spinal cord involvement, are local and radicular pain, sometimes accompanied by dermatomal sensory and motor loss. Characteristically, affected patients complain of pain when sitting or walking but usually have relief when lying down; conversely, spinal cord compression is usually associated with more pain in the lying position than when sitting or standing. MR scans should establish the diagnosis and also identify those instances in which disk herniation is caused by a vertebral body tumor.[2330]

OTHER EPIDURAL MASSES

Epidural spinal cord compression is occasionally caused by non-neoplastic masses, some of which are uncommon or rare and are listed in Table 6–9.

Table 6–9. **SOME UNUSUAL CAUSES OF SPINAL CORD SYMPTOMS**

Idiopathic vertebral hyperostosis
Hyperparathyroidism
Gout
Pseudogout
Rheumatoid nodule(s)
Epidural lipomatosis
Ossification of spinal ligaments
Calcification of arachnoid
Extramedullary hematopoiesis
Paget's disease (compression or vascular cause uncertain)
Osteomalacia
Amyloid
Nodular fasciitis
Vertebral hemangioma
Spinal cord malformations

Extramedullary hematopoiesis usually occurs in patients with severe hematologic abnormalities and only occasionally in patients with cancer who have widespread marrow destruction with compensatory hematopoiesis in the remaining vertebral marrow.[156] MR scan helps establish the diagnosis.[1628] Vertebral hemangiomas can also cause cord compression at single or multiple levels.[825,2901] The MR image differs from that of vertebral metastases in that both T_1- and T_2-weighted images are hyperintense.[2217] Radiation therapy, embolization, and decompressive surgery are all effective treatments in particular cases.[825] In patients on chronic steroid therapy, lipomatosis often develops, sometimes causing mediastinal widening or epidural cord compression.[1332,2008] Characteristically, the patient has been on steroids for a prolonged period and usually has other features of steroid excess; back pain is not prominent. The fat proliferation is often located posteriorly to the spinal cord rather than anteriorly as in most epidural tumors; MR signal of the epidural lesion is that of fat rather than tumor. Metastatic involvement of the vertebral body is absent.

Benign tumors of the spinal cord can also occur in patients with cancer. Meningiomas of the spinal canal are more common in women with breast carcinoma than in women without such cancer. MR scan or myelography can usually distinguish epidural from intradural tumors, but an exception occurs when the tumor metastasizes to a meningioma.[1175] Pachymeningeal amyloidosis from the polyneuropathy, organomegaly, endocrinopathy, monoclonal, gammopathy, and skin changes (POEMS) syndrome (see Chapter 15) also can cause spinal cord compression,[2600] as can nodular fasciitis.[2357]

Treatment

Several treatments aid in controlling symptoms of epidural spinal cord compression (Table 6–10). For most patients, definitive treatment consists of either RT or surgical decompression followed by RT. No definitive, controlled trial is available to guide the clinician toward a scientifically based decision for optimal treatment, although several studies compare the outcome of surgery with RT and other treatment modalities*; which one to choose in a specific instance is based on judgment and experience.

STEROIDS

The role of steroids in treating epidural spinal cord compression is discussed in Chapter 3, with a few additional comments here.[378,984,2679,2681] In some patients, steroids alone have salutary effects on symptoms and signs, particularly pain.[356,378,984,2679,2681] A randomized trial of high-dose steroids (96 mg dexamethasone) versus placebo concluded that steroid-treated patients were more likely to retain or regain ambulation.[2464]

Steroids have two mechanisms of action: (1) They may have an oncolytic effect on the tumor (Fig. 6–7), and (2) they ameliorate spinal cord edema. Oncolytic effects occur primarily in patients with lymphoma or breast carcinoma. In lymphoma, the effect is so rapid and dramatic that, if lymphoma is a suspected but not established diagnosis, the clinician should withhold steroids until a biopsy confirms the diagnosis.

*References 116, 511, 783, 784, 984, 1095, 1679, 2411, 2437, 2465, 2520, 2876, 2894.

Table 6–10. **TREATMENT OPTIONS FOR EPIDURAL SPINAL CORD COMPRESSION FROM METASTATIC TUMOR**

I. Treat edema
   A. Corticosteroids
   B. Possibly mannitol
   C. Possibly other agents
II. Radiation therapy
   A. External beam–high-dose per fraction
III. Chemotherapy
   A. Hormones
   B. Antineoplastic agents
IV. Surgical decompression
   A. Laminectomy
   B. Posterior-lateral approach
   C. Vertebral body resection

The length of time a clinician should wait to begin other therapy after steroids areadministered is not established. MSKCC's policy supports beginning definitive therapy, usually RT, immediately after the diagnosis is made by MR or myelography. One might argue that definitive therapy should be deferred, as it is with brain metastasis, for 12 to 48 hours to allow steroids to maximally shrink edema. Clinical data to refute or support such a position are not available. Unlike the situation in metastatic brain tumors, both experimental and clinical evidence[1768,2236,2567,2624] suggest that high doses of RT for epidural spinal cord compression do not cause immediate clinical worsening. Thus, steroids are used not to protect against potential side effects of acute RT, as with metastatic brain tumors, but to relieve pain and produce any other potential benefits that they may afford while awaiting the salutary effects of RT. Because of the rapid development of signs in cord compression, I have been hesitant to defer definitive treatment.

HYPEROSMOLAR AGENTS

Mannitol and hyperosmolar glucose[618] draw water from the normal cord at a location in which the blood–spinal cord barrier is intact. Little empiric evidence supports their clinical use.

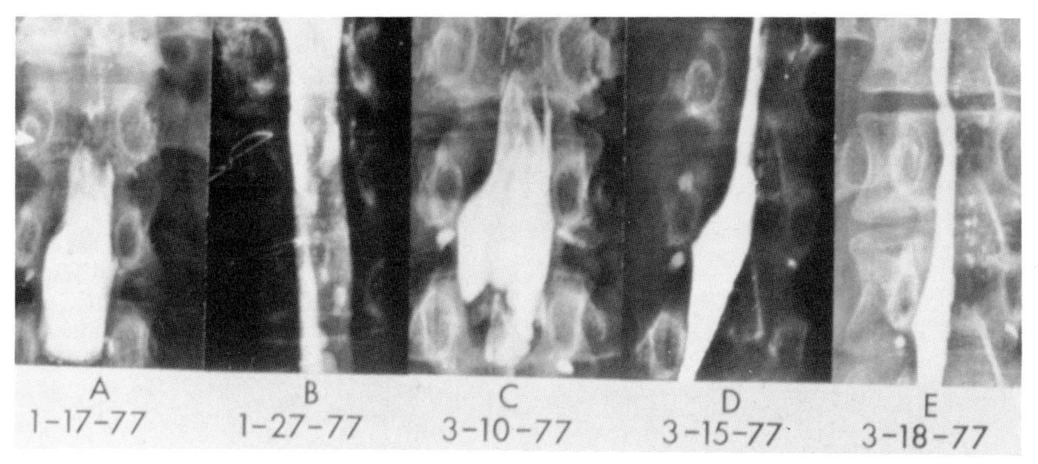

Figure 6–7. An oncolytic response to corticosteroids. This patient suffered epidural spinal cord compression from a metastatic malignant thymoma. *A,* A lumbar myelogram on January 17, 1977, reveals complete block of the contrast column at T-11. The major defect is on the right. No bone involvement is seen. *B,* On January 27, after 10 days of steroid therapy, a refluoroscopic myelogram reveals no extradural tumor. *C,* On March 10th, 9 days after steroids were discontinued, a recurrent complete block is at T-11 again with the major extradural defect on the right. *D,* On March 15, after 5 additional days of steroid therapy, the previous complete block again resolves. A small extradural defect is seen on the right. *E,* On March 18, the right decubitus view shows nearly complete resolution of the extradural tumor. (From Posner et al,[2075] p 411, with permission.)

HORMONAL AND CHEMOTHERAPEUTIC AGENTS

Only a few studies have been published regarding the effects of hormonal and chemotherapeutic agents used to treat vertebral metastases with spinal cord compression.* Because no blood–spinal cord barrier exists in epidural tumors, effective water-soluble agents should treat the spinal metastasis. In one animal study,[2644] Walker 256 tumors causing cord compression were treated more effectively by cyclophosphamide than by either decompressive laminectomy or RT. Steroids, as oncolytic agents, successfully treated some lymphomas compressing the cord, as well as some other tumors[2075] (Fig. 6–7). Occasional patients whose thyroid cancer metastasizes and compresses the spinal cord respond to thyroid suppression with thyroxin[937] and, conversely, develop spinal cord signs when thyroid suppression is withdrawn.[937,2397] Androgen suppression with orchiectomy or ketoconazole in patients with metastatic spinal cord compression from previously untreated prostate cancer may effectively relieve symptoms.[406a]

Several reports indicate that treating breast metastases with tamoxifen or treating prostate metastases with estrogens or antiandrogens ameliorates spinal cord symptoms, particularly pain. Tamoxifen may be useful even in estrogen-receptor–negative primary breast tumors because these tumors can occasionally spawn estrogen-receptor–positive spinal metastases. Carter[394] stresses the differences of methodology in reporting the outcome of spinal metastases from breast cancer treated with hormonal and chemotherapeutic agents. Usually little change is noted in radiographs of the spine, but relief of pain and survival are improved by chemotherapy. Few data report the salutary effect on other neurologic symptoms. However, one report[265] indicates that, in breast cancer with spinal cord compression, responses to systemic therapy equaled responses to RT. Positive responses to chemotherapy have also been reported in Hodgkin's disease,[342] non-Hodgkin's lymphoma,[1959] osteogenic sarcoma (either as a preoperative treatment[2521] or as sole therapy),[1923] germ-cell tumors,[496,866] Ewing's sarcoma,[1122] and neuroblastoma.[1122]

Specific hormonal and chemotherapeutic agents should be considered for treating spinal metastases and spinal cord compression

*References 342, 406a, 496, 1923, 2286, 2434.

in three settings: (1) An asymptomatic or mildly symptomatic patient with a vertebral metastasis with or without a small epidural mass might be given chemotherapy without other treatment; (2) a patient with spinal cord compression previously irradiated and who is not a candidate for further radiation or surgical therapy should be considered for chemotherapy; (3) in the acute treatment of symptomatic epidural spinal cord compression, chemotherapy probably should be used, if at all, in conjunction with either surgery or RT.

RADIATION THERAPY

Principles. RT is the mainstay of treatment even for patients who undergo surgical decompression (Fig. 6–8). Those cases in which the surgeon is generally unable to remove all or even most of the tumor require that RT follow surgery. All patients who do not undergo surgery require RT as definitive treatment except for those in whom chemotherapy is effective (see preceding). Although an optimal dose and fractionation schedule has not been established,[162,1288,1476] certain principles apply to most or all patients:

1. The smallest radiation port consistent with effective treatment should be drawn. RT to the vertebral bodies destroys bone marrow. The port is generally about 7 to 8 cm wide, but if a substantial paravertebral mass exists, the port must be modified to include that mass. The exact block site should be marked by the radiologist and carefully checked by the radiation oncologist and neurologist. Because many patients have widespread systemic cancer requiring marrow-suppressing chemotherapy, the less marrow irradiated, the better. In general, with epidural masses that involve one vertebral body, the port is centered on that vertebral body and encompasses two vertebral bodies above and below. Second lesions sometimes later compress the cord near the site of the first lesion, perhaps representing regrowth at the margin of the RT port, and arguing for a more generous initial port.[162,1329]
2. RT should begin as soon as possible after the diagnosis in patients with neu-

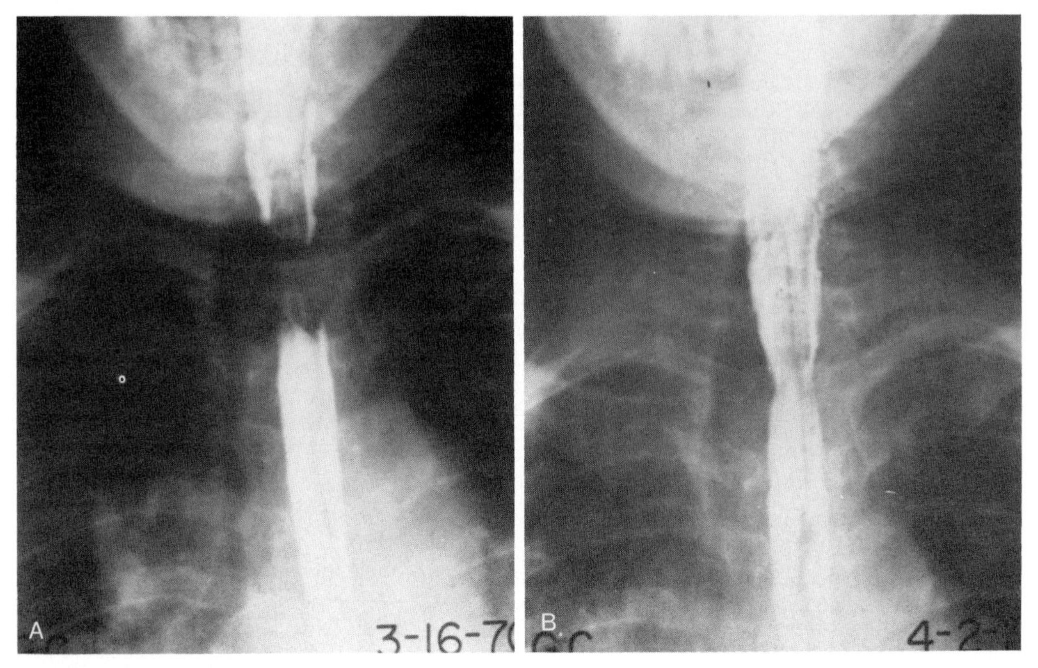

Figure 6–8. Response of tumor to RT. This patient with cervical carcinoma presented with rapidly developing myelopathy and a complete block at T-2. *A*, No bone involvement was identified on the myelogram. *B*, After 2 weeks of RT, the patient's neurologic symptoms resolved and the block largely opened. Although she was previously unable to walk, her gait returned to normal and she remained ambulatory until she died a year later of pulmonary metastases.

rologic signs or symptoms other than pain. The sooner treatment is started, the sooner it will work. Because neurologic signs and symptoms may evolve rapidly, early treatment is essential.

3. High doses of radiation should be delivered initially. One patient with paraparesis from metastatic prostate cancer was given a single tumor dose of 1000 cGy to T-8 to T-9 with resolution of pain and neurologic symptoms.[1768] Doses as high as 750 cGy have been given to children without ill effects.[2567] Protocols vary from 1000 cGy as a single dose to 200 cGy daily over a more protracted course.[1288] The usual dose is 3000 cGy in 300-cGy fractions. Based on animal experiments, which, of course, cannot be transferred directly to humans, 1000 cGy as a single dose was initially effective but led to earlier relapse when compared with animals given 500 cGy for three doses, at which dosage the response was slower but relapse occurred much later. A more protracted course of 200 cGy in eight doses was too slow; animals developed a permanent paraplegia before the RT could be effective.[2644]

   Some radiotherapists fear that radiation may lead to spinal cord swelling and exacerbate neurologic symptoms. Rubin's study[2236] in experimental animals indicates that the spinal cord did not swell when it was irradiated. Even high doses of RT failed to worsen the animals. MSKCC studies[2644] support Rubin's finding. Although animals given 1000 cGy in a single dose were worse the day following treatment, the worsening was less than in animals treated with lower doses or not treated at all, and by day 2 following treatment, the animals were substantially better. Furthermore, animals given steroids and then 1000 cGy were better the day following treatment, although the long-term outcome resembled RT alone.

4. The dose of radiation should be sufficient to treat the tumor but not enough to cause delayed damage to the spinal cord (see Chapter 13). The radiation oncologist should initially radiate patients with doses that are close to the tolerance level, hoping to eradicate the tumor for the remainder of the patient's life. Such doses may preclude early re-irradiation without a substantial risk of spinal cord damage if the patient relapses, but it appears preferable to treat the patient maximally at onset rather than to anticipate retreatment for early relapse. As indicated previously, our usual practice at MSKCC is to treat a portal encompassing two vertebral bodies, above and below the site of the block, with 10 doses of 300 cGy.

5. Worsening neurologic symptoms after apparently successful RT are not necessarily due to tumor recurrence. By eradicating tumor, RT may lead to further vertebral collapse and kyphosis, causing spinal cord compression that requires surgical decompression.[1602]

Prognosis. Patients with spinal cord compression who are ambulatory at the onset of RT are likely to maintain ambulation.* Table 6–11, from a recent series of 244 patients treated at MSKCC, indicates the likelihood of regaining or maintaining ambulation according to the initial motor score.

In most series, patients who have only pain do not become paraplegic if treated with RT.[2142] Some paraparetic patients regain ambulation, but in most series, the response of paraplegic patients is extremely poor. A recent study,[1134] however, suggests that patients who are paraplegic for hours to as long as 10 days may sometimes regain ambulation weeks to several months after RT. The rate at which the paralysis developed was more important in determining the eventual outcome of treatment than was the duration of paralysis; a slow rather than a fast rate predicted a better recovery. I have also seen delayed responses to RT but have not encountered recovery from total paralysis and sensory loss. MSKCC's policy is to treat all patients with spinal cord compression, whether paraplegic or not, recognizing that an occasional patient may have a dramatic response despite the statistics.

Patients who are not ambulatory but have reasonably good leg movement have about a 50% chance of regaining ambulation. As a

*References 265, 921, 984, 1288, 2465, 2624.

Table 6–11. **LIKELIHOOD OF REGAINING OR MAINTAINING AMBULATION ACCORDING TO INITIAL MOTOR SCORE AND TREATMENT OF 244 PATIENTS**

	STRENGTH PRIOR TO TREATMENT			
Treatment	**Ambulatory***	**Ambulatory but Weak**	**Unable to Walk (Paraparetic)†**	**Paraplegic**
Radiation therapy (N = 150)	56(96%)	40(80%)	32(47%)	22 (0%)
Vertebral body resection (N = 71)	33(97%)	20(98%)	17(47%)	1(100%)
Laminectomy (N = 23)	5(80%)	5(60%)	7(43%)	6 (0%)
Surgery (N = 94)	38(95%)	25(84%)	24(45%)	7 (14%)

*Number (%) of initial ambulatory patients who maintained ambulation after designated treatment.
†Number (%) of patients unable to walk who regained ambulation after treatment.

rule, patients with "radiosensitive" tumors respond better than do those whose tumors are less radiosensitive, but some with radiosensitive tumors fail to respond to RT, and some patients in the radioresistant group respond dramatically. One study[2130] reports complete relief of neurologic symptoms in 8 of 17 patients with cord compression from melanoma. Brachytherapy (implanting radioactive sources within the remaining tumor) has been used to treat paraspinal tumors in conjunction with partial surgical removal. The treatment appears to prevent subsequent spinal cord compression.[83]

Patients with a salutary short-term outcome, who can walk 2 to 4 weeks following RT, usually also have a satisfactory long-term outcome[984]; 75% of the patients ambulatory at the end of therapy were still ambulatory at 6 months, and 50% were still ambulatory at 1 year. Patients who do not regain or retain ambulation have a substantially shorter survival than those who do. The shorter survival results in part from the generally more advanced stage of disease of such patients and in part from complications of paraplegia, including infection, decubitus ulcers, and venous thrombosis.

BACK BRACES AND BEDREST

Back braces are prescribed for many patients with spinal cord compression, whether the spine is unstable or not. Many other patients are placed at bedrest when the initial diagnosis is made and are often kept there during the course of therapy. Neither bedrest nor back braces are indicated for most patients with epidural spinal cord compression. In the thoracic area, the ribs assist in stabilizing the spine, and back braces add little additional stability. Little or no evidence is available concerning acute damage to the spine with movement in patients with thoracic metastases, and the risks of bedrest in these patients who can be hypercoagulable (see Chapter 9) seem greater than any potential damage to the spine by ambulation. To the extent that it controls the pain when the patient is up and about, bracing the back can be tried, but the braces are cumbersome and patients rarely use them for any extended period. In the lumbar spine, bracing can also be tried for pain relief, but neither bedrest nor bracing appears necessary unless spinal instability is evident. For the cervical spine, a soft cervical collar, especially when the patient is riding in an automobile, generally is sufficient to relieve pain on motion and stabilize the spine adequately. Other, more restrictive collars, such as Philadelphia collars, are occasionally prescribed, although patients find them uncomfortable and rarely will wear them. If major instability in the cervical spine occurs, cervical stabilization should be considered.

SURGICAL THERAPY

The two surgical approaches for treating epidural spinal cord compression are posterior decompressive laminectomy and anterior vertebral body(ies) resection.

Laminectomy. Laminectomy decompresses the spinal cord and, by sectioning the denticulate ligaments, allows the cord to move backward, escaping anterior compression. Because in most instances the tumor is largely anterior to the spinal cord, the surgeon cannot remove the bulk of tumor; the purpose of the operation is to buy time for RT to take effect. When the tumor has invaded the epidural space posteriorly or posterolaterally, the surgeon can remove most or all of the tumor during laminectomy. A modified posterolateral laminectomy often allows considerable removal of tumor involving the vertebral body and has been advocated by some neurosurgeons in preference to vertebral body resection itself.[186,772,1956,2372] When a vertebral body collapse occurs (loss of 50% of vertebral body height) because of tumor, laminectomy may worsen neurologic symptoms by causing increased spinal instability.[783]

Most reports[783,921] suggest that laminectomy is not superior to RT to treat most spinal cord compression. One report suggests that in a subgroup of nonambulatory patients with lung cancer, gait was significantly better when they were treated with combined laminectomy and RT rather than with RT or laminectomy alone.[2263]

Vertebral Body Resection. Viewed as a more rational approach to treatment than laminectomy, vertebral body resection allows removal of most or all of the tumor, thus performing a "true cancer operation" rather than a simple decompression. The resected vertebra is replaced with either bone or a synthetic substance such as methyl methacrylate.[497,1095,2405,2415] Sometimes the operation is supplemented by brachytherapy. The spinal segment may be further stabilized either anteriorly or posteriorly. Usually, anterior stabilization is accomplished with Steinmann pins or plates screwed into intact bone rostral and caudal to the involved segments; posterior stabilization is achieved by instruments such as Harrington rods and hooks that engage the intact posterior elements. These stabilization procedures require intact bony elements above and below the site of compression; widespread bony metastases may preclude such surgical approaches. Using metallic instruments is disadvantageous because the metal prevents effective MR scanning of that area. Titanium instruments now being introduced may allow MR imaging with only minimal artifact.

Several reports[2011,2411] give impressive results: Harrington[1095] operated on 77 patients, many of whom were paraplegic, and reports that most regained ambulation (Table 6–12). Others have reported similar salutary outcomes. Cooper and associates[497] report stabilization or improvement in the motor function in 94% of their patients and ambulation in 88% postoperatively. Data at MSKCC (see Table 6–11) comparing patients who received laminectomy, vertebral body resection, or RT alone do not indicate statistical differences, although the number of paraplegic patients who received surgical intervention was too small for statistical analysis.

Table 6–12. **RESULTS OF ANTERIOR DECOMPRESSION AND STABILIZATION FOR METASTATIC SPINAL CORD COMPRESSION IN 77 PATIENTS[1068]**

Neurologic Status	Preoperative	Postoperative
Ambulatory	15	40
Paretic	27	24
Paraplegic	35	13

Hazards. Surgical therapy can be hazardous. Table 6–13 outlines the 30-day perioperative mortality and morbidity rates after either laminectomy or vertebral body resection and compares it with RT. Although the complication rate is greater after surgical treatment, the mortality rate is high in patients treated with RT, probably because of the poorer systemic condition of these patients. Although surgical mortality is uncommon, particularly with newer surgical and supportive care techniques, surgical morbidity can be considerable. In some series, as many as 8% to 10% of patients develop complications from the operation. Blood loss during surgery may be significant, particularly with highly vascular tumors such as renal-cell and thyroid carcinomas. Presurgical embolization may decrease operative hemorrhage.[2519] Worsening of neurologic symptoms may result either from bleeding in the epidural space or from manipulation of the compressed cord. Because most patients develop epidural spinal cord compression late in the course of their cancer when they are relatively debilitated and have often been on steroids, wound healing is poor and

Table 6–13. **30-DAY PERIOPERATIVE MORBIDITY* AND MORTALITY RATES IN 265 PATIENTS TREATED FOR SPINAL CORD COMPRESSION AT MSKCC**

	TYPE OF TREATMENT					
	RADIATION THERAPY (N = 168)		LAMINECTOMY (N = 26)		VERTEBRAL BODY RESECTION (N = 74)	
Complication	**Morbidity**	**Mortality**	**Morbidity**	**Mortality**	**Morbidity**	**Mortality**
Epidural bleed	—	—	1 (4%)	—	4 (5%)	1 (1%)
Systemic infection	10(6%)	8(5%)	7 (27%)	5 (31%)	8 (11%)	4 (5%)
Pneumothorax	—	—	1 (4%)	—	2 (3%)	—
Wound infection	—	—	4 (15%)	—	9 (12%)	—
Motor deterioration	—	—	1 (4%)	—	1 (1%)	—
Unstable spine	—	—	—	—	3 (4%)	—
Pulmonary embolism	—	—	—	—	2 (3%)	—
Total	**10 (6%)**	**8 (5%)**	**14 (54%)**	**5 (19%)**	**29 (39%)**	**6 (8%)**

*None actually deteriorated as a direct result of RT.
MSKCC = Memorial Sloan-Kettering Cancer Center.

wound dehiscence and infection are major risks. The dura mater should not be entered at the time of decompressive laminectomy or vertebral body resection, but occasionally the dura is nicked, leading to leakage of CSF. If this should happen and the dura is not repaired, it may heal spontaneously, but, in some instances, it becomes contaminated by bacteria and meningitis results.

COMPARING SURGERY AND RADIATION THERAPY

One controlled trial[2876] has been published comparing decompressive laminectomy with RT alone. The series was small and showed no difference between the two groups. Several retrospective and uncontrolled studies compare RT results with those from surgery or compare one investigator's results with those generally accepted in the literature. Interpreting these studies is fraught with difficulty because the criteria for selecting therapy were not uniform or controlled. The patients selected for surgery were usually those in the best physical condition and with the lowest tumor burden, whereas those selected for RT were often neurologically worse with more widespread systemic cancer. Conversely, many surgical series include patients who have failed RT. As might be expected, the results conflict. Early studies by Cobb and associates [465] (which addressed only breast cancer) and by Gilbert and coworkers [921] suggested that the outcome of RT alone was the same as that of decompressive laminectomy followed by RT. The Gilbert and coworkers study[921] included patients whose tumors were classified into relatively radioresistant and relatively radiosensitive tumors. No matter how the patients were classified or treated, most treated while still ambulatory maintained ambulation; about half the paraparetic patients regained ambulation, and the paraplegic patients uniformly remained nonambulatory. Sorenson and colleagues [2465] found no significant overall difference among patients treated with laminectomy plus radiation, RT alone, or laminectomy alone, but their subgroup of nonambulatory patients fared better with combined RT and laminectomy. Comparing data in a massive literature review of over 1800 patients, Findlay[783] found no substantial difference between the outcome of patients treated with laminectomy with or without RT, or with RT alone. He emphasized that the percentage of patients neurologically worse after laminectomy alone was generally higher than among those treated with RT because of instability of the spine caused by the operation. Thus, although the data conflict, most reports indicate no substantial difference between those patients who receive laminectomy as the primary treatment and those who receive RT alone.

COMBINED MODALITIES

Some investigators[2465] report that surgery combined with postoperative RT or chemotherapy is superior to either alone. Particularly gratifying long-term results have been reported with lymphoma[2014] and with myeloma,[1307] but these tumors are also often quite responsive to nonsurgical treatment.

INDICATIONS FOR SURGERY

My indications for surgery include:

1. *Unknown primary tumor.* If a patient with cord compression is not known to have cancer, a diagnosis from tissue samples is essential. An image-assisted percutaneous needle biopsy of the vertebral body is reported to give an appropriate diagnosis in 90% of instances, with a complication rate of less than 1%.[182] Results with blastic lesions are not as good.[1093,1094] Alternatively, the patient may undergo a more definitive surgical procedure, allowing both diagnosis and treatment.
2. *Relapse after RT.* If the patient cannot tolerate further RT and if the patient's general condition warrants, surgery is the only approach to relieve symptoms. In many patients, however, retreatment with RT often preserves ambulation, with low risk of radiation myelopathy.[2312a]
3. *Progression while on RT.* Perhaps the most difficult decision for the physician is that of determining what to do with a patient whose epidural spinal cord compression is being treated by RT and who seems to be getting worse. Most physicians seek surgical consultation. I often do the same, although my experience has been disappointing because surgery often fails to halt the inexorable progression of paraplegia. Persevering with RT may eventually give a satisfactory response.[1134]
4. *Rapid progression of neurologic symptoms.* Statements found in surgical literature indicate that a major indication for decompressive laminectomy is rapid progression of neurologic signs, but other statements list rapid progression of neurologic signs as a relative contraindication to decompressive laminectomy. Our own data support the latter concept. We compared surgery and RT in patients rapidly progressing and discovered that the outcome from surgical therapy was as poor or poorer than the outcome from RT.[921] Thus, although the physician's inclination in the patient who is rapidly worsening is to "do something," decompressive laminectomy does not appear to offer a satisfactory outcome.
5. *Cancer surgery as an option.* If the lesion is located in an area in which the surgeon can remove all or most of it by operative intervention, then surgical therapy appears to be the preferred treatment to debulk the tumor and allow RT to have its fullest possible effect. Such instances may include (1) tumors involving the spinous process or lamina, in which a gross total resection of tumor can be achieved, and (2) those in which only one vertebral body is involved, so that the surgeon can approach the lesion anteriorly, removing all or most of the vertebral body and the tumor in the anterior epidural space while successfully stabilizing the spine.
6. *Radioresistant tumors.* Certain tumors (e.g., renal) are highly radioresistant and a priori appear unlikely to respond to RT. However, a physician cannot be certain even when a tumor type is known to be radioresistant. If a particular patient's tumor has been irradiated previously and has not responded, the likelihood that the patient's spinal cord compression may respond to radiation is poor.
7. *Spinal instability* (see below).

Spinal Instability

In some patients with vertebral metastases, symptoms are not caused by the tumor but are secondary to spinal instability,[863] often with subluxation, as secondary effects of the tumor. Symptoms are caused by progressive kyphosis with extrusion of bone and disk into the spinal canal. Kyphosis can result not only from destruction of the vertebral body by tumor but also from successful treatment of the tumor by RT. Spinal instability, which accounts for the pain in about 10% of patients with vertebral metastases,[863] is likely to be present if (1) the tumor involves two or more adjacent vertebral bodies, (2) both anterior and posterior elements at the same level are involved, (3) involved vertebral bodies have collapsed to less than 50% of their original height, (4) the odontoid process has been destroyed, leading to possible atlanto-axial subluxation, and (5) any combination of the aforementioned occurs.

CLINICAL SIGNS

Spinal instability is characterized clinically by severe pain at the site of the lesion on attempted movement. With odontoid fractures and the atlanto-occipital dislocations, patients hold their head and neck stiffly, sometimes in a slightly awkward position, and refuse either to move it actively or to allow themselves to be moved passively. Occasionally, numbness is felt in the tongue (neck-tongue syndrome), a result of compression of afferent fibers from the lingual nerve traveling via the hypoglossal nerve to the second cervical root.[1465] The subluxed vertebral column may compress the cord, causing quadriparesis and respiratory embarrassment. In spinal instability at lower spinal levels, patients generally complain of severe pain when turning over in bed or attempting to get up. Usually, the patient is unwilling to move the affected part and exhibits tenderness to palpation or percussion over the area. The diagnosis of subluxation is easily made by plain radiographs of the spine. Spinal instability without major subluxation may be more difficult to diagnose; flexion and extension views may be required to establish the diagnosis. The patient should never be forced to move further than comfort allows.

TREATMENT

In patients whose general condition and degree of metastatic disease allow for surgery, stabilization is the treatment of choice.[497,1298,2012] Many patients with far advanced disease are poor surgical candidates, however; in others, the degree of destruction of the spine is so extensive that stabilization is not possible. These patients often benefit symptomatically from external immobilization of the spine by a cervical collar for cervical subluxation or a back brace for thoracic or lumbar involvement and by RT to the involved area. Radiation destruction of some of the tumor may allow enough healing to stabilize the spine, at least temporarily.

INTRADURAL AND INTRAMEDULLARY METASTASES

Metastatic disease within the confines of the dura constitutes fewer than 5% of all metastatic spinal cord tumors (see Fig. 2–6). These can be categorized into those that involve the subarachnoid space, predominantly causing "intradural" spinal cord compression, and those that actually invade the cord substance.[2010] Those involving the subarachnoid space represent various leptomeningeal metastases (see Chapter 7) but may present as a single mass lesion compressing the spinal cord. Intradural metastases arise when the tumor cells reach the subarachnoid space either by hematogenous dissemination or by spread of metastatic brain tumors,[1779] usually from the posterior fossa via the CSF[1780]; by perineural growth along nerve roots through the intervertebral foramen and into the subarachnoid space; or occasionally by invasion of the dura from an epidural mass. Such intradural extramedullary spinal metastases[1780,2010] cause symptoms by forming a single mass and compressing the spinal cord. Perrin and coworkers[2010] report 10 such patients with clinical features essentially identical to those of patients with epidural spinal cord compression. The primary tumors included breast (4), lung (3), melanoma (2), and uterus (1). The lesion occurred at T-5 in one patient and was found entangled in the nerve roots about the thoracolumbar junction in the remaining patients. Of the 10 tumors, 9 appeared to have spread from a brain metastasis via the CSF.

The intradural location of the tumor was identified by myelography and positive CSF cytology in two of the patients studied. Gadolinium-enhanced MR scan would probably be even more sensitive. Because the tumors are entangled in the roots within the subarachnoid space, they are not completely resectable; therefore, the treatment of choice is RT, perhaps with the addition of intrathecal chemotherapy (see Chapter 7).

Intramedullary metastases arise either from growth of subarachnoid tumor along nerve roots directly into the spinal cord or by direct hematogenous spread to the parenchyma of the cord. In 1972, Edelson and associates[708] found only 70 such cases reported in the English-language literature and added 9 cases of their own (see Table 6–14). Costigan and Winkelman[513] found 13 patients with intramedullary spinal cord lesions among 627 patients with invasive carcinoma whose spines were examined at autopsy. Of these 13 patients, 9 had hematogenous metastases to spinal cord substance; of those 9, only 4 were symptomatic; but in 3, myelopathy was the presenting symptom of systemic cancer. In the other 6 patients, leptomeningeal tumor invaded the spinal cord; two were symptomatic. In only 2 of 13 were the spinal lesions solitary central nervous system lesions; the others had brain metastases as well. The findings in all other series are similar to those of Costigan and Winkelman.[995,1281,2077,2832] Lung cancer was the most common primary tumor found (Table 6–14), representing almost 50% of the cases, equally divided between small-cell[1839] and non–small-cell tumors. Small-cell lung cancer is particularly likely to cause intramedullary spinal metastasis or leptomeningeal metastasis after prophylactic brain RT.[1192] Breast cancer accounts for about 15% of the metastases, and lymphoma (both Hodgkin's[1625] and non-Hodgkin's), for another 10%. In an occasional patient, a single intramedullary metastasis is the only site of metastatic disease. Neither the patient's symptoms nor neurologic signs distinguish intramedullary metastasis from epidural spinal cord compression.[708,2832] Those signs said to be more suggestive of intramedullary than extramedullary lesions—sacral sparing, early onset of autonomic dysfunction, and Brown-Séquard's syndrome—are not helpful in distinguishing different sites of metastases. Pain may be somewhat less common in intramedullary than in extradural lesions.[995]

Table 6–14. **PRIMARY TUMOR IN 100 PATIENTS WITH INTRAMEDULLARY SPINAL CORD METASTASES**

Tumor	No. of Patients
Lung cancer	41
Breast cancer	17
Gastrointestinal cancer	8
Malignant melanoma	7
Malignant lymphoma	7
Renal tumors	6
Adrenal tumors	3
Miscellaneous tumors	5
Unknown primary tumors	6

The tumor is often located in the ventral posterior horn and the medial lateral column, corresponding to the terminal supply of the central artery.[1105] It may be associated with hemorrhage, pencil-shaped softening, or syrinx formation.[824]

Diagnosis

Myelography demonstrates the lesion in only about 50% of symptomatic patients.[708] CT scan, whether performed postmyelographically with contrast material in the spinal canal or after IV injection of contrast, likewise may not be helpful. In those patients in whom intramedullary metastasis is a result of spread along nerve roots or from leptomeningeal metastases, the CSF often contains malignant cells. When the metastasis is hematogenous in origin, the CSF may be normal or have only a slightly increased protein concentration. The diagnosis, often impossible to make with CT or myelography, is easily made by enhanced MR scan (Fig. 6–9), in which a solid, well-circumscribed area of contrast enhancement is found in the spinal cord or subarachnoid space.[824,1558]

Once epidural lesions have been ruled out, the differential diagnosis includes primary intramedullary tumor such as glioma or

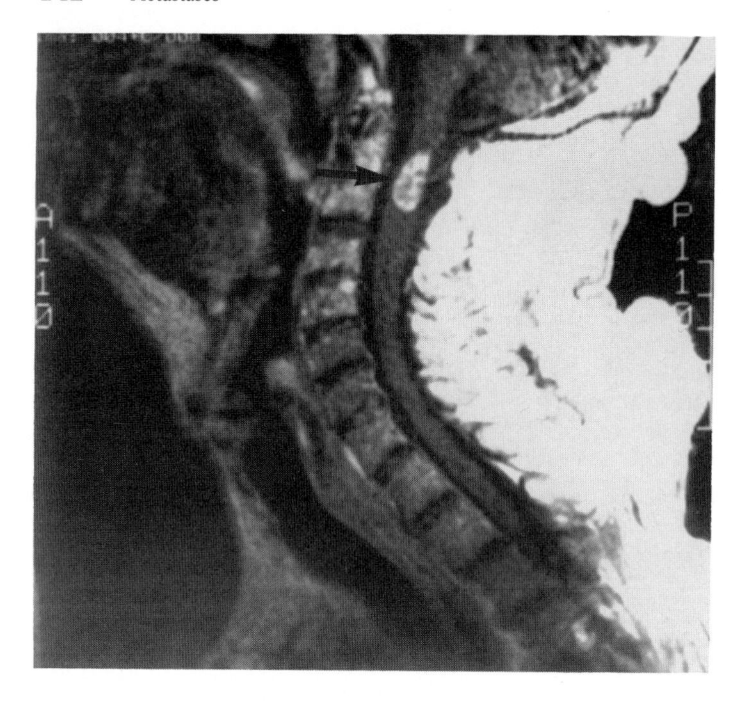

Figure 6–9. An intramedullary metastasis from lung carcinoma and an irregularly contrast-enhancing mass in the cord (*arrow*), consistent with the findings of a myelopathy at the upper cervical level.

ependymoma, radiation myelopathy in previously irradiated patients, spinal cord infarction from embolus or vascular occlusion, and paraneoplastic necrotic myelopathy. Cavernous angiomas of the spinal cord with acute bleeding can also mimic spinal cord tumors.[508] If bleeding is not evident, the characteristic MR narrows the differential diagnosis to primary and metastatic tumor. In a patient known to have cancer, particularly with widespread metastases, the diagnosis is obvious. In patients not known to have cancer, biopsy may be required to definitively establish the diagnosis.

Treatment

Most patients with intramedullary metastases develop the disorder late in the course of widespread cancer and live briefly, although they may respond temporarily to RT. In those few patients in whom the metastasis is isolated and in whom the spread has been hematogenous rather than via the subarachnoid space, the physician should consider surgical removal, particularly if the diagnosis is doubtful and surgical exploration can both establish the diagnosis and help the patient.

CHAPTER 7

LEPTOMENINGEAL METASTASES

Cancer cells that reach any portion of the nervous system in contact with the CSF are likely to be shed and float along CSF pathways to other areas of the nervous system, where they may settle and grow (Fig. 7–1). These cells may seed the meninges either diffusely or multifocally. The resulting leptomeningeal tumors may be visible grossly or only on microscopic examination. The tumor can remain within the meninges or invade the parenchyma of the brain, spinal cord, or cranial or peripheral nerves. The terms applied to this disorder have varied. When the primary disease is leukemia, the term "meningeal leukemia" is generally used. When the primary tumor is not leukemic, the general term "meningeal carcinomatosis"[890] has been applied, even if the tumor is a lymphoma or sarcoma. The terms "carcinomatous meningitis" or "neoplastic meningitis" are frequently used misnomers that suggest a leptomeningeal inflammatory response, which may or may not accompany tumor in the CSF.[1942] The terms "leptomeningeal seeding" or "leptomeningeal metastasis" seem more appropriate.

First described by Eberth[704] in 1870 and named "meningitis carcinomatosa" by Siefert[2404] in 1902, leptomeningeal metastasis was once thought to be rare, a subject of only individual case reports[963] and a diagnosis made only at autopsy. In 1974, two large clinical series of leptomeningeal metastases from solid tumors[1588,1942] could cite fewer than 125 previous reports.[1588] By this time, however, meningeal leukemia was clinically well recognized. Since the 1970s, leptomeningeal metastasis from solid tumors has assumed increasing importance in neuro-oncology because of its apparently increasing

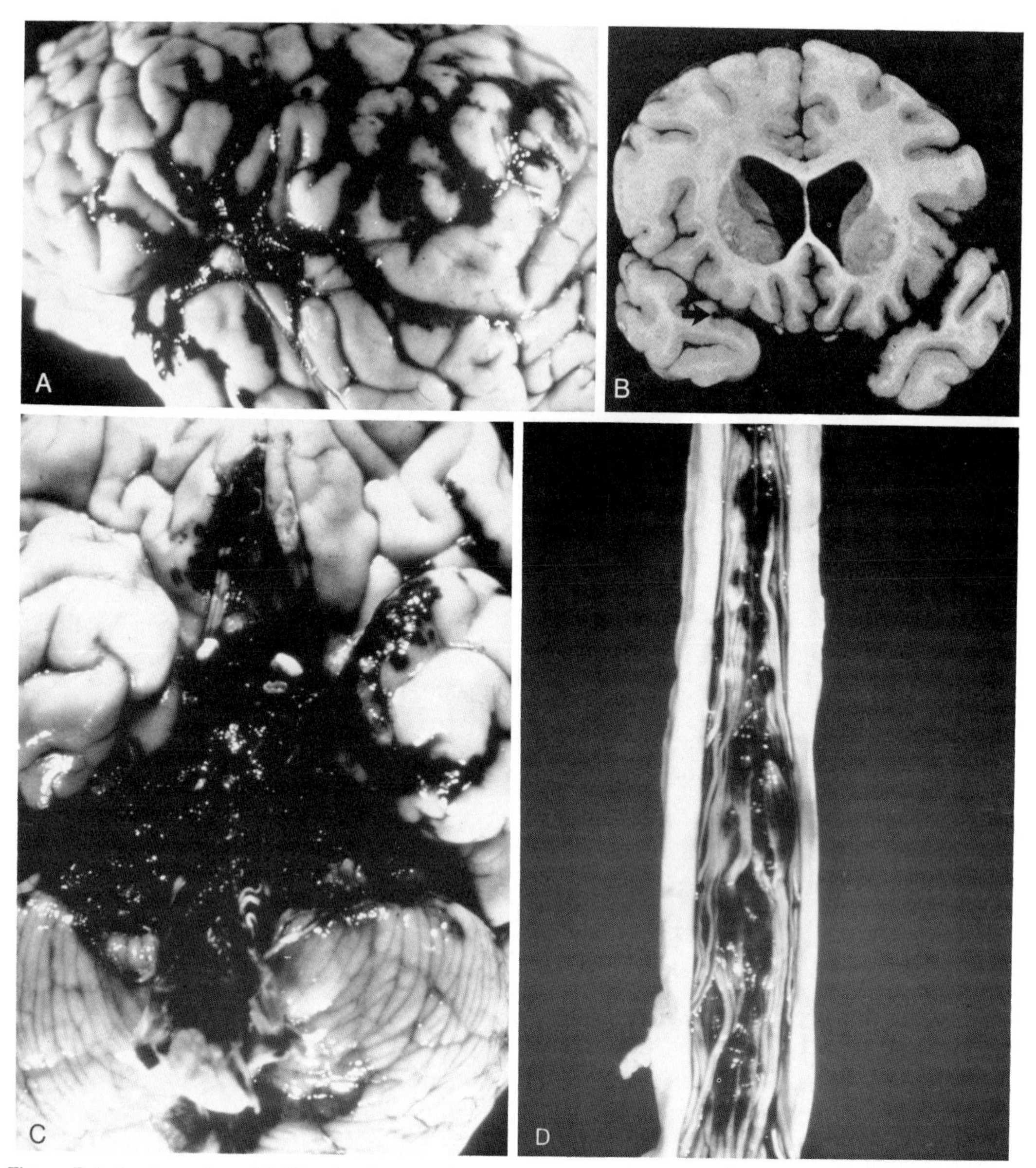

Figure 7–1. Leptomeningeal infiltration from malignant melanoma in a 23-year-old woman, demonstrating the predilection of tumor to concentrate in particular anatomic areas. *A,* Lateral view of cerebral hemisphere with tumor concentrated within the Sylvian fissure and the communicating sulci over the surface. Tumor is relatively absent near the dorsal surface. *B,* Coronal section of the hemispheres through the anterior portion of the Sylvian fissure shows the same pattern. A single, small, discrete cortical nodule is in the temporal lobe (*arrow*). Note the hydrocephalus that is due to obstruction of spinal fluid absorption pathways in the subarachnoid space. *C,* Ventral surface of the brain showing tumor concentrated within the basal cisterns, extending laterally at the optic chiasm to fill the communicating cistern of the Sylvian fissure. *D,* Ventral surface of the spinal cord showing tumor over the cord and nodular swellings along nerve roots. (From Olson et al,[1942] with permission.)

frequency and the severe neurologic disability it causes.[890]

FREQUENCY

Although the exact incidence of leptomeningeal metastasis is difficult to determine, several modern studies (Table 7–1) have found an overall incidence varying from 0.8% to 8%. The higher figure is probably the more accurate of the two. Part of the difficulty in tracking the incidence of leptomeningeal metastasis is that the tumor may be inapparent to gross inspection at autopsy, and, because it may seed the leptomeninges in a multifocal rather than a diffuse fashion, it may not be identified on microscopic examination unless the pathologist examines microscopic sections taken from several areas likely to be invaded by tumor. For example, in some patients only the spinal meninges may be involved[1987] (Fig. 7–2), and, unless the spinal cord is examined, the diagnosis may be missed. Furthermore, even easily identifiable clinical signs may be attributed to peripheral metastases or nonmetastatic disorders.

Leptomeningeal metastases from some primary neoplasms are increasing while those from other primary tumors are decreasing. Meningeal leukemia from acute lymphoblastic leukemia has decreased from as high as 66% of patients to about 5% of patients.[1590] The opposite is true of small-cell lung cancer[2205] and breast cancer,[262,2863] in which clinical evidence suggests an increasing incidence. We have encountered several patients with breast cancer whose site of relapse after high-dose chemotherapy with bone marrow rescue was in the leptomeninges. In addition, we have found a 12% incidence of isolated leptomeningeal relapse in patients whose systemic breast cancer has responded to Taxol.

Whether or not the rate of occurrence is actually increasing, reports of antemortem diagnoses of leptomeningeal metastasis causing clinical complications are more numerous than previously. Aisner and colleagues[22] report a 10% incidence in patients with small-cell lung cancer. Rosen and colleagues[2205] report an incidence of leptomeningeal metastases in 11% of patients with small-cell lung cancer. They also note that the actuarial incidence of leptomeningeal metastases rises from 0.5% at presentation to 25% if the patient survives for 3 years. Increased awareness of the problem led to an increase in antemortem diagnosis from 39% prior to 1977 to 88% after that date. Aroney and associates[86] report that 42% of patients with small-cell lung cancer who relapsed after initial treatment did so in the meninges; in 27%, the meninges were the only site of relapse. Prophylactic RT to the brain (see Chapter 5), which effectively prevents brain metastases, does not prevent leptomeningeal metastases in patients with small-cell lung cancer.[134]

The incidence of leptomeningeal metastasis from breast cancer at autopsy varies from 3% to 40%, depending on the series.[1505,2612] A recent study of leptomeningeal metastases with infiltrating lobular breast carcinoma reports a clinical incidence of 2.7%, which contrasts with a 5.2% incidence of brain metastases.[2445] As in other series, leptomeningeal metastasis was usually a late con-

Table 7–1. **INCIDENCE OF LEPTOMENINGEAL METASTASIS IN PATIENTS WITH CANCER**

Reference	Dates	No. of Autopsies	No. (%) of Patients with Leptomeningeal Tumor	No. (%) of Patients with Leptomeningeal Tumor Without Other Intracranial Masses
Posner and Chernik[2073]	1970–1976	2374	184 (8)	63 (3)
Gonzalez-Vitale and Garcia-Bunuel[946]	Before 1976	2227	—	18 (0.8)
Takakura and associates[2544]	1950–1970	3359	118 (3.5)	—

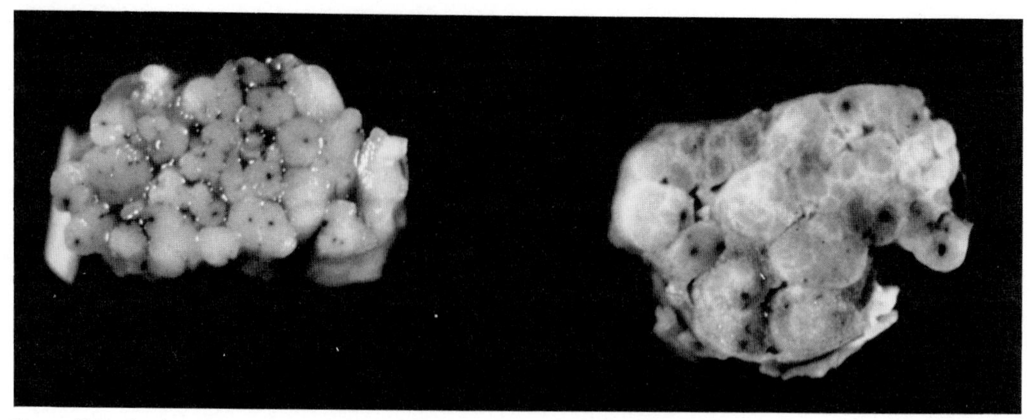

Figure 7–2. Cauda equina of a person who died without neurologic disease (*left*), and a patient who died with leptomeningeal metastasis from Hodgkin's disease (*right*). The spinal roots involved by tumor are enlarged and matted when compared with the smaller, discrete roots of the nondiseased person.

sequence of the tumor. In a Memorial Sloan-Kettering Cancer Center (MSKCC) study, we found the leptomeninges involved as the sole site of intracranial disease in 3% of patients with breast cancer. Leptomeningeal metastasis with or without other intracranial lesions was present at autopsy[2073] in 8% of all patients with cancer. Leptomeningeal metastases are usually accompanied by other metastatic CNS tumors, primarily dural or parenchymal metastases. Leptomeningeal metastasis was the sole intracranial lesion in only 40 of 2,088 patients who had cancer other than leukemia, an overall frequency of 1.9%.[2073]

Any systemic cancer can seed the leptomeninges. Several recent reports summarize the clinical incidence of leptomeningeal metastases from particular tumors, including acute nonlymphocytic leukemia (5%–15%),[598,2019] non-Hodgkin's lymphoma (6%),[734,1177] head and neck tumor (1%),[2140] breast cancer (5%),[2863] and small-cell lung cancer (15%).[2205] Gastric carcinoma, once believed to be a major cause of leptomeningeal tumor,[1789] is now rarely encountered. Carcinoma of the breast[262] and lung[2574] (particularly small-cell[2205]), melanoma,[1783] leukemia, and lymphoma are common offenders (Table 7–2). Other less common tumors that can metastasize to the leptomeninges include mycosis fungoides,[1111,1618] multiple myeloma,[1662] squamous-cell carcinoma,[2769] thyroid cancer,[148] rectal cancer,[306] carcinoid,[1850] rhabdomyosarcoma,[205] chronic lymphocytic leukemia,[398] and Hodgkin's disease.[181]

Not all leptomeningeal tumors are metastatic. Primary lymphomas,[1451] melanomas,[19,2300,2423] and rhabdomyosarcomas[2448] of the leptomeninges are less frequent than metastatic lesions but can arise as primary neoplasms confined to the leptomeninges. Most primary CNS lymphomas are parenchymal, often with leptomeningeal spread[580]; most metastatic lymphomas, on the other hand, are meningeal,[2135] but exceptions are not rare.[740,1304,1451]

Leptomeningeal metastases, although occasionally a first sign of initial or recurrent cancer, are usually a late manifestation of systemic cancer and often accompany relapse elsewhere in the body.[1942,2205,2863] Some patients develop symptoms before the primary tumor has been discovered, whereas others, particularly those with breast carcinoma, become symptomatic many years after the initial diagnosis and treatment of the primary cancer. Similar late occurrences have been reported with leukemia.[2343] Of 50 patients with solid tumors, 11 had no systemic metastases at the time neurologic symptoms occurred; the cancer appeared to have been cured in 5 patients.[1942] On a general hospital neurology service, most patients found to have leptomeningeal tumor have not been known previously to have cancer or they give only a remote history of cancer.

Table 7–2. **FREQUENCY OF LEPTOMENINGEAL METASTASIS AS THE SOLE INTRACRANIAL LESION FOR SPECIFIC PRIMARY TUMORS**

Primary Tumor	Total No. of Autopsies	No. (%) of Patients with Leptomeningeal Metastases
Leukemia	287	28 (10)
Acute lymphocytic leukemia	87*	21* (24)
Acute myelogenous leukemia	104*	5* (5)
Lymphoma	309	15 (4)
Hodgkin's	119*	2* (2)
Non-Hodgkin's	190*	13* (7)
Breast	324	11 (3)
Melanoma	125	6 (5)
Lung	297	4 (1)
Gastrointestinal	311	3 (1)
Sarcoma	126	1 (1)

*Subgroup of major category.
Source: Adapted from Posner and Chernik,[2073] p 583.

PATHOPHYSIOLOGY OF SIGNS AND SYMPTOMS

Hydrocephalus

Leptomeningeal metastases can cause CNS dysfunction in several ways. One of the most common is hydrocephalus (see Fig. 7–1B and Fig. 7–1C). The tumor invades the base of the brain and occludes the CSF outflow foramina of the fourth ventricle. It also frequently infiltrates the Sylvian fissure and, at times, the arachnoid villi. The meningeal tumor and its accompanying inflammatory response also increase resistance to CSF absorption, leading to hydrocephalus. Intracranial pressure is usually elevated, but slowly developing hydrocephalus may cause ventricular dilatation without elevation of CSF pressure (i.e., normal-pressure hydrocephalus). Conversely, rapid occlusion of the subarachnoid spaces by tumor, particularly when localized near the sagittal sinus, may elevate intracranial pressure but cause only slight to moderate dilatation of the ventricles.[1078] Both phenomena occur with leptomeningeal metastasis and may lead to diagnostic confusion, particularly when either hydrocephalus or increased intracranial pressure is the first or only symptom. Leptomeningeal leukemia may sufficiently raise intracranial pressure to cause tentorial and cerebellar herniation, sometimes leading to death.[2433]

Even in patients without evidence of hydrocephalus or increased intracranial pressure, substantial abnormalities of CSF flow dynamics often occur. Studying CSF bulk flow with a radioisotope instilled in the cerebral ventricle, Grossman and colleagues[1020] found such abnormalities in 70% of their patients with leptomeningeal metastasis. The abnormalities were of the following three types: The radionuclide tracer failed to (1) leave the ventricular system at a normal rate, (2) reach the lumbar sac at a normal rate, or (3) ascend over the cortical convexities within 24 hours. The results imply that chemotherapeutic agents injected into the ventricle of such patients may not distribute uniformly throughout the subarachnoid space. Furthermore, if ventricular outflow is completely obstructed, chemotherapeutic agents become trapped in the ventricular system and diffuse across the ependyma into the brain substance, increasing the likelihood of neurotoxicity.[1020] Chamberlain and Corey-Bloom[420] report finding unsuspected physi-

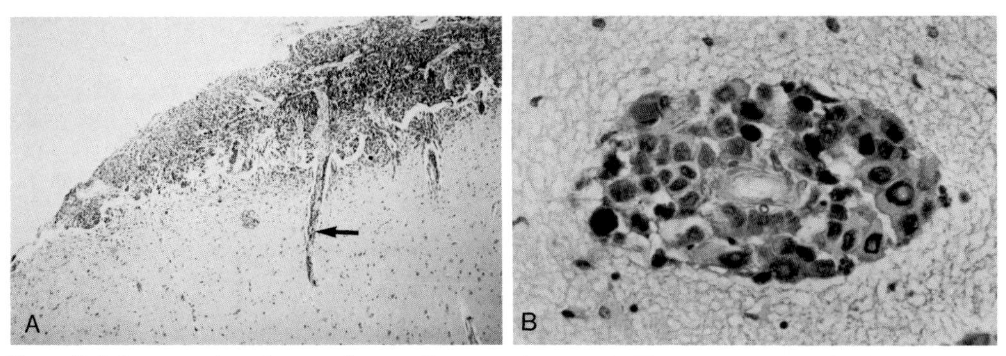

Figure 7–3. Leptomeningeal tumor from malignant melanoma. *A,* The tumor involves the leptomeninges over the brain's surface and grows down the Virchow-Robin spaces (*arrow*), but the brain parenchyma is not invaded. The area immediately underlying the tumor mass is pale, probably from ischemia. *B,* Examined at a higher power, the malignant cells can be seen localized to a Virchow-Robin space.

ologic blocks to radionuclide flow in the spinal canal of some patients with leptomeningeal metastasis. The abnormal CSF flow is due to the presence of leptomeningeal tumor because patients with leukemia or lymphoma who lack leptomeningeal disease have normal flow dynamics.[1043]

Parenchymal Invasion

Leptomeningeal tumor can grow along Virchow-Robin spaces into the brain to cause neurologic dysfunction, such as focal or generalized seizures[316] (Fig. 7–3). Such tumors may also extend widely within the perivascular spaces without actually infiltrating the brain itself. Conversely, the tumor may directly invade brain, spinal cord, and cranial and peripheral nerve roots to cause neurologic symptoms (Fig. 7–4).

Ischemia

The effect of tumor invasion into Virchow-Robin spaces down to the arteriolar level is not known, but such a tumor probably interferes with the blood supply or consumes oxygen meant for neurons. Microscopic examination of the brains of patients with leptomeningeal tumor has identified ischemic changes or frank infarction in cortical areas in which tumor has invaded (see Fig.

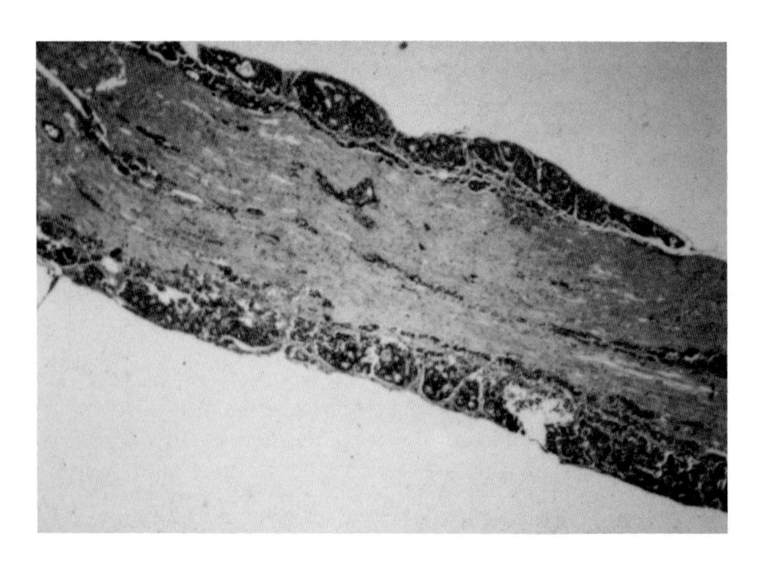

Figure 7–4. Infiltration of a cauda equina spinal root by leptomeningeal tumor. The tumor can be seen both on the surface of the root and within its depths. The area of infiltration is marked by pallor, indicating demyelination.

7–3).[1385,2750] In some patients with leptomeningeal metastases, a cerebral arteriogram will identify narrowing or obliteration of cerebral blood vessels.[1475,2750] Transient ischemic attacks[2750] and stroke[1385] are clinical consequences of these vascular changes. Cerebral blood flow is decreased in some patients with leptomeningeal tumor; the magnitude of this decrease roughly correlates with cognitive changes caused by the leptomeningeal disease.[2410]

Metabolic Competition

Symptoms may be caused by competition between the tumor and neurons for essential metabolites such as glucose.[1153] Leptomeningeal tumor invasion causes hypoglycorrhachia. In experimental animals, investigators find decreased cerebral glucose utilization in brain areas underlying leptomeningeal tumor and also at anatomically remote areas that are functionally related to structures subjacent to the tumor.[1153] The syndrome of "hypothalamic leukemia"[998,2049] can be explained by metabolic competition between neurons and infiltrating tumor cells. In this disorder, leukemic patients in systemic remission inexplicably gain weight. CSF examination reveals meningeal leukemia, and when CNS leukemia is treated, the weight returns to normal. In the few pathologically reported cases, the hypothalamus is infiltrated by tumor,[1047] presumably entering the brain from the third ventricle. Because other hypothalamic functions appear to be normal and the situation is reversible, the best hypothesis is that neurons in the hypothalamus sensitive to the glucose concentration are deprived by competition from adjacent tumor cells. An 18-year-old girl, an MSKCC patient, in remission after treatment for acute lymphoblastic leukemia, gained 20 kg during her first college semester despite being athletically active and obtaining high grades. Only when she discovered foot weakness did she return to her oncologist, who found 1000 malignant cells and a glucose concentration of 7 mg/dL in her CSF. RT to the brain and intrathecal methotrexate induced a weight loss of exactly 20 kg, returning her to her original weight.

Immune Responses

Several reports suggest that leptomeningeal metastases trigger an immune response in the CNS.[2317,2790] A recent study[2791] of 47 paired serum and spinal fluid samples from patients with leptomeningeal metastasis from a variety of carcinomas identified elevated immunoglobulin G (IgG) and immunoglobulin M (IgM) indices (CSF production of antibody), oligoclonal bands, increased CSF interleukin-6, and tumor necrosis factor-α, the last only in patients with malignant melanoma. The findings were not helpful diagnostically, and it is not clear whether they play a role in clinical symptomatology.[2789,2791,2806]

Blood–Cerebrospinal Fluid Barrier Disruption

The relationship of leptomeningeal metastases to the blood–CSF barrier[33,1887] is diagnostically and therapeutically important (see Chapter 3). Because leptomeningeal leukemia was not treated effectively by parenteral chemotherapy, the concept arose that the blood–CSF barrier remains intact when leptomeningeal metastasis develops. Clinical and experimental evidence indicate the contrary, however. Bleyer and Poplack[241] demonstrated that, after systemic injection, higher levels of methotrexate are achieved in the CSF of patients with meningeal leukemia than in those without the disease. This finding indicates that the barrier to the passage of that water-soluble chemotherapeutic agent is disrupted when the leptomeninges are infiltrated with tumor. Furthermore, leptomeningeal metastases can often be identified by contrast enhancement of the meninges in the brain or spinal cord, indicating disruption of the blood–CSF barrier. Gadolinium-enhanced MR scans are particularly effective in identifying this disruption.[828,837a] Ushio and colleagues [2646] have shown by entry of horseradish peroxidase into leptomeningeal tumor in an experimental rat model that the blood–CSF barrier appears to be disrupted through vascularization of the tumor by fenestrated capillaries. They also demonstrated that, although parenterally administered methotrexate is ineffective in prolonging survival in animals with leptomeningeal tumor when given prior to the fifth day after injection of tumor cells into the CSF, survival is prolonged if the drug is administered after the fifth day. These data suggest that leptomeningeal tumor does not substantially alter the blood–CSF barrier until the tumor's growth has been sufficient to stimulate its own vasculature. At that point, the barrier is at least partially breached, and chemotherapeutic agents can enter to a greater degree. Clinical evidence, however, indicates that the blood–CSF barrier disruption is not complete, and parenteral chemotherapy with water-soluble agents is not always effective in eradicating and certainly not in preventing leptomeningeal metastases. Nevertheless, some investigators have demonstrated good responses to systemic chemotherapy in some patients with leptomeningeal metastasis.[2404a] One report describes a good response of leptomeningeal prostate metastasis to hormonal therapy.[1744a]

CLINICAL FINDINGS

Leptomeningeal metastasis affects the CNS at more than one site, thereby causing multifocal signs and symptoms. Physicians should suspect leptomeningeal metastasis in patients with signs and symptoms indicative of nervous system dysfunction at more than one site.

For that purpose, it is useful to divide neurologic signs and symptoms into those originating from three separate anatomic areas—the brain, the cranial nerves, and the spinal roots.[1338,1942,2750] A fourth set of symptoms arises from generalized irritation of the leptomeninges induced by the tumor. Two important clues should lead the physician to suspect strongly the clinical diagnosis of leptomeningeal metastasis: (1) Careful taking of history often identifies symptoms suggesting involvement of more than one anatomic area, and (2) even if the patient's symptoms suggest involvement of a single anatomic area, careful neurologic examination may reveal multifocal abnormalities, indicating that other areas of the nervous system are asymptomatically involved. For example, a patient may complain only of focal seizures (brain), but when an absent ankle or knee jerk (spinal root) is discovered on examination, meningeal seeding becomes a likely diagnosis. Signs and symptoms indicative of meningeal irritation, such as nuchal rigidity when present in the afebrile patient, also suggest the diagnosis.

Not all patients have symptoms or signs involving the three anatomic areas. In one series,[2750] at the time of diagnosis 50% of the patients complained of symptoms in one area only, but only 25% had signs and symptoms limited to one area, suggesting unifocal disease. Another 50% of the patients had signs or symptoms suggesting the involvement of two anatomic areas, and about 25% had signs or symptoms pointing to all three anatomic regions. The earlier the diagnosis is considered, the greater is the likelihood of unifocal abnormalities. The most common site is the spinal area, involving more than 75% of patients. A little more than half have cranial nerve involvement, and half also have cerebral signs and symptoms. Leptomeningeal signs, such as stiff neck and pain on straight-leg raising, are present in only 15% of patients.[2750]

The following paragraphs summarize the symptoms and signs of leptomeningeal metastasis. The data are culled from several series of patients,* as well as some individual case reports.

Cerebral (Brain) Symptoms and Signs

Table 7–3, from MSKCC data, details the signs and symptoms in the intracranial cavity, except for cranial nerve signs.

HEADACHE

Headache affects almost 25% of the patients and is usually among the first symptoms, but the type of headache is nonspecific. In some patients it is bifrontal, while in others it is diffuse or located at the base of the skull, radiating into the neck. Headache is associated with nausea, vomiting, or lightheadedness in some patients. Rarely, the headache mimics migraine or cluster headache.[585] Severe episodic headache indicates plateau

*References 734, 1588, 1604, 1853, 1942.

Table 7–3. **CEREBRAL SYMPTOMS AND SIGNS IN 140 PATIENTS WITH LEPTOMENINGEAL METASTASES FROM SOLID TUMORS**

SYMPTOM			SIGN		
	Initially* (%)	**At Any Time (%)**		**Initially* (%)**	**At Any Time (%)**
Headache	38	40	Papilledema	12	12
Mental change	25	30	Abnormal mental state	50	50
Nausea and vomiting	12	20	Seizures	14	15
Vertigo/lightheadedness	2	4	Extensor plantar(s)	50	66
Gait difficulty	46	68	Hemiparesis	0	1
Dysarthria/dysphasia	4	12	Diabetes insipidus	1	2
Loss of consciousness	6	13			

*Total >100% because many patients had more than one symptom or sign.
Source: Data combined from Olson et al,[1942] p 125, and Wasserstrom et al,[2750] p 760.

waves associated with increased intracranial pressure (see Chapter 3).

GAIT DIFFICULTY

Many patients appear to have mild gait apraxia,[789,2513] characterized by a broad-based stance and difficulty lifting their feet from the floor when attempting to walk. Others are mildly ataxic, unsteady on turning or when attempting tandem walking, probably because of cerebellar pathway dysfunction. Some patients have leg weakness (see the following), further compromising gait. In most instances, the gait difficulty is hard to define on examination and probably has multifactorial causes.

MEMORY AND CONCENTRATION

About 25% of patients present with this complaint, and over 33% complain of cognitive dysfunction at some time during the course of their illness. In approximately 50% of patients with leptomeningeal metastasis, a careful mental status examination reveals difficulty with recent memory and sometimes with concentration.

EPISODIC LOSS OF CONSCIOUSNESS

This complaint usually results from seizures,[1338] but plateau waves are also an occasional cause. Increased intracranial pressure with resulting plateau waves may occur in the absence of identifiable hydrocephalus and may be relieved by ventriculoperitoneal shunting. Generalized or focal seizures are common. Nonconvulsive status epilepticus,[316,633] easily mistaken for a confusional state or psychosis, has also been reported.

OTHER COMPLAINTS

Other complaints include dizziness or lightheadedness and speech difficulty, either dysphasia or dysarthria. Diabetes insipidus (DI), a common complication of breast carcinoma,[2861] usually results from metastases to the sella turcica with secondary involvement of the posterior pituitary. Less commonly, leptomeningeal metastasis leads to tumor invasion of the pituitary stalk as it passes through the subarachnoid space.[2113,2572] In one series, metastatic invasion of the posterior pituitary caused DI in 20% of all patients seen in a mixed general and cancer hospital.[1214] Furthermore, DI occurs in almost 1% of patients with breast cancer.[1214]

SIGNS

Many patients have hyperreflexia and extensor plantar responses, but signs of major parenchymal dysfunction, such as aphasia, hemiparesis, hemisensory loss, or visual field defects, are uncommon. Visual field defects may occasionally arise from invasion of the optic chiasm or optic tract (see the following), but focal hemispheric signs usually suggest the presence of hematogenous parenchymal metastasis as well as leptomeningeal tumor.

Invasion of the cortex by leptomeningeal tumor can cause cortical brain dysfunction. An unusual and rare manifestation of leptomeningeal tumor with cortical invasion, the encephalitic form of metastatic carcinoma, has been identified by Madow and Alpers.[1645] In this disorder, neurologic signs result from the tumor's invading the underlying cortex.[802] The invasion is widespread, and because it is microscopic, the results of imaging studies are negative but malignant cells may be found in CSF. Patients generally present with confusion and disorientation, as well as frequent seizures and focal neurologic signs such as hemiparesis or a hemisensory defect. One report[1770] describes the triphasic waves typical of metabolic brain disease on the EEG of such a patient (see Chapter 11).

A unique patient with leptomeningeal tumor from adenocarcinoma of the lung suffered from cerebral salt wasting leading to hyponatremia.[1954] Another patient with leptomeningeal tumor presented with central neurogenic hyperventilation.[1342]

Cranial Nerve Symptoms and Signs

Cranial nerve abnormalities are not usually major presenting complaints of patients with leptomeningeal tumor, although on careful examination, mild abnormalities of ocular movement, facial weakness, or decreased facial sensation and hearing loss are often found. Both signs and symptoms of cranial nerve dysfunction become more prominent as the disease progresses (Table 7–4). Although the most common complaint is diplopia, patients also complain of hearing loss, visual difficulties, and less commonly, decreased taste, swallowing difficulty, and hoarseness. The general rule that most patients with ocular muscle dysfunction complain of diplopia before the examiner can recognize ocular paralysis does not apply to these patients, in whom eye movement dysfunction is often found without diplopia.

Blindness has been described as the first or most prominent symptom in a number of patients when tumor directly invades the optic nerves or optic chiasm.[41,1346] The phenomenon is most common in leukemias, lymphomas, and breast carcinoma. Because blindness can be a complication of chemotherapy (see Chapter 12), diagnosis may be confusing if the visual loss occurs during treatment.[263] Sudden bilateral hearing loss also has been reported.[1213] Vertigo and hearing loss resembling Ménière's syndrome can occur as a complication of subarachnoid tumor that has spread to the labyrinth and the cochlea.[1482,1952] In fact, Ménière's original patient may have had leukemic involvement of the labyrinth.[100] Isolated oculomotor weakness can be a presenting sign,[2812] but a more common finding is multiple unilateral oculomotor pareses, involving the oculomotor,

Table 7–4. **CRANIAL NERVE SYMPTOMS AND SIGNS IN 140 PATIENTS WITH LEPTOMENINGEAL METASTASES FROM SOLID TUMORS**

SYMPTOM			SIGN		
	Initially (%)	**At Any Time (%)**		**Initially (%)**	**At Any Time (%)**
Visual loss	8	12	Optic neuropathy	2	22
Diplopia	8	20	Ocular muscle paresis	30	38
Facial numbness	0	4	Trigeminal neuropathy	12	14
Hearing loss	6	9	Facial weakness	25	26
Tinnitus	0	4	Hearing loss	20	20
Dysphagia	2	4	Decreased gag reflex	0	9
Decreased taste	0	2	Hypoglossal neuropathy	8	10
Hoarseness	0	1			

Source: Data combined from Olson et al,[1942] p 125, and Wasserstrom et al,[2750] p 761.

Table 7–5. **SPINAL SYMPTOMS AND SIGNS IN 140 PATIENTS WITH LEPTOMENINGEAL METASTASES FROM SOLID TUMORS**

SYMPTOM			SIGN		
	Initially (%)	**At Any Time (%)**		**Initially (%)**	**At Any Time (%)**
Pain	25	40	Nuchal rigidity	16	17
Neck	0	2	Neck pain with movement	6	6
Back	18	50	Straight leg raising	12	16
Radicular	12	25	Reflex absence	60	76
Paresthesias	10	42	Dermatomal sensory loss	50	50
Weakness	22	50	Lower motor neuron weakness	78	78
Bladder/bowel dysfunction	2	17			

Source: Data combined from Olson et al,[1942] p 125, and Wasserstrom et al,[2750] p 761.

trochlear, and abducens cranial nerves and usually associated with meningeal invasion within the cavernous sinus (see Chapter 8). Unilateral facial palsy mimicking Bell's palsy is also a common presenting symptom.[2670]

A clue that cranial involvement is secondary to leptomeningeal tumor rather than to epidural tumor at the base of the brain (see Chapter 8) is that multiple cranial nerves are usually affected.[1246] If the involvement is bilateral, it is even more likely that the pathology lies in the subarachnoid space rather than at the base of the brain. The differential diagnosis can be difficult if only one nerve is involved.

Spinal Symptoms and Signs

Spinal symptoms affect more than 50% of patients with leptomeningeal metastases (Table 7–5). Leptomeningeal tumor frequently invades the nerve roots of the cauda equina, sometimes forming masses that can be seen on myelography or MR scan.[837a,2541] Occasionally, leptomeningeal tumor is restricted to the spinal meninges.[1987] Symptoms can be divided into two broad categories: (1) those caused by invasion of spinal roots (neural dysfunction) (see Fig. 7–4) and (2) those caused by invasion of the leptomeninges alone (meningeal irritation). Meningeal signs include pain in the neck or back, sometimes associated with nuchal rigidity, that can mimic acute meningitis in severity. When the lumbar puncture reveals increased pressure with a large number of white blood cells (WBCs) but few or no tumor cells, the differential diagnosis may be difficult, but the absence of organisms and the presence of malignant cells usually establishes the diagnosis, as discussed later in this chapter.

Direct invasion of nerve roots frequently causes radicular pain, sometimes mimicking the pain from a herniated lumbar disk. In addition to pain, patients complain of weakness, paresthesias, and bladder or bowel dysfunction. The characteristic sign of bladder dysfunction from spinal cord compression (see Chapter 6) or leptomeningeal tumor is asymptomatic bladder enlargement. The patient is unaware of the sensation of bladder or bowel fullness and often does not report a change in urination.

Spinal root signs, primarily the absence of one or more deep tendon reflexes, are found in approximately 70% of patients on initial examination. A cauda equina syndrome with bilateral leg weakness, foot numbness, absent ankle reflexes, and diminished rectal tone is relatively common.

LABORATORY TESTS

Those laboratory tests that help establish the diagnosis of leptomeningeal metastasis are examination of the CSF and MR scan of brain and spine. Myelography, cerebral arteriography, and other laboratory tests are now rarely indicated (Table 7–6).

Table 7–6. **LABORATORY ANALYSIS FOR LEPTOMENINGEAL METASTASIS**

Cerebrospinal Fluid
Routine
- Pressure
- Cell count
- Protein concentration
- Glucose concentration
- Cytologic examination

Special
- Biochemical markers
- Cellular markers—immunohistochemistry, flow cytometry
- Cell surface markers
- DNA–RNA flow cytometry

MR Scans with Contrast
Hydrocephalus
Focal masses
Meningeal enhancement

Myelography
Intradural masses

Arteriography
Extrinsic vessel narrowing

Lumbar Puncture

Examination of the CSF is the most valuable diagnostic test for leptomeningeal metastasis.[930,1338,1650] The test should be deferred if the patient is also suspected of harboring an intracranial or spinal mass lesion(s) because of the possibility of causing herniation (see Chapter 14). In this situation, an MR scan should be done first. If a mass is evident, lumbar puncture, if still clinically indicated, can wait the few days it takes to control intracranial pressure with steroids. Furthermore, the contrast-enhanced MR scan may establish the diagnosis (see the following). Patients with clinical evidence of spinal or cauda equina compression should probably have an MR first, or the lumbar puncture should be done at the time of myelography (see Chapter 6). If a block is found, treatment can be started immediately.

At the time the lumbar puncture is performed, care should be taken to procure enough CSF for full diagnostic evaluation, as will be discussed later. This includes a minimum of 4 mL for cytologic examination. (Table 10–6 details the amount of fluid required for other diagnostic tests.) Routine examination of the CSF in patients suspected of harboring leptomeningeal metastases should also include careful measurement of pressure, the counting of red blood cells (RBCs) and WBCs, and analysis of protein and glucose concentration. Culture for organisms is unnecessary unless one suspects infection.

CEREBROSPINAL FLUID PRESSURE

Because leptomeningeal metastases can obstruct CSF absorptive pathways, the CSF pressure is elevated in at least 50% of patients. Pressure elevations frequently occur without evidence of hydrocephalus on CT or MR scan. However, the physician should be careful to rule out other causes of intracranial pressure common in patients with cancer. For instance, because of its effect on cerebral blood flow and volume, elevated pCO_2 levels substantially raise intracranial pressure. An increase in pCO_2 of approximately 4 mm Hg doubles the intracranial pressure. Thus, patients with respiratory failure from lung and other cancers may have increased intracranial pressure. Also, intracranial pressure reflects cerebral venous pressure, which, in turn, reflects systemic venous pressure. Compression of the superior vena cava, congestive heart failure, and jugular vein compression raise intracranial pressure. These phenomena must be excluded for the physician to attribute an elevation of intracranial pressure, as measured by lumbar puncture, to intracranial disease.

The range of normal intracranial pressure, measured by lumbar puncture in the lateral recumbent position with the patient relaxed, varies between 90 and 250 mm H_2O or CSF.[500] In most patients, however, particularly the middle-aged or debilitated, the pressure is less than 160 mm CSF; higher levels should be viewed with suspicion. Levels greater than 180 mm CSF should enhance the clinician's suspicion that intracranial pressure is abnormal. The pressure should be measured as quickly as possible after the patient is relaxed; if one waits several minutes, leakage of spinal fluid around the needle can give a falsely low reading of a truly elevated intracranial pressure.[1617]

The only accurate indication of increased intracranial pressure is direct measurement. Some investigators report that the identification of venous pulsations on ocular funduscopic examination indicates normal intracranial pressure, but that sign is not reliable.[2671] The presence of venous pulsations usually is well correlated with normal intracranial pressure, but their absence does not correlate well with elevated pressure. Venous pulsations persist in a few patients with substantially increased intracranial pressure.

CELL COUNT

The WBC count is increased in more than half of patients with leptomeningeal metastases. The WBCs are usually lymphocytes, although occasional polymorphonuclear leukocytes are found. The cell count may vary from just a few cells to many hundreds, raising the suspicion of an infectious meningitis. Eosinophils in the CSF, usually suggestive of a parasitic infection, have been reported in a number of patients with leptomeningeal metastasis from Hodgkin's disease[1834] and lymphoma.[1373] The eosinophils may occur in the absence of malignant cells in the CSF and can be a strong clue to the presence of lymphomatous infiltration of the meninges in clinically appropriate circumstances. A patient with both eosinophilic and basophilic meningitis associated with leptomeningeal leukemia has been reported.[340] A note of caution: CSF eosinophilia can complicate therapy with ibuprofen,[2112] a drug frequently administered to patients with cancer for pain management.

RBCs associated with xanthochromia result from bleeding of leptomeningeal tumor. Bleeding can occur with any tumor invading the leptomeninges but frequently complicates leptomeningeal melanoma. The yellow color of the CSF is bilirubin and should not be mistaken for melanin which, when present in the CSF, is black. Frank subarachnoid hemorrhage is not common.[1604]

PROTEIN CONCENTRATION

The frequently elevated protein concentration is probably a combined result of breakdown of the blood–CSF barrier with exudation of serum proteins into the CSF and of tumor and WBC breakdown directly related to leptomeningeal infiltration. CSF protein concentrations of greater than 2 g/dL occur occasionally in patients with leptomeningeal metastasis and are at times sufficiently high for the fluid to actually clot.

The physician should assess CSF protein levels from Ommaya reservoirs with caution. The normal ventricular protein level of about 10 mg/dL is much lower than that in the cistern or the lumbar sac. A level of 30 or 40 mg/dL is thus a substantial elevation. In addition, a dead space is present in the reservoir. Protein appears to accumulate in this space if the reservoir is not tapped frequently. One of our patients, a 17-year-old boy with leukemia, underwent a puncture of an Ommaya reservoir that had not been disturbed for a year. The fluid in the 2.5-mL dead space of the reservoir was not discarded but was instead assayed and found to have a protein concentration of 366 mg/dL. A second procedure performed the following day revealed a normal ventricular protein concentration of 6 mg/dL.

In addition to the generalized increase in protein, increases may occur in specific proteins. Elevated CSF IgM in patients with leptomeningeal myeloma[2413] in the absence of an elevated albumin is diagnostic because IgM does not cross a relatively intact blood–CSF barrier and thus must be produced by cells within the subarachnoid space. Schipper and colleagues[2317] have reported that 8 of 22 patients with leptomeningeal metastases from various tumors had elevation of IgG in the CSF with an elevated IgG index or oligoclonal bands suggesting local production. Fractionation of CSF protein by protein electrophoresis or immunoelectrophoresis often gives additional clues in the analysis of patients with suspected leptomeningeal tumor. Elevated myelin basic protein concentration in the CSF is present in many patients with leptomeningeal metastases,[1853a] usually clearing after successful treatment, but it may follow treatment of meningeal leukemia.[1562]

GLUCOSE CONCENTRATION

Hypoglycorrhachia, although not common, is highly specific. A glucose level less than 40 mg/dL is found in 25% to 30% of patients with leptomeningeal metastases.[627,2750] In the absence of a clear-cut infection, hypoglycorrhachia strongly indicates leptomeningeal tumor. Some caveats, however, are necessary. A persistently elevated or depressed serum glucose level can alter the CSF glucose level, which generally is 50% to 60% of the serum level. Simultaneous measurement of blood and CSF glucose is not useful, particularly when the patient's serum glucose levels change rapidly, because it takes more than an hour for the CSF level to equilibrate with the serum concentration. I use an absolute level of less than 40 mg/dL as indicative of hypoglycorrhachia, recognizing that some higher levels may indicate a depressed CSF glucose in diabetic patients.

The cause of hypoglycorrhachia is unclear. Two possibilities exist: (1) diminished carrier-mediated transport of glucose across the blood–CSF or blood–brain barrier[792] and (2) glucose metabolism by malignant cells. I favor the latter hypothesis, in particular, because the close inverse correlation between the levels of glucose and lactate[2328] suggests that the glucose is being metabolized intrathecally. Glucose is metabolized not only by malignant cells, which favor anaerobic glycolysis, but also by the reactive WBCs and proliferating pial cells induced by the malignant infiltration. The degree of hypoglycorrhachia is not correlated with the density of cells found in the CSF, just as the number of malignant cells found in the CSF is not correlated with the number of cells infiltrating the leptomeninges.

CYTOLOGIC EXAMINATION

Cytologic analysis of CSF is the definitive diagnostic test and virtually the *sine qua non* for establishing leptomeningeal metastasis[48,930,1478] (Fig. 7–5). A minimum of 4 mL of CSF should be procured, immediately fixed in an equal volume of absolute alcohol, and then sent to the laboratory, where it is centrifuged, fixed on a slide with albumin, and stained. Some cytologists believe that higher yields are achieved and fewer false-negative results are encountered if CSF is filtered through a Millipore filter.[48,2340,2359] Others believe that better cytologic detail can be achieved by cytocentrifugation of unfixed CSF but only if it is delivered to the laboratory *within minutes* after its collection. Using the standard cytocentrifuge, our results appear to equal those obtained in the literature, although Kaplan and coworkers,[1338] using the Millipore filter, report a higher yield with CSF from the first lumbar puncture.

Table 7–7 indicates the results of examining CSF from 90 patients with leptomeningeal metastases confirmed by either clinical course or microscopic analysis at autopsy. Malignant cells were encountered in the CSF of approximately 50% of the patients at the initial lumbar puncture. The other 50% pre-

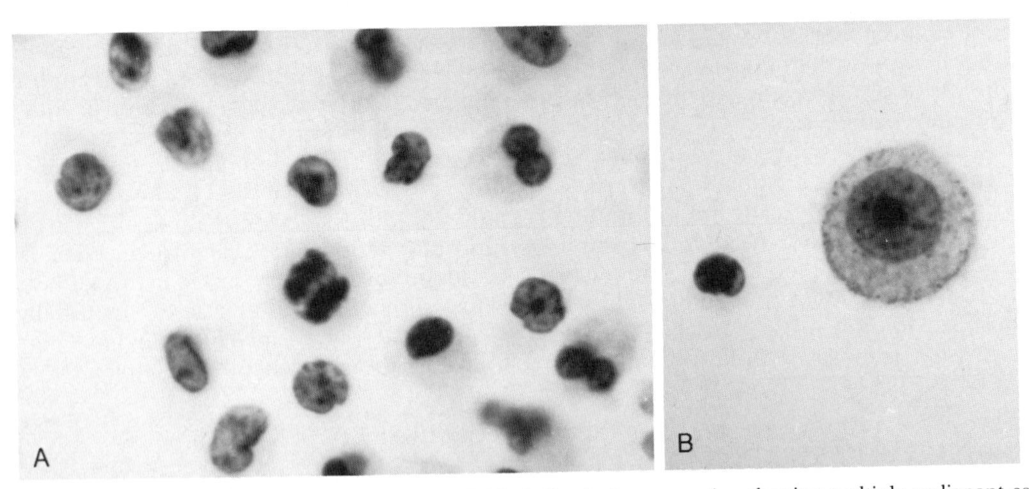

Figure 7–5. Malignant cells in the cerebrospinal fluid. *A*, Cytologic preparation showing multiple malignant cells, including one with a metastasis from a patient with small-cell lung cancer. *B*, A single malignant cell (*right*) next to a normal lymphocyte in a patient with malignant melanoma.

Table 7–7. **LEPTOMENINGEAL METASTASES FROM SOLID TUMORS IN 90 PATIENTS: CEREBROSPINAL FLUID FINDINGS**

	Initial	%	Subsequent	%
Pressure >160 mm CSF	45	50	64	71
Cells >5/mm^3	51	57	65	72
Protein >50 mg/dL	73	81	80	89
Glucose <40 mg/dL	28	31	37	41
Positive cytology	49	54	82	91
Normal	3	3	1	1

Source: From Wasserstrom et al,[2750] p 762, with permission.

sumably had "false-negative" test results. However, the CSF was virtually always abnormal in some respect. Occasionally, the CSF is entirely normal in patients with leptomeningeal metastasis identified by MR scan[837a] (see the following).

Sometimes repeated lumbar punctures are helpful; in about 90% of the patients studied, malignant cells are eventually identified. A false-negative cytologic test result is more likely when the leptomeninges are infiltrated sparsely with tumor, but sometimes a false-negative cytology occurs even with extensive infiltration of the leptomeninges of the cauda equina.[930] Apparently, in these instances, the tumor adheres tightly and does not easily exfoliate into the CSF. Our data indicate that a false-negative cytology is encountered more commonly with carcinomas than with acute lymphoblastic or other leukemias, although Kaplan and associates[1338] find no difference. Reed-Sternberg cells, the diagnostic malignant cell in Hodgkin's disease, are only occasionally found in CSF even when the meninges are heavily infiltrated.

A false-positive cytology (cells that are apparently malignant in patients who do not have leptomeningeal tumor) occurs in four settings:

1. The literature reports a 20% to 40% incidence of positive cytology in patients with metastasis in the brain but without leptomeningeal tumor.[136] This has not been our experience. When positive CSF cytology was correlated with pathologic examination of the nervous system at autopsy, not a single patient with a positive cytology was identified who did not have at least one detectable focus of leptomeningeal tumor.[930] At times, however, a patient with a brain metastasis that focally infiltrates the leptomeninges may develop a positive cytology. The incidence of such focal infiltration yielding malignant cells on CSF examination, in our experience at MSKCC, is low but must be considered. It might be wise to treat such patients because it is possible that, if untreated, diffuse leptomeningeal seeding will develop.
2. Malignant cells are sometimes found in the CSF of asymptomatic patients, especially with breast or small-cell lung cancer. These are not truly false-positive test results but represent early development of leptomeningeal tumor and are analogous to identifying malignant cells discovered on a routine lumbar puncture in patients with leukemia and lymphoma; in one series, 10% of lymphoma patients who were asymptomatic[2135] had malignant cells in the CSF. These patients probably require CNS treatment.
3. Sometimes reactive lymphocytes are misinterpreted as malignant, particularly in patients with lymphoproliferative disorders who suffer CNS viral infections (e.g., herpes zoster).[930,1340a,2135] In general, these errors can be avoided if the patient's physician reviews the cytologic slides with the pathologist, giving him or her the benefit of the full history and clinical situation.
4. The physician should always be aware of possible technical errors. At times, slides can be mislabeled.

Striking differences may be evident in both

Table 7–8. **SOME CEREBROSPINAL FLUID TUMOR MARKERS**

CSF Tumor Marker	Comments
Carcinoembryonic antigen (CEA)	Greater than 1% of serum CEA* suggests leptomeningeal tumor
Human chorionic gonadotropin (β-HCG)	Choriocarcinoma, embryonal carcinoma, germ-cell tumor
Alpha-fetoprotein	Teratocarcinoma, yolk sac tumor, endodermal sinus tumor, embryonal carcinoma
CA-125	Ovarian carcinoma
CA 15-3 (BRCA)	Breast cancer
β_2-microglobulin	Above 2.0 mg/L,* elevated by infection; carcinoma and lymphoma (not specific)
β-glucuronidase	Above 80 mU/L* (not specific)
Lactic dehydrogenase (LDH)	Isozyme V above 10% of total LDH* (not specific; elevated by infection and neoplasia)

*Values suggestive of leptomeningeal metastasis.

biochemistry and cytology between the lumbar and ventricular CSF. Often the cytology is positive in the lumbar CSF but negative in the ventricular CSF; the opposite is rare. Protein concentration, normal in the ventricle, may be grossly elevated in the lumbar space, and hypoglycorrhachia may be present in the lumbar space and absent in the ventricle. Thus, both for the initial diagnosis and after the effects of therapy, lumbar CSF samples are vital.[1840,2627] Our policy is to perform at least three lumbar punctures over several days in patients suspected of harboring leptomeningeal metastases if the cytology is initially negative. Occasionally, cisternal fluid is positive when lumbar punctures are negative.[1840,2195] Cisternal fluid can be sampled by a lateral cervical puncture at C-2 under fluoroscopic visualization.

Immunocytochemistry

Pathologic examination of the CSF using monoclonal antibodies has been reported recently to enhance routine cytologic examination.[268,464,888] In one series, combined use of routine cytology and immunocytochemistry led to a 9% increase in sensitivity for detecting malignant cells. Thus, the technique is useful only in a limited number of patients. Monoclonal antibodies against surface markers on lymphocytes can be useful to diagnose CNS lymphoma. They are particularly helpful if cytologic evaluation fails to distinguish between reactive and malignant lymphocytes. Demonstration by surface markers of a monoclonal population of lymphocytes establishes the diagnosis of tumor. Unfortunately, polyclonality does not rule out tumor because a combination of malignant lymphocytes and lymphocytes reactive to the malignancy may lead to polyclonal proliferation.[747,1420,1556]

Biochemical Markers

The markers listed in Table 7–8 have assumed more importance in the diagnosis of systemic cancer in recent years and have been analyzed in the CSF as a means of identifying leptomeningeal metastases.* Carcinoembryonic antigen (CEA), alpha-fetoprotein (AFP), beta human chorionic gonadotropin (βHCG), and other biochemical markers have proved useful not only in assisting in the diagnosis of malignant disease but also in following the course of treatment.†

Biochemical markers can be divided into specific and nonspecific categories. When found in the CSF, specific markers, such as

*References 10, 118, 119, 1080, 1664, 1710, 1842, 1852, 1882, 1955a, 2545, 2672, 2673.

†References 1384, 1664, 1710, 1955a, 2545, 2627, 2673, 2750, 2751, 2862.

CEA,[2673] AFP, βHCG, and melanin (in the case of melanoma), are virtually diagnostic of leptomeningeal metastasis from a specific tumor except when a very high serum concentration of the marker has led to seepage into the CSF across a normal blood–brain barrier or a blood–brain barrier partially disrupted by a metastatic brain tumor. To distinguish between these possibilities, the serum and CSF concentrations should be compared. For practical purposes, a rapid calculation of the expected CSF-serum ratio (1% with CEA) will determine whether the CSF is disproportionately elevated. Metastases outside the leptomeninges, such as in the brain, do not seem to have a substantial effect on the CSF concentration of these markers. Gross elevation of substances normally found at low levels in the CSF, such as IgM in patients with multiple myeloma or 5-hydroxyindoleacetic acid (5-HIAA) in patients with carcinoid,[1850] are also diagnostic. A high molecular weight, epithelial-associated glycoprotein antigen (HMFG1) has been reported in the CSF of patients with leptomeningeal tumors but not in normal CSF or inflammatory meningitis.[1822] Galactotransferases are elevated in the CSF of patients with meningeal leukemia and lymphoma and decline rapidly with intrathecal chemotherapy.[1955a]

The nonspecific markers, such as β-glucuronidase,[2545] isozyme V of lactic dehydrogenase,[2751] β_2-microglobulin,[1080] and myelin basic protein,[1651,1853a] although elevated in many patients with leptomeningeal tumors (the β_2-microglobulin particularly in leukemias and lymphomas), may also be elevated in patients with inflammatory disorders of the nervous system.[1710,2018] Elevated CSF alkaline phosphatase concentration has been reported for leptomeningeal metastasis from lung carcinoma.[1463] CSF ferritin has also been measured as a potential marker of leptomeningeal metastasis and has been found useful as a nonspecific marker of either inflammatory or neoplastic meningeal involvement by some, but not all, researchers.[1774,2887] Prostate-specific antigen may be elevated when prostate cancer involves the leptomeninges.[1744a] If a physician can confidently rule out inflammatory meningitis, striking elevations of these biochemical markers indicate the presence of leptomeningeal tumor. In general, all markers are lower in concentration in ventricular than in lumbar fluid.[2750]

Flow Cytometry

Another method used to examine CSF cells for malignancy is flow cytometry.[457,696] Flow cytometry occasionally detects abnormal cells when the results of routine cytologic analysis are negative and when biochemical markers are absent. The presence of aneuploid cells and, in particular, hyperdiploid cells in CSF strongly suggests leptomeningeal tumor. In addition, CSF cells can be examined by flow cytometry for the presence of CEA on cell surfaces, occasionally proving to be diagnostically useful. Flow cytometry's role in diagnosing leptomeningeal tumor is still being investigated.

According to one report,[966] the chromosomal analysis of cells in the CSF has helped diagnose leptomeningeal metastases from lung cancer.

Computed Tomography or Magnetic Resonance Scanning

Two findings help identify leptomeningeal metastases by CT or MR scan.* First, the scan can identify areas of disrupted blood–CSF barrier, both cerebral (Fig. 7–6) and spinal (Fig. 7–7).[1268,1429,1506,2878] These changes are not pathognomonic because similar images can be caused by acute or chronic inflammatory lesions of the leptomeninges or by lumbar puncture in the absence of tumor (see Chapter 14). When the clinical suspicion of leptomeningeal metastasis is strong, however, a CT or MR scan showing contrast enhancement in the basal cisterns, cauda equina, or ependyma provides sufficient confirmation for treatment even in the absence of identifiable malignant cells in the CSF. On the MR scan, the enhancement may be diffuse or may reveal multiple nodules, particularly in the cauda equina. Frequent false-negative findings in cytologically proved leptomeningeal metastases[2878] may be de-

*References 1417, 1568, 2185, 2334, 2591, 2630, 2878.

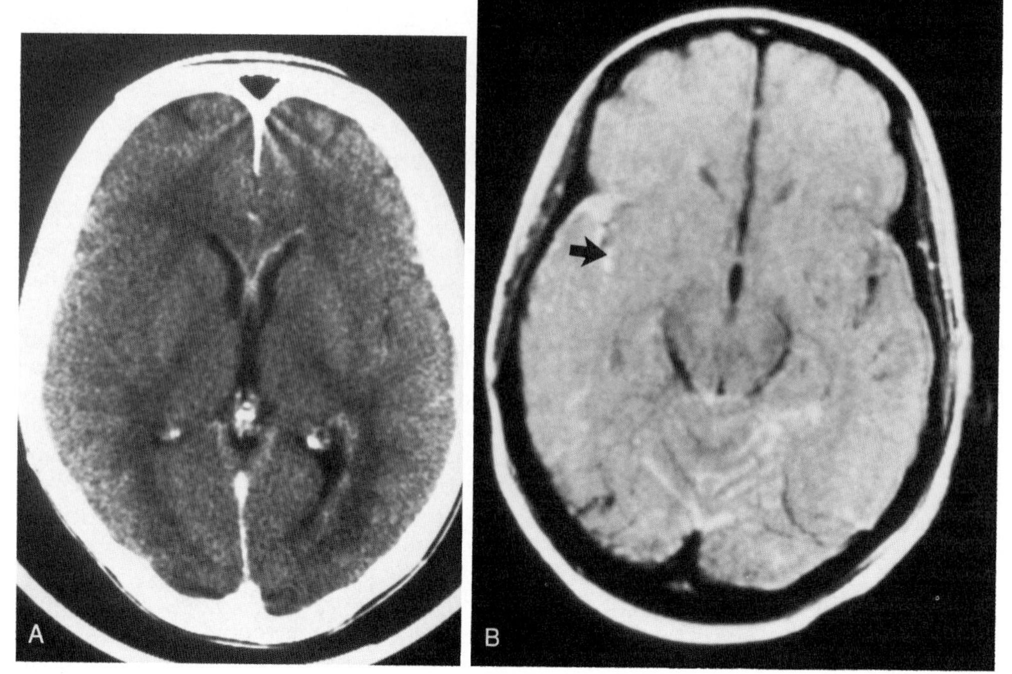

Figure 7–6. *A,* This CT scan shows enhancement of the ependyma of the lateral ventricle from metastatic breast cancer. *B,* This MR scan displays enhancement of leptomeningeal disease from breast carcinoma in the cerebellar folia as well as in the Sylvian fissure (*arrow*).

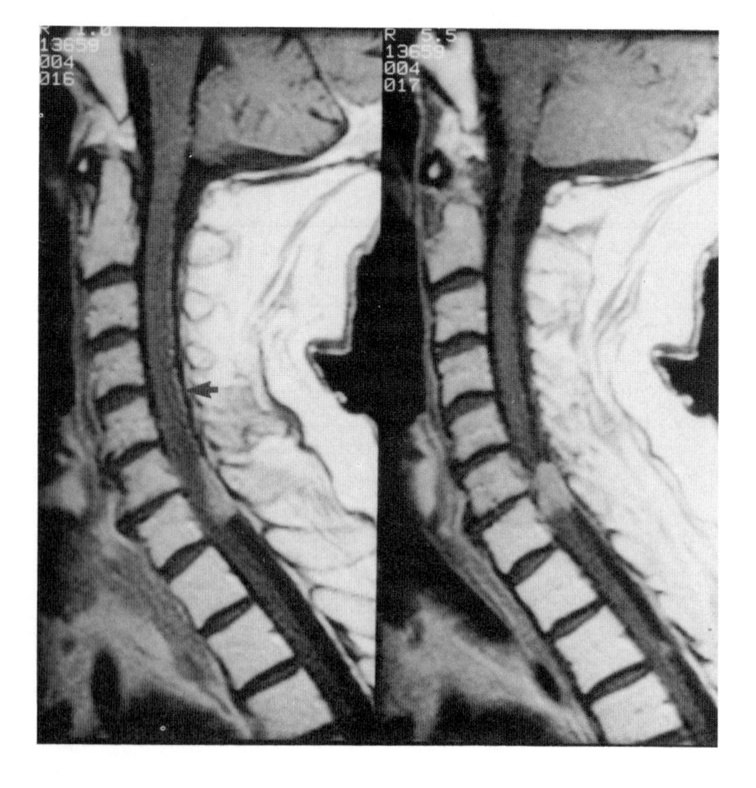

Figure 7–7. This magnetic resonance scan shows a leptomeningeal tumor in the spinal canal of a patient with small-cell lung cancer. The patient had received prophylactic whole-brain radiation and subsequently developed a metastasis in the cerebellopontine angle with a subependymal nodule as well. A large intradural extramedullary metastasis is present at the C-7 level. In addition, in the *left panel,* enhancement of the leptomeninges leading cephalad from the lesion (*arrow*) can be seen.

creased by using higher doses of gadolinium. Care must be taken when interpreting MR scans, particularly those enhanced with higher doses of contrast material. Mild enhancement of otherwise normal-appearing spinal roots may not be pathologic.

Second, in the absence of contrast enhancement of the basal meninges, communicating hydrocephalus suggesting obstruction of CSF absorptive pathways should lead one to suspect leptomeningeal tumor. This change is nonspecific because hydrocephalus can be caused by various lesions, but it may support a diagnosis of leptomeningeal metastasis in a patient strongly suspected of having this disorder.

Enlarged ventricles do not establish the diagnosis of hydrocephalus because cerebral atrophy, sometimes induced by RT or chemotherapy, likewise enlarges the ventricles, but an MR scan may help differentiate these entities, particularly if white-matter hyperintensity shows at the ventricular frontal horns, suggesting periventricular edema from transependymal absorption of CSF because of obstructed ventricles. White-matter hyperintensity can also be caused by RT and chemotherapy, but the changes tend to involve the entire white matter rather than just the periventricular area.

Myelography

When the results of the gadolinium-enhanced MR scan of the spine are negative,

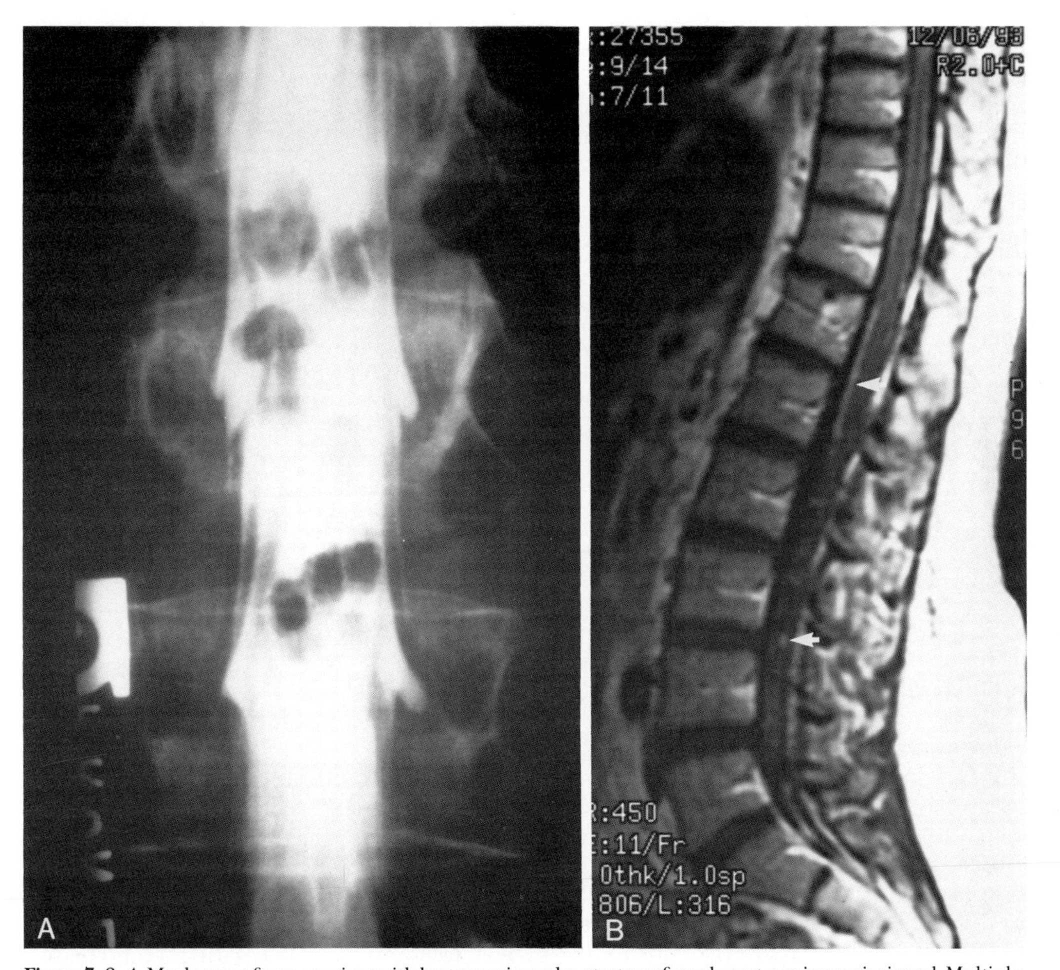

Figure 7–8. *A,* Myelogram from a patient with leptomeningeal metastases from breast carcinoma is viewed. Multiple, large filling defects, representing tumor nodules, stud the cauda equina. *B,* An enhanced MR scan from a patient with ovarian cancer metastatic to the leptomeninges is seen. The nodules and linear root enhancement (*arrows*) are more subtle in this patient.

myelography rarely identifies leptomeningeal tumor.[1429] In 49 consecutive patients[2750] with leptomeningeal metastasis, the myelogram was diagnostic in 13. A myelographic finding of small nodules along nerve roots suggests leptomeningeal metastasis (Fig. 7–8). Although this type of finding can be present in patients with primary meningeal tumors such as neurofibromas, multiple nodules along roots, particularly in a patient with systemic cancer, strongly suggest leptomeningeal metastasis.

Cerebral Arteriography

Occasionally, cerebral arteriograms help support a diagnosis of leptomeningeal metastasis.[1385,1475,2750] Multiple constrictions of meningeal blood vessels suggest invasion or compression by leptomeningeal disease. These findings are also encountered in some patients with tuberculosis and other granulomatous infections of the nervous system, including vasculitis.

Other Diagnostic Tests

The EEG is nonspecific. Results may be normal or show focal or generalized slow or sharp activity. Triphasic waves generally believed to indicate metabolic encephalopathy have been reported in leptomeningeal tumor.[1770]

Electromyography assists in diagnosing leptomeningeal metastasis in some instances. Prolonged F-wave latencies (i.e., waves that mark conduction of the most proximal portions of the motor roots[71,1339]) have been reported of value in diagnosing leptomeningeal tumor in a number of patients. I have rarely found the test necessary.

A biopsy of the leptomeninges is occasionally diagnostic when all other tests fail,[436] although I have encountered at least one negative biopsy in a patient who was later found to have extensive leptomeningeal tumor on an autopsy examination. An intriguing report of direct visualization of spinal roots through a lumbar puncture needle by fiberoptic endoscopy suggests the possibility of direct visualization to localize the site of a biopsy of leptomeningeal tumor[1937] in those rare patients in whom diagnosis cannot be made by other means.

DIFFERENTIAL DIAGNOSIS

The clinical suspicion of leptomeningeal metastasis rests on finding either multifocal neurologic symptoms or signs, signs suggestive of meningeal irritation, or both. The first finding can be mimicked by multiple brain or epidural metastases and the second by CNS infection. To differentiate leptomeningeal metastases from multiple parenchymal and/or epidural metastases requires imaging of the brain and spine to look for mass lesions and CSF analysis to search for malignant cells. If malignant cells are present, the patient has leptomeningeal tumor despite whatever else he or she may have. Differentiating leptomeningeal metastasis from CNS infection, particularly in patients with lymphomas, who are susceptible to both illnesses, is more difficult.[2350,2750] The diagnosis can often be established only by careful and repeated examination of the nervous system.

In general, patients with leptomeningeal metastasis develop identifiable neurologic signs—particularly cranial or spinal nerve dysfunction—early, when meningeal signs and even changes in the CSF such as pleocytosis and high protein are mild. Patients with CNS infections, on the other hand, tend to develop cranial and spinal nerve abnormalities late in the course, if at all. Thus, signs of meningeal irritation accompanied by fever and abnormal CSF with a normal neurologic examination suggest CNS infection, whereas cranial and spinal nerve dysfunction without meningeal signs or fever and with only modest CSF changes suggests tumor.

Diagnostic Approach

The clinical diagnosis of leptomeningeal metastasis usually suggests itself in one of four settings:

1. As indicated previously, when a patient presents with symptoms or signs of neurologic dysfunction at several levels of the neuraxis. (The patient could be suffering from multiple mass lesions, such as a combination of a brain metasta-

sis and epidural spinal cord compression, but widespread leptomeningeal metastasis is a more parsimonious explanation.)

2. When a patient has neurologic disease that may initially suggest a single CNS lesion, but imaging of the area in question does not reveal a metastatic mass. Microscopic tumor involving the leptomeninges and the brain or spinal cord must then be considered.
3. When a patient presents with headache, nuchal rigidity, and, sometimes, radicular pain suggesting an inflammatory meningitis. Such patients are usually afebrile, and a diagnosis of leptomeningeal involvement by tumor must be considered as well.
4. When an image of the brain or spine, taken to rule out a mass lesion, shows evidence of either leptomeningeal enhancement or obstruction of CSF pathways (e.g., hydrocephalus).

Whatever the setting, the first step (Fig. 7–9) is to scan the area of maximal symptomatology, preferably with a gadolinium-enhanced MR scan. If there is a strong clinical suspicion of leptomeningeal metastasis but the brain MR scan is negative, an enhanced scan of the spine, even in the

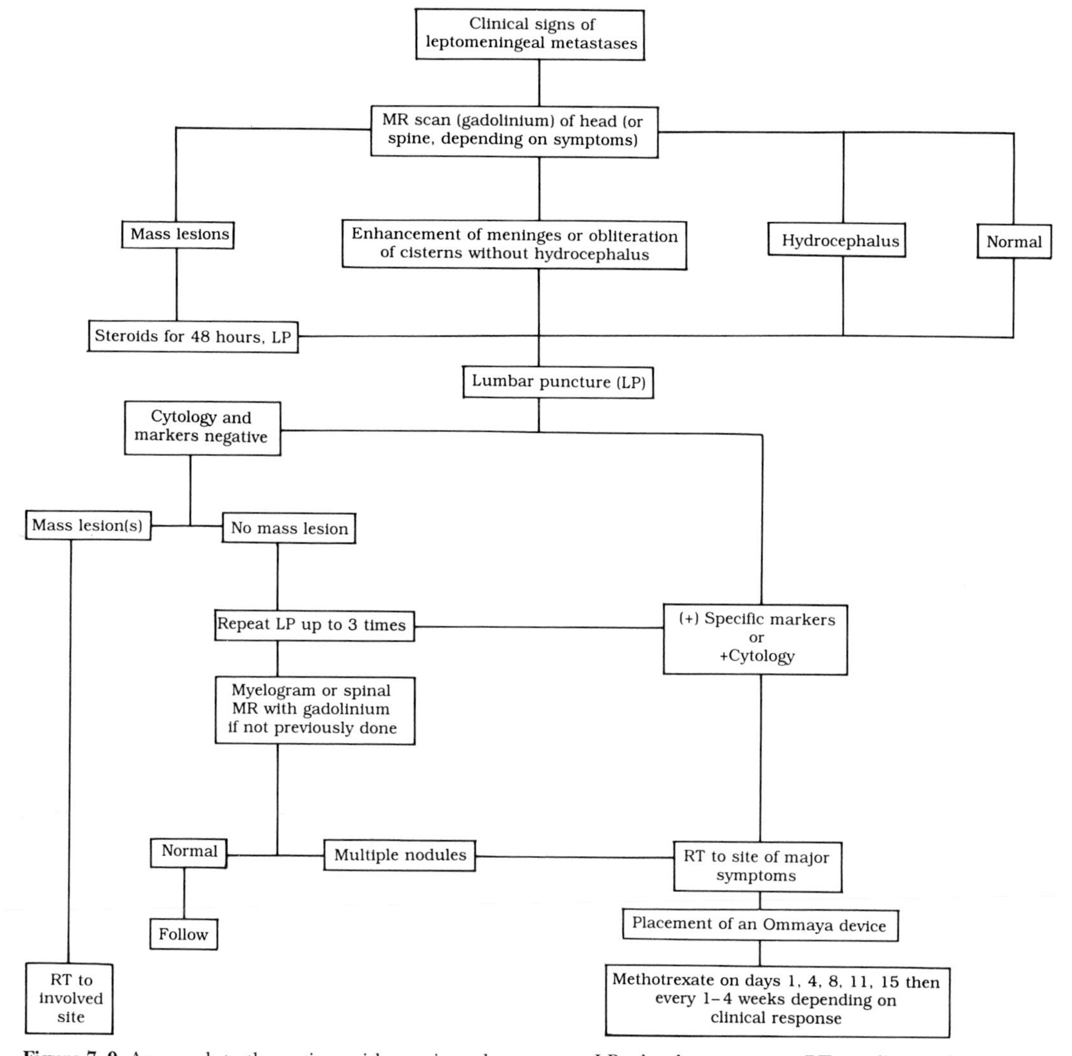

Figure 7–9. Approach to the patient with meningeal symptoms. LP = lumbar puncture; RT = radiation therapy.

absence of spinal symptoms or signs, should precede CSF examination. If the scan does not reveal an alternative diagnosis to leptomeningeal tumor, such as a brain tumor or intramedullary spinal cord tumor, lumbar puncture is the next diagnostic test. If malignant cells are found in the CSF, the diagnosis of leptomeningeal metastasis is established and treatment should be started. If the results are negative, the lumbar puncture should be repeated up to three times within the next several days to a few weeks to look for malignant cells, which are the gold standard for diagnosis.

Other laboratory tests that mandate treatment in the absence of malignant cells but in the presence of appropriate clinical findings include:

1. enhancing nodules on MR scan, if one can be certain that the patient does not suffer from multiple neurofibromas;
2. diffuse enhancement of the leptomeninges on MR scan, if infection can be ruled out; and
3. specific CSF markers (CEA, β-HCG) higher in CSF than in serum or much higher than can be accounted for by diffusion across the blood–brain barrier.

Hydrocephalus alone on the CT or MR scan does not establish the diagnosis of leptomeningeal metastasis, and that finding is not indicative for treatment; meningeal tumor is not a common cause of normal-pressure hydrocephalus.

In a few patients, even after a thorough workup, the diagnosis is uncertain; malignant cells are not identified, scans are not diagnostic, or clinical symptoms could be due to nonmetastatic disease. In those instances, it is wise to wait at least 2 weeks, repeat the lumbar puncture, consider a lateral cervical puncture to sample cisternal fluid, and repeat the scans using an increased dose of contrast. Virtually all of the problems will clarify themselves within a few weeks.

Occasionally a lumbar puncture or scan performed for other reasons suggests the presence of leptomeningeal metastasis. Even in the absence of symptoms, if the diagnosis can be established by laboratory tests, treatment should be undertaken. I usually defer RT for asymptomatic patients and treat with intrathecal drugs alone (see the following).

In rare instances, a leptomeningeal biopsy may be necessary to establish the diagnosis, particularly in patients who are not known to have an underlying neoplasm and whose clinical symptoms or laboratory results arouse suspicion of leptomeningeal tumor. Because the disorder may be multifocal rather than diffuse, the biopsy sample should be chosen on the basis of clinical symptoms and the knowledge of the loci of leptomeningeal spread (see Fig. 7–1), which is best detected at the cisterns at the base of the brain and the leptomeninges of the cauda equina.

TREATMENT

The major therapeutic modalities (Table 7–9) are RT and chemotherapy.[236,1017,2750] The major problem in treating leptomeningeal metastasis is that the entire neuraxis must be treated. If only symptomatic areas are treated, that area will rapidly be reseeded from tumor elsewhere in the meninges. Immunotoxin therapy[1846,2720a,2886a] and gene therapy[2118] are still experimental.

Radiation Therapy

External-beam RT can be delivered either to the entire neuraxis or to symptomatic sites, leaving the remainder of the neuraxis to be

Table 7–9. **TREATMENT OF LEPTOMENINGEAL METASTASES**

Surgery
Biopsy for diagnosis
Insertion of cannula and reservoir for therapy
Ventricular
Lumbar
Radiation
Whole neuraxis
Symptomatic sites
Chemotherapy
Parenteral
CSF
Lumbar
Ventricular
Immunotherapy
Monoclonal antibodies

treated by chemotherapy. Intrathecal radiation with radioactive nuclides such as gold[543,659,1754] or radiolabeled monoclonal antibodies[184,1821] is another method of delivering RT, but it is subject to the same limitations as intrathecal chemotherapy (see the following). RT is the most effective method of relieving symptoms.[1905] Ideally, the entire neuraxis should be radiated, but delivering the necessary dose to the entire neuraxis in patients suffering from carcinoma or lymphoma often compromises the bone marrow so that RT cannot be completed or no further therapy can be given for the systemic tumor.

My policy has been to irradiate symptomatic areas, using chemotherapy to treat the rest of the neuraxis.[1066,2750] Asymptomatic areas that show leptomeningeal mass lesions unlikely to be penetrated by intrathecal drugs probably should also be irradiated. Because RT and chemotherapy with methotrexate appear to be synergistic in causing CNS toxicity (see Chapter 12), I prefer not to irradiate the brain unless symptoms or signs such as hydrocephalus require it. In those patients with cranial nerve palsies as the major symptom, RT can be delivered to the base of the skull, sparing most of the brain from RT side effects. In patients presenting with weak lower extremities or bladder and bowel dysfunction, the lumbosacral spine (i.e., the cauda equina) is irradiated. Patients with hydrocephalus or focal seizures receive whole-brain RT.

Chemotherapy

ROUTE OF ADMINISTRATION

Chemotherapy can be given either systemically or directly into the CNS.[229,665] Systemic chemotherapy is sometimes helpful when the blood–brain barrier has been extensively disrupted by the tumor,[1326,2404a] when higher doses of an agent (e.g., high-dose methotrexate) yield therapeutic CSF levels,[139,1722a] or if the tumor is sensitive to a lipid-soluble chemotherapeutic agent. For theoretic reasons, it would appear that chemotherapeutic agents injected into the CNS are superior. By definition, all leptomeningeal tumor is in contact with CSF and, thus, injection into CSF should achieve high concentrations of the chemotherapeutic agent at the tumor site without excessively exposing the bone marrow or the rest of the body to toxicity. Also, because most leptomeningeal metastases are only a few cells thick and do not form mass lesions, all of the cells in contact with the subarachnoid space should be bathed in the chemotherapeutic drug. Other clinicians have objected to this theoretic postulate on the grounds that often tumor cells are buried in Virchow-Robin spaces deep in the sulci, where circulating chemotherapeutic agents might not reach. Studies to prove or refute this point are unavailable. One study concerning the distribution of radioactive methotrexate (MTX) and cytosine arabinoside (ara-C) after intrathecal injection suggests rapid and extensive penetration into spinal cord parenchyma, however.[343] Distribution of radiolabeled monoclonal antibody was likewise revealed to be widespread in a postmortem study done on one patient.[184] For these theoretic reasons, my colleagues and I usually choose to use chemotherapeutic agents injected into the CSF.

If the clinician chooses to inject chemotherapeutic agents into the CSF, a route must be determined. The agents can be injected directly into the lumbar CSF or into the lateral ventricle of the brain by the use of a ventricular cannula (Ommaya device) with a subcutaneous reservoir placed in the scalp (Fig. 7–10).[546,871,1042,2523] I prefer the latter for both theoretic and practical reasons:

1. Chemotherapeutic agents injected by lumbar puncture can inadvertently be injected into epidural or subdural spaces. In one series, this occurred 10% of the time,[1473] even though the lumbar puncture and intrathecal injection appeared successful to the physician. One is more likely to achieve a successful injection on the first lumbar puncture and to fail to do so on subsequent lumbar punctures in part because a subdural or epidural CSF collection may have developed as a result of the previous puncture. Such a collection collapses the normal subarachnoid space but yields CSF through the needle, giving the physician a false sense of security. An incorrect injection is particularly likely in a patient who, after a previous lumbar puncture, is suffering from

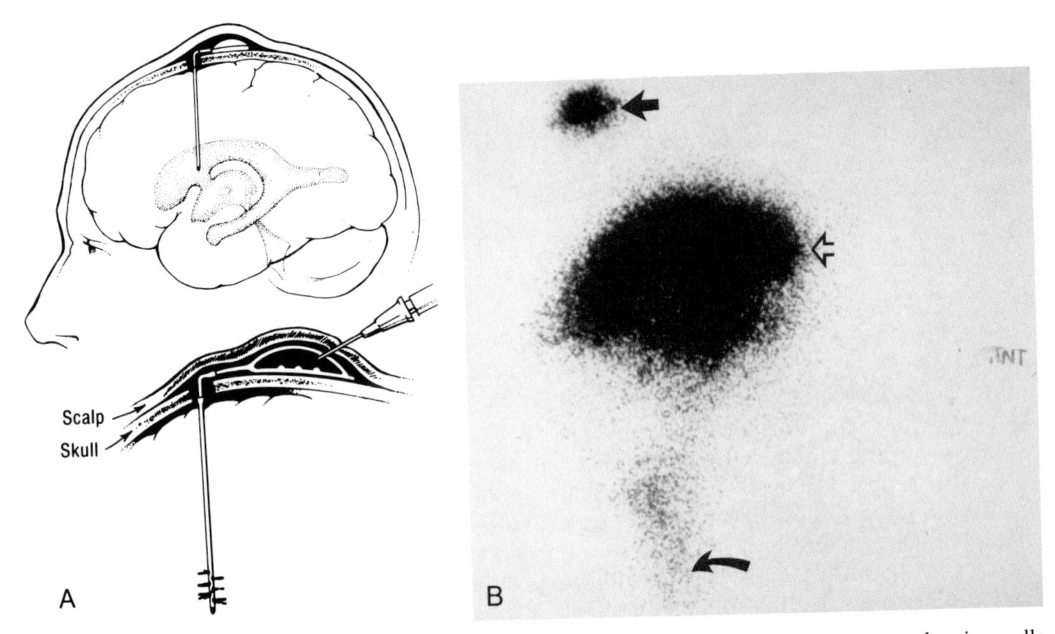

Figure 7–10. *A*, Ommaya device as modified at Memorial Sloan-Kettering Cancer Center. A 23-gauge scalp vein needle is used to enter the reservoir implanted over the bone but beneath the scalp (*bottom*) and the drug is injected into the anterior horn of the lateral ventricle to Monro's foramen. The catheter enters the brain through a burr hole, anterior to the reservoir site, so that the needle cannot penetrate the brain. *B*, Radionuclide ventriculography minutes after injection of ^{131}I albumin into an Ommaya reservoir. Residual radioactivity is present in the reservoir (*closed arrow*), and the ventricular system is uniformly filled with radionuclide (*open arrow*). Areas at the base of the brain and down the spinal cord (*curved arrow*) are beginning to accumulate the radionuclide.

post–lumbar puncture headache, indicating a CSF leak. To avoid subdural or epidural injection, some have placed lumbar catheters attached to subcutaneous reservoirs, but this has no advantage over the intraventricular Ommaya reservoir.[699]

The presence of a subdural collection of fluid, occurring either spontaneously from a tear in the dura or after a lumbar puncture, can be diagnostically confusing as well. In patients suffering from postural headache, an attempt at lumbar puncture may sample only the subdural collection, yielding a fluid that may contain WBCs but not tumor cells and an elevated protein concentration. Such fluid may not truly reflect findings in the subarachnoid space and may mislead the observer into believing that the patient has leptomeningeal infiltration with tumor or infection when, in fact, the CSF is normal. To compound the problem, some patients with intracranial hypotension and postural headache following lumbar puncture developenhancement of the meninges onMR scan, mimicking the breakdown of the blood–brain barrier that is seen with leptomeningeal infiltration[1974] (see Chapter 14).

2. Even if the chemotherapy is placed correctly into the subarachnoid space via lumbar puncture, the entire neuraxis, particularly the ventricular system, may not achieve a high concentration of the agent. Even in the absence of obstruction to CSF flow,[420,1020] lumbar injection does not guarantee therapeutic levels in the ventricle.[2369] In the absence of obstruction, intraventricular injection reliably produces therapeutic drug levels in both ventricle and lumbar sac.
3. Once an Ommaya device is placed, ventricular fluid can be sampled and the chemotherapeutic agent injected with little or no discomfort to the patient. Repeated lumbar punctures are often

uncomfortable and meet with considerable patient resistance. Occasional lumbar puncture is necessary, however, to follow the progress of the disease.

4. Empiric evidence supports the superiority of ventricular over lumbar therapy.[240,2367]
5. An Ommaya device can be used even when the platelet count is too low to safely perform a lumbar puncture (see Chapter 9).

CHEMOTHERAPEUTIC AGENTS

Figure 7–9 outlines our current treatment protocol. RT is delivered to symptomatic sites. A ventricular cannula (Ommaya device) is placed into the right frontal horn of the lateral ventricle and connected to a subcutaneous reservoir in the frontal area[871] (see Fig. 7–10).

MTX and ara-C are the most widely used agents.* Other agents include thiotepa,† which exits the CSF within minutes,[2511] diaziquone,[1326] radiolabeled monoclonal antibodies,[1474] lymphokine-activated killer cells and interleukin-2,[1783,2280,2390,198]Au-colloid,[659] and dacarbazine.[422] Experimental studies in animals have used hydroxypercyclophosphamide (the active agent of cyclophosphamide),[84,846] ACNU,‡ toxin-linked antibodies,[2639,2906] trimetrexate,[138] melphalan,[838a] MCNU,[1397a] and topotecan,[2523a] as well as others.[1410,2164,2643] Liposome-entrapped agents, particularly ara-C, have also been used experimentally to treat meningeal tumor.[421,1195]

The therapeutic level for MTX is 1 μM.[238,2512] CSF levels should be kept at 1 μM or higher for 48 to 72 hours after administration of the drug. The dose for adults is generally 12 mg twice a week, although Strother and colleagues[2512] have demonstrated that a schedule consisting of an initial dose of 6 mg followed by supplemental doses of 6 mg, 4 mg, or 2 mg at 24 and 48 hours, according to serial measurements of MTX levels in the ventricle, will maintain the therapeutic level for 72 hours. The volume of CSF reaches the adult level by the age of 4 years, so that these recommendations apply to most children as well.[238] Bleyer and colleagues[235] have shown that a dose of 12 mg of MTX intrathecally in children older than 2 years of age, given prophylactically, was more effective in preventing CNS leukemia than the previously used schedule of 12 mg/m^2. When 12 mg is used as a fixed dose, MTX levels reliably exceed and remain greater than 1 μM for at least 48 hours.[238] Higher doses are not necessary and lower doses are inadequate. Initially, MTX is administered twice a week, so that therapeutic CSF levels are maintained almost continuously, but, after five injections (see Fig. 7–9), the frequency of MTX administration is decreased; eventually, intrathecal MTX may be administered monthly. Intrathecal therapy should be continued for at least 3 to 6 months and perhaps indefinitely; the most effective duration of treatment has not been established. Some investigators combine drugs and add hydrocortisone to decrease acute toxicity (aseptic meningitis) of the MTX,[2517] but data do not demonstrate increased efficacy of chemotherapeutic combinations over single agents.[1171] MTX is not metabolized by the nervous system and is reabsorbed into the bloodstream by bulk flow and by transport via the choroid plexus from CSF to systemic circulation.

In patients being treated with intrathecal MTX, oral leucovorin is given twice a day on the day of treatment and for the following 3 days to prevent systemic toxicity (usually mucositis) from MTX reabsorbed into the systemic circulation. Leucovorin does not cross the blood–brain barrier in amounts sufficient to interfere with the effect of MTX on the CNS tumor.[1739]

Ara-C is the only widely used alternative to MTX. The drug is not metabolized by the CNS and is given in a dose of 50 mg twice a week. Some physicians who treat leukemia and lymphoma alternate MTX and ara-C to decrease toxicity. Ara-C is probably less toxic but is also less effective than MTX in most instances.

Thiotepa is administered as 10 mg twice a week. Its rapid absorption from the CSF (leaving the CSF within an hour) raises questions about its efficacy.

*References 1171, 1945, 2485, 2750, 2862.
†References 915, 1037, 1039, 2495, 2609.
‡References 79, 1224a, 1537, 2304, 2391, 2868.

Cerebrospinal Fluid–Systemic Shunts

Patients with symptomatic increased intracranial pressure caused by leptomeningeal metastases are candidates for CSF–systemic shunt. A ventriculoperitoneal shunt is the procedure of choice. Patients selected for shunting include those with severe and intractable headache, severe papilledema with potential visual loss, stupor or obtundation, or repetitive plateau waves. Occasionally, steroids will lower intracranial pressure enough so that shunting is not required, allowing time for other therapy to treat the CSF blockage.

Treatment of the patient with intrathecal chemotherapy after shunting is a dilemma. Some physicians place "on-off" valves in the shunting system, allowing the shunt to be turned off for several hours after drugs are injected into the ventricular system. The need for a shunt implies obstruction of CSF pathways. However, drugs injected into the ventricular system may not exit during the time the valve is closed off and thus will never have contact with tumor in the subarachnoid space. In addition, transependymal absorption of the chemotherapeutic agent leads to neurotoxicity. Some patients cannot tolerate valve closure for even a few hours.

My approach has been to perform the shunt when necessary and give intrathecal drugs by lumbar puncture after the shunting is complete. The chemotherapeutic agent then encounters the spinal leptomeninges and basal cisterns before entering the ventricular system and exiting through the shunt.

Some physicians are concerned about the possibility of seeding the peritoneal cavity from the shunt. This presents a theoretic but not a practical problem (see Chapter 14).

Complications

In skilled hands, complications of the placement and use of Ommaya reservoirs are uncommon.[1638,1917,2523] Hemorrhage at the time of placement occurs in fewer than 1% of patients. In addition, a small number of reservoirs fail after placement. They may have been misplaced, such as through the floor of the third ventricle into the basal cisterns, into brain substance, or, on one occasion, into the Sylvian fissure. If inappropriately placed, they may become occluded with detritus. To ensure proper placement, a CT scan should be done after Ommaya insertion but before chemotherapy is administered through the device. If the reservoir is obstructed or if the ventricular pressure exceeds tissue pressure, injected material backs up along the catheter and can form a fluid mass in the brain.[1522]

Infection complicates about 5% of reservoirs at some time during therapy.[1917] Common organisms are *Staphylococcus aureus, S. epidermidis,* and *Propionibacterium acnes.* Other organisms are occasional offenders. Most reservoir infections are asymptomatic, but a few patients develop symptoms of meningitis (i.e., headache, stiff neck, and fever). I have seen occasional *P. acnes* infections that appeared to clear without treatment, but most of the infections require therapy. Instillation of chemotherapeutic agents into the reservoir often effectively sterilizes the system.[2526] At times it is necessary to remove the reservoir, but a new one can be inserted and treatment continued.[2608] The side effects of chemotherapy are discussed in Chapter 12.

Prognosis

Evidence from retrospective analyses indicates that untreated patients, once they have become symptomatic, generally progress rapidly and succumb to their leptomeningeal tumor within 6 weeks to 2 months from the initial diagnosis.[1942,2205] In a rare patient, the disease is more indolent. Two MSKCC patients with breast carcinoma have had extraordinarily long courses. One presented with hydrocephalus that responded to shunting; 2 years later, she developed weakness in her legs. At that time, malignant cells were found in the CSF, and treatment was undertaken. The second patient complained of weakness and numbness in the lower extremities for about 18 months before clinical evaluation revealed malignant cells. Because of the patient's reluctance, another 6 months elapsed before treatment was undertaken, with only very slow progression of the illness. A third patient also had a 2-year course of leg weakness before CSF examination revealed malignant adenocarcinoma cells. The primary tumor site was never found.

Several reports detail the outcome of different treatment protocols. In general, the results with leukemia are excellent.* Because these tumors are sensitive to MTX and ara-C, leukemia, like lymphoma,[2026,2135] can often be eradicated from the nervous system, although relapse does occur.[2026] In studies with solid tumors, the results are not as good* (Table 7–10). In about 75% of patients, neurologic symptoms either stabilize or improve. In many of these patients, treatment results in several months of good-quality life. About 25% of patients grow progressively worse despite treatment. Those patients who are least neurologically damaged at the time treatment is undertaken do better than those patients with fixed neurologic deficits. Exceptions do occur, making patients with advanced neurologic symptomatology worthy of treatment. For example, marked improvement in visual or hearing loss is occasionally reported. In one of our patients with adenocarcinoma of the lung metastatic to the leptomeninges, vision improved from less than 20/200 to 20/20 and remained there. Of solid tumors, breast carcinomas and small-cell lung cancer respond best; melanomas respond worst.

Along with the clinical response, CSF findings often improve. In some patients, malignant cells disappear and protein and glucose concentrations return to normal. In others, cytology is persistently positive despite clinical improvement and improvement in other CSF variables[699,2750,2863] (see Table 7–10). Some believe that no treatment helps and that apparent benefit derives from patient selection,[459] but this view appears unduly pessimistic.

Despite initial clinical improvement, most patients have a short survival, usually only a few months. About 15% of patients with breast cancer survive more than a year, but such survival is rare with lung cancer or melanoma. Occasional patients do have long and useful survival after treatment of established meningeal metastases from solid tumors.[1411]

Despite a rather extensive literature, often consisting of reports with small numbers of patients, a general agreement does not exist on how or even whether to treat leptomeningeal metastases from solid tumors other than lymphomas. Ongerboer de Visser and colleagues[1945] report good responses of breast cancer to intensive intraventricular MTX therapy, with a 25% 1-year survival. Grossman and colleagues[1015] report no significant neurologic improvement in 59 adults with nonleukemic malignancies, 28 of whom had breast cancer. Pfeffer and coworkers [2026] report 9 complete responses and 6 partial responses in 27 patients with breast cancer following a protocol using intrathecal MTX and RT; unfortunately, treatment complications occurred in 30% of patients, with 4 deaths. Boogerd and coworkers,[262] who studied 58 patients with breast cancer and leptomeningeal metastases, report that a multivariate analysis of pretreatment characteristics showed a poor prognosis for patients older than age 55 with lung metastases, cranial nerve involvement, hypoglycorrhachia, and elevated protein concentrations. Patients with good risk factors had a better response to treatment and a longer survival rate. Siegal and colleagues[2404a] report sustained responses to systemic therapy in 31 of 137 (23%) patients with leptomeningeal metastases.

It seems obvious that leukemia and lymphomas involving the leptomeninges should be treated vigorously with intrathecal drugs. A significant percentage of patients with breast cancer respond with sufficient improvement in clinical symptoms and long enough survival to warrant their treatment as well. The same appears true of small-cell lung cancer. The prognosis for non–small-cell lung cancer, melanoma, and other adenocarcinomas affecting the leptomeninges is so poor that one might question the usefulness of vigorous treatment.[967,968]

---

*References 240, 241, 1042, 1370, 2485.

*References 262, 880, 967, 1853, 2026, 2296, 2404a, 2750, 2862.

Table 7–10. **TREATMENT OF LEPTOMENINGEAL METASTASIS FROM SOLID TUMOR**

Reference	Primary Tumor	No. of Patients	RT	IT Chemotherapy	Response (%)	Median Survival (Weeks)	1-Year Survival (%)
Shapiro and colleagues[2367]	*Total*	*67*	Yes	MTX	58	18.0	—
	Breast	15					
	Lung	7					
	Lymphoma	6					
Yap and colleagues[2862]	*Total*	*40*	Yes	MTX	67	24.0	—
	Breast						
Rosen and colleagues[2205]	*Total*	*24*	Yes	MTX	63	7.0	0
	Lung						
Wasserstrom and colleagues[2750]	*Total*	*90*	Yes	MTX	50		
	Breast	46			61 (Breast)	23.0	21
	Lung	23			39 (Lung)		
	Melanoma	11					
Trump and colleagues[2609]	*Total*	*25*	Yes	TT	76 (CSF)	23.0	—
	Breast	16		MTX	37 (Neurologic PR)		
	Lung	2					
	Lymphoma	4					
Giannone and colleagues[915]	*Total*	*22*	Yes	MTX	60 (PR)	10.0	0
	Breast	10		ara-C			
	Lung	7		TT			
	Lymphoma	2					
Stewart and colleagues[2495]	*Total*	*23*	Yes	MTX	100 (CSF)	9.0	11
	Breast	3		HC	56 (Neurologic PR)		
	Lung	7		ara-C			
	Lymphoma	7		TT			

Ara-C = cytosine arabinoside; CR/PR = complete/partial response; CSF = cerebrospinal fluid; HC = hydrocortisone; IT = intrathecal; MTX = methotrexate; NS = not significant; RT = radiation therapy; TT = thiotepa.

*All patients received some form of RT (2500–3000 rad) (cranial or symptomatic sites). Chemotherapy was administered intraventricularly twice a week. After achieving a response, the treatment interval was gradually decreased from once a week to every 8 weeks for 6 to 12 months.

†Outcome in percentage of those who received RT and ventricular MTX.

Source: Adapted from Gangji,[880] p 55.

Continued.

Table 7–10. *Continued.*

Reference	Primary Tumor	No. of Patients	RT	IT Chemotherapy	Response (%)	Median Survival (Weeks)	1-Year Survival (%)
Hitchins and colleagues[1171]	*Total*	*44*	Yes	MTX	61	12.0	15
	Breast	13				vs ($p = 0.084$)	
	Lung	13		MTX	45	7.0	
	Lymphoma	3		ara-C			
Pfeffer and colleagues[2026]	*Total*	*98*	Yes	MTX	27 (CR)	10.0	10
	Breast	33			18 (PR)		0
	Lung	8					20
	Lymphoma	36					
Boogerd and colleagues[262]	*Total*	*44*	Yes	MTX	50	12.0	11
	Breast						
Grossman and colleagues[1015]	*Total*	*59*	Yes	MTX	0 (Neurologic PR)	15.9	
	Breast	28		vs			
	Lung	13		TT		14.1	
	Lymphoma	11				($p > 0.1$, NS)	
Nakagawa and colleagues[1853]	*Total*	*29*	Yes	MTX		23.0	14
	Breast	8		or	31 (CSF)		
	Lung	14		MTX	33 (Neurologic PR)		
Ongerboer de Visser and colleagues[1945]	*Total*	*33**	Yes	MTX	79†	24.0†	25†
	Breast						
Sause and colleagues[2296]	*Total*	*27*	Yes	MTX	31	13.0	10
	Breast	17					
	Lung	4					
	Melanoma	3					

CHAPTER 8

CANCER INVOLVING CRANIAL AND PERIPHERAL NERVES

Because nerves are found everywhere in the body, it is not surprising that they are frequently invaded or compressed by tumors. Although peripheral nerve lesions generally lack the potential for neurologic devastation that occurs with brain, leptomeningeal, and spinal cord metastases, they often cause severe pain and, depending on the nerve involved, can cause substantial neurologic disability. Tumors can involve nerves either by direct extension, as when the brachial plexus is compressed by a superior sulcus tumor of the lung, or by metastases, as when cranial nerves are invaded by tumor metastatic to the base of the skull. This chapter considers those cranial and peripheral nerve lesions that occur after nerves have exited from the subarachnoid space, thus distinguishing them from leptomeningeal metastases.[506,817,818] Table 8–1 classifies the lesions by anatomic site and shows the sequence in which they will be discussed in this chapter.

FREQUENCY

The frequency of peripheral nerve involvement in patients with cancer is underrated for several reasons: (1) Even when present, peripheral nerve involvement is rarely included in the diagnostic coding of patients who have widespread cancer. (2) The most frequent anatomic sites of nerve metastases, at the skull base and in the brachial plexus, are usually not carefully dissected during autopsy examinations. (3) Pain, the most common symptom of peripheral nerve involvement, is often believed to result from local disease affecting nerve endings rather than from direct involvement of a nerve trunk or plexus.

A few studies address the incidence of peripheral and cranial nerve dysfunction in

Table 8–1. **ANATOMIC SITES AT WHICH TUMOR CAN INVADE**

Cranial Nerves
Single cranial nerve
Multiple cranial nerves
Spinal Roots (after exit from subarachnoid space)
Nerve Plexuses
Brachial
Cervical
Lumbar
Lumbosacral
Sacral
Peripheral Nerves
Mononeuropathy and mononeuropathy multiplex
Polyneuropathy
Muscles

particular tumors. For example, facial nerve paralysis occurs in 5% to 25% of patients with malignant parotid neoplasms[163]; the lower figure is associated with acinous-cell carcinomas and the higher figure with undifferentiated carcinomas. In approximately 3% of patients with lung cancer, the cancer develops in the superior pulmonary sulcus (Pancoast tumor) and involves the brachial plexus.[1335]

Even in the absence of incidence data, it is clear that cranial and peripheral nerve dysfunction is a common and important clinical problem. Certain head and neck tumors[280,463,1814] and some melanomas[1639] are known to be neurotropic, often tracking back along cranial nerves to reach the subarachnoid space or even the brainstem (Fig. 8–1). Neural invasion also occurs in prostate and colorectal cancer,[1421] in which it indicates a poorer prognosis than in cancer that does not invade nerve endings. Tumors of the lung apex frequently involve the brachial plexus, causing pain and sometimes other neurologic signs long before the initial tumor is discovered.[1335] Breast tumors metastatic to axillary lymph nodes can also affect the brachial plexus. Abdominal and pelvic tumors may involve the lumbar or sacral plexus; pain and subsequent sacral plexus dysfunction often herald recurrence of prostate and colon cancer.

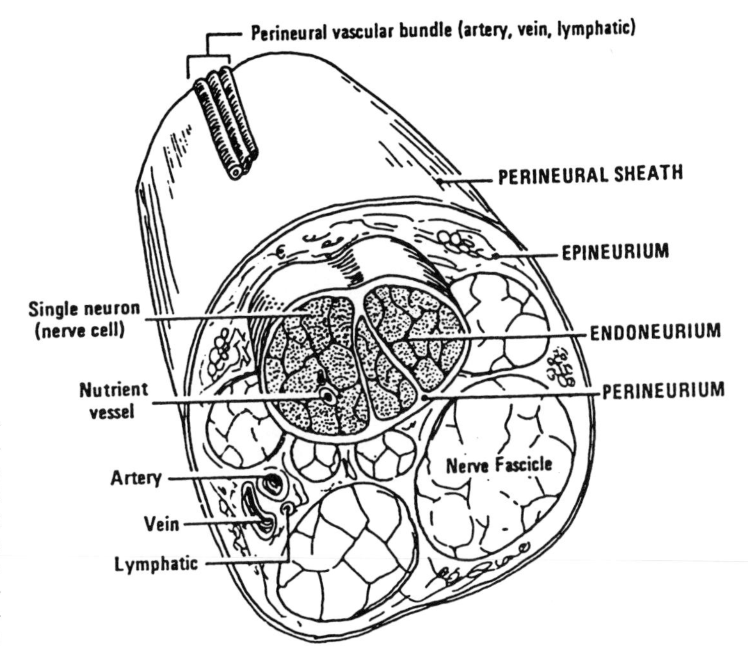

Figure 8–1. Cross-section of a cranial nerve. The only lymphatics associated with the peripheral nerve are found in the epineurium and perineural sheath. Neurotropic carcinoma may spread along these lymphatic channels but more often spreads along tissue spaces of various neural sheaths. (From Batsakis,[163] p 426, with permission.)

CRANIAL NERVES

Each of the 12 cranial nerves can be selectively involved by tumor. Table 8–2 lists common cranial neuropathies from cancer.

Tumors that involve cranial nerves usually either originate near the base of the skull or metastasize there from a distant primary site. They can then either invade the cranial nerves or compress them. Tumors also may grow into or through neural foramina of the skull. Neural foramen invasion is a common complication of nasopharyngeal carcinoma; approximately 15% to 35% of patients first present with cranial nerve palsies,[2501,2582,2621] a poor prognostic sign. A metastasis from a distant primary site (e.g., breast, lung, or prostate cancer[2122]) to the skull base can also compress cranial nerves.[978,983] Neuroblastoma has a predilection for the skull, particularly the orbit. Metastases to soft-tissue structures at the skull base or in the upper neck may also lead to cranial nerve damage. A common site is the cavernous sinus just lateral to the sella turcica.

Clinical Findings

Cranial nerve palsies either may be the first sign of cancer[2775] or may occur late in the course of the disease. In a study of 150 patients with nasopharyngeal cancer, 23 pre-

Table 8–2. **METASTATIC LESIONS CAUSING CRANIAL NEUROPATHIES**

Lesion Site	Findings	Comments
Eye	Decreased visual acuity; retinal detachment	Choroidal lesions are more common than retinal; pain, proptosis, and diplopia are rare; breast and lung cancer are common causes
Orbit	Pain, proptosis, diplopia; sensory loss V_1; decreased visual acuity in ⅓ of cases, usually late	As common as choroidal metastases; breast and prostate cancer and neuroblastoma are common causes
Parasellar	Unilateral frontal headache, oculomotor palsies (III, IV, VI), sensory loss V_1	Vision is rarely affected, no proptosis
Sella	Diabetes insipidus	Anterior pituitary insufficiency and visual loss are uncommon; when present they suggest a primary pituitary tumor
Middle cranial fossa	Facial numbness ($V_{2,3}$); abducens palsy in some (VI)	Lightninglike facial pains (trigeminal neuralgia) are rare in patients with neoplastic compression
Jugular foramen	Hoarseness, dysphagia, pain in pharynx (IX, X), sternocleidomastoid weakness (XI), occasionally tongue weakness (XII)	Papilledema may occur if a dominant jugular vein is compressed; glossopharyngeal neuralgia is uncommon
Occipital condyle	Unilateral occipital pain and neck stiffness, unilateral tongue weakness (XII)	Pain may radiate to frontal or temporal areas and may be the major complaint
Mandible	Unilateral numb chin and gum, "mental neuropathy"	Numbness also results from meningeal or calvarial metastases, breast cancer, and lymphoma
Carotid sinus or glossopharyngeal nerve	Syncope, pharynx or neck pain on swallowing	Cardioinhibitory, vasodepressor, or both; head and neck cancer; indicates recurrent tumor; may be life-threatening

Source: Adapted from Henson and Posner,[1141] p 2277.

sented with cranial nerve dysfunction as the only symptom. Symptoms included diplopia, trigeminal neuralgia, dysarthria, dysphagia, anosmia, ptosis, and hoarseness. Neurologic symptoms eventually developed in 74 other patients.[2621]

Several reports indicate that cranial mononeuropathies can be a first sign of cancer that originates elsewhere in the body[369,1701,2241] or can be the first sign of metastatic disease[2241] years after a cancer has been "successfully" treated.[1032] This last phenomenon is fairly common with neurotropic head and neck tumors, which may cause their first neurologic symptom years after their initial surgical removal.[163] One study[1065] estimates that cranial nerve dysfunction occurs in 13% of patients with breast carcinoma. The most frequently affected cranial nerves were trigeminal and facial. A cavernous sinus syndrome with visual loss as an early symptom[1193] may be the presenting sign of systemic lymphoma.[1312]

OLFACTORY NERVE (CRANIAL NERVE I)

The olfactory nerve is rarely tested in a routine oncologic or even neurologic examination. Perhaps for that reason, no reports describe isolated metastasis involving the olfactory nerve as a presenting symptom of metastatic cancer. Olfactory nerve loss, however, has been reported to affect 3% of patients with nasopharyngeal cancer.[2621] The olfactory system, which is an extension of the brain rather than a true cranial nerve, has a long intracranial course outside the cerebrum proper, along the base of the skull and through the cribriform plate to the olfactory epithelium. Metastases to the base of the anterior fossa would be expected to compress the olfactory nerve, either unilaterally or bilaterally, causing loss of odor perception. The optic nerves lie nearby and are often involved as well. Olfactory groove meningiomas[129] or esthesioneuroblastomas (olfactory neuroblastomas) are more frequently recognized as causes of olfactory nerve dysfunction. The olfactory groove is occasionally compressed and the olfactory function lost as a false-localizing sign (see Chapter 5) of a brain tumor or hydrocephalus.[541]

Direct loss of olfactory function from metastatic tumors is uncommon. Olfactory loss probably also occurs as a symptom of leptomeningeal metastases (see Chapter 7) involving the olfactory groove, but this is rarely recognized or reported. Unlike the rest of the central and peripheral nervous system, however, both taste buds and olfactory receptors have a relatively high cellular turnover rate. (Olfactory neurons are believed to be the only reproducing neurons in the adult CNS.) These rapidly reproducing cells can be damaged by radiation and chemotherapy (see Chapter 13), often leading to abnormalities of odor and taste perception that can depress appetite, leading to weight loss. Intravenous fluids have been reported to cause temporary paraosmia and parageusia (distorted sense of smell and taste).[368a]

OPTIC NERVE (CRANIAL NERVE II)

Visual loss is a common symptom of nervous system metastases,[2550] although isolated hematogenous invasion of the optic nerve itself seldom occurs.[85,1193] More common sites of metastases causing visual loss include the skull base,[2371] orbit,[253] retina (choroid),[103,660,2776] uvea,[1087a] optic chiasm, and the leptomeninges surrounding the optic nerves. Metastatic brain tumors also may cause visual loss. For example, cortical blindness can result from bilateral occipital metastases or may be a secondary effect of increased intracranial pressure compressing the optic nerves themselves or the posterior cerebral arteries that supply the visual cortex.

Bilateral ocular disease may be the initial presentation of malignant lymphoma[1392] or prostatic carcinoma.[2888] Even when they are not the presenting complaint, ocular metastases may occur when the patient's primary tumor has been "successfully" treated and he or she is believed to be cured.

In one series, 9% of children with leukemia developed ophthalmopathy, including retinal hemorrhages and infiltration of the optic nerve, retina, iris, or orbit.[2170] Direct, presumably hematogenous, metastases to the optic nerves may be the only sign of relapse in childhood acute lymphoblastic leukemia[873,2341] because the optic nerve, like the rest of the CNS, can be a sanctuary for leukemic cells. The diagnosis is usually suggested by the rapid onset of visual loss, often bilateral. The leukemic infiltrates can be identified on funduscopic examination, although the raised hemorrhagic disk may be confused with papilledema. Distinguishing papilledema caused by increased intracranial pressure from infiltration of the optic disk by tumor can be difficult, but papilledema rarely causes loss of visual acuity, except for transient visual obscurations that are common but not dangerous. Infiltration of the optic disk, on the other hand, usually causes severe visual loss and should be treated emergently. Other sites of leukemic sanctuary that may cause visual loss include the anterior chamber of the eye.[1898]

Hodgkin's disease[2401] and solid tumors, including carcinomas of the breast and lung, can also generate isolated hematogenous metastases to the optic nerve. When such tumors metastasize to the optic nerve head, they can be seen by funduscopic examination, but if the metastasis is retrobulbar, the disk may appear either normal or atrophic despite severe visual loss. Surprisingly, such metastases are often bilateral. Direct invasion of the optic nerve by nasopharyngeal carcinoma is an occasional presenting complaint of that tumor.[382]

Metastasis to the retinal choroid[103,660,2776] occurs more commonly than direct optic nerve involvement. Any tumor can involve the choroid; breast carcinoma is the most common offender.[1750] In one series, 10% of 98 asymptomatic women with breast carcinoma were found to have choroidal metastases[1755] (Fig. 8–2). In another review of 112 patients[836] with metastases to the choroid or orbit, breast cancer was the primary tumor in 50% (66) of the patients; lung cancer was primary in 15% (17). Similar metastases have been reported with carcinomas of the prostate and bladder[458,641] as well as other tumors.[28,771] Patients who have symptoms usually complain of blurred vision, visual loss, or both, depending on the choroidal lesion site. Although the lesion can often be seen on funduscopic examination as a mass elevating the retina, indirect ophthalmoscopy through dilated pupils or ocular ultrasound may be required to identify peripheral lesions. If untreated, such lesions cause secondary glaucoma with intractable pain. The metastases usually respond to treatment with either radiation or chemotherapy.[313,660]

Leukemia often affects the retina, as found in 8 of 60 children at autopsy. Choroid infiltrates were found in 26, all asympto-

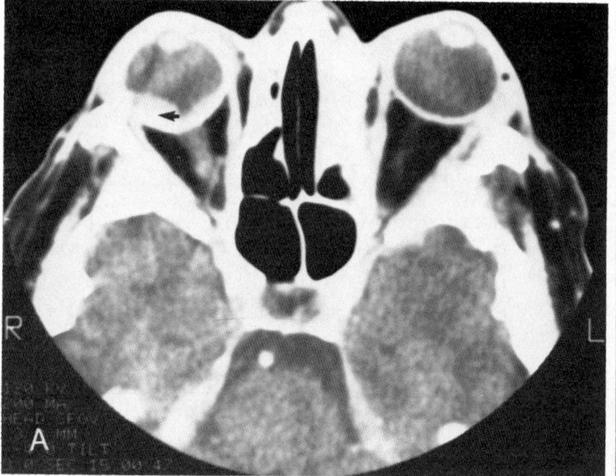

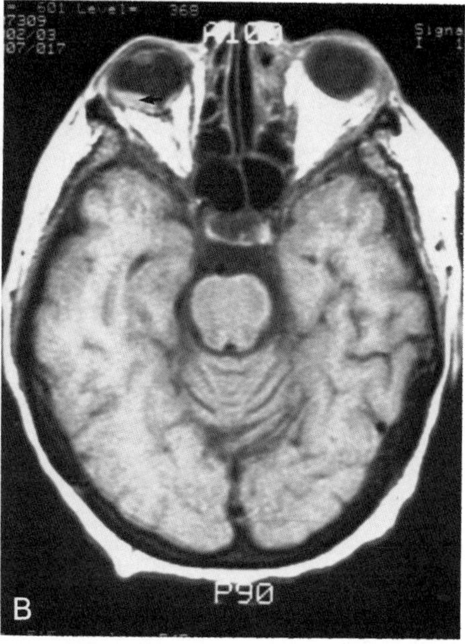

Figure 8–2. This patient with breast carcinoma presented with loss of vision in the right eye. Both the CT scan of the orbits *(A)* and the MR scan of the brain *(B)* demonstrate tumor in the choroid of the right eye *(arrows)*.

matic during life, and 4 had optic nerve involvement associated with leptomeningeal leukemia.[2181] In another series of 89 patients with acute leukemia, orbital metastases affected 7.[2396]

Symptomatic lesions of the choroid cause decreased visual acuity as the presenting complaint; retinal detachment is also common. Unlike choroid metastases, orbital tumors cause pain, proptosis, and diplopia from ocular muscle palsies, although vision may be lost if the optic nerve is also invaded or compressed. One unusual sign reported with primary optic nerve tumors is transient unilateral visual loss that occurs when the patient deviates his or her eyes in a certain direction. The sign is believed to be caused by arterial compression from the tumor.[289]

Metastases to the iris or ciliary body are uncommon and usually asymptomatic. Occasionally they bleed, causing hyphema as an initial sign of the cancer.[2257] Ciliary body metastases may simulate uveitis, but cytologic examination of the aqueous humor yields tumor rather than inflammatory cells.[1806] Breast cancer is the common offender.

Tumor need not be in the orbit or optic nerve to cause visual loss or ophthalmoplegia. Metastasis or primary carcinoma of the sphenoid sinus often presents either with visual loss when the tumor invades the anterior–superior portion of the sinus to involve the medial aspect of the optic canal, or with diplopia, usually as the result of involvement of the superior orbital fissure.[1087]

OCULAR MOTOR NERVES (CRANIAL NERVES III, IV, AND VI)

The term "ocular motor" applies to any of the three nerves supplying the ocular muscles: oculomotor (cranial nerve III), trochlear (cranial nerve IV), and abducens (cranial nerve VI). Dysfunction of individual ocular motor nerves,[1519] either alone or in combination, causes diplopia.[2250] Patients first complain of slightly blurred vision, like a "ghost" on a television set, which clears when either eye is covered. As the dysfunction progresses, the images double. The symptoms are usually progressive, although rare spontaneous remissions have been reported.[868] Paradoxically, the more severe the ocular motor paralysis, the less it bothers the patient. Images close together are much more disturbing than large deviations, in which one image can be relegated to the visual periphery. Because the binocular visual apparatus is so finely tuned, minimal dysfunction of ocular motor nerves causes symptoms. A patient often complains of diplopia undetected by the physician during a bedside examination of the ocular muscles. Conversely, diplopia found by the examiner at extremes of the patient's lateral gaze but not otherwise complained of by the patient is probably irrelevant. Patients with leptomeningeal tumor are an exception; bedside examination may reveal asymptomatic ocular motor dysfunction.

Diplopia may be caused by lesions anywhere along the ocular motor apparatus, from the orbit to the brainstem, or by lesions that infiltrate ocular muscles.[93] Orbital masses are common causes, particularly those that emanate from breast and prostate cancers[253] and from neuroblastomas. Orbital metastasis may be the first evidence of cancer or a late sign of widely metastatic disease. Affected patients usually present with diplopia with or without pain. Proptosis (exophthalmos), usually unilateral, is also an early symptom (Fig. 8–3). Occasional patients with scirrhous breast carcinoma develop diplopia associated with enophthalmos (retraction of the globe) caused by the metastatic fibrotic reaction.[2260,2586] Highly vascular metastases, such as renal-cell carcinoma, may cause pulsating exophthalmos that can be mistaken for a vascular malformation or an arteriovenous fistula.[1218] Orbital metastases are easily identified by CT or MR scan. If an orbital lesion is suspected, the physician must specifically request orbital views because routine scanning may not detect small orbital lesions. In rare patients, metastases to the orbit that originate from colon cancer or melanoma can calcify, confusing the diagnosis.[843]

Direct involvement of ocular nerves by tumor often provides the presenting complaint of patients whose cancer has metastasized to the bones of the skull base or has grown from outside the skull into the intracranial cavity through foramina. Because of its long intracranial course along the skull base, the abducens nerve is often the first affected. Two common sites of metastasis, the

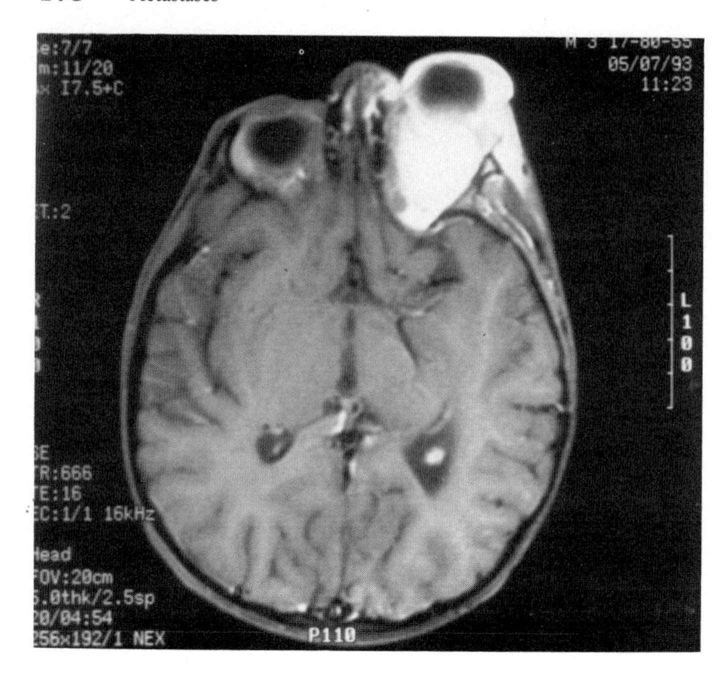

Figure 8–3. Orbital metastasis causing massive proptosis.

cavernous sinus and the parasellar area (see the following), are symptomatically characterized by diplopia, usually involving more than one ocular motor nerve.

Although ocular motor palsies are commonly symptomatic of metastatic tumor, tumor is not the most frequent cause. One series of 49 patients, age 15 to 50, with isolated sixth-nerve palsies revealed only 2 patients with metastatic tumors, 1 from breast carcinoma and 1 from cylindroma.[1828] Even when the paralysis lasted more than 3 months, as in another series of 38 patients, only 3 instances of paralysis were due to metastasis.[2299] In 1000 unselected patients with paralysis of one or more ocular motor nerves, neoplasms caused 14% (143). Of these, 69 were metastatic and another 6 were due to nasopharyngeal carcinomas. Of the 75 patients with metastatic or nasopharyngeal tumors that caused ocular motor paralysis, cranial nerve VI alone was affected in 35 patients, III alone in 12, and IV alone in 4. Combinations included III and IV in 3 patients, III and VI in 7 patients, and all three nerves in 14 patients.[2250]

Ocular Motor Syndromes. The orbital, parasellar, and cavernous sinus syndromes are caused by direct extension of cancer from the skull base or by metastases to this area. Each has characteristic signs and symptoms.

The orbital syndrome occurs with carcinomas of the breast, lung, and prostate, and with non-Hodgkin's lymphoma[128] and neuroblastoma. Tumor metastasizes to the skull and grows into the orbit or, rarely, metastasizes to the soft tissues of the orbit itself.[1591a] Whichever the cause, the syndrome is usually characterized initially by a dull, continuous supraorbital ache. The first neurologic symptom other than pain is generally blurred binocular vision, soon followed by frank diplopia. Initially, the examination shows proptosis of the involved eye, accompanied by a degree of external ophthalmoplegia. Many patients also have decreased sensation in the ophthalmic division of the trigeminal nerve. Rarely is endophthalmos present.[2260] When the orbit is palpated, the tumor sometimes can be felt either as a discrete mass or as increased resistance to orbital displacement. At other times, a striking tenderness is noted when bone surrounding the orbit is palpated. Because the tumor generally stays outside of the sheaths surrounding the optic nerve, decreased vision, visual field deficits, and papilledema rarely occur until very late in the course, when failing vision and optic atrophy appear. One of our patients with Ewing's sarcoma developed an orbital metastasis characterized by diplopia and, later, optic atrophy. The lesion responded to radiation.

A year later, he presented with headache and contralateral papilledema, or Foster Kennedy's syndrome, and was found to have a skull metastasis compressing the sagittal sinus. The atrophic optic nerve could not develop papilledema.

Orbital metastases are an unusual complication of systemic cancer. Ferry and Font[771] report only 28 patients with orbital metastases from a series of 235 patients with metastatic disease of the eye; the remainder involved the choroid. Nevertheless, in 17 of these 28 patients, orbital metastases were the initial sign of malignancy.

Parasellar metastases either arise in the sella turcica and extend into the cavernous space[2583] or metastasize directly to the cavernous space.[1773,2134,2525] The parasellar syndrome is characterized by unilateral frontal headaches and ocular paresis, usually without proptosis. Because the veins draining from the orbit empty into the cavernous sinus, they may be compressed, leading to striking periorbital edema. Thus, edema is usually more prominent in the parasellar syndrome than in the orbital syndrome, but proptosis, if present, is less. The unilateral headache is localized to the supraorbital frontal areas and generally is characterized as a dull, aching pain; some patients complain of episodic, sharp shooting pains that are not, however, typical of trigeminal neuralgia. Diplopia results from involvement of the ocular motor nerves as they traverse the cavernous sinus. Among our seven patients, four had oculomotor nerve paresis, one had trochlear paresis, and five had abducens paresis.[983] Some patients complained of paresthesias over the forehead, and sensory loss was detectable in one. Two patients had papilledema; none complained of visual loss.

The metastatic parasellar syndrome is relatively common. Roessmann and colleagues,[2190] in an autopsy study of 60 consecutive cases of carcinoma, report 16 parasellar bony lesions, of which 9 were due to breast cancer. Conversely, in 102 patients whose parasellar syndrome was diagnosed clinically, 23 cases were caused by metastases, usually from cancers of the breast, prostate, or lung.[2583] Most investigators agree that parasellar lesions usually begin with metastasis to the bone, either the petrous apex or the sella turcica, rather than with direct extension to the cavernous space. Cavernous sinus involvement is usually unilateral but may be bilateral.[1773] MRI is the best diagnostic test because CT may fail to detect small but symptomatic lesions.[2076,2245] Sometimes a radionuclide bone scan is helpful. Occasionally, a biopsy is necessary to establish the diagnosis.[2226,2634]

Carcinomas arising in the face, usually squamous but occasionally basal cell, may cause the cavernous sinus syndrome by growing microscopically along the first or second division of the trigeminal nerve to the cavernous sinus. In such instances, facial pain or sensory loss is the first symptom. Diplopia occurs later. A mass lesion may not be identifiable on MR, and diagnosis may require biopsy. The specimen should be taken from nerve endings at the site of the original lesion (Fig. 8–4).

TRIGEMINAL NERVE (CRANIAL NERVE V)

Facial pain, with or without numbness, is a common symptom of tumor involving the trigeminal nerve. Facial pain without numbness can also be a symptom of a nonmetastatic lung tumor[220,260] (see page 182). When facial pain is caused by a metastasis, the site can be anywhere from the most peripheral branches of the trigeminal nerve in subcutaneous tissues of the face, as when squamous-cell carcinomas of the skin invade cutaneous branches of the nerve,[280,393,902] to the entry of the trigeminal nerve into the brainstem. When the nerve is involved in the cavernous sinus or parasellar area, it is usually associated with oculomotor abnormalities as described previously.

Pain, numbness, or both may occur as isolated symptoms. In one series of 64 patients presenting with isolated numbness of the face, 3 had metastatic tumors to the skull base.[1204] Characteristic syndromes related to metastatic cancer are the gasserian ganglion syndrome and the numb chin syndrome.

Gasserian Ganglion Syndrome. Numbness, paresthesias, and usually pain referred to the trigeminal distribution are the typical presenting complaints.[983] The symptoms may be present for 2 weeks to 1 year (median = 3 weeks) before diagnosis. Painless numbness

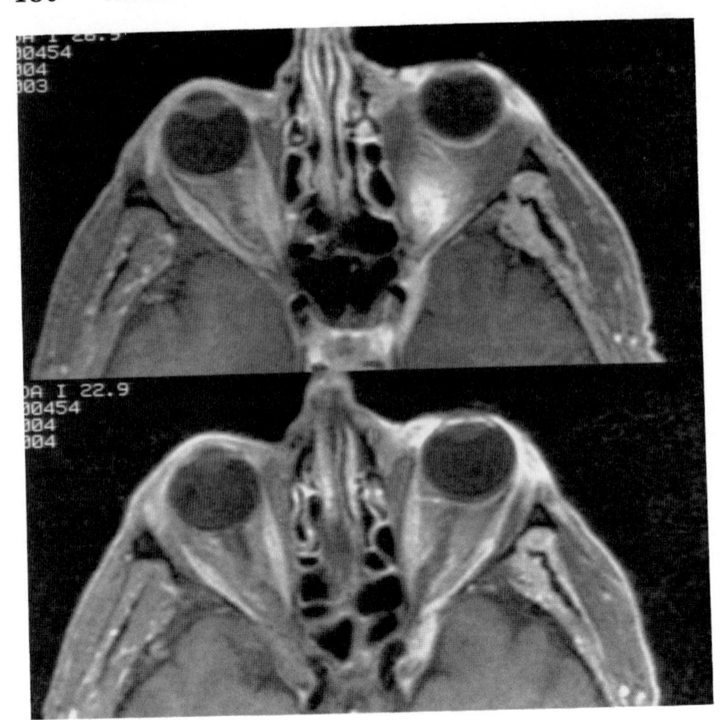

Figure 8–4. Neurotropic skin tumor involving the cavernous sinus. This patient developed diplopia several years after treatment of a squamous-cell carcinoma of the forehead. In addition to ocular palsies, pain and sensory dysfunction were present in the first division of the trigeminal nerve. The cavernous sinus on the left (right side of figure) is thickened and hyperintense after administration of gadolinium. Slight proptosis of the left eye is noted but no tumor is discernible in the orbit.

or facial paresthesias are common. The numbness begins close to the midline on the upper lip or chin and progresses laterally to the anterior part of the ear. Although uncommon, sensory symptoms, usually a gritty feeling in the eye, may occur in the first division of the trigeminal nerve. Pain consists of either a dull ache in the cheek, jaw, or forehead or lightninglike pain similar or identical to trigeminal neuralgia but unaccompanied by trigger points. Although lightninglike pain may temporarily be the only symptom, numbness and sensory loss rapidly appear, differentiating this entity from idiopathic trigeminal neuralgia, which is not associated with sensory loss. Headache is uncommon, in contrast to the parasellar syndrome, in which most patients suffer headache as an early and severe symptom.[983]

By the time of diagnosis, examination reveals sensory loss in the distribution of one or more trigeminal nerve roots in almost all patients, and often some evidence of dysfunction of the motor root as well. Obvious weakness of the pterygoid or masseter muscles may be absent, with no deviation of the jaw visible on jaw opening, but the physician may see or feel slight atrophy of the temporalis and masseter muscles and note a delay in contraction and less palpable bulk of the ipsilateral masseter when the patient bites down. Even in the absence of clearly defined weakness or atrophy, electromyography often reveals denervation. Motor loss distinguishes involvement of the gasserian ganglion and trigeminal nerve by tumor from trigeminal sensory neuropathy (a non-neoplastic syndrome[1051]). In addition, because the tumor often spreads beyond the area of the ganglion, other motor nerves, particularly the abducens, may also become involved.

In patients with hematogenous metastases directly to the ganglion, radiographic evaluation may be normal, although MR scans sometimes suggest enlargement of the gasserian ganglion and the tumor may enhance. A fine-needle biopsy can establish the diagnosis.[677] If the ganglion is secondarily involved from tumor metastasis to the petrous bone, a CT or a radionuclide bone scan usually establishes the diagnosis. The gasserian syndrome is so characteristic in patients known to be suffering from an underlying neoplasm, in particular breast or lung carcinoma, that focal radiation is indicated even in the absence of radiographic findings. A lumbar puncture should always be performed to evaluate for leptomeningeal metastases (see Chapter 7).

Numb Chin Syndrome. The numb chin usually results from dysfunction of the inferior alveolar nerve compressed by metastases to the mandible.[2360] It may also be caused by metastases to the skull base[348,369,1208,1603] or leptomeninges. Patients complain of numbness, almost always painless, over the chin and lower lip. The symptoms are usually unilateral; occasionally they occur on both sides simultaneously and, in rare cases, alternately. Signs consist of sensory loss over the chin and a contiguous area on the inside of the lip and gum. The loss may be mild or severe, and the symptoms may persist or may disappear spontaneously after a few weeks or months. In one series[1701] of 19 patients, chin numbness was the presenting symptom of a neoplasm in 9 of them. Lymphoma and leukemia were the most common causes. Breast cancer is also a relatively common cause.[369] Panoramic radiograms of the mandible identify bone metastases in fewer than 50% of the patients, but an MR scan is more often positive. The CSF may contain malignant cells, suggesting leptomeningeal tumor. The diagnosis is usually made clinically. The disorder often responds to treatment of the metastasis: RT is directed to the mandible after leptomeningeal metastases are excluded. Chemotherapy can be given either systemically or intrathecally, depending on the site and nature of the lesion. The importance of the numb chin syndrome is that it may be the first sign of cancer[369] or metastasis. In a patient not known to have cancer, it should prompt a search for an occult neoplasm, particularly a lymphoma or a breast cancer. It is unclear why the symptoms sometimes remit spontaneously. The disorder has also been reported as a complication of sickle cell anemia,[1409] presumably because of infarction of the nerve, and of mandibular atrophy in the elderly.[858]

FACIAL NERVE (CRANIAL NERVE VII)

Like the trigeminal nerve, the facial nerve may be involved by metastasis anywhere along its course. Facial paralysis is particularly likely to be an isolated finding when neurotropic carcinomas of the skin and salivary glands invade branches of the nerve and grow perineurally.[163,280,298,393,902] Although the facial nerve is predominantly a motor nerve, facial pain may be an early symptom, followed by partial or complete facial paralysis. The onset is usually gradual and progressive, differentiating it from the more common, acute Bell's palsy. Depending on where along its course the nerve is damaged, other facial nerve branches (such as those subserving taste, hearing acuity, and tearing) may be involved. Loss of taste is unilateral, unlike the bilateral distortion of taste that is fairly common in patients with cancer, and reflects systemic rather than direct nerve involvement.[632] The facial nerve may be damaged during surgery for malignant parotid tumors.[355,2119] Leptomeningeal metastases may cause unilateral facial paralysis as a first sign, but other cranial nerve dysfunction soon appears. Acute Bell's palsy, either idiopathic or secondary to herpes zoster (see Chapter 13), may cause enhancement of the seventh cranial nerve on MR scan, suggesting leptomeningeal tumor.[1401a]

Facial nerve paralysis accompanied by pain and otorrhea is usually infective in origin, but metastatic tumor occasionally causes symptoms of otitis.[1693] Malignant external otitis, an infection (see Chapter 10), may be mistaken for metastatic tumor.[425,637]

ACOUSTIC AND VESTIBULAR NERVES (CRANIAL NERVE VIII)

Loss of hearing (acoustic nerve) and vertigo (vestibular nerve) can result from leptomeningeal tumor or from metastases to the temporal bone, which are easily identifiable with MR scan. Cerebellopontine angle metastases can mimic acoustic neurinoma, causing hearing loss, vertigo, and tinnitus as well as facial and trigeminal involvement. Isolated metastases to the temporal bone or to the soft tissues of the inner ear occur by hematogenous spread from leukemias, lymphomas, and solid tumors; by direct extension of carcinomas of the head and neck region; or by invasion by nasopharyngeal tumors.[191] Symptoms are usually unilateral and evolve over days or weeks. Sudden bilateral hearing loss has been reported with bilateral temporal bone metastases.[1238] The labyrinth and cochlea also can serve as a sanctuary for leukemic cells.[1976]

GLOSSOPHARYNGEAL AND VAGUS NERVES (CRANIAL NERVES IX AND X)

Several clinical disorders can be associated with metastatic tumor involving these lower cranial nerves. Metastases in the subarachnoid space or at the skull base usually cause dysfunction of other cranial nerves (e.g., hypoglossal) as well as the glossopharyngeal and vagus nerves (see "Jugular Foramen Syndrome" following). More distal metastases may damage the two nerves either together or individually. Metastatic involvement of the glossopharyngeal nerve in isolation usually does not cause a motor deficit. Afferent fibers of this nerve are involved in blood pressure control, however; glossopharyngeal tumors may stimulate baroreceptor reflexes, causing hypotension and syncope. Motor fibers of the vagus nerve innervate palatal muscles (on the ipsilateral side) and larynx muscles; their dysfunction leads to dysphagia and hoarseness from vocal cord paralysis. Involvement of afferent vagal fibers may also cause cardiovascular dysfunction and syncope (see the following). Unilateral facial pain can be an unusual symptom of involvement of the vagus nerve in the chest by lung cancer. Recent reports[220,260,1871] describe 14 patients with unilateral aching facial pain in and around the jaw and ear, usually on the right side because of the close anatomic relationship of the vagus nerve to mediastinal lymph nodes, in whom investigation eventually revealed an ipsilateral lung tumor. The pain had been present as long as 4 years in some patients, and treatment directed at the lung tumor relieved the pain. The hypothesis is that the pain is referred to the face by the vagus nerve.

Patients in whom the motor portion of the vagus nerve is affected by tumor usually complain of dysphagia and hoarseness. If the involvement is proximal, examination usually reveals flaccidity of the ipsilateral palate and shift of the uvula to the contralateral side when the gag reflex is elicited or when the patient vocalizes. The gag reflex is absent on the ipsilateral side. More distal involvement of the vagus nerve can selectively involve only the larynx muscles. Hoarseness and a weak cough follow. Even with involvement of the larynx alone, dysphagia with repeated aspiration of liquids is often present. Sometimes the aspiration can be relieved by Teflon injection of the paralyzed vocal cord.[2741]

Dysphagia is such a common problem when tumor metastasizes to lower cranial nerves that the physician sometimes fails to recognize dysphagia resulting from esophageal or cervical lesions rather than from neural involvement. Neural dysphagia presents more difficulty in swallowing liquids, whereas esophageal or pharyngeal compression or obstruction makes solids more difficult to swallow.[2548] Non-neural dysphagia may be a presenting symptom of metastatic breast cancer.[938]

Jugular Foramen Syndrome.[983,2531] Patients with most tumors involving the jugular foramen present with either hoarseness or dysphagia.[983] A dull, unilateral, aching pain localized behind the ear on the involved side usually is a prominent feature. Rarely, the metastasis causes glossopharyngeal neuralgia with very brief throat pain followed by syncope. Signs include weakness of the palate, vocal cord paralysis, weakness and atrophy of the ipsilateral sternocleidomastoid muscle and the upper part of the trapezius, and sometimes Horner's syndrome. Compression by the tumor of the transverse sinus or the jugular vein within the jugular foramen sometimes causes papilledema.[978] Some patients have ipsilateral weakness and atrophy of the tongue, indicating extension of the tumor to the hypoglossal nerve. The diagnosis is usually easily established with an MR scan.

Syncope. With or without pain, syncope may be the only symptom of metastatic involvement of the glossopharyngeal or vagus nerve[1635,1948] (Fig. 8–5). This condition commonly accompanies head and neck tumors and is particularly likely when the tumor recurs after initial treatment, especially after radical neck dissection. The tumor affects the carotid sinus nerve fibers on the carotid artery or the more proximal nerve fibers at the skull base. Affected patients complain of severe paroxysms of pain lasting from a few minutes to 30 minutes. The pain may be in the neck, the ear, or the side of the head and

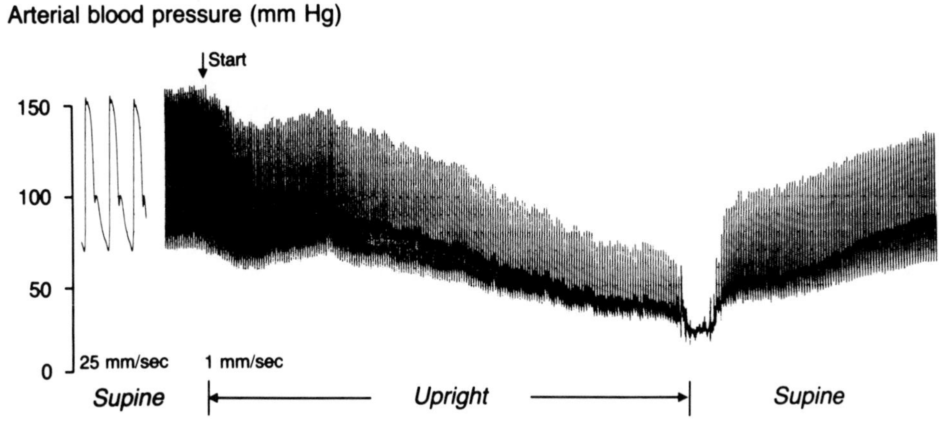

Figure 8–5. A 72-year-old woman with breast cancer that had metastasized to the glossopharyngeal region had recurrent episodes of sudden lightheadedness, diaphoresis, and syncope. A dual-chamber pacemaker was implanted, but syncope recurred, always preceded by severe neck pain. During a tilt-table test with the pacemaker inactivated, the results of which are shown here, the patient's usual symptoms developed. She lost consciousness and had a seizure but regained consciousness immediately after she was returned to the supine position. The study shows a profound vasodepressor reaction with minimal slowing of the sinus rhythm. Treatment with disopyramide, 150 mg three times a day, eliminated the syncopal episodes over a period of 5 months of follow-up care. (From Osswald and Trouton,[1953] p 30, with permission.)

is accompanied by syncope, the result of sudden hypotension. The hypotension is sometimes, but not always, accompanied by bradycardia and occasionally by cardiac arrest. The disorder may occur once every few weeks to several times a day. The patient usually recovers from each episode promptly, although the cardiac arrest may be life-threatening. This disorder is probably a result of aberrant discharge of the damaged nerve, which stimulates brain nuclei to inhibit sympathetic vasoconstrictor tone.[1948] Sometimes the condition resolves spontaneously as the tumor progresses to completely destroy the nerve.

Treatment is difficult. If the underlying tumor can be treated successfully, the syndrome may resolve. Bradycardia or cardiac arrest is the primary cause of the syncope in only a few instances so that, although a pacemaker may help, the severe hypotensive episodes usually continue to cause syncope despite the pacemaker. Several drugs, including anticonvulsants and sympathomimetic drugs,[1635,1948] have been used to treat the disorder but none have been entirely successful. Sectioning of the involved glossopharyngeal or vagus nerve usually cures the disorder but may cause transient hypertension.

Another cause of syncope related to metastatic tumor is swallow syncope.[1534] This rare syndrome can also result from involvement of glossopharyngeal or vagal afferents or from metastatic tumor in the esophagus. The patient suddenly loses consciousness during a hard swallow, usually because of intense bradycardia caused by stimulation of baroreceptor nerves. This disorder can often be blocked by atropine or similar drugs.

SPINAL ACCESSORY NERVE (CRANIAL NERVE XI)

The spinal accessory nerve innervates the trapezius and sternocleidomastoid muscles on the ipsilateral side. It arises from upper cervical segments, enters the skull, and then exits through the jugular foramen. Rarely is it involved alone by tumor, although it is often sectioned during radical neck dissection[2536] (Chapter 14). Involvement of the nerve leads to drooping of the shoulder, aching pain, shoulder and arm discomfort, and a little weakness of the head's turning to the opposite side. On examination, weakness usually is not prominent; instead, the physician finds atrophy of the superior portion of the trapezius muscle and the sternocleidomastoid, particularly when the patient tries to contract those muscles. Electromyography settles the issue of whether the muscles are denervated.

HYPOGLOSSAL NERVE (CRANIAL NERVE XII)

The hypoglossal nerve leaves the skull through the hypoglossal foramen of the occipital bone and travels in the neck to as low as the second or third cervical vertebral body before curving back to innervate the tongue. Thus, ipsilateral tongue paralysis can occur when nerve is involved by tumor in the subarachnoid space, at the hypoglossal foramen, or in the upper neck. Because the twelfth nerves are close together at the lower end of the clivus before leaving the skull, metastases to that bone can cause bilateral hypoglossal palsies. Bilateral hypoglossal paralysis can also complicate RT to the upper neck[1297] (see Chapter 13).

Occipital Condyle.[983] A syndrome caused by metastatic tumor involving the occipital condyle is more common than the jugular foramen syndrome and somewhat more difficult to diagnose. The clinical picture is quite uniform. Patients complain of continuous, severe, localized, unilateral occipital pain made worse by neck flexion and often associated with a stiff neck. Sometimes the pain radiates anteriorly toward the ipsilateral temporal area or eye. About half of the patients complain of dysarthria, dysphagia, or both, specifically related to difficulty in moving the tongue. Symptoms usually appear weeks to months before a diagnosis is made. On neurologic examination, patients hold their necks stiffly and are sometimes tender to palpation over the occipital area on the involved side. The ipsilateral tongue is atrophic, and sometimes fasciculations are evident. The tongue deviates toward the weak side when it is protruded but cannot be deviated toward that side when in the mouth.[2173] When the tongue is resting in the mouth, the ipsilateral side is higher, giving the appearance of deviation to the other side.

Diagnosis and Treatment

When tumors invade the base of the brain, MR is the diagnostic test of choice.[2079] It is particularly useful in evaluating tumor encasement of the arteries, invasion of the cavernous sinus, and the relationship of tumor to cranial nerves such as the optic nerve and optic chiasm. Bone destruction, however, is more easily observed on CT scan.[1971] In that regard, radionuclide bone scans are often helpful as well.[312] At times, diagnosis requires biopsy.

The treatment depends on the nature of the underlying tumor. RT and chemotherapy are usually the treatments of choice.[431,2000,2696] Recent improvements in surgical therapy for primary tumors of the skull base occasionally make such approaches feasible in patients with single metastases.[1252,1274] Monitoring of sensory-evoked potentials has been reported to be helpful during surgery.[900] Radiosurgery[406a,1337] and brachytherapy[200,1437] may also be useful.

SPINAL ROOTS

Metastatic tumor can involve spinal roots in two ways. The less common way is by direct hematogenous metastasis to the nerve root or dorsal root ganglion; more common is invasion or compression of roots by tumor in the paravertebral space. In the first instance, one or two roots are usually involved. In the second, tumor may grow longitudinally in the paravertebral space to involve multiple roots. A metastasis to a single dorsal root ganglion or spinal root may be asymptomatic because the sensory distribution of dorsal roots usually overlaps enough that damage to a single root does not cause either sensory or motor loss. On the other hand, hematogenous metastases to dorsal root ganglia can cause pain and paresthesias in the distribution of the dermatome(s) supplied by that root.

Patients usually suffer symptoms when nerve roots or their sympathetic fibers are compressed or invaded by paravertebral tumors. The first symptom is usually that of chronic and aching pain in the sensory distribution of the root. The pain sometimes has the lightninglike characteristics of trigeminal neuralgia or tabes dorsalis. Pain may be the only neurologic symptom for a variable time, but eventually, other signs of either hyperfunction or loss of function appear. Paresthesias usually tingle but may occasionally burn. Numbness and loss of sensation also eventually occur in the involved dermatomes. Loss of autonomic function leads to diminished or absent sweating and increased redness and warmth of the skin.

When upper thoracic segments and the stellate ganglion are involved, as occurs with Pancoast tumors, Horner's syndrome develops. It is characterized by miosis, ptosis, and diminished sweating over the ipsilateral half of the face and (depending on the sympathetic roots involved) the upper extremity. When the arm is affected, the skin of the fingers fails to wrinkle after immersion in warm water because the sympathetic fibers that cause the wrinkling are nonfunctioning.[290] Less common are signs of autonomic hyperfunction with focal hyperhidrosis,[2043,2734] piloerection, and sometimes coolness and pallor in the involved dermatome. Intermittent or continuous mydriasis may be evident, as well as gustatory sweating[839] (i.e., hemifacial ipsilateral sweating when eating spicy foods).

Motor signs of nerve root involvement by tumor include weakness and atrophy in the distribution of the involved root. Occasionally, fasciculations may be observed. Muscle cramps are often an early sign of nerve root or peripheral nerve damage in patients with cancer,[2484] and the muscle innervated by the involved nerve root is sometimes paradoxically enlarged.[498]

When nerve roots in the cervical and lumbosacral areas are involved, the diagnosis is usually fairly obvious because weakness and loss of reflex function or Horner's syndrome are associated with typical radicular pain in the upper or lower extremity. When thoracic and abdominal roots are involved, the diagnosis is more difficult. Involvement of a few dermatomes may cause only pain and paresthesias. Autonomic dysfunction, weakness, and sensory loss may be absent or inapparent. Sometimes one superficial abdominal reflex is absent, or an observant clinician may note failure of the abdominal muscles to contract symmetrically. A careful sensory examination of the trunk and inspection for autonomic dysfunction are mandatory. In patients complaining of shoulder or upper extremity pain, the presence of even a mild Horner's syndrome may be helpful in establishing the diagnosis. In one series[922] of 216 patients with Horner's syndrome, the symptoms in 58 were caused by malignant neoplasms involving sympathetic fibers. Involvement of sympathetic fibers reaching the lower extremities is characterized by redness, increased temperature, and dryness of the leg. In one report, 2 of 15 patients with tumors involving the lumbosacral plexus and associated sympathetic fibers complained of a hot, dry foot with or without pain as the first symptom of a lumbar plexopathy.[553] Conversely, patients with paravertebral tumor involving nerve roots may present with signs of sympathetic overactivity.[2734]

Diagnosing nerve root involvement may be difficult. If microscopic metastasis has occurred by hematogenous spread to a root, the diagnosis is virtually impossible except at autopsy or during the course of ganglionectomies for pain treatment. If a tumor in the paravertebral space compresses the root, resulting changes are often apparent radiographically. The best test is the MR scan, which identifies a paravertebral mass and also may reveal that the tumor has grown through the intervertebral foramen to compress the spinal cord. Radiation is often effective in relieving symptoms, particularly pain.[2460]

NERVE PLEXUSES

The three major nerve plexuses are the brachial, lumbar, and sacral. The latter two are often affected together by tumor, producing a disorder known as lumbosacral plexus dysfunction. Brachial plexus involvement by tumor is more common than the others and is also more serious because it affects the hand rather than the leg. Also, pain and neurologic dysfunction of the brachial plexus are often more severe and difficult to treat.

Brachial Plexus

The brachial plexus is commonly compressed or invaded by tumors arising at the lung apex (Pancoast tumor)[622] (Fig. 8–6) or by lymph node metastases arising from breast carcinoma.[1412] In both instances, because of the anatomy of the brachial plexus, tumor tends to compress or invade the plexus from below, involving those fibers that begin as the

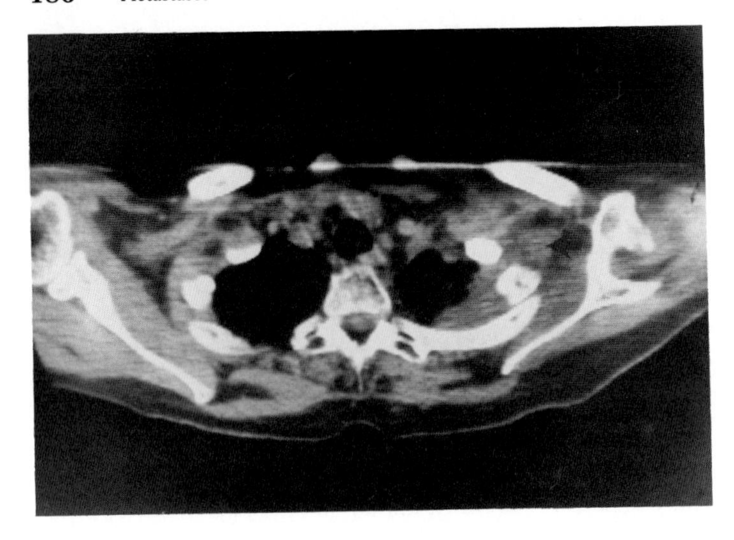

Figure 8–6. A CT scan showing invasion of the brachial plexus by Pancoast tumor of the lung *(arrow)*. The patient presented with a typical history of pain radiating down the medial arm, preceding discovery of the tumor by several months.

C-8 and T-1 root and end as the ulnar nerve. Wherever the plexus is involved along its course, the primary symptom is pain. The pain usually begins as posterior or lateral shoulder pain of a dull, aching quality and rapidly expands to include the medial aspects of the upper arm, the elbow, and frequently the forearm. In many patients, the pain localizes to either the posterior shoulder or around the elbow; the local pain may so overshadow the other areas of the nerve's distribution that the physician is tempted to investigate the bony or soft-tissue structures around the shoulder or elbow rather than the more proximal nerve plexus. Even when nerve compression is suspected, the diagnosis of cervical intervertebral disk disease is often made and cervical traction applied. Involvement of the C-8 and T-1 roots by cervical disks is uncommon,[2869] but it is the characteristic symptom of tumor involving the brachial plexus.

Paresthesias and numbness, and less often pain, are commonly perceived in the ring and little fingers. Significant sensory signs are rarely present unless the patient complains of sensory symptoms; even then, they are less striking. Pre-existing sensory signs in the medial upper arm may have been unrecognized by the patient, however, and their discovery may confuse the diagnosis. For example, radical mastectomy sacrifices the intercostobrachial nerve, causing sensory loss in the posterior and medial aspect of the arm.[95,2684,2757] Patients are often not aware of this, although phantom sensation in the breast after mastectomy is frequent, and phantom pain is common.[1431] If the sensory loss is discovered by a physician who suspects new brachial plexus dysfunction, the apparent new sensory loss may be misleading.

Accompanying the loss of sensation and the paresthesias of brachial plexus tumors is weakness, which usually begins in the small muscles of the hand, making it difficult to hold small objects, such as pencils, or to oppose the thumb and fifth finger. Later, the weakness extends to involve finger (grip) flexors, wrist flexors and extensors, and elbow extensors (triceps muscle). Biceps, brachioradial, and deltoid muscles are often spared until later. Initially normal, the triceps reflex diminishes and finally disappears as the disease progresses. The biceps and brachioradialis reflexes are usually spared until later. An early and useful sign of lower plexus involvement is ipsilateral absence of the finger-stretch reflex, especially if the reflex is present on the contralateral side. Bilaterally, absent finger-stretch reflexes in a patient with otherwise brisk reflexes are often an early sign of T-1 vertebral body and root involvement with cord compression. If the tumor is medial, the sympathetic trunk may be involved, and the observant patient may note the ptosis and hypohidrosis of Horner's syndrome.

In typical patients, the results of the neurologic examination may be normal early in the development of the illness, when pain and paresthesias are the only symptoms. Inspection of the chest may reveal fullness of the supraclavicular or infraclavicular fossa on the involved side, so that the sharp lines of the clavicle are effaced. Sometimes, an increased venous pattern over the anterior chest represents collateral circulation from an axillary or subclavian vein compressed by tumor. Palpation of the supraclavicular fossa and axilla may reveal adenopathy or diffuse thickening of tissues, suggesting tumor. Firm palpation or percussion, particularly in the supraclavicular area, may cause pain or paresthesias in the arm, suggesting demyelination of the brachial plexus in that area. Tumor can decrease the size of the thoracic outlet, leading to changes in pulse and blood pressure in the involved arm. Furthermore, as the involved plexus is stretched, pain is likely to be exacerbated and paresthesias appear. Thus, the shoulder should be examined through a full range of motion to determine in which position pain is increased, whether a bruit develops over the subclavian artery, or whether the blood pressure and pulse in the arm diminish. Except that pain is uncommon with radiation fibrosis, these findings of brachial plexus involvement do not distinguish tumor from radiation fibrosis (see Chapter 13), however, or even from a benign thoracic outlet syndrome.[1092,1412,1494,2580]

LABORATORY TESTS

The first diagnostic laboratory test is a chest radiograph. The film should be examined to be sure that the apices of the lungs are well seen and that one can determine if tumor is present in the superior portion of the lung or in the supraclavicular area. Apical views sometimes help when the results of routine chest radiograph are normal. If this test is unrewarding, a CT or MR scan through the brachial plexus, with particular attention to the paravertebral area, may reveal evidence of tumor not otherwise seen.[396] The scan also reveals any intravertebral extension of the brachial plexus lesion. If a Horner's syndrome is present or if a tumor is found close to the vertebral body, an MR of the cervical spine may be helpful. If nodes are palpated in the supraclavicular area or axilla and the diagnosis is uncertain, biopsy may document evidence of tumor, strongly suggesting that the pain and brachial plexus dysfunction result from tumor compression. Electromyography can identify the distribution of denervation and suggest the site of plexus involvement.[1092] Myokymia on electromyography suggests radiation fibrosis rather than tumor (see Chapter 13).[1092]

In some patients, laboratory tests yield evidence of brachial plexus dysfunction but fail to reveal the cause; exploration of the plexus with biopsy of surrounding tissues may be necessary. Kline and his colleagues[688,1391] propose a posterior exploration to examine the entire plexus. If one finds fibrous bands compressing the plexus instead of tumor, these can be removed. The widest possible exploration is necessary to be certain of the presence or absence of tumor. Even with exploration, the diagnosis may not be possible if the tumor does not cause a discernible mass that can be biopsied but instead invades the nerves, yielding no grossly visible evidence of its presence.

COURSE

Untreated pain will grow progressively more severe. Similarly, neurologic dysfunction will spread from the lower to the upper plexus and eventually will paralyze the entire upper extremity. Lymphedema and an increased venous pattern are often late accompaniments. The pain is usually completely disabling and overshadows the functional disability. Often the pain develops into a reflex sympathetic dystrophy (or sympathetically maintained pain) with trophic changes in the hand and nails. This particular painful complication requires specific treatment (see Chapter 4).

DIFFERENTIAL DIAGNOSIS

The major problem in differential diagnosis occurs in patients previously irradiated to the upper thorax or axilla (e.g., after mastectomy for breast cancer). The development of a brachial plexopathy usually indicates tumor recurrence or radiation fibrosis; several clinical clues help distinguish the conditions (Table 8–3). Pain is a more common presenting complaint and is usually much more severe[1092,1412,1494,2580] in patients with tumor that invades the plexus than in patients with radiation fibrosis. Increasing lymphedema suggests radiation involvement[806,1412] rather than tumor. Radiation plexopathy often in-

Table 8–3. **CLINICAL FEATURES OF BRACHIAL PLEXUS SYNDROMES IN PATIENTS WITH BREAST CANCER**

	Tumor Infiltration	Radiation Fibrosis	Reversible Radiation Injury	Acute Ischemic Brachial Plexopathy
Incidence of pain	89%	18%	40%	Painless
Location of pain	Shoulder, upper arm, elbow, medial forearm	Shoulder, wrist, hand	Hand, forearm	—
Nature of pain	Dull aching in shoulder; lancinating pain in elbow and ulnar aspect of hand; occasional dysesthesias, burning, or freezing sensations	Aching pain in shoulder; paresthesias in C5, C6 distribution in hand	Pain in shoulder; paresthesias in hand and forearm	Paresthesias in hand and forearm
Severity of pain	Severe in 98% of patients	Usually absent or mild (severe in a few patients)	Mild	—
Course	Progressive neurologic dysfunction, atrophy, weakness C7–T1 distribution; pain persistent; Horner's syndrome	Progressive weakness in C5–C6 distribution; pain stabilizes with appearance of weakness	Transient weakness and atrophy in C6–C7, T1; complete resolution of motor findings	Acute nonprogressive weakness and sensory changes
CT	Circumscribed mass with diffuse infiltration of tissue planes	Diffuse infiltration of tissue planes	Normal	Normal; angiography shows subclavian artery segmental obstruction
MRI	High signal intensity in circumscribed mass on T_2-weighted images; may enhance with gadolinium	Diffuse low signal intensity on T_2-weighted images; no change with gadolinium	No available data	Normal
Electromyographic findings	Segmental slowing, no myokymia	Myokymia	Segmental slowing, no myokymia	Segmental slowing, no myokymia
Lymphedema	May be stable or increase	Usually increases	No change	No change

Source: Adapted from Foley,[806] p 728, with permission.

volves muscles of the shoulder girdle before it involves the hand, is painless, and is associated with lymphedema, whereas tumor involving the plexus often begins in the C-8 and T-1 roots, affects the hand before the shoulder, is painful, and is not associated with lymphedema. Horner's syndrome is more common with tumor recurrence than with radiation plexopathy.[1412] Other investigators have not found the motor distribution helpful in distinguishing between these two entities,[1092,1494,2580] but all agree that myokymia on electromyography is virtually pathognomonic of radiation fibrosis.[1092]

An acute reversible brachial neuritis syndrome has been reported in a few patients shortly following RT for breast carcinoma.[2278] Symptoms generally occur about 4 months after RT and are characterized by mild shoulder pain and arm paresthesias. Weakness may be severe but is reversible. The pathogenesis of the syndrome is unknown.

Acute ischemic brachial neuropathy results from occlusion of the subclavian artery, a late complication of RT (see Chapter 13). The disorder is predominantly motor, sudden in onset, and painless.[905] Paresthesias may be felt in the forearm and hand.

The thoracic outlet syndrome rarely causes diagnostic difficulties because the pain it generates is usually intermittent rather than continuous, is related to the position of the arm, and rarely is associated with severe motor or sensory dysfunction, other than paresthesias, in the extremities.

Primary nerve sheath tumors are distinguished by their history,[807] and the diagnosis is made with biopsy.[688]

In patients not known to have cancer, the most common error in differential diagnosis is to assume that the brachial plexus involvement is caused by cervical osteoarthritis or cervical disk disease. This common error can usually be avoided by remembering that most cervical osteoarthritis involves the C-5, C-6, or C-7 roots, causing pain in the outer aspect of the arm and lateral aspect of the forearm, and usually causes paresthesias in the thumb, index, and middle fingers rather than in the fifth finger. If weakness is present, it usually involves the triceps, deltoid, biceps, or brachioradialis; hand muscles are spared. Reflex loss affects triceps, biceps, and brachioradialis; finger-stretch reflexes are usually spared. It is unusual for brachial plexus tumor to involve these structures first. Although radiation plexopathy may involve more proximal muscles early, it can be distinguished from cervical disk disease by the absence of pain; cervical disk disease is rarely painless.

Another problem in differential diagnosis is distinguishing acute brachial neuritis from tumor involvement of the plexus. Acute brachial neuritis is characterized by the sudden onset of severe pain referred to the tip of the shoulder, followed in several days by marked weakness, particularly of muscles around the shoulder girdle but sometimes of arm muscles as well. The deltoid and serratus anterior muscles are most commonly involved. Biceps, brachioradialis, and supraspinatus can also be involved. Motor changes are usually much more striking than sensory changes. After one to several weeks, the pain tends to clear spontaneously, and strength usually returns to normal without treatment after weeks to months. The acute onset, rapid progression, and relative absence of sensory changes, as well as the distribution of the muscle weakness, exclude the diagnosis of brachial plexus tumor and suggest brachial neuritis. Acute brachial neuritis is more common in patients with Hodgkin's disease, as is Guillain-Barré syndrome, than it is in the general population. In patients with Hodgkin's disease, brachial neuritis may occur early during RT,[1666] after the first or second treatment, or it may be unassociated with radiation.

TREATMENT

Two general approaches are used to treat brachial plexus tumor. The first is to try to diminish or eradicate the tumor by RT or chemotherapy. RT often can effectively relieve the pain and diminish the tumor size.[46,1403] It is usually less effective in restoring neurologic function, particularly if severe weakness or sensory loss is already present. If only mild changes in neurologic function have occurred, RT often restores full function. When RT or chemotherapy cannot relieve pain, it must be treated directly. Pain from brachial plexus involvement is particularly intense and intractable. A vigorous trial of analgesic agents is essential, using opioids in adequate doses with adjuvant analgesic agents (see Chapter 4). If these fail, the physician should consider a high cervical cordotomy[1249] or rhizotomy. If, as is often the case, the pain is in part sympathetically maintained, a stellate ganglion block may relieve the pain; repeated blocks may give prolonged relief. The management of cancer pain has been reviewed recently.[1077]

Lumbar Plexus

Tumors that frequently affect the lumbar plexus include colorectal carcinomas; retroperitoneal sarcomas; or metastatic tumors from breast, lymphoma, cervix, bladder, or prostate.[1270,2704] The plexus may be involved by local extension of the tumor along lymphatic channels into the vertebral bodies or paravertebral space. Isolated lumbar plexus involvement is less common than sacral plexus involvement, although both often occur together as a lumbosacral plexopathy (Fig. 8–7). The tumor generally is bulky and compresses the plexus, but it may invade neural structures without causing a mass. The severity and type of pain vary with the site of plexus involvement but is generally of two types (Table 8–4): (1) If the lumbar plexus is involved, dull, aching back pain occurs near the costovertebral angle. This local pain may be absent or completely overshadowed by a radicular distribution of pain involving the groin and anteromedial aspect of the thigh. (2) If the lower plexus is involved, the back pain is usually somewhat lower, often near the iliac crest, radiating into the buttocks and down the posterior aspect of the thigh and leg toward the ankle. Sometimes the entire plexus is involved. The aching pain extends anteriorly and posteriorly in the thigh and leg. Usually exacerbated either by sudden movement or, at times, by lying in the supine position, the pain is sometimes relieved by standing or walking, a phenomenon that helps distinguish plexus lesions from bony disease of the pelvis or hip. This pain may be present without other neurologic signs or symptoms. When neurologic symptoms other than pain occur, they usually appear first as motor weakness with mild sensory complaints. If the upper lumbar plexus is involved, the patient complains of difficulty climbing stairs and walks with his or her leg held in rigid extension to avoid knee buckling. The patient may also note atrophy of the anterior thigh and muscle tenderness in the quadriceps. If the lower lumbar plexus is involved, the patient may complain of foot drop.

On examination, focal findings are usually minimal. Sometimes the tumor mass can be felt on rectal examination. The hip can generally be moved through a full range of motion without substantial pain, although extreme external rotation may cause pain, perhaps from irritation of a branch of the sciatic nerve to the capsule of the femoral head. Palpation of the pelvic bones usually has likewise negative findings. If the lower lumbar plexus is involved, straight-leg raising

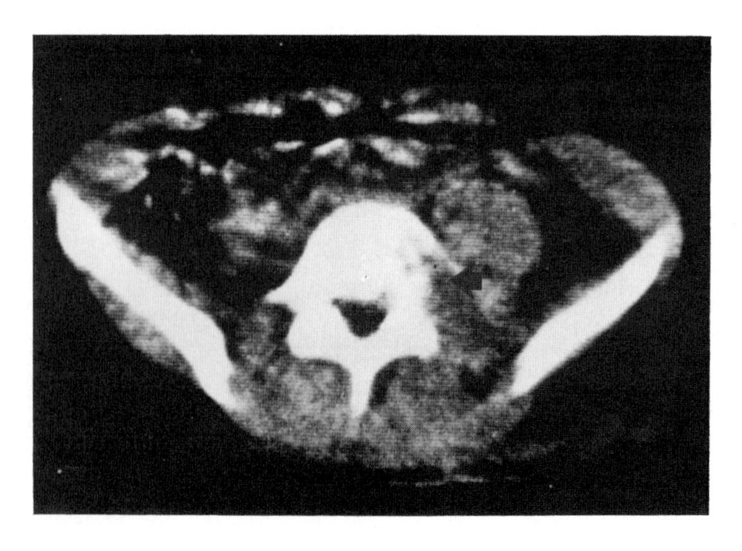

Figure 8–7. A CT scan showing left lumbosacral plexopathy resulting from recurrence of pelvic cancer. The transverse process of the vertebral body and the lateral portion of the vertebra are infiltrated by tumor *(arrow)*. The patient had a painful lumbar plexopathy involving the ipsilateral lower extremity.

Table 8–4. **SYMPTOMS AND SIGNS OF TUMOR INVOLVING LUMBOSACRAL PLEXUS**

Clinical Level	Upper	Lower	Pan-Plexus
Number of patients	12	16	6
Most common tumor	Colorectal	Sarcoma	Genitourinary
Pain distribution			
Local	Lower abdomen	Buttock, perineum	Lumbosacral
Radicular	Anterolateral thigh	Posterolateral thigh, leg	Variable
Referred	Flank, iliac crest	Hip and ankle	Variable
Numbness/paresthesias	Anterior thigh	Perineum, thigh, sole	Anterior thigh, leg, foot
Motor and reflex changes	L-2–L-4	L-5–S-1	L-2–S-2
Sensory loss	Anterolateral thigh	Posterior thigh, sole	Especially anterior thigh, leg
Tenderness	Lumbar	Sciatic notch, sacrum	Lumbosacral
Positive SLRT			
Direct	6/12	8/16	5/6
Reverse	2/12	8/16	5/6
Leg edema	5/12	6/16	5/6
Rectal mass	3/12	7/16	1/6
Sphincter weakness	0/12	8/16	0/6

STLR = straight-leg–raising test.
Source: From Jaeckle et al,[1270] p 10, with permission.

may reproduce the patient's pain. In patients with upper plexus lesions, pain may be absent on straight-leg raising, but severe pain often occurs when the leg rapidly descends after it has been raised either voluntarily or passively, probably because the iliopsoas muscle is also affected by tumor, making sudden stretching painful. If the upper plexus is involved, the physician finds weakness of the iliopsoas and sometimes of the quadriceps muscle as well. The patellar reflex may be diminished or absent, but sensory changes are usually few and mild. If the lower lumbar or upper sacral plexus is involved, the weakness is generally most marked in the hamstring muscles and the dorsiflexors and plantar flexors of the foot; the achilles reflex is absent. The proximal muscles that are supplied by the lower lumbar plexus, including adductor magnus, gluteus maximus and medius, and tensor fasciae latae, also are weak. The focal weakness of proximal muscles suggests that the plexus is involved rather than more peripheral structures in the thigh or leg, such as the sciatic or peroneal nerve.[2288]

LABORATORY TESTS

The laboratory approach indicated for brachial plexus lesions can be applied here. MR scan is probably the best diagnostic test for identifying tumor involvement of the lumbar plexus. At times, when the plexus is invaded rather than compressed, radiographic tests are not revealing. On occasion, particularly with very difficult diagnoses, surgical exploration of the plexus is necessary.

DIFFERENTIAL DIAGNOSIS

Metastatic disease of the hip is identified on examination by severe pain on hip movement and evidence of tumor on a bone scan. Compression by tumor of the femoral, obturator, or sciatic nerve in the pelvis can be distinguished from plexus involvement by the distribution of muscles involved and also by location of the radiographic mass identified.[2193] Remember, however, that referred pain may cause local tenderness in muscles and bone, often leading the clinician to misinterpret the tender area as being the lesion site.

Another source of possible misinterpretation is osteitis pubis, an illness that is sometimes misdiagnosed as peripheral nerve or plexus tumor. Infection of the symphysis pubis and pubic bone may follow genitourinary surgery.[517] Symptoms do not appear for several weeks after the operation but then begin as severe pain down the medial aspects of both thighs, often with surprisingly little pubic pain. The pain is frequently so severe that the patient cannot walk. Neurologists are sometimes asked to consult in such instances because of suspected lumbar plexus or nerve root involvement. The neurologic examination is normal insofar as can be determined; patients frequently are unwilling to move their legs. The symphysis pubis, when palpated, is very tender; the pain produced by palpation is often perceived both locally and in the areas where the patient feels the spontaneous pain. Radiographs of the pubic bone may reveal inflammatory changes, or the results may be normal. The diagnosis is made with biopsy specimen and bone culture. Symptoms are relieved completely by appropriate antibiotic treatment. The organism is usually *Staphylococcus* or *Pseudomonas.*

Other bone and joint disorders complicating cancer and sometimes confused with nerve or plexus lesions are avascular necrosis (see Chapter 4) and diffuse bone and joint pain accompanying acute leukemia.[1690] Osteoporotic fractures of the pelvis may simulate metastatic disease.[1112]

RT delivered to tumors in the lumbosacral area can cause radiation plexopathy, which generally begins a year or more after the original radiation was begun (see Chapter 13). Radiation damage is usually characterized by bilateral, indolent leg weakness, often accompanied by lymphedema, whereas patients with tumors involving the lumbosacral plexus usually have severe unilateral pain and weakness without lymphedema.[2579]

TREATMENT

The principles applied to treating brachial plexus involvement also apply to the lumbar and sacral plexuses. RT is delivered to the area and analgesic agents are administered for the pain. If this regimen is ineffective, cordotomy should be considered.

Sacral Plexus

The sacral plexus is usually involved by tumor from the colon, prostate, bladder, or uterus, which extends directly to the sacrum (Fig. 8–8). The sacral plexus is closer to the midline than is the lumbar plexus, and because the involvement of the sacral plexus is usually secondary to bony invasion of the sacrum, bilateral (albeit asymmetric) changes are common. The symptoms usually begin as dull, aching, midline pain, often exacerbated by lying in a supine position or sitting, and sometimes relieved by lying in a

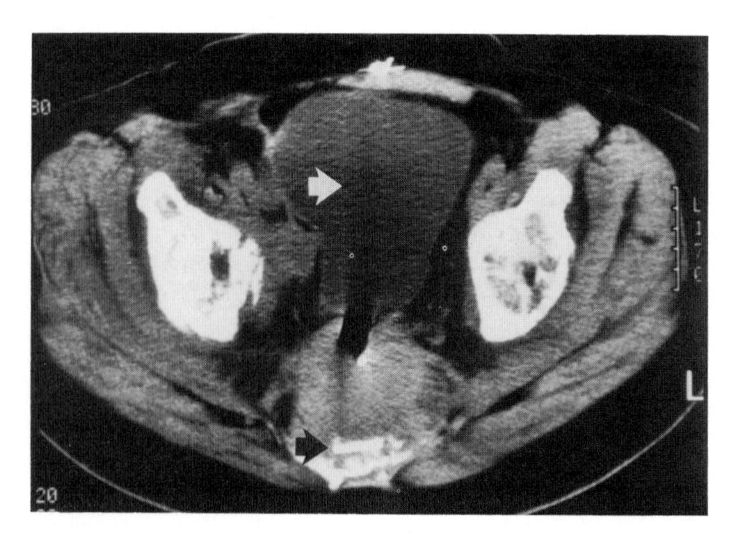

Figure 8–8. A CT scan of bilateral sacral plexopathy caused by recurrent rectal cancer. The sacrum is infiltrated and partially destroyed by the tumor *(black arrow).* The bladder is grossly enlarged because of denervation *(white arrow).*

prone position or by standing or walking. The pain sometimes radiates into the buttocks but not into the posterior aspects of the thigh or leg. The pain is usually followed by numbness in the perianal region, beginning unilaterally but rapidly becoming bilateral. Numbness and paresthesias may involve the entire buttocks and often extend to involve the posterior aspect of the thigh. Associated with the numbness is loss of sensation of evacuating bladder and bowel; constipation is followed by urinary retention or incontinence. On examination, pain may occur if the sacrum is palpated. At times the tumor can be felt, or pain is stimulated by rectal or pelvic examination with the finger palpating posteriorly. The rectal sphincter is often lax, and the bulbocavernosus and anal wink reflexes are absent. Sensory loss to pinprick and touch also are found over the penis, portions of the scrotum or labia, and the perianal area.

LABORATORY TESTS

Laboratory tests to identify sacral plexus involved by tumor are the same as those described previously for brachial and lumbar plexus involvement. CT and MR scans are excellent tools to indicate presacral masses and sacral destruction.[2704]

DIFFERENTIAL DIAGNOSIS

The major difficulty in differential diagnosis is distinguishing leptomeningeal metastases from sacral plexus involvement. Leptomeningeal metastases are usually more bilaterally symmetric from onset and characterized by less pain than with sacral plexus involvement, in which pain is an early and prominent symptom and the findings are usually asymmetric until late. In patients suspected of harboring sacral plexus metastases, however, enhanced MR should be performed to examine the distal subarachnoid space. CSF should also be examined.

TREATMENT

The principles of treatment resemble those for other plexus involvement. RT, both external and internal, is the treatment of choice. In many instances, although patients have already received the maximum external RT, the tumor has recurred. If the pain is severe and does not respond to RT, pain relief using analgesics should be considered first; if drugs fail, consider other approaches, such as spinal opioids, chemical neurolysis, or cordotomy.[1077]

PERIPHERAL NERVES

Peripheral nerves can be involved by tumor either focally or diffusely. Peripheral neuropathy that is due to tumor is much less common than that which is due to chemotherapy (see Chapter 12). Diffuse involvement by tumor, causing a sensorimotor polyneuropathy, is rare and is usually caused by leukemia, lymphoma, or myeloma.* Also rare are tumors that are metastatic to individual peripheral nerves,[1716,2107,2500] also usually caused by leukemia or lymphoma.

Mononeuropathies

The most common cause of peripheral nerve involvement is tumor that invades a contiguous bone and compresses a nerve, usually located at a point at which it either passes directly over a bone (such as the radial nerve at the humerus) or through a bony canal (such as the obturator nerve through the obturator canal).[2193] Other nerves sometimes affected include the ulnar nerve, affected by metastatic disease around the elbow or nodal metastases within the axilla; intercostal nerves, by rib metastases; the sciatic nerve, by involvement in the pelvis at several sites; and the peroneal nerve, as it passes behind the head of the fibula.

The signs and symptoms are pain at first and then sensory and motor loss in the distribution of the involved nerve. Careful neurologic evaluation with attention to the particular muscles and the distribution of the sensory loss involved easily distinguishes involvement of the peripheral nerve from that of more proximal structures such as plexuses and roots. In addition, radiating paresthesias can occur when the nerve is percussed near the site of tumor involvement (Tinel's sign).

---

*References 153, 640, 911, 1044, 1282, 1423, 1732, 1899, 2518, 2701.

The mass involving or compressing the nerve may be palpable, and palpating adjacent bones often reveals tenderness in those structures. Once the nerve involvement has been identified clinically, MR scans of the area will define the mass. Even when a mass lesion is absent, new MR techniques allow direct visualization of nerves.[781] Occasionally, no mass lesion can be clearly defined; instead, a metastasis is present within the nerve itself. I have encountered this problem in breast carcinoma and melanoma. The diagnosis can often be difficult. Usually, in addition to sensory and motor loss, the physician can identify severe tenderness at a single point along the distribution of the nerve, which sometimes indicates an area invaded by tumor. Mononeuritis multiplex, the simultaneous involvement of several individual nerves but not of all nerves as occurs in polyneuropathy, suggests a vasculitis but may result from multifocal invasion by tumor.[1521a]

DIFFERENTIAL DIAGNOSIS

Considered in the differential diagnosis are entrapment or compression neuropathies.[879] Sometimes an entrapment neuropathy is caused by cancer, as when lymphedema causes brachial plexus entrapment or carpal tunnel syndrome. Compression neuropathies, such as peroneal nerve palsy, are associated with weight loss because the nerve, no longer protected by soft tissue, is compressed against bony prominences. The nerves involved by entrapment and compression are frequently the same nerves as those involved by tumor. Also to be considered in the differential diagnosis are secondary effects of chemotherapy (see Chapter 12) and paraneoplastic vasculitis leading to mononeuritis multiplex (see Chapter 15).

A problem in differential diagnosis is distinguishing a peroneal nerve palsy from more proximal involvement of the sciatic nerve or the L-5 root. The sciatic nerve and the L-5 root control foot inversion; the peroneal nerve does not, so foot inversion should be spared with a peroneal nerve palsy. Furthermore, the hamstring muscles, which are supplied by the sciatic nerve and L-5 and S-1 roots, should not be weak when the peroneal nerve is the culprit. If the lesion is more proximal, an electromyogram should show weakness and denervation. It is also sometimes difficult to distinguish femoral nerve involvement from lumbar plexus dysfunction. The distribution of the lumbar plexus includes the adductor thigh muscles as well as the iliopsoas and quadriceps; with femoral involvement, only the iliopsoas and the quadriceps are involved.

Painless peroneal nerve palsy of sudden onset in a patient who has recently lost weight and habitually sits with his or her legs crossed—the leg with the nerve palsy on top—suggests that the patient suffers a compression neuropathy. Rarely, similar compression neuropathies occur as the radial nerve passes behind the humerus (i.e., the Saturday night palsy), leading to painless wrist drop with little sensory change. Compression neuropathies of several other nerves can occur at the time of surgery for cancer (see Chapter 14).

Polyneuropathy

Direct invasion of multiple nerves by a neurotropic tumor occasionally causes acute or subacute sensorimotor polyneuropathies, often painful. Although rare, the disorder has been reported* in a number of patients with leukemias and lymphomas and may appear before the onset of other symptoms or when the patient is in remission. On some occasions, successful treatment of leptomeningeal leukemia with intrathecal drugs may be followed by a painful polyneuropathy that appears to be the result of a tumor's infiltrating nerve roots or peripheral nerves after they exit the leptomeninges. Whether it is the tumor in the leptomeninges that spreads along nerve roots outside the CNS is not certain.

It may be almost impossible to distinguish polyneuropathy caused by direct neoplastic involvement from the more common paraneoplastic polyneuropathies (see Chapter 15) or from idiopathic polyneuropathy. Even the finding of steroid responsiveness does not help, because lymphoma and leukemia sometimes are sensitive to steroids and the drug may cause a remitting and relapsing course.

*References 911, 1044, 1423, 2395, 2500, 2518.

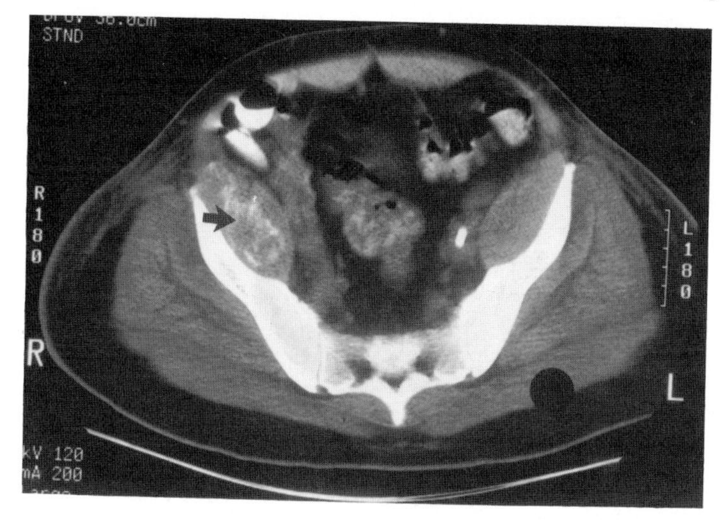

Figure 8–9. A CT scan showing a hemorrhagic metastasis in the psoas muscle on the right *(arrow)*. The patient complained of severe pain in the groin and leg. Weakness of the iliopsoas and quadriceps muscles presumably resulted from femoral artery compression. Paresthesias occurred in the anterior aspect of the thigh and medial aspect of the leg. On attempted extension of the hip, pain was present. The patient preferred to lie with flexed hip. As the hemorrhage resolved, pain and neurologic deficit improved.

The only certain diagnostic test is biopsy. If the underlying problem is leukemia or lymphoma, lymphocyte markers must be used to distinguish an inflammatory neuropathy from a neoplastic one.

Accurate diagnosis of the cause of peripheral nerve dysfunction in the patient with cancer is often difficult. These patients are susceptible not only to peripheral nerve lesions associated with their cancer but also to the far more common causes of peripheral neuropathy such as diabetes and alcoholism. Because smoking and alcohol intake are risk factors for head and neck cancer and because diabetes is such a common disorder, these factors should always be considered in patients presenting with peripheral neuropathy. In patients with known cancer under active therapy, chemotherapeutic complications are more likely to be the cause than is cancer invasion. In patients not known to have cancer, particularly those without weight loss, paraneoplastic polyneuropathy (see Chapter 15) requires careful consideration.

Because the disorder is unusual and other causes of polyneuropathy are much more common, the diagnosis of tumor invasion by metastases is infrequently made. Patients who have or have had leptomeningeal invasion, particularly if successfully treated, who then develop a painful polyneuropathy should be suspects. In patients such as those with rapidly developing, painful polyneuropathy in whom a cause is not immediately clear (especially if they have not received neurotoxic chemotherapeutic agents), nerve biopsy is usually the best diagnostic approach.

MUSCLES

Occasionally, muscles as well as peripheral nerves can be involved by leukemia or lymphoma and, sometimes, by solid tumors[674,770] (Fig. 8–9). In one systematic study of 82 autopsy cases, foci of leukemia or lymphoma[341] were found in one or more muscles in 50% (41) of the cases. The tumor can present as a mass lesion, as diffuse enlargement of one or more muscles,[996] or simply as focal weakness.[1331] Occasionally, diffuse infiltration of proximal muscles by tumor can mimic a paraneoplastic myopathy.[674] The differential diagnosis of individual nerve or muscle lesions may be difficult if the tumor is not apparent on MR study. Careful neurologic examination and electromyography can often reveal the distribution of nerve damage and distinguish myopathy from neuropathy.

PART III

Nonmetastatic Complications of Cancer

CHAPTER 9

VASCULAR DISORDERS

CNS vascular disease is common in patients with cancer.[2191] Autopsy data indicate that cerebrovascular lesions are found in about 15% of the patients who die from cancer; 50% of these had symptoms of the vascular disease while alive.[976] Cerebrovascular lesions in these patients are usually either a direct effect of tumor or its treatment on blood vessels, or an indirect effect of coagulation abnormalities generated by the neoplasm. Hemorrhagic and ischemic lesions are equally frequent (Fig. 9–1). Arteriosclerosis, save for that induced by RT (see Chapter 13), is not as common a cause of symptomatic cerebrovascular disease in patients with cancer, as it is in the general population, because severe coronary, aortic, and cerebral arteriosclerosis is less frequent in patients who die from cancer than in others (see the following)[440,1383,2488,2489] (Table 9–1). A recent retrospective analysis has suggested that, despite the data, conventional atherosclerotic stroke is the most common cause of cerebral ischemia in adult patients with cancer.[431a]

Cerebrovascular lesions complicating cancer are important to the clinician for three reasons:

1. A cerebrovascular event may precede identification of the cancer and be the first evidence that the patient suffers from disease of any kind.[505] In this situation, the physician must not only find the cause of the cerebrovascular event but also must consider an occult and potentially curable neoplasm. Although thrombotic or embolic cerebral infarction as a herald of an underlying occult neoplasm is too rare to warrant such a search in all patients who suffer a stroke, investigation of peripheral vas-

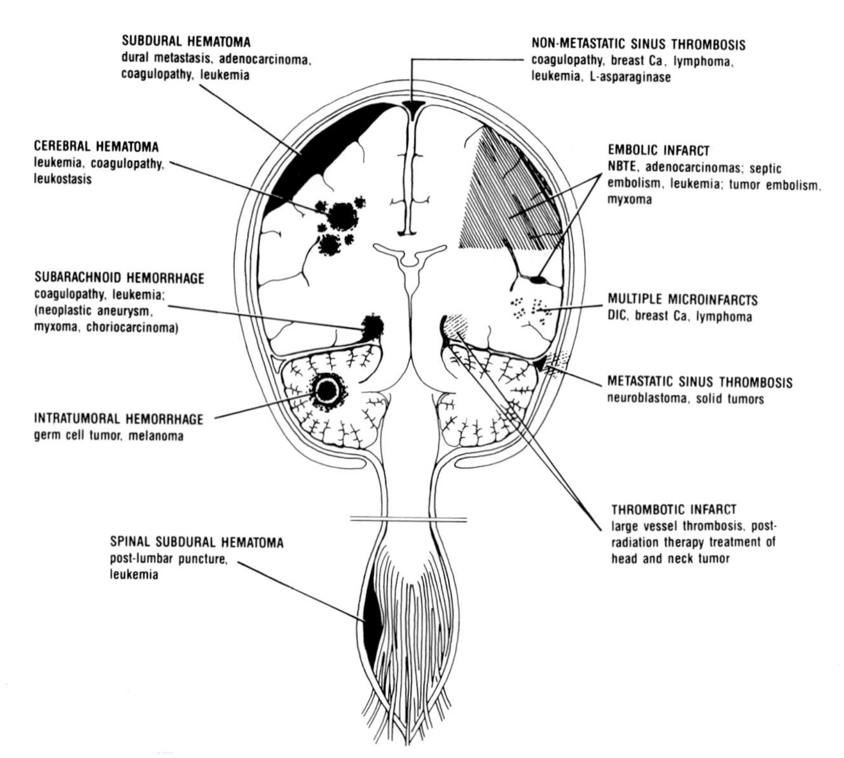

Figure 9–1. Cerebrovascular disorders encountered in patients with cancer. The left side of the figure illustrates hemorrhagic lesions and the right portion illustrates ischemic lesions.

cular events is more rewarding.[1861] Some studies suggest that an unexplained pulmonary embolus[951] or deep vein thrombosis (DVT)[15] reflects a substantially increased risk of cancer appearing within the next 2 years, particularly in patients older than age 65. One study found a 10% incidence of cancer in patients with DVT; some tumors were quite small. In patients with "idiopathic" DVT, a malignancy was found in 23%.[1799] In another series, 16% of patients with idiopathic DVT were found to have cancer within 2 years of the vascular event.[2087] Especially at risk are patients with recurrent thromboembolism. Other studies[1001] have not found such an increased incidence, however, leaving the issue of whether to pursue an extensive evaluation for cancer unresolved. Less controversy exists concerning the importance of searching for an occult malignancy in patients with migratory superficial thrombophlebitis (Trousseau's syndrome)[176,2258,2607] or nonbacterial thrombotic endocarditis (NBTE), in whom the incidence of underlying cancer is even higher. In addition, a recent report[1860] indicates that ischemic heart disease may also be precipitated by occult neoplasms.

2. Cerebral neoplasms may be mistaken for vascular events either because their symptoms develop suddenly, such as hemorrhage into a brain metastasis, or because CT or MR images initially resemble an infarct or a hemorrhage rather than a neoplasm.[2774]
3. CNS vascular disease can be a major cause of disability in an otherwise functioning patient with cancer. The patient may benefit from an accurate diagnosis and appropriate treatment, such as anticoagulation, or at least by prevention of inappropriate treatment, such as RT for a cerebral infarct mistaken for a brain metastasis. Peripheral vascular lesions, such as DVT, also cause significant disability in some pa-

Table 9–1. **CNS VASCULAR DISORDERS FOUND AT AUTOPSY IN PATIENTS WITH CANCER**

Disorders	No. of Patients	No. of Patients with Symptoms
Cerebral Hemorrhage	244	138
Intracerebral hematoma		
Intratumoral	60	47
Secondary to coagulopathy	88	57
Hypertensive	9	8
Subdural hematoma	63	16
Subarachnoid hemorrhage	24	10
Cerebral Infarction	256	117
Atherosclerosis	73	17
Intravascular coagulation	39	28
Nonbacterial thrombotic endocarditis	42	32
Septic occlusion	33	22
Tumor embolus	12	4
Venous occlusion	33	6
Miscellaneous	24	8
TOTAL	500	255

Source: Adapted from Graus et al,[976] p 17.

tients with cancer[2312] and can be difficult to treat.[1794]

PATHOPHYSIOLOGY OF CEREBROVASCULAR DISEASE

Patients with cancer experience two types of hemostatic abnormalities[212]: deficient coagulation, usually related to thrombocytopenia, which can cause cerebral hemorrhage[745]; or excessive coagulation (hypercoagulable state),* which can cause either CNS hemorrhage, infarction, or both[130,483] (Table 9–2). Even an occult cancer can precipitate a coagulopathy and lead to cerebrovascular disease.[505,1040]

Over 90% of patients with cancer develop laboratory evidence of a coagulation abnormality during the course of the cancer or its treatment.[212] In children with untreated acute leukemia, 3.1% with acute lymphoblastic leukemia (ALL) and 13.8% with acute myeloid leukemia (AML) developed laboratory evidence of a coagulation disorder. In children with AML, the existence of a coagulopathy at the time of diagnosis worsens prognosis for a complete remission.

*References 697, 1624, 1857, 1997, 2162, 2168.

Table 9–2. **COAGULATION ABNORMALITIES THAT CAUSE BLEEDING DISORDERS IN PATIENTS WITH CANCER**

Platelet Abnormalities
Thrombocytopenia
Thrombocytopathia
Antiplatelet aggregation drugs
Vascular Defects
Infiltration by tumor
Hyperviscosity/leukostasis
Extramedullary hematopoiesis
Coagulation Factor Abnormalities
Liver dysfunction
Drugs
Fibrinolysis
Von Willebrand's disease (acquired)
Disseminated intravascular coagulation

Source: Adapted from Bick,[212] p 359.

Hypocoagulation

The incidence of hemorrhage as a result of deficient clotting mechanisms[745,976] is high in patients with cancer. Approximately 15% to 25% of patients with myeloproliferative syndromes experience bleeding, usually associated with platelet dysfunction.[745] In a review of 718 patients with solid tumors, all of whom received myelosuppressive agents, 10% experienced one or more hemorrhagic episodes.[180] The most common cause, thrombocytopenia, occurs in three settings: when bone marrow is replaced by the cancer, when chemotherapy or RT damages the bone marrow, or when disseminated intravascular coagulation (DIC) develops.[180]

In general, spontaneous CNS hemorrhage occurs only when the platelet count falls lower than about 10,000 platelets/mm^3. Patients with such low platelet counts are also susceptible to intracranial hemorrhage following minor trauma or to spinal hemorrhage after lumbar puncture.

A second common cause of CNS bleeding in patients with cancer is direct involvement of blood vessels by the tumor. Certain primary cancers metastatic to brain (e.g., malignant melanoma, germ-cell tumors, renal-cell carcinoma, leukemia, and lymphoma) may invade and destroy small vessels in the tumor mass. More rarely, a tumor embolus causes an aneurysm.[1837] The damaged vessels then cause potentially fatal cerebral hemorrhages. Similar cerebral bleeding from fungal infections of the brain is discussed in Chapter 10.

Leukostasis can lead to hemorrhage but is no longer a common cause. Its incidence has declined because acute leukemia is now more rapidly diagnosed and effectively treated.

Other causes of intracranial hemorrhage[745] include DIC, particularly from acute promyelocytic leukemia (APML). The tumor releases procoagulants from the large granules in the leukemic cells and activates the extrinsic clotting pathway, consuming both platelets and other clotting factors faster than they can be replaced.[2746] The release of procoagulants is enhanced by chemotherapy-induced cell lysis. These complications usually occur in the first week of therapy. In one study[503] of 57 patients with APML, 6 suffered early death from intracranial hemorrhage.

Hypercoagulation

Several causes of excessive coagulation lead to CNS infarction (Table 9–3). Laboratory evidence for a hypercoagulable state can be found in many patients with cancer and is most marked in those with widespread cancer.[2354,2589a,2629] The hypercoagulable state may result from the cancer's production of coagulation promoters, destruction of vital organs, or cancer therapy. Injection of Walker 256 carcinoma cells into the vein of an experimental animal causes hypercoagulability, including histologic evidence of small-vessel occlusion, consumption of platelets and fibrinogen, and the appearance of fibrin-split products in the serum.[1160] When the liver is involved with cancer, production of coagulation cascade proteins is decreased, leading in turn to either excessive coagulation or deficient fibrinolysis. Liver dysfunction is a common cause of coagulopathy.[1856,2194] Malnutrition engendered by widespread cancer and its treatment has also been associated with coagulopathic abnormalities, perhaps through secondary involvement of the liver. Therapy also may cause abnormal coagulation.[1543,2249] A striking example is superior sagittal sinus occlusion associated with treating acute leukemia using L-asparaginase.[760] The mechanism of the hypercoagulable state is believed to be decreased production of antithrombin III. The venous occlusion can

Table 9–3. **THROMBOTIC DISORDERS IN PATIENTS WITH CANCER**

Platelet Aggregation
Tumor-induced thrombin formation
Tumor-ADP production
Arachidonate activation
Tumor-Cell Procoagulants
TF production
Factor X activators
Monocyte Procoagulants

ADP = adenosine diphosphate; TF = tissue factor.

result in hemorrhage, infarction, or both. Abnormal coagulation, similar to that sometimes following head injury, may develop or worsen after intracranial surgery.[2662]

Table 9–4 summarizes the usual pathophysiologic events leading to cerebrovascular disorders in patients with cancer.

CENTRAL NERVOUS SYSTEM HEMORRHAGE

Hemorrhages can occur in any part of the central or peripheral nervous system[1913] and can be classified by anatomic distribution as well as by pathophysiologic cause (see Table 9–1). In most patients, the site of CNS hemorrhage is the brain parenchyma. Subdural[1776] and subarachnoid hemorrhages are less common. Spinal hemorrhages are even rarer; they may be epidural (usually into tumor) as well as subdural, subarachnoid, or intraparenchymal (see the following). The three most common causes of CNS hemorrhage are thrombocytopenia, metastatic tumor, and leukostasis. Hypertensive hemorrhages are uncommon and can be easily distinguished from those related to cancer because they occur in the basal ganglia rather than in subcortical white matter.[976] Most subdural hematomas are related to a coagulopathy, including anticoagulant therapy, sometimes exacerbated by very minor trauma; others can develop within subdural

Table 9–4. **PATHOPHYSIOLOGY OF CEREBROVASCULAR DISEASE IN PATIENTS WITH CANCER**

Mechanism	Pathology	Typical Tumors
Direct Effect of Tumor		
Tumor embolism	Embolic infarction	Myxoma, lung cancer
	Neoplastic aneurysm	Myxoma, choriocarcinoma
Dural metastasis	Sagittal sinus thrombosis	Adenocarcinoma, neuroblastoma
	Subdural hematoma	Breast, prostate
Neoplastic infiltration of a cerebral vessel	Intratumoral hemorrhage	Melanoma, germ-cell tumors
Leukostasis	Cerebral hemorrhage	Leukemia
Related to Sepsis		
Septic embolism	Embolic infarction	Leukemia
Vasculitis	Thrombotic microinfarction	Leukemia, lymphoma
Related to Coagulation Disorders		
Sinus thrombosis	Hemorrhagic infarction	Lymphoma, breast cancer
DIC	Thrombotic infarction	Leukemia, breast cancer
NBTE	Embolic infarction	Any tumor
Thrombocytopenia	Cerebral hemorrhage	Leukemia, lymphoma
Hyperviscosity	Thrombotic infarction	Myeloma, lymphoma
Related to Treatment or Diagnostic Procedures		
Lumbar puncture	Subdural hematoma (spinal)	Leukemia
Lymphangiography	Embolic infarction	Lymphoma
Radiation therapy	Thrombotic infarction	Head and neck
Chemotherapy		
L-asparaginase	Sinus thrombosis	Leukemia
Mitomycin, bleomycin, platinum	Cerebral infarcts	Solid tumor

DIC = disseminated intravascular coagulation; NBTE = nonbacterial thrombotic endocarditis.
Source: From Graus et al,[976] p 25, with permission.

metastases. Also, patients with cancer experience typical traumatic subdural hematomas because of their increased tendency to fall.[1776] Spinal subdural hemorrhage usually occurs in patients with thrombocytopenia who undergo lumbar puncture.[707]

Spontaneous subarachnoid hemorrhage occasionally complicates hypocoagulable states, particularly thrombocytopenia, but epidural hematomas are rare in either the brain or spinal canal. The low incidence of spinal epidural hematomas in patients with cancer is surprising because this lesion is more common in the noncancer population, complicating lumbar puncture in anticoagulated patients and appearing spontaneously in patients with coagulation abnormalities resulting from liver disease.

Most patients with cancer in whom a cerebral hemorrhage is encountered at autopsy have been symptomatic during life, which is true of all hypertensive hemorrhages and most hemorrhages into tumor. Because many patients who suffer nonhypertensive cerebral hemorrhage do not succumb to it (and most who do are not examined postmortem), the actual number of cerebral hemorrhages clinically encountered is greater than the autopsy numbers indicate.

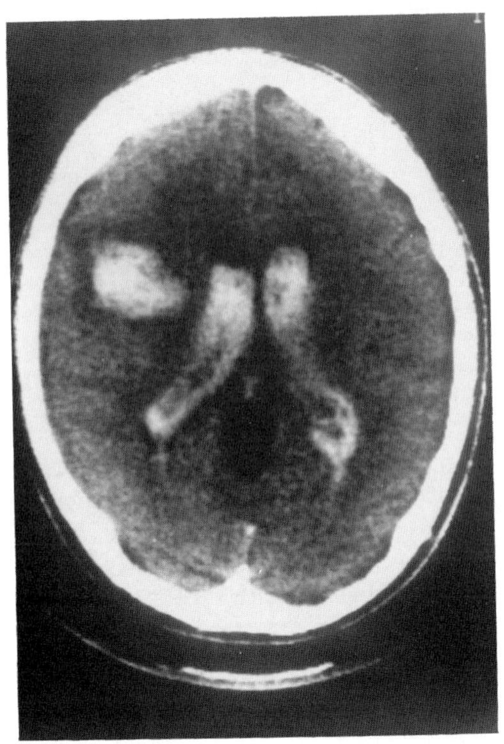

Figure 9–2. An unenhanced CT scan illustrating acute cerebral hemorrhage in a brain metastasis from lung cancer. The patient was neurologically asymptomatic until the silent metastasis bled massively and ruptured into the ventricle. The patient died; small remnants of the underlying tumor were encountered at autopsy.

Hemorrhage into Brain Metastases

The most common cause of intracranial hemorrhage in patients with nonhematologic malignancies is hemorrhage into a metastatic tumor[976,1673] that lies either within the brain substance or in the subdural space.[1776] Leptomeningeal metastases, particularly from melanomas, sometimes cause an asymptomatic hemorrhage that is detected only by lumbar puncture. Any brain metastasis has the potential for hemorrhage. The metastatic tumor most often causing intracerebral hemorrhage is lung cancer, simply because so many brain metastases are from lung cancer[1673] (Fig. 9–2). Metastatic malignant melanoma and germ-cell tumors are more likely to bleed than lung cancer, but their fewer overall numbers make them less common causes of hemorrhage.[976] Other cancers that commonly cause hemorrhage within the substance of the brain are listed in Table 9–5.

Subdural hematomas are common in patients with breast and prostate cancer because these tumors commonly metastasize to the subdural space.[2073] Bleeding, probably resulting from tumor-induced neovascularization and tumor infiltration, occurs within inner dura mater layers.[1059] As in metastatic brain tumors, the subdural metastasis may be small, so that virtually all its symptoms are caused by the hemorrhage.

CLINICAL FINDINGS

When hemorrhage occurs in a brain metastasis, symptom onset is almost always sudden, beginning with severe headache; focal neurologic signs such as hemiparesis follow within minutes. Many such patients were previously neurologically well, although usually, but not always, known to be suffering from cancer. Sometimes the history reveals subtle neurologic symptoms preceding the

Table 9–5. **ONSET OF CLINICAL SYMPTOMS IN 60 PATIENTS WITH HEMORRHAGIC METASTASIS**

			SYMPTOMS	
Type of Tumor	**No. of Patients**	**Asymptomatic**	**Gradual Onset**	**Abrupt Onset (Strokelike)**
Melanoma	22	2	14	6
Germ cell	19*	4	6	9
Other†	19	7	7	5
TOTAL	60	13	27	20

*Choriocarcinoma component in 12 of 19 (63%) patients.
†Sarcoma 4 (3 with sudden onset), lung 8 (1 with sudden onset), kidney 2, breast 1, lymphoma 2, unknown 2 (1 with sudden onset).
Source: From Graus et al,[976] p 17, with permission.

hemorrhage by days or weeks, suggesting that the sudden ictus is hemorrhage into a pre-existing lesion. The focal signs progress over minutes to hours, with massive hemorrhage; signs of increased intracranial pressure and cerebral herniation may follow. Although death may occur within several hours, usually symptoms stabilize and the patient presents to the hospital with a headache and a focal neurologic deficit. The hemorrhages are usually hemispheral and in white matter, leading to sensory or visual abnormalities or hemiplegia with or without aphasia. Hemorrhages are less common in the cerebellum or brainstem, but the latter are usually fatal.

DIAGNOSIS

The diagnosis is suspected from the clinical history and findings and confirmed by CT scan. With acute hemorrhage (see Fig. 9–2), the unenhanced CT scan is more sensitive than the MR scan, although signal heterogeneity on an MR scan identifies nonhemorrhagic tissue within the hemorrhage and suggests an underlying tumor.[101] The unenhanced CT scan reveals an area of hyperdensity surrounded by edema. The presence of significant edema around an acute hemorrhage suggests that tumor is underlying the hemorrhage because, with uncomplicated hemorrhage, edema does not develop for days. The density is greater than that usually seen in nonhemorrhagic metastases from colon carcinoma and melanomas but less than in heavily calcified tumors. An enhanced CT scan may also be helpful in the following circumstances:

1. Lack of enhancement indicates the absence of a pre-existing metastasis or obliteration of the tumor by the bleed.
2. Contrast enhancement contiguous with the hemorrhage suggests the bleed has occurred within a metastasis.
3. Areas of enhancement elsewhere in the brain suggest that the patient has multiple metastases, only one of which has bled.

Enhancement around the hemorrhage seen acutely on the CT or MR scan suggests an underlying tumor because hypertensive cerebral hemorrhages do not enhance for days to weeks after the ictus. Furthermore, enhancement of a hemorrhagic metastasis is usually irregular and thick and can be easily distinguished from the serpiginous enhancement associated with an underlying vascular malformation.

DIFFERENTIAL DIAGNOSIS

The differential diagnosis includes nonhemorrhagic tumor with apoplectic onset mimicking a vascular event (see Chapter 5), hemorrhagic infarction from vascular occlusion, and brain hemorrhage not associated with metastatic tumor. Multiple cryptic venous angiomas of the brain have been mistaken for hemorrhagic metastases.[2157,2839]

Cerebral infarction, like cerebral hemorrhage, may be sudden in onset, but increased intracranial pressure signs are uncommon because of less mass effect. Both CT and MR scans may be normal during the first 24 hours; contrast enhancement of the involved gyri develops several days later. A hemorrhagic infarct may be dense on the precontrast CT scan but not as dense as a cerebral hemorrhage; the increased density is absent at the symptom onset but develops slowly over several days as the infarct turns from an ischemic to a hemorrhagic lesion. Hemorrhagic infarcts can sometimes be distinguished by combining the clinical and radiographic findings; in patients with either bland or hemorrhagic infarction, neurologic signs are usually greater than suspected from the CT scan because the scan does not reveal the entire area of ischemia or infarction. Cerebral hemorrhage is the opposite; clinical findings are often equal to or less than expected from the CT abnormality. Exceptions occur, however, when edema or shifts of tissue cause symptoms at a distance from the hemorrhagic site.

TREATMENT

The initial medical treatment of a hemorrhage occurring in a brain metastasis is directed at the mass and is the same as treatment of increased intracranial pressure or cerebral herniation in patients suffering from brain metastases without hemorrhage (see Chapter 3).[1316] Lumbar puncture should be avoided because of the increased risk of herniation. If a coagulopathy is present, it should be treated (see the following). When the cerebral hemorrhage is unrelated to metastatic brain disease, corticosteroids are ineffective,[2080] but in patients with metastatic hemorrhages corticosteroids are useful in treating edema caused by the metastasis. Hyperosmolar agents, particularly mannitol, can increase cerebral blood volume,[2132] thus possibly exacerbating the hemorrhage. In patients with marked increased intracranial pressure and cerebral herniation, however, the effectiveness of mannitol in decreasing intracranial pressure probably outweighs the theoretic risk of increasing the hemorrhage. Hyperosmolar agents should be administered only to patients with progressive signs of increased intracranial pressure and cerebral herniation. A patient with a cerebral hemorrhage who arrives with a stable neurologic deficit is treated only with corticosteroids for the tumor edema and is closely observed.

Treatment is also directed at the metastasis itself. The criteria used to choose either surgery or RT as the primary arm for treating metastatic brain tumors apply here (see Chapter 5). RT should be delayed until the patient stabilizes, however, or increased edema associated with RT may worsen the clinical state. In a stable patient, RT is usually begun after 2 to 3 days of corticosteroid treatment. Surgery is indicated when the hemorrhage fails to respond to conservative therapy. These lesions are often relatively superficial. Many of their symptoms are caused by shifts of brain structure rather than destruction by hemorrhage; thus, the hemorrhage and its surrounding tumor can often be removed successfully, and the patient can make a good functional recovery.

A more difficult therapeutic decision exists in patients with cancer who suffer a cerebral hemorrhage but in whom the CT scan or the clinical findings do not establish the presence of a metastasis. In this instance, the patient is usually followed carefully, and the MR scan is repeated every few weeks. If the hemorrhage resolves without further evidence of cerebral metastasis, the patient is not treated. If clear evidence of a cerebral metastasis appears on the scan as the hemorrhage resolves, treatment of the metastasis should be initiated.

The prognosis of a cerebral hemorrhage from tumor is similar to that of the metastatic tumor itself; that is, radiosensitive and chemosensitive tumors such as germ-cell tumors have a good prognosis, whereas resistant tumors such as melanoma have a poor prognosis unless they can be surgically removed. If the tumor can be successfully treated and the hemorrhage has not caused severe neurologic disability, good recovery and long-term survival are possible. Because brain metastases usually bleed from veins or small arterioles and the site is often fairly superficial, the prognosis for immediate survival and functional recovery is better for metastasis-associated hemorrhage than for hypertensive basal ganglia hemorrhages.

Subdural Hemorrhage

Subdural hematomas in patients with cancer can result either from metastases to the subdural space or from bleeding that is due to trauma, cancer-induced coagulopathy, or anticoagulant therapy. In one series, 26 of 38 patients with subdural hematomas complicating solid tumors had a history of either head trauma or anticoagulant therapy, suggesting that metastasis was the cause of the subdural hematoma in only a minority. Conversely, only 4 of 32 patients with hematologic neoplasms gave a history of either trauma or anticoagulant therapy, suggesting that either metastasis or cancer-induced coagulopathy played a major role.[1776]

Tumors that metastasize to the subdural space probably reach it via Batson's plexus (see Chapter 2). The symptoms are caused by subdural hematomas or hygromas, which stem from leaking tumor neovessels or from rupture of friable vessels by minor trauma.[976,1776] Coagulation abnormalities and increased capillary pressure caused by tumor-induced venous occlusion may exacerbate the bleeding.

Neurologic symptoms from subdural lesions usually develop more slowly than do those caused by hemorrhage into a brain metastasis. The first symptom is generalized or localized headache over the hematoma, sometimes associated with tenderness to percussion over that site. The patient then develops one of several progressive clinical pictures that marks the growth of the subdural hematoma:

1. Progressive neurologic dysfunction characterized by hemiparesis and hemisensory loss may develop over days to weeks, mimicking a brain metastasis.
2. Delirium or stupor with absent or only minor focal signs may suggest a metabolic disorder (see Chapter 11), often with unilateral asterixis (contralateral to the lesion) as the only focal sign.
3. Acute bleeding into the subdural space may cause false-localizing signs (see Chapter 5) because of brainstem shift. Headache and acute encephalopathy are accompanied by hemiparesis or hemiplegia ipsilateral to the subdural hematoma. The ipsilateral hemiplegia results from shift of the brainstem away from the site of the hematoma, compressing the cerebral peduncle (which carries motor fibers from brain to spinal cord) against the contralateral tentorium cerebelli (Kernohan's notch) (see Fig. 1–3). Compression of the ipsilateral third nerve causes first a dilated pupil and, subsequently, a complete third-nerve palsy. The third-nerve palsy lies on the appropriate side (ipsilateral) to the subdural hematoma, establishing the lesion site, even in the presence of an ipsilateral hemiparesis.
4. Rarely, subdural hematomas may cause unusual clinical symptoms mimicking transient ischemic attacks,[88] Parkinson's disease,[2605] chorea,[1415] or internuclear ophthalmoplegia.[619]

PATHOGENESIS

Focal signs, when present, can reflect direct compression of the brain by the overlying hematoma, compression of vascular structures, or brain edema. The last mentioned is greater in the hemisphere underlying a subdural hematoma than in the opposite, less-compressed hemisphere.[322] The pathogenesis of the metabolic-encephalopathy–like picture is not clear.

DIAGNOSIS

The diagnosis of subdural hematoma or hygroma is made by CT or MR scan. Even when the subdural space is isodense with brain on CT scan, effacement of the normal gyral pattern is usually sufficient to suggest the diagnosis. MR scans clearly delineate subdural hematomas of any age, particularly on T_2-weighted images. Contrast injection may reveal tumor presence in the subdural space as well as the subdural blood.

TREATMENT

Subdural hematoma that is due to tumor usually requires surgical evacuation. Often it can be evacuated through a burr hole, making craniotomy unnecessary. Occasionally, placing a temporary drain or an Ommaya device (see Chapter 7) into the subdural space allows drainage of reaccumulated fluid; subdural shunts are rarely required. The fluid drained should be examined cytologically or the subdural membrane should be biopsied to determine whether tumor is causing the subdural blood, although cytologic examination may sometimes be negative even when tumor is present. If the subdural hematoma has resulted from subdural tumor, surgical evacuation of the hematoma should be followed by RT to the whole brain to treat the neoplasm and thus prevent reaccumulation of the subdural fluid.

Coagulopathic Hemorrhage

INTRACRANIAL HEMORRHAGE

Cerebral hemorrhage because of coagulopathy occurs more commonly in patients with hematologic malignancies than in patients with solid tumors. Most patients with hematologic malignancies suffer from myelocytic leukemias (Table 9–6). Patients with myeloproliferative syndromes such as polycythemia and plasma-cell dyscrasias also bleed occasionally,[1885] although transient neurologic symptoms from hyperviscosity are more common. In patients with acute promyelocytic leukemia, disseminated intravascular coagulation (DIC) with intracranial hemorrhage is a common cause of death.[503] Intracranial hemorrhage is less common in other myelocytic leukemias, and clearly defined DIC is rarely encountered. Instead, the hematologic defect is usually thrombocytopenia, with platelet counts of fewer than 10,000/mm^3. Thrombocytopenia alone is not the entire explanation for the bleeding, however. Intracranial hemorrhage much more commonly accompanies acute myelogenous leukemia with thrombocytopenia than it does lymphocytic leukemia or solid tumors that cause equal thrombocytopenia. Nor does leukostasis explain the difference in the frequency of intracranial hemorrhage in these groups.

The most common pathologic finding in leukemia is a large hemorrhage, usually found in the centrum semiovale. A single

Table 9–6. **FACTORS LEADING TO INTRACRANIAL HEMORRHAGE IN PATIENTS WITH LEUKEMIA**

Factors	HEMORRHAGE WITHOUT CNS LEUKEMIC INFILTRATION	HEMORRHAGE WITH CNS LEUKEMIC INFILTRATION	
		Parenchymal Infiltrates with Leukostasis	**Arachnoidal Infiltrates without Leukostasis**
No. of patients	50	13	6
No. of symptomatic patients	38 (76%)	8 (61.5%)	3 (50%)
Histologic type*			
ALL	5 (2)*	3 (2)	1 (1)
AML	19 (16)	2 (1)	3 (1)
APML	9 (7)	—	1 (1)
CML	5 (5)	3 (2)	1
Other	12 (8)	5 (3)	—
Hemorrhage at time of diagnosis of leukemia	7	5	—
Fever	68.4%	37.5%	100%
WBC count (per mm^3)	8,000	260,000	36,000
	100–104,000	70,000–730,000	1000–97,000
Platelet count (per mm^3)	13,500	36,000	32,000
	2000–52,000	10,000–50,000	3000–65,000
Multiple hematomas	12%	62.5%	16.6%

*Total number and ( ) number of symptomatic patients.

ALL = acute lymphoblastic leukemia; AML = acute myelogenous leukemia; APML = acute promyelocytic leukemia; CML = chronic myelogenous leukemia.

Source: From Graus et al,[976] p 19, with permission.

ruptured vessel is usually not identified, and the rather slow onset of clinical symptoms suggests that veins or small arterioles have bled. At times, leukemic infiltrates surround blood vessels within or adjacent to the hemorrhage, but most often the pathologist finds only a hematoma without an excessive number of WBCs and often with little or no inflammatory reaction. A careful search at a distance from the massive hemorrhage site often discloses microscopic perivascular hemorrhages.

CLINICAL FINDINGS

The signs and symptoms depend partially upon the compartment into which the bleeding has occurred (i.e., subdural space or brain parenchyma) and partially on the rapidity of bleeding. Headache and neurologic signs usually develop more gradually than with hemorrhage into a metastatic tumor, but otherwise the signs are essentially identical. The usual setting is an APML patient who is undergoing treatment and has profound thrombocytopenia but no neurologic symptoms until headache and neurologic signs prompt hospitalization. A CT scan establishes the diagnosis.

TREATMENT

Medical treatment aims to reduce brain edema and incipient herniation (see Chapter 3) and is also directed at the coagulopathy. In patients with documented DIC (a minority), heparin has been used to reverse the consumption of coagulation factors. I have no experience with heparin to treat intracerebral hemorrhage, but reports[964] suggest that heparin can stop GI and other bleeding abnormalities caused by DIC. Also, intracerebral hemorrhages appear to be fewer in patients with DIC who are treated with IV heparin.[1242] Tranexamic acid may also control hemorrhage in patients with APML.[105] All-*trans*-retinoic acid usually rapidly corrects APML's coagulopathy. Platelet transfusion for thrombocytopenia and replacement of coagulation factors with fresh-frozen plasma and cryoprecipitate to maintain fibrinogen levels of greater than 100 mg/dL are helpful.

If the patient deteriorates neurologically while receiving optimal medical treatment, the physician should consider surgical evacuation of the lesion. Despite the threat of continued bleeding because of the coagulopathy, subdural hematomas can be successfully evacuated in some thrombocytopenic patients. The platelet count must be restored to greater than 100,000/mm^3 before and after the operation by the transfusion of platelets and other coagulation factors. Continued bleeding may be a problem in these patients despite platelet transfusions, however; the physician should approach surgical extirpation only as a last resort when medical treatment has failed.

SPINAL HEMORRHAGE

Spontaneous spinal hemorrhages are rare in patients with cancer, but spinal subdural hematomas can follow lumbar puncture in thrombocytopenic patients[707] (Fig. 9–3). The hematoma probably results from damage by the needle to small radicular vessels as they pass through the subdural space to supply the cauda equina.[1698] Unlike intracerebral hemorrhage, spinal subdural hemorrhage is as common in patients with lymphoblastic leukemia as it is in patients with myelogenous leukemia, suggesting that thrombocytopenia and the lumbar puncture are sufficient cause for the hemorrhage and that additional coagulation deficits are not required.

Characteristically, patients with spinal hemorrhage either have a stable platelet count of fewer than 10,000/mm^3 or a rapidly dropping count rarely as high as 50,000/mm^3. Several hours following a lumbar puncture, the patient develops back pain radiating down the legs, followed by leg weakness and sensory changes indicating either cauda equina or spinal cord dysfunction. If paraplegia occurs, it usually appears within 24 hours of the lumbar puncture but sometimes is delayed for several days. The bleeding may dissect upward in the subdural space (see Fig. 9–3) to affect the spinal cord as high as the upper thoracic level. Some patients with paraplegia recover, particularly when the cauda equina rather than the spinal cord has been involved. Subdural bleeding should be suspected whenever severe back pain follows a lumbar puncture. Unfortunately, our experience is that the patient's complaint of pain is often ignored until weakness develops. The diagnosis can usually be confirmed by CT or MR scan.

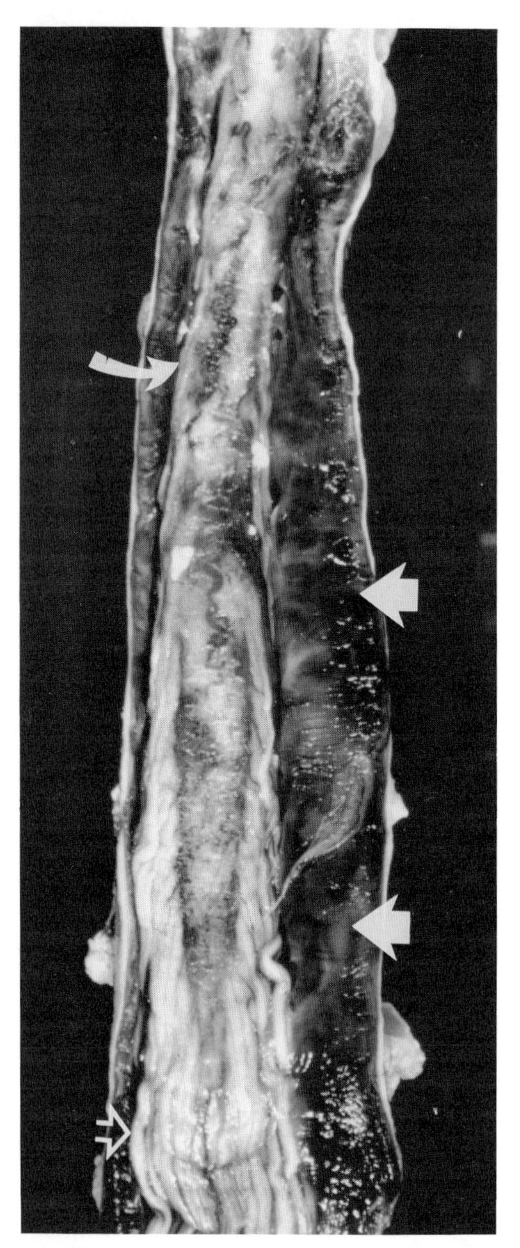

Figure 9–3. A spinal subdural hematoma in a patient with thrombocytopenia from acute lymphoblastic leukemia. Lumbar puncture was performed to instill methotrexate. The patient complained of pain and weakness in the legs within hours following the lumbar puncture. Over the next 48 hours the patient became paraplegic, with a sensory level at T-4. She remained paraplegic until her death from leukemia a year later. The hematoma mass (*closed arrows*) compresses both the cauda equina roots (*open arrow*) and the spinal cord (*curved arrow*).

The best treatment is prevention. Patients with rapidly dropping platelet counts, or those with fewer than 20,000/mm^3, should be transfused before and during lumbar puncture. The puncture should be performed with a No. 20 or smaller needle by the most skilled physician available (see Chapter 14). Since we have adopted this policy, the frequency of clinically significant subdural hematomas has dropped. We still find small subdural hematomas at autopsy in a number of thrombocytopenic patients who have undergone lumbar puncture shortly before death. Some of these small hematomas probably correlate with the clinical symptom of mild-to-moderate back pain unassociated with neurologic dysfunction that sometimes follows lumbar puncture. Patients with other hemostatic abnormalities seldom have similar problems, but special care should be taken when performing the lumbar puncture.

When patients develop post–lumbar puncture weakness, we give them platelet transfusions, but we have not tried to evacuate the hematoma because of their severe thrombocytopenia. If medical treatment fails, a case might be made for evacuation of the hematoma[227]; needle aspiration might also be considered.[2458] The decision must be made rapidly, however. Once patients become paraplegic, they are unlikely to recover function even if the hematoma is successfully treated.

I have encountered only a few spontaneous epidural hemorrhages in thrombocytopenic patients.[1034,1706] The patient complains of sudden onset of severe back pain; neurologic signs develop over minutes to hours and sometimes lead to paraplegia. In contradistinction to cord compression from metastatic tumor (see Chapter 6), spinal radiographs are usually unrevealing. MR scans typically indicate an epidural mass longer than that encountered with spinal cord compression from most tumors. The mass density on CT or MR scan is that of blood rather than tumor. Bleeding into an epidural tumor may be impossible to differentiate from spontaneous hematoma.

Intraparenchymal spinal hemorrhage rarely complicates cancer, although intramedullary metastases may occasionally bleed. Intramedullary spinal hemorrhages may be a late result of RT (see Chapter 13).

LEUKOSTASIS

Leukostasis refers to leukemic cells accumulating in small vessels of the brain[109] and in the perivascular spaces surrounding them. Leukostasis occurs in patients with either lymphocytic or nonlymphocytic leukemia[1226] who have a high circulating WBC count.[1727] Leukocytic counts greater than 300,000/mm^3 create a 60% risk of intracerebral hemorrhage if not treated promptly. Leukostasis is more likely to occur at lower counts with granulocytic blast cells than with lymphocytic cells; the granulocytic blast increases blood viscosity more than the lymphoblast, is more rigid, and occludes small vessels more readily. Leukostasis also leads to vessel-wall damage, although the mechanism is unclear. Hypotheses regarding possible mechanisms include ischemia caused by high oxygen consumption by leukemic cells in the cerebral microcirculation, mechanical disruption of the vessel wall by invasive tumor, or damage by thrombosis. Whatever the mechanism, when the vessel wall is sufficiently damaged, either microscopic or gross hemorrhage occurs. In some patients, the hemorrhages are large enough to cause death.[523] Previously, leukostasis was a common cause of cerebral hemorrhage in patients suffering from leukemia, occurring more commonly in patients with acute myelogenous leukemia than in those with lymphoblastic leukemia. With better therapy, both the overall incidence of intracerebral hemorrhage and its incidence in patients suffering from myelocytic leukemia have diminished.

Clinically, leukostatic hemorrhages are indistinguishable from hemorrhages that are due to coagulation defects, and the difference can be identified only by the presence of leukostatic changes at autopsy. Leukostasis should be suspected when a patient with intracranial hemorrhage suffers from nonlymphocytic leukemia, when severe thrombocytopenia or other coagulation abnormality is absent, and when the WBC count is or has been greater than 200,000/mm^3. Nevertheless, patients with leukostatic lesions often do have underlying abnormalities of coagulation, including thrombocytopenia, and sometimes they do not have high circulating WBC counts. Hyperviscosity, often suggested clinically by retinal hemorrhages and encephalopathy, probably also causes symptoms in some patients.[122]

Patients with high WBC counts may develop multiple small hemorrhages that are sometimes too small to be identified on CT scan. Such lesions cause delirium and focal or generalized convulsions resembling the syndrome of intravascular coagulation (see the following).

The treatment of hemorrhages that are due to leukostasis is similar to that of other intracerebral hemorrhages except that whole-brain radiation in doses of 1200 to 2400 cGy should be given if the patient survives the acute episode. RT is given to eliminate the abnormal white cells from the brain to prevent future hemorrhages. Leukostatic hemorrhages can often be prevented by radiation (e.g., 600 cGy in one dose) and by lowering the number of blast cells in the blood with hydroxyurea or leukapheresis.

HYPERVISCOSITY

Blood hyperviscosity occurs in leukemia, paraproteinemias including multiple myeloma,[1831,2103,2459] Waldenström's macroglobulinemia, and polycythemia vera. The hyperviscosity syndrome can occur in leukemia when the WBC count exceeds 200,000/mm^3. Measurable hyperviscosity is found in about 5% of patients with IgG myeloma and in 22% of patients with IgM components greater than 5 g/dL. Clinical symptoms usually occur only when the serum relative viscosity exceeds 4.0 cp. Patients may complain of headache, lethargy, dizziness, vertigo, and visual disturbances. As the viscosity rises, they may develop hemiparesis, seizures, and acute confusional states that progress to coma, so-called coma paraproteinemia.

Although the neurologic examination is usually not specific, clues to hyperviscosity or venous thrombosis include retinopathy (Fig. 9–4), characterized by tortuous and congested veins that probably represent compensatory dilatation in response to high viscosity; sometimes papilledema; and multiple retinal hemorrhages. The patient's history may also relate easy bruising, mucosal bleeding, or bleeding from the nose or uterus. The disorder is usually treatable with plasmapheresis or with phlebotomy for poly-

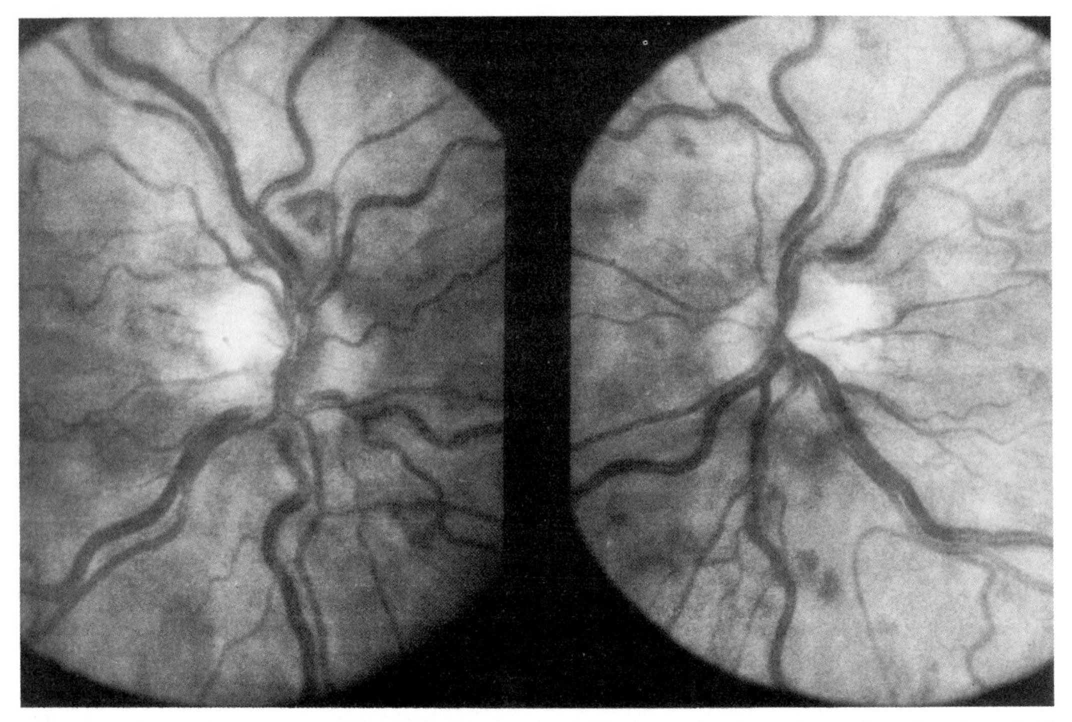

Figure 9–4. Abnormal appearance of blood vessels in a patient with a hyperviscosity syndrome from chronic myeloid leukemia. Hemorrhages in both eye grounds, grossly dilated retinal veins with arterioles of normal size, and blurred disk margins are noted. (From Russell and Wade,[2254] p 471, with permission.)

cythemia vera, or the underlying disorder is treated with chemotherapy.*

HYPERTENSION

Hypertensive intracranial hemorrhages sometimes affect patients with cancer. The patient may suffer hypertension either as a coincidental disease or as a result of renal dysfunction associated with the cancer. A common setting is a patient with cervical carcinoma who develops a pelvic recurrence leading to ureteral obstruction, hydronephrosis, renal damage, and hypertension. The neurologic findings in such patients are those of hypertensive hemorrhages and hypertensive encephalopathy, the same as with severe essential hypertension. Hypertensive ischemic lesions have been reported to complicate induction chemotherapy of acute lymphoblastic leukemia (ALL).[2039]

The symptoms begin suddenly with headache and focal neurologic signs. A hypertensive hemorrhage is usually more acute in onset, rapid in progression, and serious in outcome than other intracranial hemorrhages. The hemorrhages typically affect the basal ganglia, obviating surgery as a therapeutic option. Patients are treated conservatively, and the prognosis is poor.

*References 1571, 1831, 2090, 2254, 2456.

CENTRAL NERVOUS SYSTEM INFARCTION

CNS infarcts, whether bland or hemorrhagic, may result from arterial or venous occlusion. Arteries may be occluded either by thrombus in situ or by embolization from a distant site. Venous occlusions are almost always due to in situ thrombus formation, although I have encountered one instance of tumor embolization from the neck to cerebral veins. Table 9–1 lists the causes of cerebral infarction, and Table 9–4 classifies the pathophysiologic mechanisms of CNS infarction in patients with cancer; the following paragraphs detail these causes.

Atherosclerosis

Cerebral atherosclerosis is usually less severe in patients dying from cancer than in those dying from other causes.[440,1383,2488,2489] The reason is not entirely clear. It may be an artifact of the phenomenon that the two most common causes of death are cancer and heart disease. If all patients dying in a general hospital are studied, more atherosclerosis will likely be found in the noncancer population because patients dying from heart disease usually have relatively severe cerebral atherosclerosis. A second possibility is that the genetic or biochemical defect underlying the cancer also reduces atherosclerosis. A third possibility is that, when the patient develops cancer, tumor-generated substances or malnutrition associated with cancer may reverse previously established atherosclerosis so that the lesion is less severe by the time the patient dies from cancer.[1137] Whatever the cause, at all ages patients with lung and breast carcinomas, malignant melanoma, and hematologic malignancies have significantly less atherosclerosis in the circle of Willis than do patients dying from noncancerous causes. Between ages 50 and 70, this reduced incidence of atherosclerosis in the circle of Willis is also true for patients suffering from colon cancer and from head and neck carcinomas.[440] After the age of 70, the incidence of cerebral atherosclerosis with colon cancer and cancers of the head and neck exceeds that of the control population, whereas the incidence remains low in patients with other cancers.[440]

The clinical implication is that atherosclerotic occlusion is an uncommon cause of stroke in patients with cancer. As Table 9–1 shows, of 256 patients with cerebral infarction, only 73 were atherosclerotic and only 17 of 117 with symptomatic infarcts were due to atherosclerosis. When atherosclerotic occlusions are responsible for cerebral ischemia or infarction, accelerated atherosclerosis caused by RT delivered to a blood vessel is often the culprit (Fig. 9–5) (see Chapter

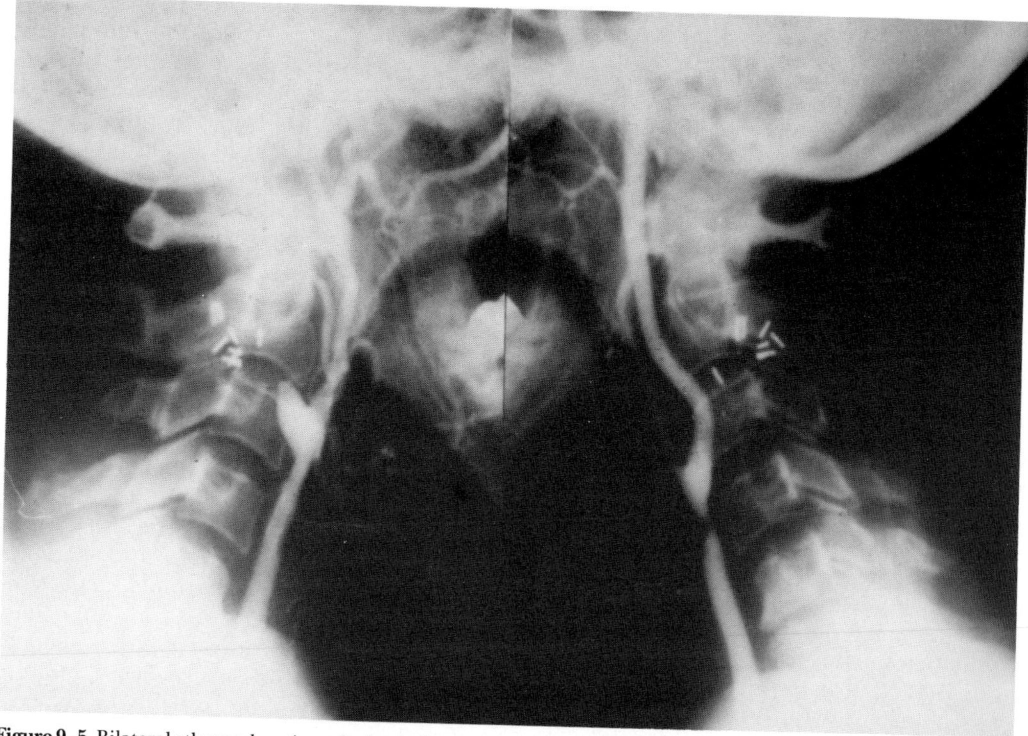

Figure 9–5. Bilateral atherosclerotic occlusions of the carotid arteries in a patient radiated 15 years previously for head and neck cancer. The patient suffered transient ischemic attacks. Both carotid arteries are occluded. Note the occlusion on the right, well below the bifurcation, an unusual place for an arteriosclerotic occlusion.

13).[717] Accelerated atherosclerosis and infarction have been reported in patients with head and neck tumors, nasopharyngeal carcinomas, and lymphomas.[717] It sometimes occurs in children whose brains have been radiated and results in the moyamoya disease.[211] Cerebral infarcts that are due to large-vessel atherosclerosis do occur in patients with cancer and in one retrospective series accounted for 33% of ischemic events in such patients. Hypercoagulable states accounted for 30% and cardioembolism for 21%. In 15% the cause was uncertain.[431a]

Disseminated Intravascular Coagulation

DIC, a common hematologic abnormality in patients with cancer,[493,1223,1675] is more common in the leukemias, particularly APML, in which its appearance with induction therapy is almost the rule. The disorder may complicate cancer at any time during its course, sometimes appearing when the underlying disease is occult[1675] or as a response to disseminated[1367] or terminal cancer. Up to 75% of patients with disseminated cancer develop chronic DIC.[130] DIC may hinder the neurosurgical treatment of brain metastases[2301] and be stimulated by other cancer complications, including sepsis[1533] (particularly with Gram-negative organisms), RT therapy or chemotherapy, and liver disease.

A strict definition of DIC requires a coagulation profile showing active coagulation and fibrinolysis. Characteristically, in acute DIC, thrombocytopenia, hypofibrinogenemia, an elevated prothrombin time (PT), and fibrinogen degradation products (FDP) are noted. DIC can be chronic, however, existing even when the platelet count, fibrinogen level, and PT are normal. The diagnosis rests on the demonstration of FDP and, more specifically, D-dimer, which is formed only when intravascular coagulation occurs. Severely ill hospitalized patients may suffer vitamin-K deficiency that can be mistaken for or may complicate DIC.[39] DIC as defined hematologically may be entirely asymptomatic and may wax and wane, at times ceasing spontaneously. Its exact pathogenesis is unknown.

PATHOLOGY

Two pathologic abnormalities occur in patients with DIC. The first, as the name implies, consists of small, fibrin-platelet thrombi that occlude arterioles or venules. Larger fibrin accumulations may at times cause local thrombus formation in veins, including those as large as the superior sagittal sinus (see the following), or vegetations on heart valves (i.e., nonbacterial thrombotic endocarditis [NBTE], a discussion of which follows[1367,2516]). DIC does not cause arterial thrombi, but valvular vegetations may embolize to large arterial vessels such as the carotid artery. Associated with the small-vessel occlusion are small infarcts. The infarcts can appear in any organ, but the most common site of both vascular occlusion and infarction is the brain. In pathology series[1366,2388] from general hospitals, the brain is involved in about 70% of patients with DIC, followed in order by the heart, kidneys, and spleen. The disorder may be unsuspected during life.

The second pathologic change is hemorrhage. When intravascular coagulation is severe, consumption of coagulation factors leads to spontaneous bleeding. The bleeding commonly occurs in the GI tract, associated with local erosion,[1675] but hematuria, subcutaneous bleeding, and bleeding into other organs can also occur. Gross bleeding into the brain is rare except with APML, in which massive cerebral hemorrhage is a usual cause of death. Microscopic bleeding in the brain in the form of hemorrhagic infarction or petechial hemorrhages surrounding occluded vessels is relatively common.[482]

Pathologic changes in the brain are interesting and unusual.[482] Grossly, the brain may appear entirely normal or may show small, scattered petechial hemorrhages in either gray or white matter. Characteristically, the petechiae occur in white matter, often the corpus callosum. In some patients with the same clinical syndrome, small hemorrhages may select gray matter rather than white matter. The causes of this selection are uncertain. Occasionally, bland infarcts can be seen grossly, but usually the infarcts and occluded blood vessels can be identified only microscopically.

Microscopically, the disease is characterized by fibrin platelet occlusions of small arterial and venous vessels of less than 50 μ. The venous occlusions permit the pathologist to conclude that the disorder is thrombotic and not embolic. Occlusions, surrounded by bland or hemorrhagic infarction, are scattered throughout both hemispheres, not concentrated in the distribution of a single large cerebral vessel. In some instances, the infarcts are all of the same age, but in others, the disease process appears to have waxed and waned, causing some old and some recent infarcts. The vessel wall appears unaffected.

Because the occluded vessels are small and the resulting infarctions are of millimeter size, no symptoms appear in most organs. Small infarcts at strategic sites in the brain, however, can be responsible for clinical symptoms. When many infarcts are scattered throughout the brain, the symptoms reflect diffuse rather than focal brain disease.

Vascular occlusions and infarcts begin when ample concentrations of clotting factors are still present in the blood. Since the substances have considerable reserves, neurologic symptoms often precede thrombocytopenia and hypofibrinogenemia. The first abnormalities are the presence of FDP and D-dimer, indicating that widespread clotting has occurred and that fibrinolysis is active. These tests are particularly helpful when platelet counts, PT, and partial thromboplastin time are normal.[460a,2798a]

INCIDENCE

DIC affecting the brain is not rare. Pathologic changes may be found in 1% or 2% of autopsy studies in a general hospital,[1366] and the clinical syndrome is encountered commonly, particularly in patients suffering from severe and widespread disease such as sepsis or cancer.[1367,2354] In a cancer hospital, DIC usually complicates the course of lymphomas rather than solid tumors, although it may occur in both conditions, and it is the single most common cause of thrombotic infarction in the brain. In our pathologic study,[976] nearly 25% (28 of 117) brain infarcts in symptomatic patients occurred as a result of DIC. This figure excludes other complications of intravascular coagulation, such as NBTE or cerebral venous sinus occlusion.

CLINICAL FINDINGS[2301,2342]

A patient suffering from advanced cancer, usually leukemia or lymphoma that is often complicated by sepsis, suddenly becomes confused. All of our patients (Table 9–7) were confused and disoriented, divided almost equally between agitated and lethargic delirium. The confusion, sometimes associated with asterixis or multifocal myoclonus, is complicated by generalized seizures in about one-third of patients. The confusion may be episodic but, if untreated, usually progresses to stupor or coma, although sometimes it spontaneously clears.

In more than half of our patients, evidence of diffuse brain disease was accompanied by additional evidence of focal brain disease (see Table 9–7), characteristically mild and fleeting. Usually, each focal neurologic abnormality lasted several hours or a day or two but then cleared, only to be replaced by evidence of neurologic disease

Table 9–7. NEUROLOGIC SIGNS AND SYMPTOMS OF INTRAVASCULAR COAGULATION IN PATIENTS WITH CANCER

Signs and Symptoms		No. of Patients
Generalized brain disease	12	
Confusion or disorientation		12
Agitated delirium		4
Lethargy or stupor		6
Coma		4
Asterixis or multifocal myoclonus		2
Generalized seizure		4
Focal brain disease	7	
Hemiparesis		2
Cortical blindness		2
Aphasia		1
Focal seizures		4
Epilepsia partialis continua		2
Ataxia		2
Cranial nerve abnormalities		1

Source: From Collins et al,[482] p 797, with permission.

elsewhere in the brain. The episodes are usually longer than transient ischemic attacks but rarely as prolonged or severe as a large-vessel occlusion.

Because sepsis is a common inciting factor in intravascular coagulation, patients may be febrile. Petechial hemorrhages in the skin are rare. Because small hemorrhages are occasionally encountered in the eye grounds, a careful funduscopic examination through dilated pupils may give a clue to the cause of a mysterious delirium. Otherwise, the physical examination is of little help.

LABORATORY TESTS

Patients are often anemic and slightly thrombocytopenic, but these changes are usually attributable to previous chemotherapy or the effects of the tumor itself. Coagulation profiles may initially be entirely normal but become abnormal during the course of the neurologic illness. The first abnormality to appear is usually elevation of FDP and D-dimer. Blood cultures may be helpful because many patients suffer from sepsis by either Gram-negative organisms or fungi. At autopsy, 2 of our 12 patients had fungal infections in the brain.

Other laboratory tests are rarely valuable. Hemorrhagic infarcts more than 5 mm in diameter are identifiable on CT or MR scan. Such large lesions, however, suggest NBTE rather than DIC. One report[1348] suggests that in a similar (but not cancer-related) disorder, thrombotic thrombocytopenic purpura (TTP), an abnormal CT scan portends a poor outcome whereas a normal scan, even in the presence of severe neurologic signs, portends a good outcome. In TTP, biopsy of skin or gum has helped to establish the diagnosis,[948] but the utility of systemic biopsy has not been examined in DIC.

DIFFERENTIAL DIAGNOSIS

Metabolic brain disease is usually the major consideration. If the patient has fleeting and episodic focal signs, the clinician should suspect DIC rather than metabolic brain disease, particularly if no underlying metabolic defect can explain the patient's encephalopathy. Opportunistic CNS infections can resemble intravascular coagulation, but headache is more common with infection, and fleeting focal signs are more common with DIC. Sometimes the two complications of cancer accompany each other because infection may cause DIC. The clinical picture of DIC differs from that of metastasis; an MR scan establishes the presence of a metastasis. In NBTE, which is part of the DIC picture, larger cerebral arteries are occluded, usually leading to a stroke rather than an encephalopathy (see the following).

TREATMENT

Because the disorder is excessive coagulation with microthrombi, anticoagulation with heparin has been recommended by many investigators as the treatment of choice.[2258] In systemic DIC, particularly when it occurs with APML, heparin has at times been valuable in reversing the hematologic defect and improving clinical signs and symptoms. The physician should fear increasing the bleeding, particularly because many of the infarcts in the brain are already hemorrhagic, but it is probably safe to heparinize most patients. Unfortunately, except in ALL, the clinical diagnosis is often established too late or the patient's underlying disease is so severe that treatment is not useful. We have treated only a few patients with heparin; the treatment appeared to ameliorate the neurologic symptoms.[460a,2798a] The chronic use of warfarin is probably ineffective.

Arterial Occlusion by Extrinsic Tumor

In rare patients, an extrinsic tumor occludes a large artery by either compressing or invading the vessel wall, causing cerebral infarction associated with thrombus formation.[1808] A review of the literature describing 40 patients with arterial compression by tumor notes that only 4 suffered from metastatic tumor.[1480] Most patients with arteries compressed by tumors have meningiomas growing in the cavernous sinus, compressing the carotid artery. Arteries embedded in tumors lose smooth muscle and eventually become amuscular tubes. In addition, such arteries are often deformed into aneurysmal or crumpled shapes. These phenomena may make arteries incapable of normal blood flow regulation even if they are not occluded by the tumor.[2857] Tumors do not often invade the walls of large arteries, so that arterial rupture or occlusion from tumor growing into the vessel is uncommon. Arterial rupture sometimes occurs in the carotid blow-out syndrome, but this is usually a result of surgery and radiation rather than tumor growing directly in the wall. Veins are much more commonly occluded by extrinsic tumor compression; the superior vena caval syndrome is a frequent presenting complaint of mediastinal tumor, and the cerebral sagittal or lateral sinuses can be occluded by skull metastases (see Chapter 5).

CLINICAL FINDINGS

When tumor involves the carotid artery, particularly with head and neck tumors and metastatic breast cancer, the patient may complain of severe headache or pain in the eye, nose, scalp, teeth, or gums; the syndrome resembles the migraine variant called carotodynia.[2128] Similar phenomena have been reported after internal carotid artery dissection and carotid endarterectomy. In some patients, syncope (usually but not always associated with headache) occurs as the carotid sinus is invaded (see Chapter 8). Characteristically, arterial compression is otherwise asymptomatic unless the patient suffers an acute vessel occlusion, leading to cerebral infarction. The diagnosis is usually not suspected in life. The MR scan shows only the cerebral infarct, although in some instances a contrast-enhancing mass can be identified at the base of the brain surrounding the carotid or vertebral artery. A cerebral or MR arteriogram is more likely to yield useful information, demonstrating not only the occluded vessel but the site of extrinsic compression from the tumor. The differential diagnosis is that of any of the other causes of cerebral infarction. The treatment should be directed at the tumor.

Cerebral Emboli

Emboli to cerebral vessels are common causes of bleeding or hemorrhagic infarction in patients with cancer (Table 9–8).[909]

Table 9–8. **CAUSES OF EMBOLIC CEREBRAL INFARCTION IN PATIENTS WITH CANCER**

Atheromatous plaques
Infected material
Bacterial or fungal endocarditis
Fungal lung lesions
Nonbacterial thrombotic endocarditis
Tumor
Mucin
Fat
Bone marrow
Calcified valves
Silicone particles
Lymphangiography
Talc
Air

NONBACTERIAL THROMBOTIC ENDOCARDITIS

NBTE is characterized by uninfected fibrin vegetations on one or more heart valves. The underlying heart valves are usually free of other pathologic abnormalities. The disorder is common in patients with cancer but also occurs in patients who die from other systemic disorders and, rarely, in those with no systemic illness.[217,335] NBTE can happen at any time in the course of the cancer and may be the first evidence of it. More commonly, NBTE occurs late, when patients have disseminated cancer. Its overall incidence at autopsy in general hospitals is about 1%.[217,615]

In most patients, emboli are detected in more than one organ, such as spleen, kidney, and heart; about 50% have emboli in the brain with or without infarction[217,615] (Fig. 9–6). Approximately 7% of patients with adenocarcinoma of the lung have identifiable vegetations on their valves at autopsy.[2204] Other cancers, including carcinoma of the pancreas, have a lesser incidence of NBTE. Contrary to former belief, mucin-secreting adenocarcinoma does not tend to cause NBTE or cerebral embolization,[335,2194] although mucin itself may embolize to cerebral vessels.

Kearsley and Tattersall[1350] report 8 patients with acute cerebral emboli among

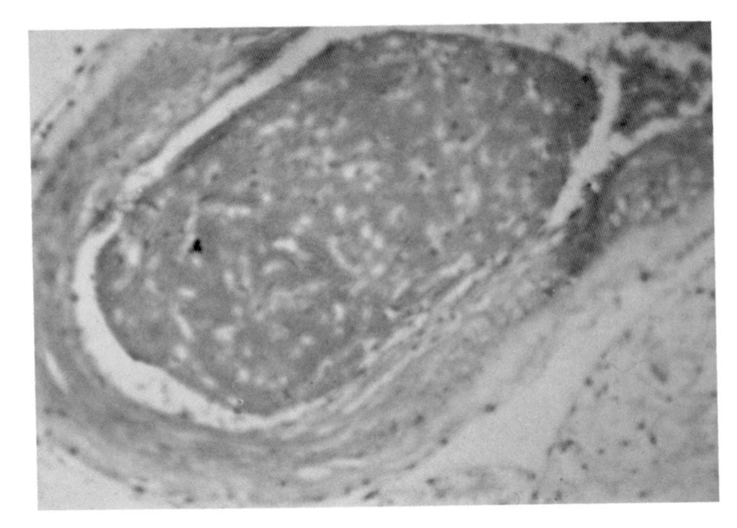

Figure 9–6. Embolus from a nonbacterial vegetation. This patient with known colon cancer suffered the sudden onset of a right hemiplegia and aphasia. She died within a matter of days and was found to have a massive infarct in her left hemisphere. Leptomeningeal and parenchymal vessels were filled with fibrin clots. A single vegetation was found on a cardiac valve.

3000 patients with cancer. Of the patients examined at autopsy, 5 had NBTE. In another study,[2152] valvular vegetations were found by echocardiogram in 5 of 30 patients with myeloproliferative disorders (i.e., polycythemia and thrombocythemia).

Most patients suffering from cancer-associated NBTE have identifiable coagulation abnormalities. Only 6 of 42 patients whom we studied with cerebral infarction from NBTE had an entirely normal coagulation profile.[976,2194] The coagulation abnormalities may be relatively mild and not reflect the extent of the clotting present in the patient. Many patients with NBTE also have other evidence of hypercoagulability, including deep-vein thrombosis or fulminant DIC. Not all patients with NBTE, however, are symptomatic. Because the heart valve disease is usually asymptomatic, the abnormality is recognized clinically only when emboli occlude vessels supplying important organs. Arteries of any size may be occluded. Medium-sized vessels, such as the middle cerebral artery and its branches, are common occlusion sites. In one of our patients, the internal carotid artery was occluded by an embolus. The brain is a common site of cerebral embolization and infarction from NBTE, but of 86 such patients examined at autopsy, only 47 had identifiable cerebral infarcts, and in only 42 of these could the infarct be attributed with certainty to embolization from the heart valve.[2194]

Clinical Findings. Although occasionally children are affected,[2877] the patients are usually adults who suffer from solid tumors, most commonly non–small-cell lung cancer. The clinical syndrome usually occurs late in the course of cancer. Of our 42 patients, 27 suffered from progressive cancer and were being actively treated, 6 had widespread disease but were clinically stable, and 7 were in the early stages of cancer. In 2 patients, neurologic symptoms preceded the diagnosis of malignancy,[2194] a phenomenon probably much more prominent in a general hospital than in a cancer hospital. By the time our patients died, the tumor was widely disseminated in most of them, but 6 had only localized tumor, 3 had carcinoma restricted to the lung, and 3 had carcinoma restricted to the cervix.

Neurologic findings can be divided into the following three groups (Table 9–9):

1. those suggesting focal brain disease, probably resulting from a single large embolus;
2. those suggesting diffuse brain disease, probably resulting from multiple small emboli scattered throughout the brain;
3. those with a combination of focal and diffuse abnormalities.

Of our 32 patients with clinical symptoms, 18 suffered from focal brain disease suggesting a stroke. The onset was usually sudden and caused fixed neurologic symptoms, usually hemiparesis or hemiplegia (Fig. 9–7). In four patients, the disease was clearly multifocal, suggesting occlusion of vessels in more than one major arterial distribution. In a minority of patients, the symptoms were transient,

Table 9–9. **INITIAL NEUROLOGIC SIGNS IN 32 PATIENTS WITH NBTE AND CEREBRAL INFARCTION**

Focal only			**18**
Aphasia		13	
With right hemiparesis	6		
With right hemiparesis and sensory loss	2		
With right hemiparesis and hemianopia	1		
With hemianopia	1		
Without other signs	3		
Focal seizures		3	
Hemiparesis, hemihyperesthesia		2	
Herniation		1	
Monocular blindness		1	
Diplopia, vertigo		1	
Cortical blindness		1	
Diffuse only			**9**
Confusion		5	
Coma		3	
Lethargy		1	
Focal and diffuse			**5**

NBTE = nonbacterial thrombotic endocarditis.

similar to transient ischemic attacks, rather than fixed. Some patients with focal signs at onset subsequently developed evidence of more generalized brain dysfunction (see the following).

Nine patients showed evidence of diffuse brain dysfunction, including confusion, stupor, or coma without focal abnormalities; the disorder resembled either metabolic brain disease or DIC. Five patients suffered combined diffuse brain dysfunction plus the sudden onset of focal symptoms suggesting major vascular occlusions, which is virtually pathognomonic.

Findings outside the nervous system sometimes suggest NBTE, including occlusive disease of vessels elsewhere in the body, such as DVT with pulmonary embolization, arterial embolization to the extremities, acute myocardial infarction, central retinal artery occlusion, and bleeding abnormalities such as GI bleeding, hematuria, and bleeding from venipuncture sites. Unlike infective endocarditis, NBTE does not cause a cardiac murmur.

Laboratory Tests. Transthoracic echocardiography (Fig. 9–8) is often negative[61,736,1183,2194]; transesophageal echocardiography may be more rewarding.[1362a,1503,2144] CT or MR scans frequently reveal evidence of infarction. If the infarcts are multiple and in the distribution of more than one cerebral vessel, the diagnosis is obvious. Bilateral carotid arteriograms may reveal evidence of multiple embolic occlusions in more than one vascular distribution even in the absence of infarction, showing that the emboli must have come from the heart. In the appropriate clinical setting, this result is virtually pathognomonic of NBTE. MR angiography, a non-

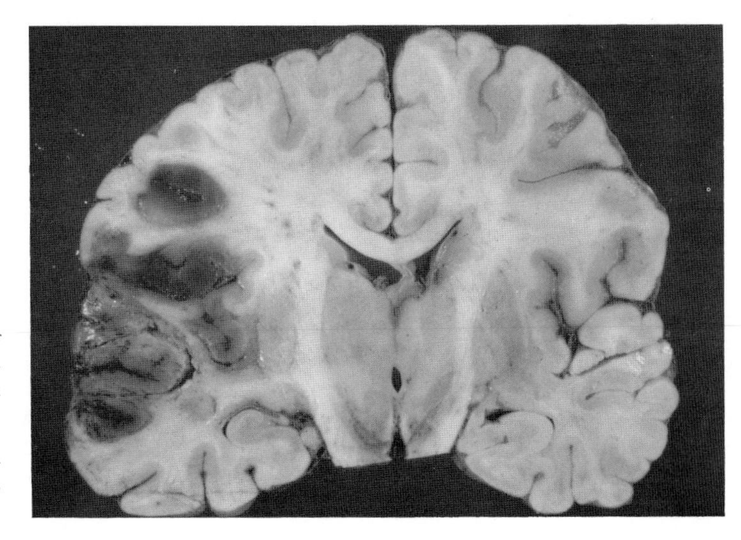

Figure 9–7. Multiple hemorrhagic infarcts in the right hemisphere of a patient with nonbacterial thrombotic endocarditis and malignant melanoma. Most of the infarcts are in the distribution of the middle cerebral artery, causing hemorrhagic infarction of cortex as well as white matter.

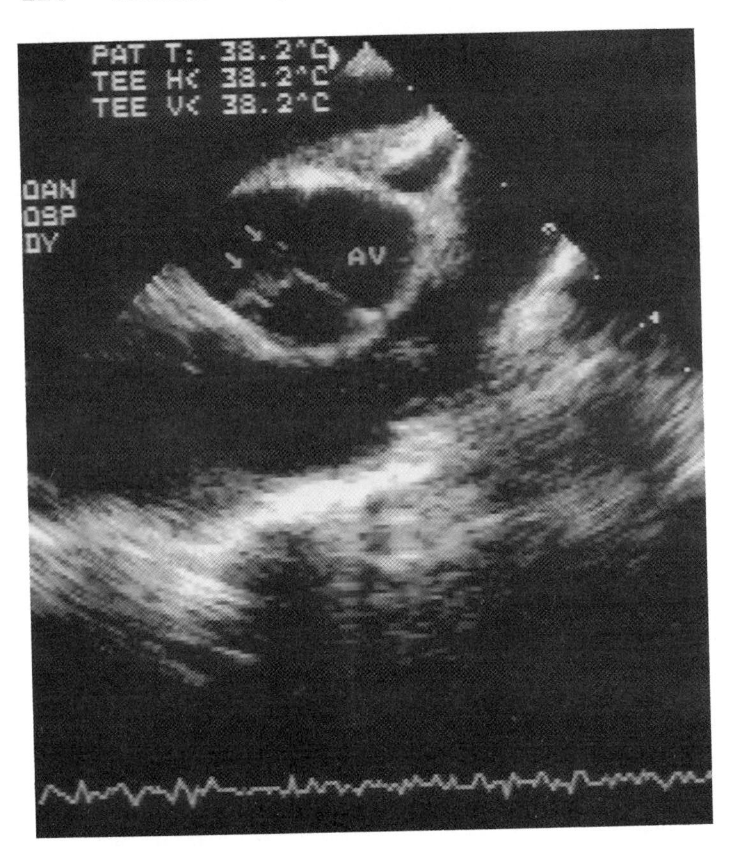

Figure 9–8. A transthoracic echocardiogram showing vegetation on a valve in a patient with nonbacterial thrombotic endocarditis. The patient suffered from leukemia and presented with multiple seizures. Bilateral posterior cerebral infarcts were found on the MR scan and large vegetations on the aortic valve (*arrows*).

invasive test, also may identify embolic occlusion of large vessels.

Pathology. The pathologic examination usually reveals vegetations on the valves.[2194] In some patients, however, all of the vegetative material has embolized and the valves appear normal. I have encountered at least one instance of a patient with multiple embolic infarctions in the brain in whom a vegetation seen at the time the heart was opened was accidentally dislodged by the prosector. The results of subsequent gross and microscopic examination of the valves were entirely normal. Some clinical evidence indicates that the disease may either wax and wane or be self-limited. Thus, the patient may have suffered a stroke in the distant past but have no evidence of disease on the heart valves at autopsy. Microscopically, the heart valves may be entirely normal or may show some evidence of microscopic vegetations in place of previously larger ones.

The brain usually shows evidence of multiple, grossly visible infarcts that are bland in approximately half of patients and hemorrhagic in the other half.[2194] In occasional patients, only a single infarct is discovered. Careful search of medium-sized blood vessels reveals platelet-fibrin thrombi in almost all patients. At times, vessels are occluded in areas without infarction and vice versa. The disease often occurs in conjunction with other neurologic complications of cancer, including DIC. We found pathologic evidence of that disorder in 11 of the 42 brains examined in our NBTE series.

Treatment. Although no controlled studies validate the treatment of this disorder, most observers consider anticoagulation to be beneficial. In two patients, transient neurologic symptoms resolved with anticoagulation; in one, neurologic symptoms recurred on two occasions when heparin doses were subtherapeutic, and the symptoms promptly disappeared when appropriate anticoagulation was achieved.[2194] Anecdotal evidence similarly suggests that anticoagulation with warfarin is ineffective in NBTE and other coagulopathies associated with cancer.[176] Thus, we have treated patients with IV heparin for 10 days to 2 weeks and then attempted subcutaneous heparin maintenance on an outpatient basis.

The possibility that anticoagulation increases hemorrhagic infarction seems to be more theoretic than real. We compared brain hemorrhages in patients treated with anticoagulants with those not so treated; no difference was found in either the number of patients with hemorrhagic infarctions or the degree of hemorrhage.[2194] Interestingly, fewer cases of DIC were noted in the treated patients than in the nontreated group.

SEPTIC ARTERIAL OCCLUSIONS

Arterial or arteriolar occlusions caused by infectious organisms, sometimes bacteria but especially fungi, with resulting bland or hemorrhagic infarction of the brain, are encountered relatively frequently. Such infarcts are the third most common symptomatic cause of cerebral infarction in the cancer population, after DIC and NBTE (see Chapter 10).

Clinical Findings. The clinical signs and symptoms depend on the number and size of vessels occluded. In most instances, small vessels of arteriolar size are occluded, and the vascular occlusions are scattered throughout both hemispheres. When this occurs, symptoms are usually those of a diffuse encephalopathy, sometimes accompanied by fleeting and mild focal signs resembling the clinical picture of DIC. Frequently, the patients are febrile, but the fever is often attributed to systemic infection, for which most patients are already being treated.

Because larger vessels are occluded and the area of infarction is large, about 33% of patients develop the acute onset of relatively severe and fixed focal neurologic deficits with or without delirium, similar to that described for NBTE. One of our patients suffered a septic occlusion of the anterior spinal artery, causing paraplegia; in another, occlusion of the basilar artery caused brainstem infarction.

The general physical evaluation may help with the diagnosis. Septic occlusion of small vessels may lead to hemorrhagic skin lesions, particularly in *Pseudomonas* infections. A biopsy of these lesions may yield the organism. Blood cultures are occasionally positive, particularly when the offending organism is a bacterium. The chest radiograph usually shows bilateral lesions, particularly with *Aspergillus* fungi; aspiration may yield the organism that is causing the neurologic symptoms. Lumbar puncture seldom helps. Occasionally, pleocytosis is present, and sometimes a few RBCs. The CSF protein is usually increased, and the CSF glucose is usually normal. Organisms are rarely identified. CT or MR scan usually reveals multiple infarcts, often hemorrhagic.

Pathology. The pathologic changes result in part from the size of the vessel occluded and in part from the duration of the occlusion. The organisms promote coagulation locally and thus generally become enmeshed in a fibrin clot. They then invade the vessel wall, usually causing an inflammatory vasculitis and sometimes causing a bland infarct to become hemorrhagic. After the vessel wall is invaded, the organism may grow freely within the substance of the brain, producing abscesses of varying size. Disseminated microabscesses are the most common pathologic feature of Phycomycetes and *Candida* infection, as well as of *Pseudomonas* infection. *Aspergillus* organisms often form one or only a few large infarcts; thus, the *Aspergillus* organism is more likely to cause severe focal neurologic disability (see Chapter 10).

The pathogenesis of the lesions is not fully established. The vascular occlusions could be caused by either thrombosis or embolization. If thrombosis is the mechanism, the circulating organisms probably lodge in small arterioles and trigger a focal coagulation process. The organisms that cause vascular occlusions in the brain are also those that have a predilection to be associated with DIC. In favor of in situ thrombosis is the absence of vegetation on valves or in heart chambers that might lead to embolization and the occasional occlusion of venules and arterioles.

An embolic pathogenesis is suggested by (1) the frequent presence of pulmonary lesions that may serve as a source for embolization, (2) infectious vasculitis that is much more prominent on the arterial than the venous side of the circulation, and (3) the occasional occlusion of large blood vessels (e.g., carotid siphon) by what appear to be fungal emboli. Both thrombosis and embolism are probable mechanisms in some patients.

Treatment. The best treatment is prevention. If the offending organism can be treated while the infection is limited to systemic organs, CNS infection and vascular occlusion may be prevented (see Chapter 10). In a Memorial Sloan-Kettering Cancer Center (MSKCC) series collected from 1970 to 1973, 18% of the patients suffering from CNS vascular disease had septic occlusions of cerebral vessels. Between 1977 and 1979, equal numbers of patients with CNS vascular disease were encountered, but only 5% suffered from septic occlusions because of the earlier use of antibiotics.[976] The incidence as a percentage of autopsies showed a similar decrease.

TUMOR EMBOLIZATION

Embolization of tumor from a primary or metastatic site outside the nervous system to the cerebral vasculature is a rare cause of cerebral vascular occlusion and may also cause pulmonary symptoms.[2331] Mucin-secreting tumors may embolize to brain. Large or small arteries are occluded by mucin or a mucin and fibrin clot with or without tumor cells.[44,589] Tumor emboli are not necessarily restricted to the brain. Major peripheral arterial occlusions can also be due to malignant tumor embolism.[2099,2588] Atrial myxomas are a rare but well-recognized cause of cerebral or spinal infarction.[1168] O'Neill and colleagues[1914] found seven adults with clinical symptoms and pathologically proved tumor emboli to the brain at the Mayo Clinic between 1951 and 1984. Three presented with cerebral infarction as the initial manifestation of cancer.

Tumors that embolize usually come from the lungs. The primary pulmonary tumor or metastasis invades a pulmonary vein, where a portion of the tumor breaks off and travels through the heart to enter the cerebral circulation. In one patient, an embolus appeared to come from a metastasis on cardiac valves. How non–lung-tumor emboli reach the arterial circulation in other patients is not clear. Paradoxic embolization is one possible route. One patient suffered a middle cerebral artery occlusion from testicular carcinoma not metastatic to the lungs. The occlusion was found at autopsy along with a tumor thrombus sitting astride a patent foramen ovale, indicating that the embolus had reached the cerebral circulation via that route.[2588] Paradoxic embolization is a relatively common cause of stroke in the general population. If a DVT first causes a pulmonary embolus, the sudden rise in right atrial pressure can open a potentially patent foramen ovale, allowing a second embolus to cross from the right to the left atrium. Because cerebral blood flow is 15% to 20% of total blood flow in the resting state, a high likelihood exists that an embolus will reach the CNS once it has entered the arterial circulation. Furthermore, the probability that an embolus of any size that reaches the cerebral circulation will cause clinical symptoms is high, whereas a small embolus in a systemic organ is often asymptomatic. Tumor emboli may be large enough to occlude large vessels, including the middle cerebral, basilar,[1914] or angular artery.[1854] The result is a bland or a hemorrhagic infarction. A fibrin reaction may be set up within the vessel, but usually the tumor does not appear to invade the vessel wall. On occasion, cerebral embolization occurs during a thoracotomy for removal of a pulmonary tumor.[1914]

Clinically, the patient suffers the sudden onset of a focal neurologic defect, which may remain unchanged until death. In a few instances, repetitive showers of small emboli cause either transient focal neurologic defects or a diffuse encephalopathy much like DIC.

Although the diagnosis may be suspected from the clinical history and clinical findings closely resembling NBTE, the correct diagnosis is rarely initially considered. The absence of coagulation abnormalities and the presence of a large primary tumor or metastases in the lung may lead one to suspect the diagnosis. Cerebral or MR arteriography will reveal the arterial occlusion but not its source. No treatment helps.

Thrombotic Microangiopathy

Several other causes of cerebral infarction (Table 9–10) are occasionally encountered in the cancer population.[976] Among these is thrombotic microangiopathy, which can occur as a complication of cancer, especially gastric, breast, lung, lymphoma,[381,1904] Hodgkin's disease and myeloma,[575] or of

Table 9–10. **OTHER CAUSES OF INFARCTION IN PATIENTS WITH CANCER**

Disorder	Association
Thrombotic microangiopathy	Malignancy (gastric, breast, lung) Chemotherapy (mitomycin, *cis*-platinum)
Vasculitis	Hairy-cell leukemia, Hodgkin's disease
Neoplastic angioendotheliomatosis	Lymphoma
Thrombocytosis	Myeloproliferative disorders
Miscellaneous (Due to decreased cerebral blood flow)	
Hypotension	Anesthesia, sepsis, chemotherapy
Carotid artery rupture	Head and neck cancer, radiation therapy
Carotid-cavernous fistula	Surgical complication
Arteriovenous shunt	Thyroid adenoma (not malignant)
Other	
Bone marrow embolus	
Undetermined cause	

cancer therapy[575,1838,2729] (Table 9–11). Occasionally, it may develop in patients apparently cured of cancer.[381] Mitomycin is the most common chemotherapeutic culprit, although other agents, including 5-fluorouracil, carboplatinum, and *cis*-platinum–based multiagent chemotherapy, have also been implicated (see Chapter 12). Clinical symptoms resemble DIC and are characterized by encephalopathy and fleeting multifocal neurologic deficits. In one patient, progressive brainstem dysfunction culminated in coma and respiratory arrest.[2729] Thrombotic microangiopathy is believed to

Table 9–11. **THROMBOTIC MICROANGIOPATHY IN THE PATIENT WITH CANCER**

Distinguishing Features	Carcinoma-Associated MAHA	Chemotherapy-Related HUS
Three most common tumors	Gastric, breast, lung	Gastric, colon, breast
Tumor status	Usually widely metastatic	Clinical remission common
Male:female ratio	1:2.1	1:1.9
Principal site of microvascular lesions	Lung	Kidney
Renal failure	Unusual	Characteristic
Severe hypertension	Uncommon	Common
Pulmonary edema	Unusual	Common
Adverse reactions to RBC transfusion	Not described	Common
Leukoerythroblastic picture	Common	Unusual
Laboratory evidence of intravascular coagulation	Common	Frequently absent
Proposed initiating factor(s)	Tumor emboli–derived factors	Chemotherapy toxicity + circulating immune complexes
Recommended treatment	Specific antitumor therapy ± heparin	Immunoperfusion or plasma exchange ± antiplatelet agents

MAHA = microangiopathic hemolytic anemia; HUS = hemolytic-uremic syndrome.
Source: From Murgo[1838] p 173, with permission.

result from the formation of circulating immune complexes or autoantibodies. It mimics microangiopathic hemolytic anemia, TTP, and the hemolytic uremic syndrome not associated with cancer. Pathologic examination reveals widespread multivascular thrombosis with platelets and fibrin, associated with microinfarction. The heart, kidneys, and brain are the most severely affected organs. The diagnosis can be suspected from blood evaluation, which shows a hemolytic anemia; the peripheral smear shows the characteristic RBC changes of a microangiopathic process with schistocytes, burr cells, and helmet cells. The platelet count decreases, and platelet survival is shortened. Evidence of DIC may coexist,[1838] but often the coagulation profile is normal. The MR scan may show on T_2-weighted images multiple, small, hyperintense lesions corresponding to the areas of microangiopathy. Immunoabsorption of plasma by protein A may be an effective treatment.

Cerebral Vasculitis

A cerebral vasculitis sometimes complicates hairy-cell leukemia. In one patient, neurologic and pathologic abnormalities were limited to the cerebral vasculature. The disorder pathologically resembles polyarteritis nodosa.[719,753,1608] Granulomatous angiitis restricted to the nervous system may complicate the course of Hodgkin's disease,[1248] perhaps related to herpes zoster vasculitis (see Chapter 10). The disorder is characterized by remitting and relapsing focal neurologic signs involving either brain or spinal cord. Patients often have headache, fever, and delirium. The MR scan reveals evidence of multiple small infarcts, particularly in the white matter of the brain; angiography may show beading or occlusion of small arterial vessels. White cells may be found in the CSF, although frequently the diagnosis can be made only by biopsy. Corticosteroids are said to be helpful in some instances, but most patients progress and then die from the neurologic disorder.[1248] The combination of cyclophosphamide and corticosteroids may be more effective than corticosteroids alone.[8a]

Neoplastic Angioendotheliomatosis (Angiotropic Lymphoma, Intravascular Lymphoma)

This systemic disorder involving the CNS and peripheral nervous system is now recognized to be an intravascular lymphoma that occludes small blood vessels in the brain, spinal cord, and peripheral nerves.[611,681,929,2126] Symptoms may include a subacutely developing dementia with or without focal neurologic signs. When signs are focal, they may suggest brain, spinal cord, or peripheral nerve involvement. The diagnosis is rarely made antemortem. A biopsy of skin lesions or cerebral vasculature may show small vessels occluded by lymphoma cells. As with other widespread small-vessel disease, even when the disease is disseminated, signs and symptoms tend to be restricted to the nervous system.[664,1271,1396] Plasmapheresis[1097] and antilymphoma chemotherapy may be useful.

Thrombocytosis

Platelet counts of more than 1,000,000/mm^3 sometimes occur in patients with severe myeloproliferative disorders, including chronic myelogenous leukemia, myelofibrosis, polycythemia vera, and primary thrombocythemia.[351] Some patients with severe thrombocytosis suffer from thrombotic or hemorrhagic complications. Neurologic symptoms include headache, paresthesias, transient ischemic attacks in anterior or posterior circulation or both, and, occasionally seizures. The clinical symptoms are usually fleeting but may be associated with small, hyperintense lesions on a T_2-weighted MR scan. A single patient has been reported with a lateral sinus thrombus related to thrombocytosis.[1781]

VENOUS OCCLUSION

Occlusion of the large venous sinuses can result from compression or invasion by metastatic tumor (e.g., tumor in the skull overlying the sagittal sinus [see Chapter 5]) or from a coagulopathy.[760,1152,1444,2418] The most commonly involved sinus is the superior sagittal sinus, although other large cerebral veins may be affected.[1053] Occlusion of cerebral venous sinuses is bland and not a part of the systemic venous septic thrombophlebitis sometimes associated with indwelling venous catheters.[2689]

Compressive Venous Sinus Occlusion

Compressive occlusion of the venous sinuses can be caused by any tumor that metastasizes to the skull vault,[2042] most commonly neuroblastoma and breast carcinoma. The tumor may occlude or compress the sinus anywhere along its course, but symptoms are unlikely unless the posterior portion of the sagittal sinus or the larger of the two lateral sinuses is compressed or occluded. Accordingly, in symptomatic patients the lesion is usually found overlying the torcular Herophili.

CLINICAL FINDINGS

The typical clinical picture can be called "pseudo-pseudotumor." Patients with known cancer and bony metastases present to the physician either complaining of headache or sometimes with florid papilledema without complaints of either headache or visual alterations.

Cancer-associated cerebral venous sinus occlusion seldom causes seizures or infarction because it develops slowly, allowing ample time for collateral circulation to develop and prevent infarction but not enough to maintain normal intracranial pressure. The diagnosis is suspected by the clinical picture and usually established by an MR scan. The sinus need not be totally occluded. Substantial but incomplete compression can raise intracranial pressure enough to cause papilledema. If lumbar puncture is performed, the pressure is markedly elevated, but the fluid is otherwise normal.

DIFFERENTIAL DIAGNOSIS

The differential diagnosis includes brain metastases and leptomeningeal metastases, but florid papilledema in the absence of other neurologic signs effectively rules these out. Rarely, sinus occlusion accompanies leptomeningeal cancer.[324] Idiopathic true "pseudotumor cerebri" must be considered if the patient is an obese, middle-aged woman.[900] In a very young or very old woman or in any man, the diagnosis of idiopathic pseudotumor is unlikely. The MR changes of skull metastasis and sinus compression are conclusive.

TREATMENT

Treatment is whole-brain RT or appropriate focal radiation therapy to the lesion site. Either electron-beam or photon therapy can be used. If the tumor is radiosensitive, it shrinks and decompresses the venous sinus. Even if the tumor does not shrink substantially, collateral circulation eventually decreases intracranial pressure, and the papilledema resolves. I have not encountered any such patients with substantial visual loss from the papilledema.

Venous Sinus Thrombosis

Spontaneous thrombosis of a venous sinus is often a more serious illness than external compression. This complication of hypercoagulability can occur in patients with carcinoma of the breast and lung and other solid tumors, but is more common in those with hematologic malignancies. The disorder can occur when the patient's cancer is relatively quiescent and need not represent a terminal disease phase.[2418,2450] The usual clinical setting is in patients with newly diagnosed leukemia or lymphoma who are receiving chemotherapy with L-asparaginase. Sinus occlusion appears to result from antithrombin III deficiency caused by the asparaginase[760,1434] and can be prevented by administering clotting factors.[1705]

CLINICAL FINDINGS

The clinical picture depends upon the size of the vessel occluded, the potential for rapidly developing collateral circulation, and whether the initial occlusion extends from its original site. The disease occurs in the following three forms:

1. A sudden onset of headache is associated with seizures and focal neurologic signs, often more striking in the legs than in the arms, followed by rapid progression to stupor, coma, cerebral herniation, and death (as in Fig. 9–9).
2. In its less florid form, a sudden onset of headache is sometimes associated with focal seizures and mild focal neurologic signs that rapidly resolve.
3. A sudden onset of headache occurs without other neurologic signs, followed by progressive neurologic symptoms that begin suddenly or gradually. These indicate extension of the thrombus from its original site. In one of my patients with breast cancer, pain behind the ear suggested a lateral sinus thrombosis; in the succeeding 3 weeks, the clot progressively occluded the rest of her venous sinus system, leading to coma and death from large, bilateral cerebral infarcts.

The diagnosis can be suspected by the clinical setting and findings confirmed by MR scan.[1250] If sinus occlusion is suspected, a gradient echo MR study should be performed. Coagulation abnormalities, if present, are relatively mild.

The CSF occasionally has a few RBCs or WBCs but usually is normal. The lumbar spinal fluid pressure typically is increased, but in some patients it remains normal, even with papilledema and unequivocal sinus occlusion. In these patients, there has probably been enough molding of the temporal lobes through the tentorium and the tonsils through the foramen magnum to isolate the

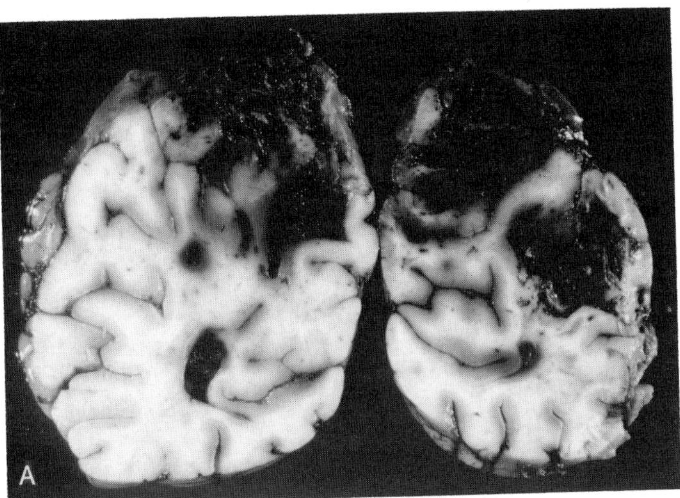

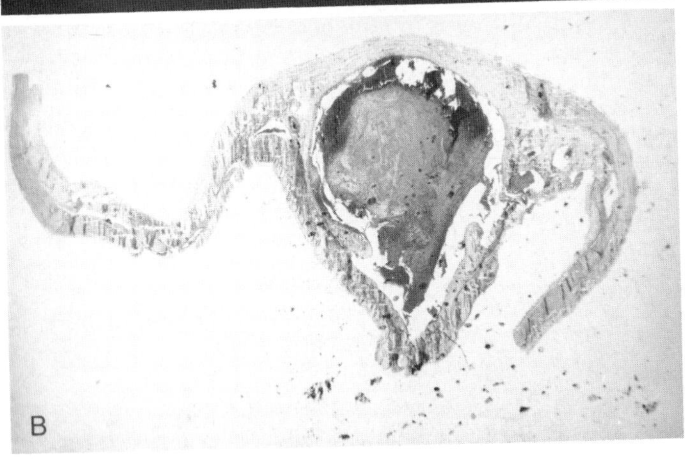

Figure 9–9. *A,* Multiple hemorrhagic infarcts from sagittal sinus occlusion. This patient had just completed the induction phase of treatment for acute myelogenous leukemia and was about to be discharged when she suffered sudden headache and collapse. She was found unconscious with bilateral cortical spinal tract signs most marked in the lower extremities. She died following herniation. A fresh occlusion of the sagittal sinus was found, with bilateral (largely parasagittal) hemorrhagic infarcts. *B,* The occluded sinus.

intracranial compartment from the spinal compartment and give an artificially low pressure in the lumbar sac. Such a phenomenon could lead to cerebral herniation, although I have not encountered it. It is probably wise not to perform lumbar punctures in these patients if the diagnosis can be made by other means and if meningeal tumor or infection is not suspected.

TREATMENT

The best treatment is not established. Usually, the disease takes a benign course whether or not it is treated. Patients who suffer the acute onset of severe neurologic disability are probably destined to herniate and die no matter what the treatment. The only ones likely to benefit from treatment are those who have a mild onset and then progress. Such patients cannot be identified in advance, raising the question of whether treatment with its attendant risk should be delivered to all patients.

The treatment has two aspects. The first is dealing with the increased intracranial pressure. I have not used steroids in most patients because the pressure signs are usually not disabling. When infarction has occurred and threatens to cause cerebral herniation, I have used hyperosmolar agents and steroids in the same manner as for metastatic tumors, but these agents have not been very helpful. One patient with intractable headache required steroids for several weeks to keep the headache under control; in this situation, they appeared to be beneficial.

The second aspect of treatment is lysis of the clot or preventing it from propagating. Some physicians recommend anticoagulant therapy with heparin. Patients at MSKCC who have been heparinized have not experienced severe cerebral hemorrhage or a change of a bland infarction to a hemorrhagic one.[281,713] On the other hand, whether these patients would have recovered under any circumstance is not clear. The use of IV heparin might very well prevent the clot from propagating, but it is doubtful that it can effectively deal with the clot already present. To complicate this issue, heparin-induced thrombocytopenia has been reported to cause a sagittal sinus occlusion.[1444] Clot-lysing agents such as streptokinase have not been tried.

PROGNOSIS AND SEQUELAE

The prognosis is generally good. Most patients fully recover after the acute episode and have no continuing neurologic disability. In one instance, an arteriogram repeated 3 weeks later revealed a patent sinus. One patient had severe headaches for a number of weeks, and another had early-morning headaches for several weeks following her occlusion. One patient developed pulmonary emboli, possibly from the sagittal sinus occlusion, and required late heparinization. With these exceptions, the course has been benign. I have followed two patients for more than 10 years who have had no further neurologic disability.

Tumor Emboli

Tumor emboli could theoretically reach the cerebral venous system either via Batson's plexus or by retrograde movement up a jugular vein invaded by head and neck cancer. I have only once encountered such a case.

Other Causes of Cerebral Infarction

Because many patients with cancer are desperately ill, they can suffer from systemic hypotension. Of 256 infarcts encountered during autopsy examinations, 4 were located in watershed areas, presumably owing to systemic hypotension from the patient's underlying illness.[976] Carotid artery rupture in patients with head and neck cancer led to 4 additional infarcts. One patient endured a hemorrhagic infarct after a surgically caused carotid cavernous fistula (Fig. 9–10); another unusual patient suffered cerebral infarction from a bone marrow embolus. Highly vascular tumors can compete with the nervous system for blood in much the same way as an arteriovenous malformation does. One unusual patient with an asymptomatic carotid artery occlusion[2515] had transient ischemic attacks when a highly vascular thyroid ad-

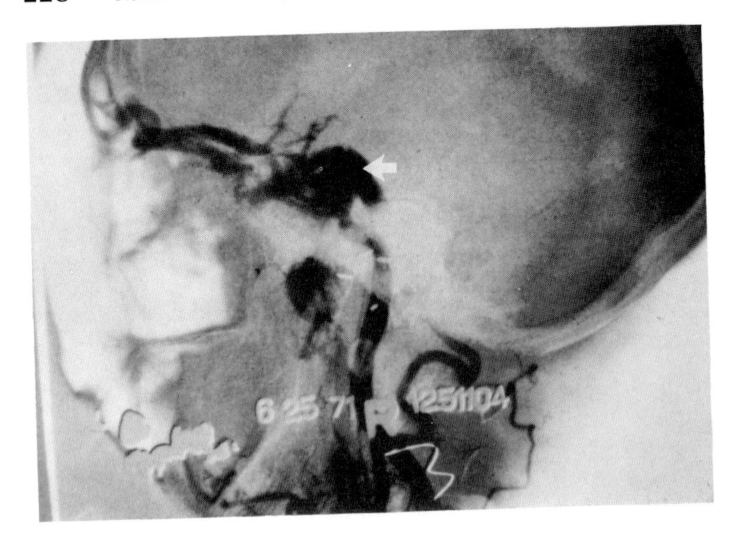

Figure 9–10. An angiogram showing a carotid cavernous fistula in a patient who had recently undergone surgery for carcinoma of the ear. During the course of the operation, the temporal bone was fractured. A bone spicule entered the cavernous sinus and carotid artery. A carotid cavernous fistula was created (*arrow*). The entire carotid blood flow emptied into the cavernous sinus, depriving the cerebral hemisphere of blood. Pressure in the sinus caused proptosis and ocular muscle paralysis. The large cerebral infarct caused the patient's death.

enoma apparently took enough cardiac output to decrease blood flow to the brain. Cerebral infarcts related to chemotherapy[661,663] are discussed in Chapter 12.

OTHER DISORDERS

Systemic Thrombophlebitis

Peripheral thrombophlebitis with or without pulmonary embolization is a common manifestation of both occult and established cancer.[2312] The disorder is particularly common following surgery for primary or metastatic brain tumors.[443,2302,2303]

Episodic Neurologic Dysfunction in Patients with Hodgkin's Disease[765]

Although it is not certain that this disorder has a vascular pathogenesis, it is discussed here because its symptoms mimic those of transient ischemic attacks. Some patients, mostly women believed to be cured of

Table 9–12. **CEREBROVASCULAR DISEASE IN LEUKEMIA/LYMPHOMA**

CNS Lesion	Primary Cancer	Mechanism
At the Time of Diagnosis or Initial Therapy		
Cerebral hemorrhage	Acute promyelocytic leukemia	Disseminated intravascular coagulation
	Acute nonlymphoblastic leukemia	Leukostasis
Sinus thrombosis	Acute lymphoblastic leukemia	L-asparaginase
At the Time of Relapse/Progressive Disease		
Cerebral hemorrhage	Acute nonlymphocytic leukemia	Coagulopathy
Thrombotic microinfarcts	Lymphoma/leukemia	Intravascular coagulation
Embolic infarct	Lymphoma/leukemia	Septic (fungal) embolism
Sinus thrombosis	Lymphoma	Coagulopathy

Table 9–13. **CEREBROVASCULAR DISEASE IN SOLID TUMORS**

CNS Lesion	Primary Cancer	Mechanism
At the Time of Diagnosis/During Remission		
Cerebral hemorrhage	Lung, melanoma, germ-cell tumor	Intratumoral bleeding
Embolic infarct	Adenocarcinoma	NBTE
	Myxoma	Tumor embolism
Subdural hematoma	Prostate	Dural metastasis
Thrombotic infarct	Head and neck carcinomas	Atherosclerosis
At the Time of Relapse/Active Disseminated Disease		
Cerebral hemorrhage	Melanoma, germ-cell tumor	Intratumoral bleeding
Subdural hematoma	Adenocarcinoma—breast, prostate	Dural metastasis
Thrombotic microinfarcts	Breast carcinoma	Intravascular coagulation
Sinus thrombosis	Breast carcinoma	Coagulopathy
Embolic infarct	Lung carcinoma	NBTE

NBTE = nonbacterial thrombotic endocarditis.

Hodgkin's disease, suffer transient episodes of neurologic dysfunction lasting 15 seconds to 45 minutes. Most have been in remission for months to years before developing the neurologic disorder. The unilateral or bilateral attacks are usually visual, with scintillating scotomata or transient visual loss. Other symptoms include focal weakness, sensory loss, or aphasia. Some patients develop weakness or sensory changes in their extremities. The episodes recur at intervals of days to weeks; they may be identical but more often they vary from episode to episode. In most patients, the attacks clear after months or years, either spontaneously or in response to taking low-dose aspirin.[765]

The pathophysiology of these transient episodes is unknown. It is not even certain that they are related to the underlying Hodgkin's disease. Levy[1549] has reported similar transient neurologic episodes in healthy people without a history of cancer. No epidemiologic study has been done to determine the frequency of such episodes in the general population or in the Hodgkin's disease population.

Whether or not these episodes are vascular is also uncertain. Migraine variants, as described by Fisher,[788] are another possible pathophysiologic mechanism. Although the episodes are usually benign, careful examination of the arterial system to look for a source of emboli is probably indicated when a patient treated for Hodgkin's disease presents with such symptoms.

APPROACH TO THE PATIENT

Table 9–12 details the most likely cerebrovascular lesions to be found in patients with hematologic neoplasms. The lesions differ depending on whether the vascular disorder appears at the time of diagnosis and initial treatment of the neoplasm or during progressive disease or relapse.

Table 9–13 details the likely cerebrovascular lesions in patients with solid tumor. As with leukemia and lymphomas, the lesions differ depending on whether they appear early or late in the course of the cancer.

CHAPTER 10

CENTRAL NERVOUS SYSTEM INFECTIONS

CNS infections are an uncommon complication of cancer and are probably decreasing in frequency as a result of earlier and more vigorous antibiotic use in patients with systemic infection.[1025] Nevertheless, CNS infections are more common in patients with cancer than in the general population and are more challenging to treat. In 1970, 0.2% of all admissions to Memorial Sloan-Kettering Cancer Center (MSKCC) had CNS infection (i.e., positive CSF cultures).[438] Beginning in 1971, the number of infections decreased, so that by 1974 the incidence was about 0.05%.[439] This figure has remained essentially unchanged, discounting CNS infections in AIDS patients, not considered here.

Patients with specific types of cancer are more likely than others to develop a CNS infection. About 85% of intracranial infections occur in the 12% of patients with cancer hospitalized with lymphoma, acute leukemia, or a surgically induced communication between the subarachnoid space and the surface of the body. CNS infections other than herpes zoster strike 2.7% of patients with Hodgkin's disease, 0.5% of patients with non-Hodgkin's lymphoma, and 2.5% of patients with chronic lymphocytic leukemia.[1198]

The usual florid symptoms apparent in immunocompetent patients with CNS infection often are absent in patients with cancer. Instead of severe headache, high fever, nuchal rigidity, and focal neurologic signs, patients may be afebrile or have only a slight increase in body temperature. Increasing confusion or lethargy may be the only additional signs to suggest a CNS infection.[1198,1615] For example, in a recent series[2801] of 13 patients with cryptococcal meningitis, only 8 had headache, 2 had nuchal rigidity, and 2 had fever. The diagnosis of brain abscess may be even more difficult because headache and fever are characteristically absent and focal neurologic signs may be absent as well.

The organisms causing CNS infection in the cancer patient are common in the environment but are uncommon causes of infection in the normal host.[82] Cryptococcal and listerial organisms are the major causes of meningitis in patients with cancer, and *Toxoplasma* and *Aspergillus* organisms are the major causes of brain abscess. *Haemophilus influenzae, Neisseria meningitidis,* and, surprisingly, *Mycobacterium tuberculosis* rarely cause CNS infections in patients with cancer.

Because most CNS infections in patients with cancer result from an abnormality of host defense mechanisms and because the particular abnormality is often characteristic of the underlying cancer or its treatment, the clinician can often predict with reasonable confidence the likely invading organism.[438, 1198, 1615, 2057] For example, acute meningitis in a patient with Hodgkin's disease with a normal WBC count is likely to result from a *Listeria* or *Cryptococcus* infection. If that patient has undergone a splenectomy as part of treatment, *Streptococcus pneumoniae* is also a likely cause of meningitis. If, however, that same patient has been under intensive chemotherapy and if the absolute neutrophil count is fewer than 1000/mm^3, Gram-negative organisms such as *Pseudomonas aeruginosa* or *Escherichia coli* are likely offenders.[438,1198]

Once the organism is known, vigorous antibiotic treatment often eradicates the infection. The same host factors that led to the patient becoming infected make treatment difficult, however; relapse and superinfection are frequent. Furthermore, in one study,[1198] in 39% (19) of 49 patients with CNS infections that were associated with systemic infections, the CNS was infected by different organisms from those infecting the rest of the body, or multiple organisms infected the CNS, either simultaneously or sequentially.

On the following pages, I discuss the pathophysiology, diagnostic approach, and common causes of CNS infection in patients with cancer. Many considerations that apply to cancer-associated infections also apply to infections complicating other immune disorders such as organ and bone-marrow transplantation, autoimmune diseases being treated with immunosuppressive drugs, and the immunosuppression caused by AIDS. Several recent reviews[82,2100,2101,2123] address CNS infections in patients with cancer as well as the broader topics of systemic infections in these patients,[2238] infection in the immunocompromised host,[490,1989a,2829] and CNS infections in general.[2308,2628]

PATHOPHYSIOLOGY OF CENTRAL NERVOUS SYSTEM INFECTION

Host Defenses

PHYSICAL BARRIERS

For an offending organism to reach the nervous system, it must penetrate two barriers, one between the body's surface and its interior and the second between the body's interior and the CNS (Table 10–1). The first

Table 10–1. **STEPS IN THE DEVELOPMENT OF CENTRAL NERVOUS SYSTEM BACTERIAL INFECTION**

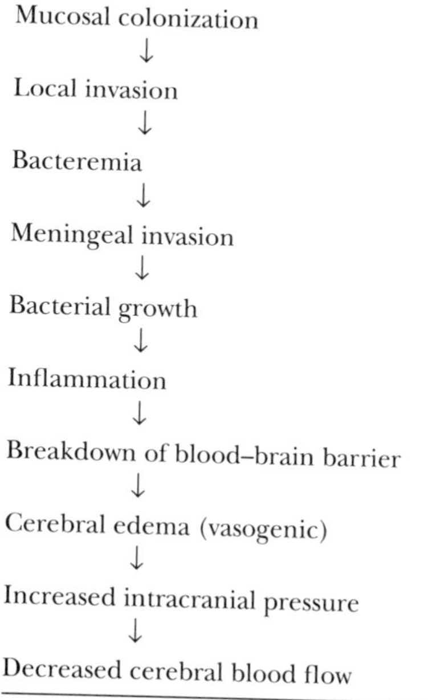

Mucosal colonization
↓
Local invasion
↓
Bacteremia
↓
Meningeal invasion
↓
Bacterial growth
↓
Inflammation
↓
Breakdown of blood–brain barrier
↓
Cerebral edema (vasogenic)
↓
Increased intracranial pressure
↓
Decreased cerebral blood flow

Source: Adapted from Tunkel et al,[2619] p 611.

barrier includes skin, mucous membranes, and epithelium of the GI, respiratory, and genitourinary systems. Several factors affecting patients with cancer make it easier for organisms to penetrate the first barrier, including:

1. Tumors, wounds, or mucosal erosion (e.g., from chemotherapy) may disrupt the integrity of the barrier.
2. Previous antimicrobial therapy may have altered normal flora, yielding organisms better able to penetrate the barrier.
3. The body's normal ciliary action may be damaged by chemotherapy, preventing mechanical clearing of organisms.
4. Diagnostic or therapeutic procedures such as indwelling venous, epidural (for pain), or urethral catheters provide a conduit for organisms to bypass normal barriers.

The CNS–surface barrier sometimes is directly penetrated by surgery on the head or spine that creates a direct communication between the surface and the CSF, but more often the invading organisms reach the CNS via the arterial circulation. Because organisms that penetrate surface barriers enter the venous circulation before the arterial circulation, they are likely to infect liver or lungs before the brain. Thus, brain abscesses caused by *Nocardia* or *Aspergillus* organisms usually develop after similar lesions have formed in the lung and can be identified on chest radiograph. Blood cultures are commonly positive in patients with cancer suffering from bacterial meningitis, except for meningitis caused by *Nocardia* organisms. Nevertheless, as already mentioned, in about 40% of patients, the organisms infecting the CNS differ from those causing concomitant systemic infection[1198]; sometimes the organism reaches the CNS via the bloodstream without evidence of infection elsewhere in the body.

IMMUNOLOGIC DEFENSES

Even when epithelial barriers are penetrated, normal host defenses usually eradicate the organisms. In patients with cancer, the following five abnormalities of host defense mechanisms predispose the patient to CNS infection[82,438] (Table 10–2):

1. Impaired cellular immunity from T-cell and mononuclear phagocyte abnormalities may occur as a result of the cancer or its treatment. This defense mechanism is particularly impaired in patients with lymphoma, especially those with Hodgkin's disease, and in patients receiving corticosteroids or other cytotoxic drugs.
2. Impaired neutrophil function (abso-

Table 10–2. **HOST DEFENSE ABNORMALITIES IN PATIENTS WITH CANCER**

Major Host Defect	Usual Cancers	Other Risk Factors
T-lymphocyte, mononuclear phagocyte defects	Hodgkin's disease Non-Hodgkin's lymphoma Chronic lymphocytic leukemia	Steroids Alkylating agents Antimetabolites Antitumor antibiotics
Neutrophil defects (granulocytopenia)	Acute leukemias Solid tumors	Chemotherapy
Abnormal immunoglobulins	Chronic lymphocytic leukemia Multiple myeloma	Steroids
Splenectomy	Chronic myelogenous leukemia Hodgkin's disease Hairy-cell leukemia	
Communication between CSF and surface	Spinal column tumors Skull tumors Head and neck cancer	Head and spine surgery Cerebroventricular reservoirs, shunts

lute neutropenia of <1000 cells/mm^3) is common in patients with acute leukemia and during the chemotherapy of many cancers. Qualitative abnormalities of neutrophil function can also follow chemotherapy even when neutrophils are not quantitatively depressed[1148]; examples include steroid therapy and several specific diseases of neutrophil function.[1513] The absence of neutrophils may also prevent the CNS from mounting a cellular response to the infection, causing a falsely reassuring "benign" CSF.[1615]

3. Low immunoglobulin production occurs in patients with multiple myeloma, chronic lymphocytic leukemia, or congenital hypogammaglobulinemia. Such patients cannot mount an immunoglobulin response to an antigenic challenge.[450] A similar phenomenon often occurs following combined radiation therapy (RT) and multidrug chemotherapy in advanced Hodgkin's disease or following bone marrow transplantation. Opsonizing and bactericidal antibodies decline and susceptibility to infection with encapsulated bacteria increases.
4. Splenectomy was once part of the treatment of some patients with Hodgkin's disease.[450,2739] The result was low immunoglobulin production in response to an antigenic challenge, inability to produce IgM-opsonizing antibodies, and loss of the spleen as a filter of organisms.[1188] The combined effects heightened vulnerability to bacterial organisms, particularly the pneumococcus.[1a]
5. An anatomic communication between the CNS and an epithelial surface occurs in patients with tumors of the skull or spine, either when the tumor erodes into the CNS or a surgical procedure creates a fistula between the CNS and the surface. Deliberate disruption of the barrier is more common, as when a ventricular cannula is placed for the injection of chemotherapeutic agents or a ventriculoperitoneal or ventriculoatrial shunt is used to divert obstructed CSF (see Chapter 14).

MULTIPLE DEFECTS

Many patients with cancer suffer a multiplicity of immune system abnormalities. For example, a splenectomized patient with Hodgkin's disease who is being treated with chemotherapeutic agents may have abnormalities of both T- and B-cell function as well as neutropenia. Many agents used for cancer treatment have multiple effects on the immune system. Corticosteroids are probably the most frequent and serious offenders encountered in neuro-oncology. They suppress antibody production, decrease both the acute and chronic inflammatory response, interfere with T-cell–mediated immunity, reduce interferon production, impair wound healing, and interfere with the clearance of foreign materials. They also attenuate the inflammation of meningitis[1398] and appear to interfere with the entry of antibiotics into the CSF.[861] Some cytotoxic drugs also have such multiple effects.

Infection Sites within the Central Nervous System

Compartmentalization of infection within the nervous system is common (Table 10–3).

Some organisms, such as *Listeria* and *Cryptococcus,* usually attack only the leptomeninges, causing either acute or chronic meningitis. These organisms can on occasion cause encephalitis, cerebritis, or brain abscesses.[120,592,849,1815] Others, such as *Nocardia* and *Toxoplasma,* settle focally within the parenchyma, causing focal encephalitis or brain abscesses. Organisms such as varicella-zoster virus invade the brain diffusely; they cause a diffuse encephalitis with or without an accompanying meningitis, that is, a meningoencephalitis. Finally, some organisms with a predilection to thrombose blood vessels of the brain (e.g., *Aspergillus*) can cause either cerebral infarction or hemorrhage. Varicella-zoster can also cause a vasculitis without other evidence of CNS infection.

Secondary involvement of the cerebral vasculature in infection is also common. Even without an inflammatory response, necrosis and occlusion of small vessels within the brain

Table 10–3. **INFECTION SITE WITHIN CENTRAL NERVOUS SYSTEM AND RESULTANT COMPLICATIONS**

Primary Site	Infections	Causal Organisms	Complications
Leptomeninges	Meningitis	*Listeria*	Hydrocephalus, arachnoiditis
		Cryptococcus	Cranial nerve palsies
		Listeria	Vasculitis (infarcts)
Brain parenchyma	Focal cerebritis Abscess	*Nocardia* *Toxoplasma*	Cerebral edema, herniation, dementia, intraventricular rupture
Cerebral cortex ± meninges	Encephalitis Meningoencephalitis	Varicella-zoster Herpes simplex	Seizures
Cerebral blood vessels	Vasculitis	Varicella-zoster *Aspergillus* *Mucorales*	Cerebral infarction or hemorrhage

sometimes occur with acute bacterial meningitis[1615] (Fig. 10–1). Vasculitis may narrow or occlude major arteries at the base of the brain, small vessels within the brain parenchyma, sulcal veins, and venous sinuses. Patients with meningitis who show such abnormalities on an angiogram have an unfavorable prognosis.[2027]

MENINGITIS

Bacteria reach the leptomeninges and cause meningitis by crossing the blood–CSF barrier, probably at the choroid plexus as well as other sites. Some cerebral capillaries possess specific adhesion receptors that bind and transport bacteria into the CSF.[2109,2619] Once in the CNS, bacteria can multiply rapidly because many host defense mechanisms found elsewhere in the body, such as complement and immunoglobulins, are present only at very low levels in CSF. Bacteria reaching the subarachnoid space evoke hyperemia in meningeal vessels, leading to the migration of polymorphonuclear leukocytes, if the patient has any, into the subarachnoid space[259,694,990,2109] (see Table 10–1). The WBCs and the engulfed invading organisms form an exudate that surrounds the blood vessels in the Virchow-Robin spaces, but the organisms rarely enter into the brain parenchyma except in areas in which a con-

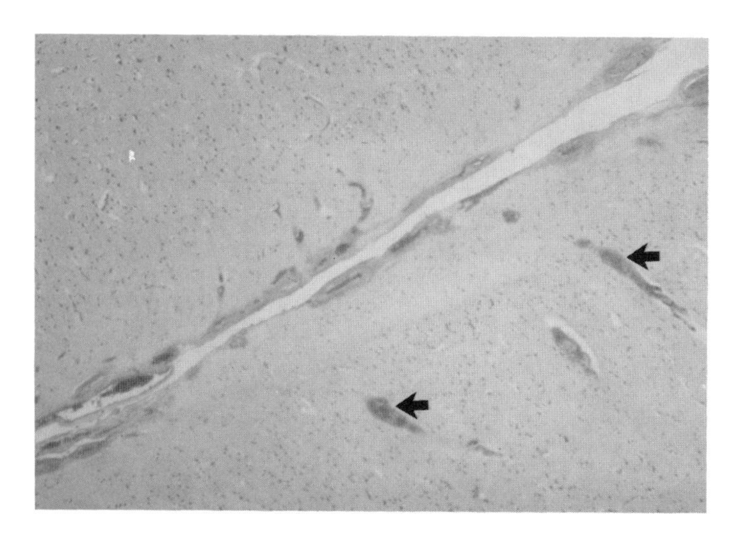

Figure 10–1. Photomicrograph of a brain section from a neutropenic patient who died of Gram-negative meningitis. The cortical section shows a bacterial vasculitis. The areas surrounding the blood vessels are all bacteria; white cells were absent in the field. The patient died despite antibiotic treatment.

comitant vasculitis has led to infarction. Nevertheless, the brain is not spared in meningitis. The exudate at the base of the brain may impede CSF absorption, causing hydrocephalus with increased intracranial pressure. Vasculitis produced by the organism may cause cerebral infarction with secondary abscess formation.[2027] Toxic substances secreted by the organisms and the WBCs responding to them may cause cerebral edema[796,2619,2620] or other forms of CNS damage.[2556,2557] The combined insults occasionally cause cerebral herniation and death.[1211]

The combined bacterial invasion and inflammatory response, particularly the production of cytokines, have several deleterious consequences. The blood–brain barrier breaks down as both tight junctions open and vesicular transport increases, leading to vasogenic brain edema.[2108] An initial increase in cerebral blood flow is followed by a decrease.[2028] The combination of brain edema and increased blood flow causes intracranial hypertension and can lead to cerebral herniation. Autoregulation of cerebral blood flow ceases[2620] so that the blood flow rate varies passively with the systemic blood pressure. Thus, hypertension increases blood flow, causing cerebral edema, whereas hypotension may lead to focal or generalized cerebral ischemia and sometimes infarction. An increase in resistance to CSF absorption across the arachnoid granulations contributes to the increased intracranial pressure and perhaps causes the late development of hydrocephalus.[283] Many of these changes are believed to be cytokine-related and can be prevented or ameliorated by corticosteroids.[925,1921] Thus, although the clinician may be loath to use corticosteroids in an infected, already immunosuppressed patient, judicious use can prevent permanent brain damage associated with bacterial meningitis.

CEREBRITIS AND BRAIN ABSCESS

Brain abscess[80,2834] and cerebritis[2273,2758,2834] differ from meningitis. Most of the organisms causing them, like those causing meningitis, are blood-borne and lodge in small distal vessels at the gray-matter–white-matter interface, similar to blood-borne tumor emboli (see Chapter 2). The organisms and accompanying WBCs breach the vascular wall and cause an area of local infection or cerebritis. The brain responds with an intense vascular proliferation; the vigor of this response depends on the type of organism and the patient's immune status. The neovascularization at the edge of the cerebritis does not possess a normal blood–brain barrier, so a ring of enhancement can be seen on an MR or CT scan. The ring enhancement does not necessarily mean that a capsule has formed. With time, a collagenous capsule does form, effectively walling off the abscess from the normal brain. The capsule is characteristically thicker near the cortex, where oxygenation is better, and somewhat thinner near the ventricular surface.[2834] Thus, abscess rupture, when it occurs, is usually into the ventricle rather than into the subarachnoid space. Spinal epidural abscess can result either from contiguous infection of vertebrae or from blood-borne organisms.[562]

MENINGOENCEPHALITIS

In encephalitis or meningoencephalitis, the invading organism may affect the entire brain and the leptomeninges as well. The pathologic picture depends on the nature of the organism and the patient's immune response. The inflammatory response of the leptomeninges and the cortex may be widespread, with microabscess formation, but if the organisms invade without a response by the patient's immune system, little inflammation may occur.

CLINICAL FINDINGS

Signs and Symptoms

The signs and symptoms of CNS infection in patients with cancer (Table 10–4) are determined by the lesion's anatomic site, the virulence of the infecting organism, and the host's reaction to the infection. In general, the signs and symptoms are less fulminant, less severe, and often more slowly evolving than in the general population. They are also more likely to be lethal, however, because the immune system of the patient with cancer is usually compromised. The most common symptoms are as follows:

1. Headache occurs in most but not all

Table 10–4. **SIGNS AND SYMPTOMS OF CNS INFECTIONS IN PATIENTS WITH CANCER**

Frequent
Headache—typically mild to moderate
Fever—new or increased in an already febrile patient
Personality changes, delirium
Seizures
Uncommon
Nuchal rigidity
Focal neurologic deficit

patients with meningitis, encephalitis, and brain abscesses.[438,1615] Because the headache may be mild, patients with other pain from their cancer may not notice or volunteer the complaint. To complicate the issue, many patients are febrile from the cancer or systemic infection, and the fever can cause mild-to-moderate headache.

2. A body temperature greater than 38.5°C (101.5°F) is the most common sign of CNS infection.[1615] Particularly with brain abscess, however, fever may be absent. Many patients with meningitis and meningoencephalitis are already febrile from systemic infection. An increase in an already-present fever, when accompanied by headaches, suggests CNS infection.
3. Personality change is often the only clue to CNS infection.[1198,1615] Behavioral changes may be mild, characterized only by lethargy and irritability, or severe, with delirium, stupor, or coma. Because such patients are often severely systemically ill, mild changes in behavior may pass unnoticed.
4. Seizures are common in some series of patients but uncommon in others. They were present only in 7 of 55 infections in immunocompromised hosts[1198] and in none of 15 patients with cryptococcal meningitis in a recent MSKCC series.[2801] In another series,[1615] 40% of neutropenic patients with meningitis had seizures. When seizures do occur, they are as likely to be a manifestation of meningitis or meningoencephalitis as of brain abscess.
5. Nuchal rigidity is surprisingly uncommon in patients with CNS infection, even those who have meningitis. In one series[1198] of immunocompromised patients, only 6 of 10 patients with *Listeria* meningitis and only 4 of 11 with meningitis caused by more conventional bacteria had nuchal rigidity.
6. Focal neurologic signs, such as hemiparesis or aphasia, are more common in cerebritis and brain abscess than in meningitis but can occur in the latter as a result of cerebral infarction from vasculitis.[692,2455] Rarely, vasculitis may lead to aneurysm formation with subarachnoid hemorrhage.[2013] The particular focal neurologic signs in a given patient depend on the locus of the lesion. In patients with meningoencephalitis, in which the infection is diffuse, focal signs are often mild and fluctuating; they more closely resemble the neurologic findings in disseminated intravascular coagulation (see Chapter 9) than in metastasis.
7. The evolution of symptoms and signs is usually subacute or chronic rather than acute. For example, in 6 of 10 patients with *Listeria* meningitis, symptoms evolved over 2 to 10 days and, in 2 patients, for more than 10 days.[1198] Only 2 patients developed their symptoms in less than 48 hours. Slow evolution is particularly common in cryptococcal or toxoplasmal infection. Unless seizures or cerebral infarction causes acute symptoms, the course may be indolent, even in patients infected with organisms that cause acute symptoms in the normal host.

Meningitis

The clinical picture of meningitis in patients with cancer varies from an acute, fulminant infection with headache, fever, stiff neck, and stupor to an indolent infection causing only malaise at the time of discovery by CSF examination.[1615] The diagnosis is easiest in a patient with lymphoma who is in remission and not under active treatment but presents with sudden headache, fever, stiff neck, and delirium. If the patient has not had a splenectomy, the most likely cause is *Listeria* organisms; if he or she has had a splenectomy, the cause is either *Listeria* or *S. pneumoniae*. Even the pneumococcal vaccine does not always prevent pneumococcal infection.[2425] Generally speaking, pneumococcal infections are usually more fulminant, evolving over just a few hours.[68] *Listeria* infections tend to evolve over days, although by the time the patient reaches the hospital, both infections may be equally severe. A less likely diagnosis is cryptococcal meningitis; although this is a common cause of meningitis in the lymphoma population, the symptoms tend to evolve more slowly. A rare cause of acute meningitis in these patients is toxoplasmosis.

The diagnosis is more difficult in patients under active treatment for cancer. Such patients are frequently symptomatic from the underlying disease or its treatment when CNS infection develops, so that often the early symptoms are attributed to the underlying disease rather than to a new and superimposed illness. The major manifestations of meningitis, however, are usually the same and only partially masked by the underlying illness. Most patients who are alert enough to give an adequate history complain of headache. Fever is almost always present, but many patients are already febrile from the underlying illness. The onset of meningitis is usually heralded by a fever spike of 0.5°C to 1.0°C (1–2°F) higher than the patient's baseline temperature. Most patients are delirious, and many become stuporous or comatose within the first 24 hours of symptoms. Nuchal rigidity is frequently absent, particularly in patients with low peripheral WBC counts, possibly because the meninges do not mount an adequate inflammatory response to the invading organisms.

GENERAL PHYSICAL EXAMINATION

Evidence of infection elsewhere in the body may suggest not only the source but also the nature of a CNS infection. For instance, most patients with *Nocardia* or *Aspergillus* meningitis have evident pulmonary disease at the time symptoms of meningitis develop. Patients with *Candida* meningitis usually also have systemic evidence of candidiasis elsewhere, such as a nodular rash. Gram-negative organisms generally cause septicemia before meningitis develops, unless a fistula connects the CSF to the surface.

NEUROLOGIC EXAMINATION

The neurologic examination rarely helps with the diagnosis. Sometimes the optic fundi reveal evidence of infection in the form of Roth's spots.[1280] These retinal hemorrhages with a white center are nonspecific and are found in many embolic and thrombotic disorders and even in the retinitis of toxoplasmosis.[1176] Cranial nerve palsies, lower motoneuron weakness, and absent reflexes are uncommon. When they are present, the clinician should suspect that the meninges have been invaded by tumor rather than by organisms (see Chapter 7).

DIAGNOSIS

Lumbar Puncture. The diagnosis of meningitis is established by examining the CSF.[259] The quandary is when to perform a lumbar puncture in a patient with cancer suspected of CNS infection (Table 10–5). CSF examination is essential for appropriate diagnosis and treatment, but if the neurologic symptoms result from a mass lesion, a lumbar puncture may do more harm than good. Rarely, a lumbar puncture performed in a patient without a mass lesion but with meningitis[2156] or even pseudotumor cerebri causes death from herniation of a swollen brain. The decision to perform a lumbar puncture should be based on the acuteness and nature of the patient's symptoms. A patient with the acute onset of headache, delirium, and fever, in whom the suspicion of acute meningitis is strong, should undergo lumbar puncture[986] immediately, regardless of signs of increased intracranial pressure or mass lesion. In no instance should a lumbar puncture be deferred for a CT or MR scan if the patient is suffering from symptoms of acute meningitis; the time between onset of symptoms and death may be only a few hours if treatment is not begun. Furthermore, beginning antibiotic therapy empirically for suspected CNS infection may preclude definitive diagnosis and be deleterious to patient care in the long run.

Table 10–5. **CONSIDERATIONS FOR PERFORMING A LUMBAR PUNCTURE IN PATIENTS WITH CANCER***

INDICATIONS FOR TEST
Absolute
Suspicion of meningitis
Relative
Suspicion of nervous system disease, especially encephalitis or meningoencephalitis
Intrathecal therapy for meningeal leukemia or fungal meningitis
Symptomatic treatment of severe headache from subarachnoid hemorrhage or leptomeningeal metastases
Before anticoagulant therapy for cerebrovascular disease
CONTRAINDICATIONS
Absolute
Tissue infection in region of puncture site
Relative
Brain tumor or abscess
Spinal cord tumor
Thrombocytopenia or coagulopathy
Increased intracranial pressure
COMPLICATIONS OF TEST*
Common
Headache
Backache
Less common
Lumbar radicular pain
Hearing abnormalities (hearing or sensation of echoing in the head)
Diplopia (sixth-nerve palsy)
Enhanced meninges on MR scan
Rare
Transtentorial or foramen magnum herniation
Worsening of spinal tumor symptoms
Spinal hematoma (patients with bleeding tendency)
Herniated or infected disk
Reaction to anesthetic agent
Meningitis (contaminated needle, children with sepsis)
Subdural effusion

*See also Chapter 14.

CSF should be removed slowly in quantities sufficient to establish a definitive diagnosis (Table 10–6). Most complications of lumbar puncture occur not because of the fluid removed at the time of the lumbar puncture but because of a further leak of fluid through the dural tear made by the needle. If the CSF pressure is very high, the patient should be placed under constant observation after the lumbar puncture and an indwelling IV line should be placed. Corticosteroid treatment should be considered.[1921] A hyperosmolar agent such as mannitol should be available at the bedside to treat herniation if warning symptoms develop (see Chapter 3).

When the situation is less acute and a CT or

Table 10–6. **CSF VOLUME FOR COMMON DIAGNOSTIC TESTS**

Microscopy and Test	Volume of CSF Required
Culture	5–10 mL*
Cytology (malignant cells)	4 cc
Cell count and differential	0.5–1.0 mL
Glucose and protein	0.5 mL†
Serologic test for syphilis	0.5 mL†
Cryptococcal antigen	0.5 mL†
Oligoclonal bands	2 mL†

*Larger volumes are better.
†These tests can be done on supernatants from culture.

MR scan can be performed quickly, a mass lesion should be ruled out before the patient undergoes lumbar puncture (but see reference 68). Some patients have both mass lesions, such as brain metastases, and acute meningitis. These patients should be given steroids and mannitol to treat the edema associated with the mass lesion at the time the lumbar puncture is performed.

If the CSF from a patient suspected of acute meningitis is cloudy, therapy should be started immediately, even before the spinal fluid is fully evaluated (Table 10–7).

Cerebrospinal Fluid Evaluation. The CSF of most patients with bacterial or fungal meningitis resembles CSF from patients without cancer: the pressure is elevated, the fluid is cloudy with both neutrophils and lymphocytes, the protein concentration is elevated, and the glucose concentration is depressed.[986,1570] In many patients with severe leukopenia, and even in occasional otherwise-healthy individuals, the expected CSF pleocytosis is not found, at least initially.[1947] Of 26 patients with a peripheral WBC count fewer than 1000 cells/mm^3, 12 had 5 or fewer WBCs/mm^3 in the CSF at the time of clinical onset[1615] (Fig. 10–2). Organisms were cultured from all 12. An additional 3 patients with peripheral WBC counts in the normal or elevated range also had fewer than 5 WBCs/mm^3 in the CSF. Meningeal infections with normal CSF WBC counts occurred in patients with meningitis from *Pseudomonas, Listeria, S. pneumoniae, E. coli,* and *Proteus.* Of 15 patients with normal CSF WBC counts, 3 had hypoglycorrhachia.

It is not certain why hypoglycorrhachia sometimes occurs in the absence of a CSF pleocytosis. Carrier-mediated glucose transport could be diminished by the infection, but Fishman[793] has shown that diffusion of glucose into the CSF is increased by acute meningitis because the blood–brain barrier is disrupted. Glucose metabolism probably is increased partly by organisms and partly by WBCs, but Petersdorf and colleagues[2017] showed that an extraordinarily large number of organisms are necessary to metabolize glucose to hypoglycorrhachic levels. Activation and proliferation of pial and arachnoid cells responding to the inflammation may also promote increased glucose metabolism.[1868]

Sufficient fluid must be sent to the laboratory to ensure growth of even a few organisms in CSF. If meningitis is suspected and the initial fluid is not purulent, send 10 mL to the laboratory for smear, and culture for aerobic and anaerobic bacteria and fungi. Cell count and differential requires 1 mL (see Table 10–6). The rest of the specimen should be centrifuged to concentrate the organisms. The supernatant fluid can then be used for chemical and serologic assays and the sediment placed in culture. An additional 4 mL of CSF should be analyzed cytologically for tumor cells because the major alternate diagnosis to acute or subacute meningitis is leptomeningeal infiltration.

The treating physician should examine the CSF himself or herself. By holding a tube of CSF to natural light and shaking it, as few as 25 to 50 WBCs/mm^3 can be identified by the naked eye.[2427] Identification of this small number of cells in the CSF depends on the Tyndall phenomenon, that is, light rays refracted by their encounter with the cells. Opalescent or turbid spinal fluid suggests the presence of several hundred or a few thousand cells. A few hundred RBCs may lend turbidity to the spinal fluid without altering its color.

A cell count should be performed in a counting chamber and a spun specimen stained with both Gram's and Wright's stain. A careful search for bacterial and fungal organisms, as well as malignant cells or parasites, should be made on the Gram's- and Wright's-stained slides. Organisms that can

Table 10–7. **EMPIRIC TREATMENT OF CNS INFECTION IN PATIENTS WITH CANCER**

Primary Immune Defect	Blood Leukocyte Count	CSF Findings	Recommended Therapy	Alternate Therapy
T-lymphocyte, mononuclear phagocyte defect	Normal	Pleocytosis, no organisms, negative cryptococcal antigen	Ampicillin for listerial or pneumococcal organisms	Trimethoprim-sulfamethoxazole (cotrimoxazole)† or vancomycin or chloramphenicol and erythromycin
	Normal	No organisms ± pleocytosis, cryptococcal antigen positive	Obtain more CSF consider amphotericin B + 5-FC for cryptococcus	Fluconazole or itraconazole
	Low	No organisms ± pleocytosis	Ampicillin + ceftazidime: + gentamicin IV + IT for Gram-negative meningitis	Ampicillin + imipenem
Neutrophil defect	Low	No organisms ± pleocytosis	Ceftazidime plus gentamicin IV ± IT	Imipenem
	Normal	No organisms ± pleocytosis	Ceftazidime plus gentamicin IV ± IT	Imipenem
Splenectomy	Normal	No organisms, pleocytosis	Cefuroxime ± vancomycin	Ampicillin or cotrimoxazole or both
Surgery	Normal	No organisms, pleocytosis	Ceftazidime + gentamicin IV ± IT and oxacillin	Vancomycin can be substituted for oxacillin

5-FC = 5-fluorocytosine (flucytosine); IT = intrathecal or intraventricular administration (see text).

*Other semisynthetic penicillins, such as methicillin or nafcillin, may be substituted for oxacillin; aminoglycosides, such as amikacin or tobramycin, may be substituted for gentamicin.

†Cotrimoxazole is the same preparation as trimethoprim-sulfamethoxazole.

be identified on Gram's stain include most of the bacteria, some parasites such as *Trichomonas* or *Amoeba*, and cryptococci; the latter are also identified by an india ink preparation (Fig. 10–3).

Serologic tests of CSF should include cryptococcal antigen, which is virtually always positive in the presence of cryptococcal meningitis and is diagnostic whether or not the organism grows in culture or is seen on Gram's stain. When bacterial meningitis is suspected, antigens for pneumococcus, meningococcus, and haemophilus can be measured in CSF. IgM toxoplasmal antibodies are occasionally positive in infection of the nervous system from *Toxoplasma* organisms even when the IgG serology is negative. *Aspergillus* and *Candida* antibodies are rarely but occasionally positive and sometimes yield a clue when organisms are not otherwise seen. Certain enzymes in the CSF (e.g., β-glucuronidase) are increased in infection, but they do not help to differentiate the kind of infection or even to distinguish between infection and leptomeningeal metastases (see Chapter 7).

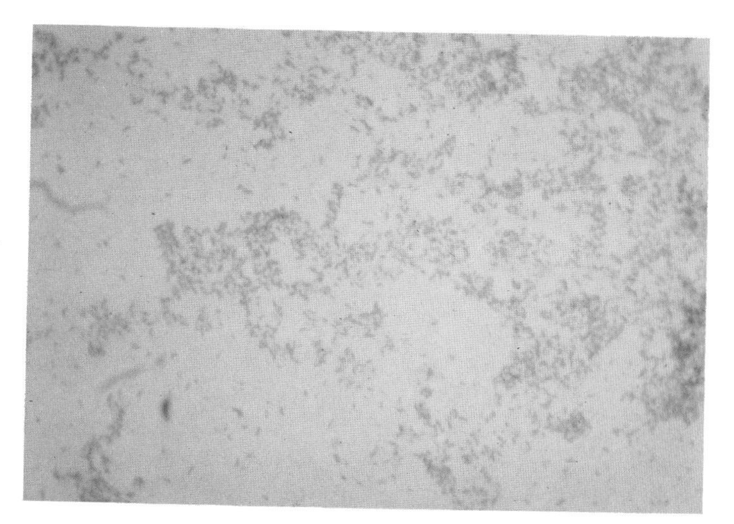

Figure 10–2. A photomicrograph of an uncentrifuged specimen from the CNS showing Gram-negative rods (*E. coli*) in the cerebrospinal fluid of a neutropenic patient with acute lymphocytic leukemia. No white blood cells are seen in the field. The patient had an elevated protein and a depressed glucose concentration in the cerebrospinal fluid. He died despite antibiotic therapy.

Imaging. In patients with meningitis, the CT or MR scan may show multifocal enhancement of the leptomeninges.[283,2900] This finding is indistinguishable from that of leptomeningeal metastases and hard to distinguish from meningeal enhancement following lumbar puncture (see Chapter 14). Features suggesting meningitis include loss of definition of cerebral sulci and evidence of hydrocephalus.[283]

Meningoencephalitis

The clinical pictures of encephalitis and meningoencephalitis vary with the pathology and the offending organism. In general, when the organisms cause meningitis with secondary encephalitis, the signs and symptoms (fever, headache, and stiff neck) resemble those of meningitis alone, but delirium is more prominent and focal signs, particularly focal and generalized convulsions, are more frequent. Seizures and focal signs that occur early with meningitis are probably caused by direct invasion of the brain by the organism. When such signs occur late, particularly after treatment is well under way, vasculitis with thrombosis and infarction is a more likely cause. Such vascular changes may lead to permanent neurologic impairment despite successful treatment of the underlying infection.

Contrast enhancement of the basal cisterns and cortical sulci on CT or MR scan may attest to the intensity of the inflammation.[283] Contrast enhancement of cortical gyri suggests that infection and inflammation involve the brain as well as the meninges.

When the process is primarily encephalitic (i.e., without important meningeal involvement), the usual signs of meningitis may be absent. Instead, the illness begins with focal or generalized convulsions, or both, accompanied or followed by delirium often associated with asterixis and multifocal myoclonus (see Chapter 11). Fixed focal signs, such as hemiparesis or visual field deficits, may be present as well. The differential diagnosis includes metabolic encephalopathy (see Chapter 11) and focal brain lesions such as metastases. A severe and sustained delirium preceding seizures, especially when associated with intense multifocal myoclonus, can occur with either CNS infection or metabolic encephalopathy, but metabolic encephalopathy usually does not cause fever, and prominent focal signs are uncommon. When focal signs predominate in a delirious patient, they suggest encephalitis rather than a metabolic process. Cerebral infarcts or metastases can cause the focal signs but they cause delirium less often.

CSF changes may or may not be helpful diagnostically. Pleocytosis is usually but not always present. The protein and glucose concentrations are frequently normal; cultures are negative because the infection is usually viral. Serologic examination of the spinal fluid may help. The diagnostic approach, differential diagnosis, and treatment are the same as with meningitis.

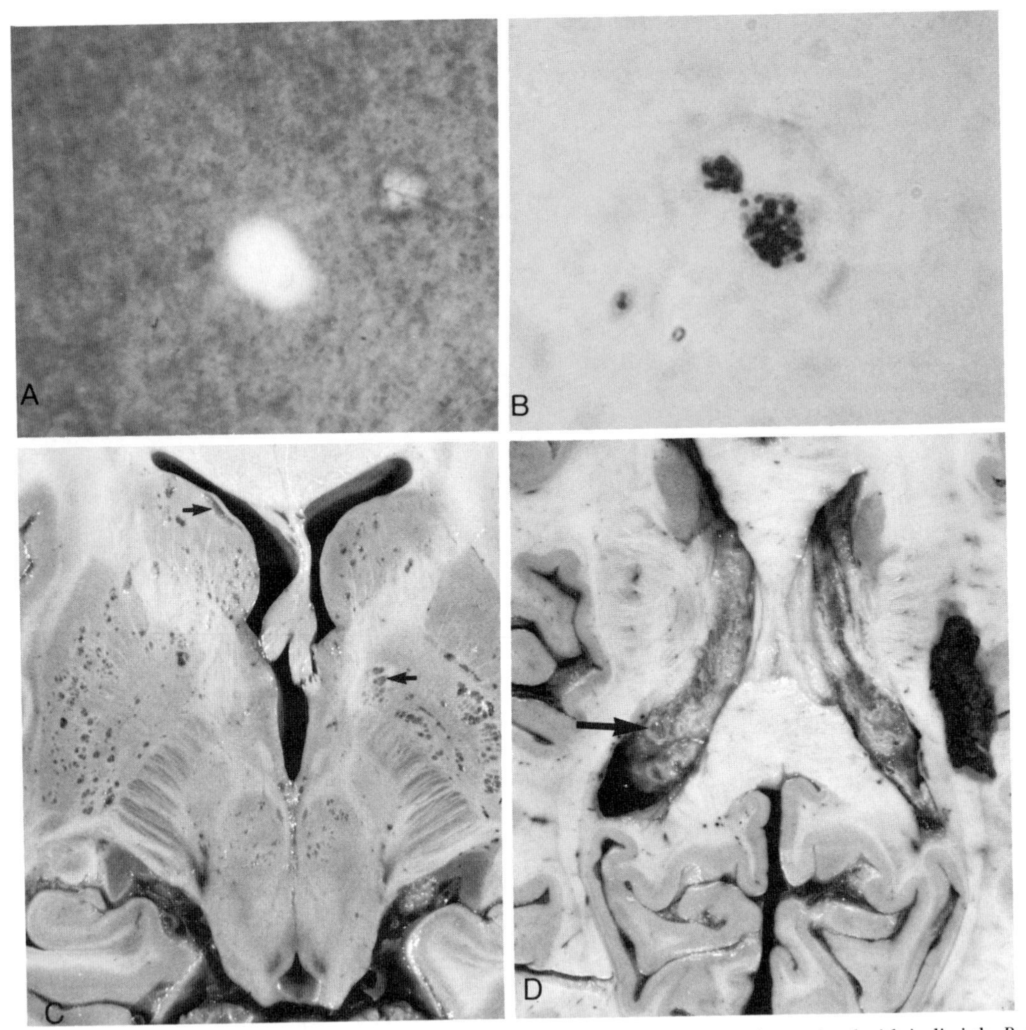

Figure 10–3. Cryptococcal organisms in the cerebrospinal fluid. *A,* A budding organism stained with india ink. *B,* A Gram stain. The patient had lymphoma and cryptococcal meningitis. *C* and *D,* Two pathologic examples of cryptococcosis. *C,* The typical soap-bubble appearance of *Cryptococcus* involving the basal ganglia (*arrows*). *D,* The fibromucoid appearance of the choroid plexus involved by *Cryptococcus* (*arrow*).

Brain Abscess

The symptoms and signs of brain abscess depend on the causal agent. *Toxoplasma* abscesses have a predilection for the basal ganglia and may lodge there as a single mass. The subacute development of neurologic signs, especially hemiparesis, is indistinguishable from that of brain metastasis. *Nocardia* abscesses are often multifocal and cause either slowly progressive multifocal signs, similar to those of multiple metastases, or focal or generalized seizures. Although the diagnosis of brain abscess may be suspected based on the underlying cancer, differentiation from a brain metastasis may be possible only with biopsy. PET scanning with glucose may differentiate a hypermetabolic lymphoma from a hypometabolic toxoplasmal abscess.[1180]

CT and MR scans help identify brain abscesses.[2900] Typically, scans reveal a hypointense area before contrast and a ring of enhancement after contrast.[283] Some small abscesses appear as a solid mass, and occasional abscesses are hyperintense before contrast. An abscess can sometimes be differentiated from tumor by the nature of the ring enhancement. The enhancing ring of an abscess is generally thinner and more uniform than the ring of a tumor.

With suspected toxoplasmal abscesses, the diagnosis is best determined by the results of a therapeutic trial (see page 255). With other suspected abscesses, stereotactically directed needle biopsy performed early in the diagnostic workup both establishes the diagnosis and reveals what organisms the abscess contains so that appropriate antibiotic therapy may be instituted.

Vascular Lesions

Vascular lesions caused by infection produce sudden focal neurologic signs, usually in a patient known to be suffering from systemic infection[2203] or meningitis[1239,2013] (Fig. 10–4). The clinical and arteriographic picture resembles nonbacterial thrombotic endocarditis (NBTE) or other causes of cerebral infarction.[1305,2194] After a delay of several hours to days, the CT and MR scans reveal abnormalities characteristic of cerebral infarction (see Chapter 9). CSF examination often fails to help, although pleocytosis may be present and organisms occasionally can be grown, especially *Aspergillus* and Zygomycetes, and less often *Candida*. The diagnosis is usually easy because vascular disorders typically occur late in patients with overwhelming bacterial or fungal infection; many are being treated for the infection at the time the stroke occurs. Varicella-zoster vasculitis may cause a stroke after other signs of infection have resolved (see below).

APPROACH TO THE PATIENT

The physician must consider both the primary cancer and the impaired host defense mechanisms that are likely to lead to CNS

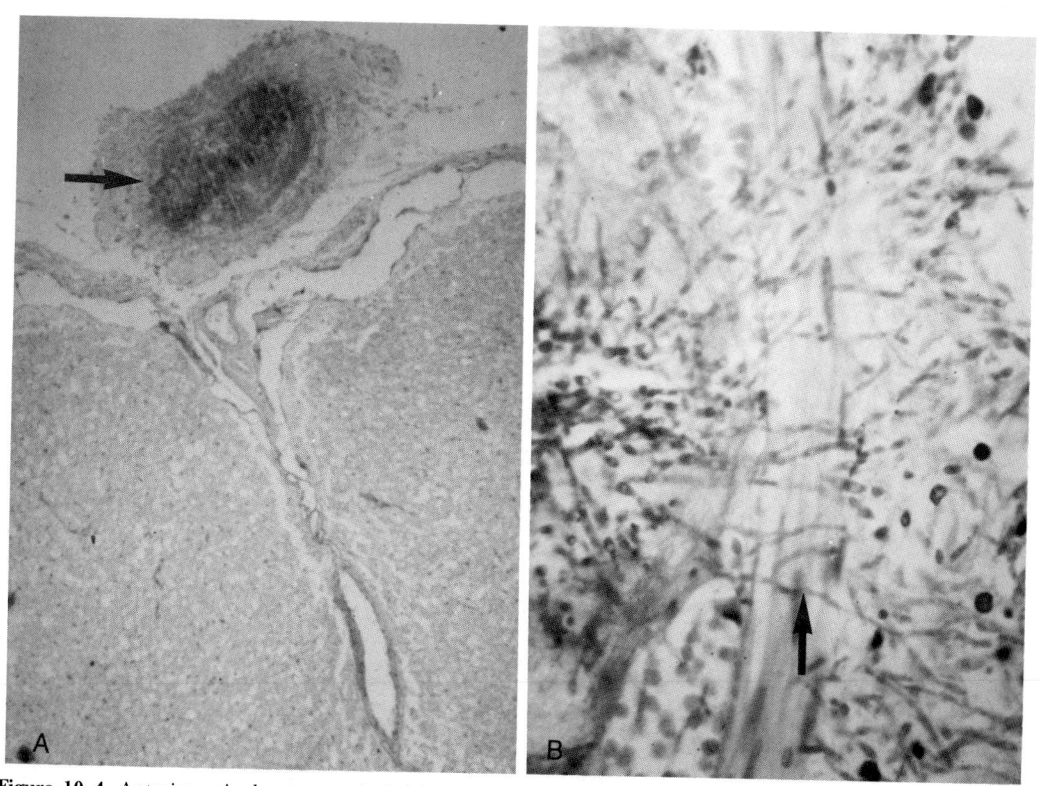

Figure 10–4. Anterior spinal artery occluded by aspergillosis in a neutropenic patient with acute lymphocytic leukemia. The patient suffered sudden onset of paraplegia days before death. *A*, At autopsy, the anterior spinal artery was occluded (*arrow*). *B*, The fungi can be seen growing through the vessel wall (*arrow*).

infection, as shown on Table 10–2. Infections are most likely to occur in patients who are least likely to have other forms of neurologic dysfunction from cancer. For example, infection in Hodgkin's disease is common but CNS metastases are rare; by contrast, CNS infections are rare in patients with solid tumors but metastases are common. The major factors predisposing to infection are as follows:

1. Hodgkin's disease or non-Hodgkin's lymphoma (Fig. 10–5);
2. leukopenia either from disease or chemotherapy;
3. long-term immunosuppressive drugs, particularly corticosteroids;
4. a surgical or tumor-induced communication between the CNS and an epithelial surface.

A scrupulous search for a systemic nidus of infection is essential. Skin lesions are sometimes found with *Nocardia* infections[2825,2875] and also may complicate *Pseudomonas* sepsis.

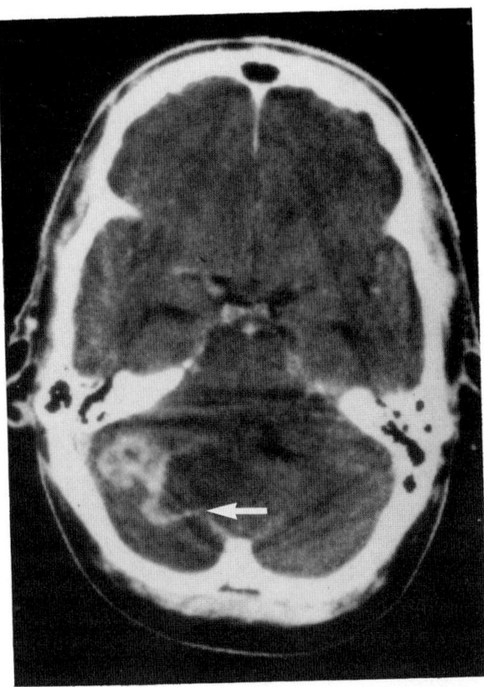

Figure 10–5. A CT scan showing a nocardial abscess in a patient with chronic lymphocytic leukemia. The patient presented with headache and acute cerebellar signs but no fever. The vascular structure draining the abscess (*arrow*) led initial consideration to a highly vascular tumor. The abscess was discovered on resection. The patient made a complete recovery.

Chest radiographs or CT scans may reveal *Aspergillus,* Zygomycetes, or *Nocardia* abscesses that can be diagnosed with lung biopsy. Examination of blood, urine, or other bodily fluids may either identify the organism on culture or identify antibody titers that strongly suggest an active infection. In patients suffering pain, a bone scan may reveal an increased area of isotope uptake in the skull or spine, the first visual change of osteomyelitis. A gallium scan may detect a deep-seated systemic abscess, or a CT scan may identify an abscess in the paravertebral region potentially communicating with the subarachnoid space.

The physician should search for communications between the CNS and the outside environment.[1536,1669] CSF otorrhea or rhinorrhea in patients suffering from a cancer involving the skull may presage CNS infection, and CSF may sometimes leak from poorly healing back wounds in patients who have undergone laminectomy. In one of our patients, a careful examination of an exenterated eye socket detected an infected CSF fistula that explained the patient's delirium.

The neurologic examination usually does not help either to establish a diagnosis of CNS infection or to determine its specific cause. Instead, the physician must rely on laboratory test results. When clinical evidence indicates acute meningitis, the CSF must be examined. CT or MR scans with and without contrast should be performed to look for meningitis, encephalitis, or abscess.[2880] When clinically indicated, a CT scan with "bone windows" will identify erosion of the skull base or the orbits that may form a communication between the CNS and the surface. If the diagnosis cannot be made in any other way, a brain biopsy may be necessary.

Table 10–7 outlines an empiric approach to treating patients suffering from an acute CNS infection before the organism is identified. The physician first attempts to identify the underlying immune deficit, usually determined by the patient's primary illness and blood neutrophil count, and then chooses antibiotics based on the likely organism causing CNS infection in that setting. Antibiotics that cross the blood–brain barrier easily are more effective than those that do not.[2326]

In patients with T-lymphocyte or mononuclear phagocyte defects caused by lymphoma but with normal blood neutrophil counts, *Listeria* is the most common infecting organism, particularly if cryptococcal antigen is absent from CSF. Because so many patients are acutely ill, antibacterial antibiotics (e.g., ampicillin) should be started immediately after spinal fluid is sampled, even before the outcome of the Gram's stain is known. Although *Cryptococcus* is a common offending organism, antifungal agents can be deferred safely for a few hours until the the cryptococcal antigen determination or the Gram's or india ink stain implicates a cryptococcal infection. Once this meningitis is identified, amphotericin B and 5-flucytosine should be added to ampicillin as initial treatment. In patients suffering from T-cell defects with low peripheral neutrophil counts, ceftazidime and gentamicin should also be administered. Because gentamicin crosses the blood–brain barrier relatively poorly, the physician should consider intrathecal or intraventricular gentamicin in a dose of 5 to 8 mg/day.

If the underlying abnormality is a defect of neutrophil function, ceftazidime and gentamicin are the drugs of choice as initial therapy, whether the blood neutrophil count is normal or low. Other third-generation cephalosporins and imipenem are successful against enteric Gram-negative meningitis and appear to be reasonable alternatives.

In patients suffering from immunoglobulin abnormalities or who have been splenectomized, cefuroxime should be started immediately, along with penicillin, pending the outcome of the cultures. In areas of the world in which penicillin resistance is common among the pneumococci, vancomycin should be added until susceptibility studies are available. In those with a suspected CSF–surface communication, a combination of drugs, including oxacillin (for staphylococcal infection), ceftazidime, and gentamicin, is the initial treatment of choice. If methicillin-resistant infections or coagulase-negative staphylococcal infections are common, vancomycin should be used instead of oxacillin. Whether quinolines, such as ciprofloxacin, will be equally effective remains to be seen.

The antibiotic agents mentioned are designed to treat the common bacterial and fungal infections that begin acutely or subacutely in patients with cancer. Modifications of the regimen are necessary when the physician suspects other organisms, when a different offending organism such as a toxoplasmal or viral agent is identified, or when careful monitoring of the patient indicates that the selected treatment is not working. More detailed guidelines for the treatment of specific CNS infections have been published recently.[1524,1719,2285,2803]

SPECIFIC ORGANISMS CAUSING CENTRAL NERVOUS SYSTEM INFECTION IN PATIENTS WITH CANCER

T-Lymphocyte and Mononuclear Phagocyte Defects

Table 10–8 lists the organisms likely to cause CNS infections in patients with impaired cellular immunity. These patients either have underlying disorders, such as lymphoma or chronic leukemia, or are taking steroids or other immunosuppressive agents such as azathioprine. Neutrophil function may be normal, and patients generally have a normal (or even elevated) WBC count.

BACTERIA

Listeria. This organism is the most common cause of bacterial meningitis in patients with cancer; virtually all patients are taking steroids or have recently done so. An aerobic Gram-positive rod, *Listeria* is widespread in the environment, being found in tap water, sewage, milk products, and stools of healthy people. *Listeria* has been implicated in foodborne outbreaks involving milk products and processed meats, and it affects patients with poor cellular immunity, including patients with cancer, the elderly, neonates, patients with cirrhosis, pregnant women,[898,1084,1363] and occasionally people who are otherwise healthy. Between 1972 and 1979, 53 cases of infection caused by *Listeria* organisms were reported to the New York City Health Department.[442]

Listerial meningitis is usually associated with lymphoma or chronic leukemia. The peripheral WBC count may be normal or

Table 10–8. **CENTRAL NERVOUS SYSTEM INFECTION WITH T-LYMPHOCYTE, MONONUCLEAR PHAGOCYTE DEFECT**

Infection	Bacteria	Fungi	Parasites	Viruses
Meningitis or meningoencephalitis	*Listeria*	*Cryptococcus* *Coccidioides* *Histoplasma*	*Toxoplasma* *Strongyloides*	Varicella-zoster Papovavirus (progressive multifocal leukoencephalopathy) Cytomegalovirus
Brain abscess or encephalitis	*Nocardia* *Listeria*	*Cryptococcus* *Histoplasma*	*Toxoplasma*	Cytomegalovirus Herpes simplex

elevated. The usual clinical signs are of acute or subacute meningitis,[1079] slightly less fulminant than pneumococcal meningitis but more than cryptococcal meningitis. In some instances, the illness may begin indolently with mild headache and personality change, but generally severe headache, nausea, vomiting, fever, and stiff neck dominate the picture; patients look quite ill.

The organism induces an intense inflammatory reaction in the leptomeninges, which may occlude CSF absorptive pathways and lead to hydrocephalus. *Listeria* also tends to invade brain parenchyma, causing a focal cerebritis, a diffuse encephalitis, or an abscess. Any portion of the brain or spinal cord[1815] can be involved, but the organism has a peculiar tendency to invade the brainstem, causing focal brainstem signs.[120,926,934] The clinical course of the brainstem infection is usually biphasic; headache, vomiting, fever, and leukocytosis precede the brainstem signs by 4 to 10 days.[2758]

The diagnosis of *Listeria* meningitis is suspected from the clinical findings and is confirmed by CSF examination. The CSF contains several hundred WBCs with a neutrophilic predominance, despite the organism's name. The glucose concentration is usually low, and the protein concentration is elevated. Organisms are identified by Gram's stain of CSF sediment in only about 10% of cases.[1079] Even when organisms are found, destaining may cause them to appear to be Gram-negative rather than Gram-positive rods, leading to an incorrect diagnosis. They may also mimic Gram-positive cocci. Because the illness is potentially lethal, a patient with a T-lymphocyte or mononuclear phagocyte defect who has a normal or elevated peripheral WBC count and symptoms of meningitis should be considered to have *Listeria* meningitis and be treated empirically with ampicillin.[1079] Isolation from culture may take 2 to 3 days, so it is not helpful in acute treatment. Acute or subacute development of focal signs of brain or brainstem dysfunction may result from cerebral infarction, bacteria-induced vasculitis, or direct invasion of brain by the organisms. If the organisms reach the brain hematogenously, the meninges may be spared and the CSF can be entirely normal. In such patients, blood cultures are usually positive for *Listeria*. All patients with *Listeria* infections, including septicemia from *Listeria monocytogenes* without neurologic signs, require both CSF examination and an MR brain scan. The latter usually suggests brain invasion.[926]

The drugs of choice are ampicillin, 2 g every 4 hours, or penicillin, 2×10^6 U every 4 hours, for at least 3 to 4 weeks. Patients treated for a shorter period often relapse, particularly if they have cerebritis. For severely ill patients, gentamicin may be added because of synergism with penicillinlike drugs. It is given both systemically and intrathecally, in doses of 2 to 10 mg once or twice daily. Trimethoprim-sulfamethoxazole, vancomycin, erythromycin, and chloramphenicol or tetracycline have been used successfully in patients allergic to penicillin.[1545]

If *Listeria* meningitis is diagnosed early, it can usually be treated effectively. Those who succumb typically are either terminal from their cancer or have suffered a delay in the diagnosis of meningitis. Most respond rapidly to appropriate antibiotics, but an occasional patient, particularly if stuporous or comatose on admission, may respond more slowly (e.g., after 72 hours). Slow recovery suggests direct invasion of the brain by the bacteria or, more likely, meningitis-induced hydrocephalus. If the patient's mental state has not returned to normal within a week and if the ventricles are obviously enlarged, shunting should be considered before the hydrocephalus causes irreversible brain damage.

Nocardia asteroides.[2825,2875] This aerobic, filamentous-branching, Gram-positive rod, which may be weakly acid-fast, belongs to the same family as the actinomycetes and mycobacteria. In patients with impaired cellular immunity, infection spreads from the lung to cause either brain abscesses[82,273] (usually multiple) or, less commonly, meningitis. Up to 50% of patients with *Nocardia* pulmonary infection develop CNS lesions.[150] The abscesses are usually indolent, presenting with the clinical symptoms of single or multiple mass lesions resembling metastases rather than infection. Chorioretinitis also occurs.[1758] Organisms are infrequently identified in the spinal fluid. Even when present, they grow slowly; the microbiology laboratory should be alerted to the possibility of nocardial infection so that they will keep the culture for several days.

Nocardia infection in the CNS is suspected when lymphoma or chronic lymphatic leukemia patients or those receiving steroid therapy[273] develop focal neurologic signs associated with one or more contrast-enhancing lesions in the brain. The patient usually also has lung or skin lesions diagnosed by culturing these organs. Infection with multiple organisms can occur, however, so if the brain lesions do not respond clinically and on scan within 7 to 10 days, the physician should consider stereotactic needle biopsy of a brain lesion. Treatment is with sulfadiazine at 120 mg/kg per day for 1 or 2 weeks and 60 mg/kg per day for several months. Trimethoprim-sulfamethoxazole has also been used with success, although no comparative clinical trials have been reported. It is very important to identify the sensitivity of the organism from at least one site because as many as 20% of patients may be resistant to the trimethoprim-sulfamethoxazole combination. Cefuroxime has been effective for pulmonary disease.

FUNGI

Fungal infections now rival bacteria as a cause of death in patients with cancer[1816,2272,2736] and those undergoing bone marrow transplantation.[1816] The common pathogen in patients with T-cell defects is *Cryptococcus.*[1340,2801] In some geographic areas, histoplasmosis[2046] and coccidioidomycosis[1448,2616] are also culprits. Cryptococcal infection usually causes a subacute or chronic meningitis[1445,2592,2879] but may cause local abscess formation[882] or ventriculitis without meningitis. During the past 11 years, 14 patients without AIDS but with cryptococcal meningitis have been treated at MSKCC; 6 had Hodgkin's disease, 5 had non-Hodgkin's lymphoma, and 3 had chronic leukemia. Twelve received steroid therapy.

The cryptococcal organism is ubiquitous in soil and generally spreads to the CNS via the lung. The disorder may affect seemingly healthy individuals as well as the obviously immunosuppressed. In patients with cancer, the clinical course is usually subacute with headache and fever. In occasional patients, the disorder develops insidiously and may last months to years before the diagnosis is made. Nuchal rigidity is uncommon. The onset is usually slower than with pneumococcal or *Listeria* meningitis but more rapid than in patients suffering from leptomeningeal metastases. Usually patients do not have neurologic signs other than mild encephalopathy, although cranial nerve palsies (especially facial and acoustic) and papilledema occur occasionally. Cranial nerve palsies, especially when accompanied by absent deep tendon reflexes, should lead the physician to suspect leptomeningeal metastasis instead of, or in addition to, cryptococcal meningitis.

Intracerebral lesions occur either as nonenhancing gelatinous pseudocysts not surrounded by edema or as contrast-enhancing granulomas surrounded by edema.[882] Occasionally, lesions may be mixed. The intracerebral lesions can be diagnosed with certainty only by biopsy. In an appropriate clinical setting, high titers of serum cryptococcal antigen or positive blood cultures may prompt the physician to treat the brain lesions empirically.

The diagnosis of cryptococcal meningitis is made by a CSF examination that reveals elevated CSF pressure, an increased number of lymphocytes, a low glucose, and a high protein concentration. The india ink preparation identifies an organism with a clear halo due to the polysaccharide capsule surrounding the yeast, but the inexperienced observer may mistake RBCs, lymphocytes, and occasional inanimate debris in spinal fluid for fungi and should consider an india ink preparation positive only if budding yeast forms are clearly identified. Gram's stain reveals an irregularly stippled Gram-positive organism with a faintly Gram-negative capsule. Organisms are visible in the CSF in only about half the cases, and growth in culture may not be apparent for several days. Testing the CSF for cryptococcal antigen is highly reliable. A titer of greater than 1:4 establishes the diagnosis; a titer greater than 1:256 carries a poor prognosis. Cryptococcal antigen tests may take 2 to 6 weeks to become positive after the infection begins, and test results may be negative if the patient is infected with unusual, small capsular forms of the organism. If the patient has a cryptococcal abscess rather than meningitis, the CSF may be normal and the diagnosis can be established only by stereotactic needle biopsy.

The organism usually responds to IV amphotericin B, 0.7 to 1.0 mg/kg per day and flucytosine, 75 to 100 mg/kg per day.[82] A lipid complex of amphotericin B is under investigation.[2007] In severe or fulminant cases, intrathecal amphotericin B (administered intraventricularly through an Ommaya reservoir) may be life-saving.[2058] In one series,[2058] 6 of 7 recent patients with cryptococcal meningitis so treated responded to therapy, whereas 5 of 6 patients who were less severely ill and did not receive intrathecal drugs died of the infection. Intrathecal amphotericin B has also proved helpful in coccidioidal meningitis.[1448] For intrathecal treatment, begin with 0.01 mg of amphotericin B and escalate at 12- to 24-hour intervals up to 0.5 mg/day as long as the CSF antigen remains positive. Administration by intraventricular reservoir rather than by lumbar puncture is preferred for the reasons given in Chapter 7 and also because intrathecal administration of amphotericin B by lumbar puncture can cause severe leg and back pain. Fluconazole, 200 to 400 mg/24 hours, should be considered for maintenance in patients with sustained immunocompromise.[287] The role of other antifungal agents is less certain.[949,2524]

The sequelae of cryptococcal meningitis include cranial nerve palsies (particularly deafness), occasionally visual loss,[2161] and hydrocephalus that may require shunting. With early and aggressive treatment, most patients, even those suffering from lymphoma, do well if their underlying disease remains in remission.

VIRUSES

The herpesviruses (varicella-zoster, herpes simplex, or cytomegalovirus) may invade the CNS of patients with T-cell deficiencies.[2508] The latter two are particular problems after bone marrow transplantation,[1989a,2829] as is *Herpesvirus* 6.[682]

Varicella-Zoster. A major cause of nervous system dysfunction in patients with cancer, varicella-zoster virus also occurs in the apparently immunocompetent. The disorder may affect over 50% of those with Hodgkin's disease.[1028] Concomitant bacterial infection is common.[1652] Table 10–9 shows the range of neurologic complications of varicella-zoster infection.

Varicella. Chickenpox is a more severe infection in children with cancer than it is in healthy children. In one study[763] of 77 children with cancer who developed varicella, visceral dissemination occurred in 19 and fatal encephalitis in 2. The most common neurologic complication of chickenpox is an acute ataxic meningoencephalitis, more likely to occur in the immunosuppressed than in the general population. It is characterized by sudden ataxia, sometimes with dysarthria and nystagmus. Neurologic symptoms may precede or follow the rash by days or, rarely, weeks. More widespread evidence of encephalitis may include lethargy, seizures, and other focal signs. Most patients recover fully. The pathogenesis of the disorder is not known, but is hypothesized to be either direct invasion of the CNS by the virus or an immune encephalomyelitic response to the viral infection. Recent evidence[2322] sug-

Table 10–9. **NEUROLOGIC COMPLICATIONS OF VARICELLA-ZOSTER VIRUS INFECTIONS**

Associated with Varicella
Meningoencephalitic syndromes
Primary viral encephalitis
Postinfectious encephalomyelitis
Acute cerebellar ataxia
Intracerebral hemorrhage secondary to coagulation disorders
Myelitis
Aseptic meningitis and suppurative meningitis
Guillain-Barré syndrome
Reye's syndrome
Congenital varicella syndrome
Associated with Herpes Zoster
Postherpetic neuralgia
Segmental motor weakness
Encephalomyelitis
Aseptic meningitis
Myelitis alone
Cranial nerve palsies
Guillain-Barré syndrome
Cerebral vasculitis
Multifocal leukoencephalitis syndrome
Myositis

Source: Adapted from Kennedy,[1358] p 178.

gests that varicella-zoster virus can reach the nervous system by either neural or hematogenous spread.

Reye's Syndrome. A metabolic disorder that follows viral infection, usually varicella or influenza,[1563] Reye's syndrome is characterized by the sudden onset of severe, recurrent vomiting and the rapid development of irritability, confusion, and coma. Intracranial pressure is increased, and death is caused by cerebral herniation. At autopsy, acute fatty changes are found in the liver, and the brain is edematous. The disorder is much more common in children but has also been reported in adults.[2652] It does not appear to be more common in the immunosuppressed than in the immunocompetent population. Hypoglycemia from the liver disorder is a common complication. Ingestion of aspirin during the acute viral infection appears to be a risk factor for the development of Reye's syndrome, but the exact cause of the metabolic disorder is not established.[1405,1563,2652]

Herpes Zoster. This disorder is much more common in the immunosuppressed patient. Within 36 months after treatment for Hodgkin's disease, about 30% of patients treated with chemotherapy and RT and about 10% of those receiving RT alone have developed herpes zoster.[1028,2315] The attack rate is higher in children than in adults, whereas in the immunocompetent population, the elderly are much more likely to be affected.[1028] The peak incidence occurs within 6 months following RT and chemotherapy. In some instances, the zoster infection erupts at the site of a developing neoplasm or an RT portal. Herpes zoster is somewhat more likely to disseminate in patients with cancer than in the immunocompetent, but in both groups the disorder usually runs a benign course. Cutaneous herpes zoster typically begins with pain, itching, or paresthesias in the distribution of dermatomes in which the virus, latent in dorsal root ganglion neurons, reactivates. A rash follows in 3 to 7 days. The dermatome involved occasionally indicates metastatic disease of that dorsal root, but this phenomenon is so uncommon that it does not warrant extensive evaluation such as myelography or MRI unless other suspicion indicates neoplastic involvement of that site. The rash usually begins as patchy erythema in a dermatome, but after about 12 to 24 hours, vesicles appear that become pustules in a couple of days and then dry up within a week. Usually, the rash is mild and clears within a few weeks, but in patients with cancer the local rash may be severe, leading to ulceration and sloughing of the skin, which may require grafting. Many patients with herpes zoster have a few vesicles outside the involved dermatome, but dissemination of the rash is more likely in cancer patients. The pain is usually maximal before and at the time the rash is present; it diminishes as the rash clears, leaving areas of hyperpigmentation or depigmentation with variable degrees of sensory loss in the dermatomal area.

COMPLICATIONS. The virus may also spread proximally along the dorsal root into the spinal cord to cause a myelitis, may disseminate into the subarachnoid space to cause meningitis, or may seed the bloodstream with secondary spread to the nervous system, causing an encephalitis.[1227] Rarely, particularly when the ophthalmic division of the trigeminal ganglion is involved, the virus may cause a local vasculitis with carotid occlusion and cerebral infarction.[712,2843]

Several distinct neurologic syndromes are associated with herpes zoster:

POSTHERPETIC NEURALGIA. In as many as 4% of patients with cancer and herpes zoster, severe pain outlasts the resolution of the rash. Postherpetic neuralgia is more common in those with cancer but is not directly related to the severity of the initial rash. The pain has two components: (1) lancinating or lightninglike pains in the dermatome, which usually clear spontaneously, and (2) a constant, burning pain, which may be incapacitating. Carbamazepine and other anticonvulsants relieve the lancinating component but usually have little effect on the burning pain. Early treatment with corticosteroids (see the following) may prevent the neuralgia.

MOTOR NERVE DYSFUNCTION. A few patients develop motor paresis involving neighboring spinal or cranial nerves. When weakness occurs, it usually appears a few days to a few weeks after the rash, although on occasion it precedes the rash. The weakness usually begins suddenly, reaching its maximum within a day or so. The muscles paralyzed are those supplied by the spinal root affected by the herpes, although motor weakness may be more widespread than the cutaneous abnormality and occasionally is distant from the cutaneous change. Most patients recover fully, but a few are left with permanent paralysis. Muscle paralysis, which affects about 0.5% of herpes zoster patients, appears to be no more frequent or severe in those with cancer.[2581] The facial nerve and geniculate ganglion are commonly involved in Ramsay Hunt syndrome. Auditory and vestibular symptoms may accompany this syndrome.[1358] Paralysis of ocular or jaw muscles may complicate herpes involving the ophthalmic division of the trigeminal nerve.

In rare instances, either the pain of herpes zoster or motor loss associated with a rising herpes zoster titer has been reported without a cutaneous rash (zoster sine herpete).[689,701,921a,1714]

MYELITIS. The virus may directly invade the spinal cord, causing a local inflammatory response. Symptoms usually appear several days (median = 12 days) after the rash; rarely, the rash may be absent.[1133] Myelitis begins with ipsilateral weakness and progresses over several days. The course may be remitting and exacerbating.[921b] Neurologic dysfunction varies in severity from minor long-tract signs to a complete transverse myelopathy[625] resulting from spinal cord necrosis. The major pathologic alterations are in the dorsal root ganglia and adjacent posterior horn. Abnormalities include demyelination and necrosis, the latter from vasculitis. Viral particles are found in oligodendroglia, some astrocytes, and ependymal cells. The virus may spread vertically in the cord, causing symptoms and signs rostral to the dermatome with the cutaneous rash.[2322] Detection of persistent viral DNA in CSF may aid in the diagnosis.[921b]

ENCEPHALITIS.[1283] Encephalitis is characterized by fever, headache, and delirium, sometimes with nuchal rigidity and pleocytosis. Pleocytosis is found in as many as 50% of uncomplicated cutaneous zoster infections, indicating that minor, clinically inapparent meningitis, myelitis, or encephalitis may be frequent. Antibodies have been found in CSF,[54,210] suggesting intrathecal synthesis.

CEREBRAL VASCULITIS. Two overlapping syndromes result from cerebral vasculitis. One is characterized by headache and confusion progressing to stupor or coma, sometimes with multifocal or generalized convulsions. Focal neurologic signs, including hemiplegia, are sometimes present. Pleocytosis is characteristic. Pathologically, vasculitis involves small vessels in the hemisphere ipsilateral to a trigeminal herpes, or it may be more diffuse in patients whose herpetic rashes have been elsewhere in the body and in whom the virus presumably reached the cerebrovascular structures by hematogenous spread. Pontine infarction may follow cervical zoster,[2218] or thalamic infarction may follow lingual zoster[901] (Fig. 10–6). Viral particles have been identified in the vascular structures.[712,1572] The infection may be associated with either an intense inflammatory reaction[1572] (i.e., granulomatous arteritis) or little or no inflammation.[712] The relationship, if any, between zoster vasculitis and the granulomatous angiitis associated with Hodgkin's disease is unclear (see Chapter 9).

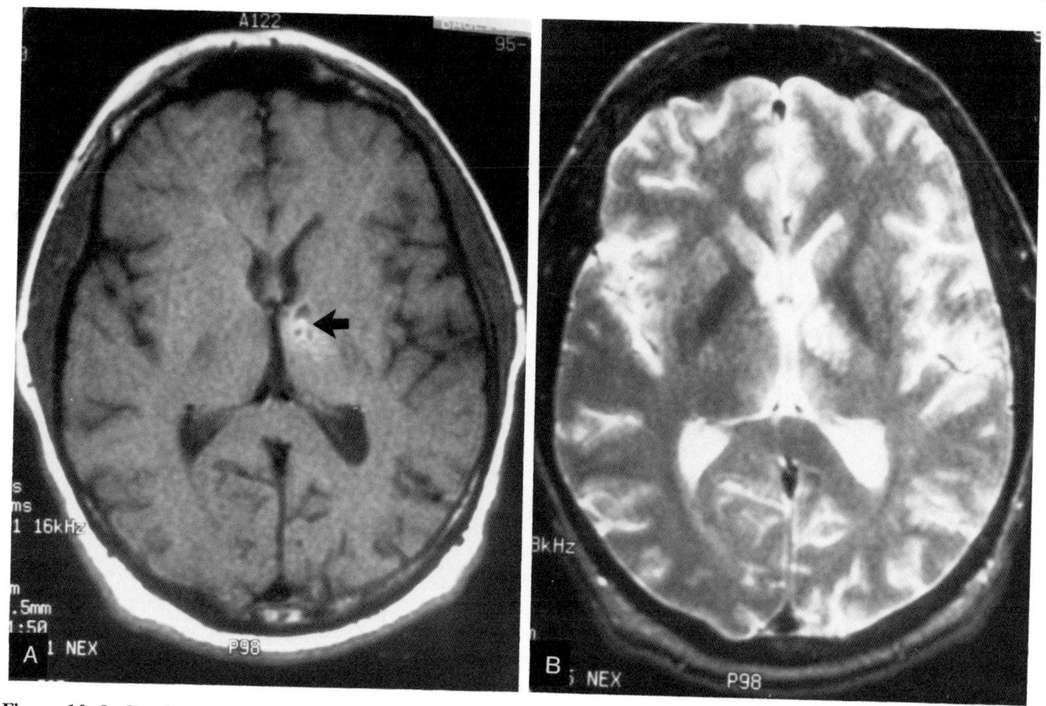

Figure 10–6. Cerebral infarct from herpes zoster vasculitis. This 38-year-old man with non-Hodgkin's lymphoma suffered a sudden hemiparesis while recovering from cervical (C-2,C-3) herpes zoster. *A,* A T_1-weighted MR scan demonstrated a basal ganglia infarct (*arrow*). *B,* A T_2-weighted image confirmed findings suggesting that the infarct had resulted from a vasculitis involving penetrating vessels at the middle cerebral artery.

A second clinical syndrome, which occurs when large- or medium-sized arteries are infected, is characterized by the sudden onset of headache and contralateral hemiplegia following ophthalmic-division trigeminal herpes.[1161] Confusion, stupor, and coma are less common in this disorder than in the more diffuse form. An occlusion of the carotid artery is visible on MR arteriography. A similar angiitis has been reported following primary varicella infection.[2344]

SLOWLY DEVELOPING MULTIFOCAL BRAIN DYSFUNCTION. Clinically similar to progressive multifocal leukoencephalopathy (a discussion of which follows), this disorder affects patients with lymphoma or Hodgkin's disease who have suffered from herpes zoster in the remote past. The diagnosis can be established only with brain biopsy and identification of the virus at the lesion site.[1206] On MR scan, it may resemble a bacterial brain abscess with ring enhancement.

DIAGNOSIS. Diagnosing herpes zoster infection is usually easy. In the first few days, the pain is dermatomal without rash. The clinician might suspect tumor in a spinal root, but the sudden onset without preceding vertebral pain suggests herpes zoster. The diagnosis may be more difficult if motor changes precede the rash or if the rash develops in an inconspicuous area. The sudden onset of Bell's palsy with or without eighth-nerve dysfunction in a lymphoma patient also suggests leptomeningeal metastasis, and a modest pleocytosis encourages that diagnosis. Nevertheless, a careful examination of the auditory canals, palate, and the scalp under the hair may yield evidence of sensory loss or a few herpetic vesicles. Serum titers for varicella-zoster virus should be drawn in the acute state and repeated a couple of weeks later. A fourfold rise suggests herpes zoster infection. Occasionally, the rash of herpes simplex may also appear in a dermatomal distribution and be mistaken for herpes zoster. If doubt persists, the virus can usually be recovered from cutaneous vesicles.

The diagnosis of herpes zoster complications is usually not difficult if the patient has had a recent cutaneous viral infection. Cerebrovascular involvement or delayed encephalitis are more difficult diagnoses. In the appropriate clinical setting, cerebrovascular involvement can sometimes be established by arteriography, but encephalitis requires biopsy, appropriate cultures, and immunofluorescent stains.

All immunosuppressed patients with herpes zoster infections should be treated with acyclovir administered intravenously in a dose of 12.4 mg/kg every 8 hours for 7 days. Whether the drug is as efficacious when given orally has not been established, but if given it requires a dose of 800 mg five times a day for 5 to 7 days. The drug appears to decrease late complications, including postherpetic neuralgia. Corticosteroids also reduce the incidence of postherpetic neuralgia if given in the acute stage of the rash, but they probably should not be given to immunosuppressed patients suffering from the disorder. The treatment of postherpetic neuralgia is often frustrating for both the physician and the patient. Various approaches are discussed in detail elsewhere.[867]

Herpes Simplex. Systemic herpes simplex infections are common in the immunosuppressed host. After cytoreductive therapy for bone marrow transplant, 70% to 80% of seropositive patients develop herpes simplex infection, usually characterized by ulcerative mucositis.[352,2829] Herpes simplex encephalitis appears to be increased in the immunosuppressed population. We have encountered several patients who have developed this disorder when they have lymphoma[2220] or primary or metastatic brain tumors[1676] that are being treated with corticosteroids. Characteristically, an otherwise stable patient suddenly exhibits altered behavior and consciousness and possibly headache or language disturbances, sometimes associated with focal or generalized seizures but usually without fever. In most, the disease course appears no different from that of herpes simplex encephalitis in the immunocompetent population.[2802] A single patient with herpes simplex type-2 encephalitis complicating the management of brain metastases has been reported.[1676] Abnormalities in the medial temporal lobe on MR scan resembled those in the immunocompetent patient[2900] (Fig. 10–7). A single case report[2092] describes a patient with Hodgkin's disease and impaired

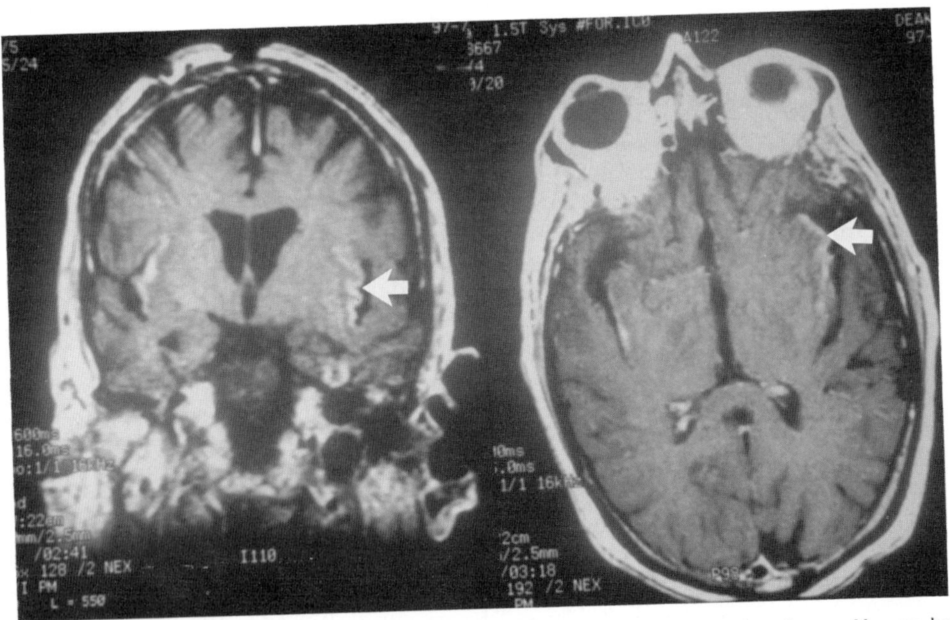

Figure 10–7. A contrast-enhanced MR scan of a man with stage IV non-Hodgkin's lymphoma. He was being treated for epidural spinal cord compression and suddenly became confused and disoriented. Lumbar puncture revealed white cells in the spinal fluid, and the contrast-enhanced MR scan showed enhancement with bilateral involvement of the medial temporal cortex (*arrow*). An initial diagnosis of leptomeningeal tumor was made. At autopsy, the patient was discovered to have herpes simplex encephalitis.

immunity who had an atypical slowly progressive clinical course leading to death. The pathologic features consisted of widespread neuronal destruction, astrocytic proliferation, and inclusion bodies without the typical inflammatory changes or hemorrhagic necrosis generally found in the medial temporal lobes.

The diagnostic problem is recognition that the sudden change in behavior in a patient with a chronic neurologic disease associated with cancer is the result of a new acute viral encephalitis rather than cancer involving the CNS. Clinical suspicion of that diagnosis should lead to immediate acyclovir treatment.[2802] The CSF may contain RBCs and WBCs. Cultures are negative, but polymerase chain reaction (PCR), which identifies herpes simplex virus DNA in the CSF, allows an early diagnosis in most instances.[104] Depending on the clinical situation, a brain biopsy may be necessary to establish a definitive diagnosis. Histologic changes at autopsy are usually typical of those found in the immunocompetent host, with inflammation and necrosis primarily in the medial temporal lobes. Both meningitis and myelitis may accompany herpes simplex type-2 infections.[812a] The diagnosis can be made by CSF culture.

Progressive Multifocal Leukoencephalopathy. An infection of oligodendrogliocytes, progressive multifocal leukoencephalopathy (PML) is caused by the JC virus, a papovavirus.[2323] The virus is acquired by most people in childhood and is not associated with a significant illness. The virus remains latent, and with impaired cellular immunity, particularly with lymphoma or chronic lymphocytic leukemia, it may reactivate and cause a rapidly progressive demyelinating illness characterized by multifocal signs (usually hemispheral but sometimes cerebellar) that progress during 3 to 6 months to bilateral paralysis and stupor or coma. The diagnosis should be suspected in patients with depressed cellular immunity from disease or prolonged chemotherapy who develop progressive neurologic dysfunction, particularly when the signs are multifocal and unaccompanied by headache, seizures, or changes in the CSF. The CT or MR scan[2900] may be normal very early in the course of the illness but eventually reveals multifocal (occasionally single), punched-out lesions of the white matter that usually do not contrast enhance and rarely cause mass effect (Fig. 10–8). Occasionally, the scan of nonenhancing lymphomas may be similar. A definitive diagnosis can be established only by biopsy. Uniformly effective treatment is unavailable, although some[314,315] have reported responses to IV or intrathecal cytarabine (but see reference 63a). Recent reports of JC viral genome[25] detected by PCR in CSF[319,2767] or blood[2598] lymphocytes give promise of a diagnosis without biopsy. Some studies, however, suggest that the JC viral DNA may be found in the brain of patients without PML, raising a question about the meaning of positive results from PCR studies.[1809,2800] In a rare patient, especially one who can mount an inflammatory response, the disease remits spontaneously or stabilizes for long periods.[2321] The MR scans of such patients may reveal mass lesions that contrast enhance.

Cytomegalovirus. Cytomegalovirus (CMV) infects about 50% of persons by the time they are 50 years of age, but more than 90% of these are asymptomatic.[135] The virus in the nervous system may reactivate in patients with depressed cell-mediated immunity, particularly after bone marrow transplantation.[1989a,2829] The symptoms are of subacute encephalitis, with headache, confusion, and lethargy. One of our patients had focal brainstem signs only, accompanied by a contrast-enhancing lesion on MR scan.

The virus has a predilection for ependymal cells of the lateral ventricles[135,2530] and may be suspected when MR scanning shows contrast-enhancing lesions as streaks surrounding the lateral ventricles in a patient with clinical encephalitis.[678] CMV also causes a retinitis characterized by large yellow or white exudates, as well as perivascular hemorrhage.[2054] Seroconversion, or an increase in the already positive CMV antibody titer, supports the diagnosis. The virus can sometimes be cultured from the urine, saliva, or buffy coat, although rarely from CSF or brain tissue. Brain biopsy specimens reveal periventricular necrosis and giant cells, fused macrophages for which the virus, found in intracellular inclusions, is named. Treatment with ganciclovir, 10 mg/kg per day (in two divided doses) for 4 to 6 weeks, may be effective.

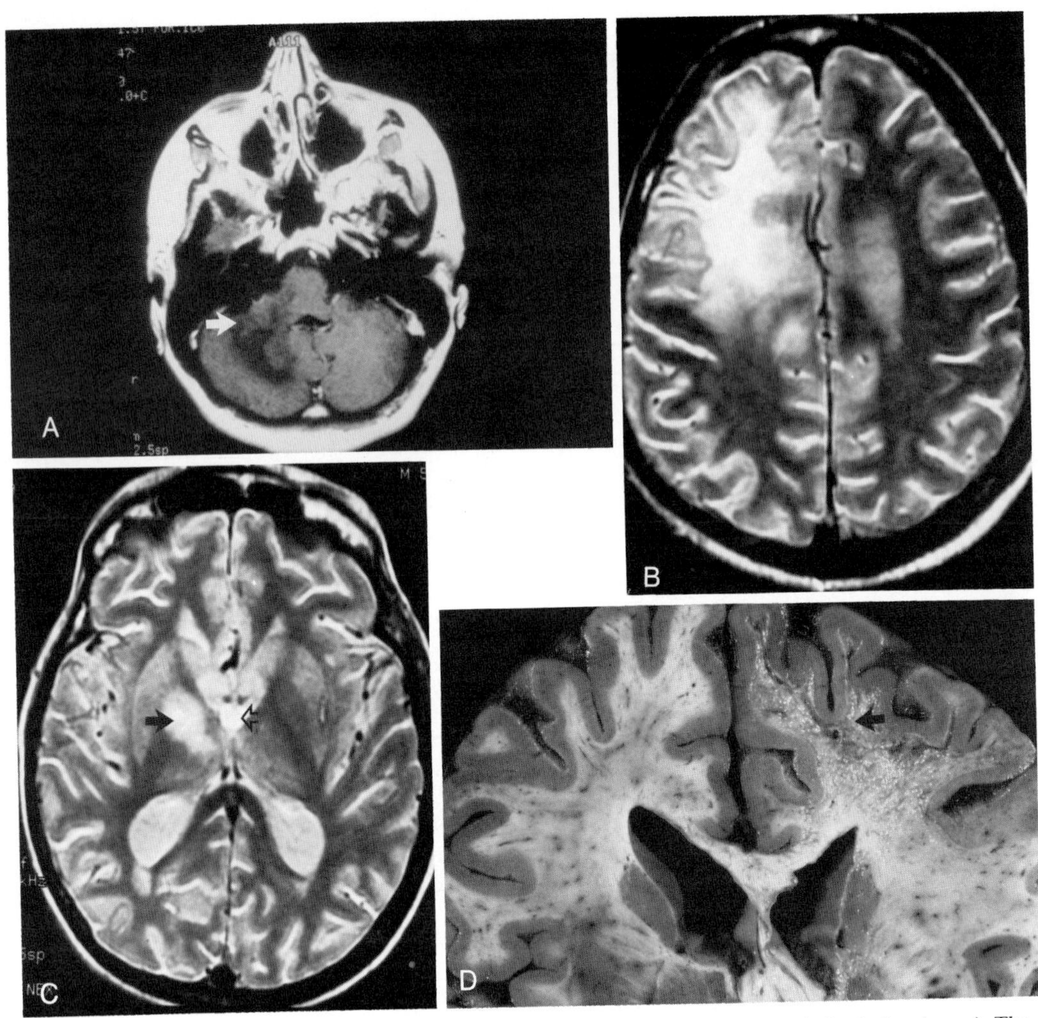

Figure 10–8. *A,* A patient with chronic lymphocytic leukemia presented with a single cerebellar lesion (*arrow*). The lesion was hypointense on T_1-weighted images and did not enhance. The spinal fluid examination was normal. The patient's only symptom was progressive cerebellar dysfunction, which was originally thought to be paraneoplastic. A needle biopsy specimen revealed progressive multifocal leukoencephalopathy (PML). *B,* Another case of PML with the typical hyperintense T_2-weighted MR image restricted to white matter, sparing the cortex. *C,* In this patient, however, the virus also involved basal ganglia (*solid arrow*) and brainstem. An incidental colloid cyst (*open arrow*) caused mild hydrocephalus. *D,* The autopsy specimen shows the typical white matter abnormality (*arrow*) that spares the cortex.

Foscarnet, 60 mg/kg every 8 hours for 15 days, has been effective in the treatment of CMV retinitis.

The virus has also been associated with a Guillain-Barré–like polyneuritis in both immunocompetent and immunosuppressed hosts.[2268] The polyneuropathy sometimes resembles a cauda equina syndrome with urinary retention and lower extremity sensory loss. The CSF contains WBCs and virus; PCR may identify viral DNA in CSF.[2838]

Other Viruses. Although their incidence is unknown, several other viruses have been reported to infect the CNS in patients suffering from cancer. They include measles, enteroviruses,[17,2841] and adenoviruses.[567]

PARASITES

Toxoplasma gondii. The most common parasitic CNS infection in patients with cancer with impaired cellular immunity, *Toxoplasma* *gondii* is also especially prevalent in AIDS patients.[1114,1864] In patients with Hodgkin's disease, *Toxoplasma* brain abscesses are more common than brain metastases, but the reverse is true in non-Hodgkin's lymphomas. Toxoplasmosis also sometimes affects those with other cancers who are treated with steroids or chemotherapy. The pathologic changes of CNS toxoplasmosis may consist of (1) a meningoencephalitis with multiple small necrotic abscesses scattered throughout the cortex and subcortex, with a diminished inflammatory response so that often they are not visible on CT or MR scan, or (2) one or more large mass lesions with a predilection for the basal ganglia.[207,910,2082] Clinically, the disorder is characterized either by focal neurologic signs, usually in the absence of headache and fever, or by a diffuse encephalopathy accompanied by seizures. The CT or MR scan, when results are positive, reveals one or more ring-enhancing lesions with a predilection for basal ganglia and cerebral cortex (i.e., gray matter rather than white matter). Occasionally, the lesion is hypodense without contrast enhancement or is homogeneously enhancing; the latter resembles CNS lymphoma. MR is more sensitive than CT for detecting small lesions. The presence of a deep-seated mass lesion in a Hodgkin's disease patient is almost pathognomonic of toxoplasmal abscess, and the patient can be treated on that basis.

Acquired *Toxoplasma* retinitis that causes acute visual loss has been reported[1696] in several patients with depressed immunity. The organism may also cause an acute or subacute meningitis. If the patient has meningitis, the CSF has a lymphocytic pleocytosis with high protein and sometimes low glucose concentrations.[1004] The organism is usually not isolated from the spinal fluid.

Whether the brain infection is a reexacerbation of an old asymptomatic infection or a new one is not clear. Usually, IgM and IgG antibodies are positive and rise during the infection; some exceptions occur, particularly in patients with severe hypogammaglobulinemia or with AIDS. Because treatment with sulfadiazine and pyrimethamine usually has a rapid response and is quite safe, the therapy often establishes the diagnosis without biopsy. Biopsy should be considered only if this treatment does not lead to improvement in the clinical and scan pictures within a week to 10 days. Antibody titers should be measured in both blood and CSF; they may be positive in CSF when absent from blood. Treatment includes sulfadiazine, 1 g po qid, and pyrimethamine, 100 mg/day for 1 day and then 25 to 50 mg each day thereafter. The optimal duration of treatment is unknown. Folinic acid, 10 mg/24 hours, prevents pancytopenia.

Strongyloides stercoralis. A worm that resides in the upper intestine of individuals in the Southeastern and South Central United States,[899] *Strongyloides stercoralis* causes CNS infection in patients with impaired cellular immunity, particularly those who have been on high-dose corticosteroids.[530] The larvae escape from the bowel and disseminate hematogenously to the CNS, causing a meningoencephalitis, sometimes with a concomitant bacterial meningitis and pneumonitis from enteric bacteria carried by the worms. The clinician should suspect this disorder when a patient on corticosteroids develops upper abdominal cramping pain associated with a headache and stiff neck. If several Gram-negative organisms are found in CSF or blood, the diagnosis is more strongly suspected. The worm itself has been found in the CSF[695,1743] in a few patients, but the diagnosis is usually established by finding larvae in the stool, sputum, or duodenal contents. The patient is treated with thiabendazole, 25 mg/kg bid, for 7 days. Prevention is far better than treatment. Examination of stool or duodenal aspirates should be performed in patients from endemic areas who are about to be given immunosuppressive drugs. If the results of one of these tests are positive, the patient should be treated prophylactically.

Eosinophilic Meningitis. Eosinophils in the CSF are usually caused by parasitic CNS infections.[276,1432] Nevertheless, in some patients with Hodgkin's disease,[1990] lymphoma,[1373] or leukemia,[340] eosinophils appear to be a reaction to meningeal tumor. One report[340] describes basophilic meningitis in a similar situation. Eosinophilic meningitis may also complicate foreign bodies such as shunt tubing in the CSF.[2601,2618] Other causes of "eosinophilic" meningitis include sarcoidosis,[2346] nonsteroidal anti-inflammatory drugs,[2112] and the hypereosinophilic syndrome.[2773] Eosinophils may cause CNS dysfunction,[2763,2792] presumably by cytokine release.

Neutrophil Defects

Table 10–10 lists the organisms that commonly invade the CNS of patients with granulocytopenia or other defects of neutrophil function. These defects account for about 25% of CNS infections in patients with cancer. The most common cause of neutrophil defects in patients with cancer is neutropenia that is due to cytotoxic chemotherapy or bone marrow replacement by tumor, as in leukemia. Corticosteroids also impair neutrophil function and, when used to treat such patients, may enhance the likelihood of CNS infection. Although certain organisms, such as *Listeria,* do affect patients with neutrophil defects as well as those with T-cell deficits, by and large different organisms affect the two groups. The major offenders in those with neutrophil defects are enteric bacilli and several fungal organisms that are usually nonpathogenic. Parasitic and viral infections are not a specific complication of neutrophil defects.

CNS bacterial infections develop when the absolute neutrophil count falls lower than $1000/mm^3$.[1615] *Pseudomonas* and *E. coli* are the major offenders.[1615] About 50% of neutropenic patients who develop CNS infections have also been receiving steroid therapy, and a few have ventricular catheters in place. The underlying disorder is usually acute leukemia or lymphoma. Patients present with either a new fever or an increasing body temperature if already febrile. Most develop acute or subacute changes in mental state, with confusion, lethargy, and occasionally coma. Some have headache, and about 40% have seizures, but few have nuchal rigidity.

The diagnosis is difficult because most patients are already seriously systemically ill. Even when the clinician suspects infection because of increasing confusion and fever, examining the CSF for cells may not be useful because many patients lack pleocytosis, but the results of Gram's staining and culture are usually positive.

ENTERIC BACILLI

Neutropenic patients and those with abnormal communication between the CSF and an epithelial surface, particularly the bowel, are susceptible to CNS infection caused by enteric Gram-negative bacilli that reside in the patient's own GI tract.[254] On occasion, Gram-negative meningitis complicates the course of patients with cell-mediated immune disorders.[254] At MSKCC, *P. aeruginosa* is the most common offending organism, followed by *E. coli* and *Klebsiella, Enterobacter,* and *Proteus* species. *Salmonella* is a rare offender.[254] The organisms may cause either meningitis or a brain abscess, which may contain more than one organism. *P.*

Table 10–10. **CENTRAL NERVOUS SYSTEM INFECTIONS IN PATIENTS WITH NEUTROPHIL DEFECTS (GRANULOCYTOPENIA)**

Infection	Bacteria	Fungi
Meningitis	Enteric bacilli	*Candida* sp.
	Pseudomonas aeruginosa	
	Escherichia coli	
	Klebsiella pneumoniae	
	Listeria monocytogenes	
	Streptococcus pneumoniae	
	Staphylococcus aureus	
Meningoencephalitis	Same	
Abscess	Same	*Aspergillus* sp.
		Mucoraceae
		Candida sp.

aeruginosa often causes a vasculitis that may, in the septic patient, lead to multiple small cerebral infarcts.

CNS infection from enteric Gram-negative bacilli is usually an acute meningitis. The CSF is usually purulent but may be devoid of WBCs, particularly when the patient is severely neutropenic. Despite the absence of WBCs, the glucose concentration is usually low and the protein concentration high. Organisms are readily apparent in the Gram's stain specimen.

Treatment is outlined at the end of this chapter (Table 10–11). In some patients whose initial response is unsatisfactory, treatment may be improved by the placement of an Ommaya device and direct intraventricular injection of the antimicrobial agents. Nevertheless, the prognosis is poor. Survival rates at MSKCC vary between 20% and 40%. Many patients, however, are desperately ill from cancer, other side effects of its therapy such as thrombocytopenia and anemia, and systemic infection. In those patients who are in relatively good condition at the time the Gram-negative meningitis develops, vigorous treatment usually yields a satisfactory outcome without significant sequelae.

Treating Gram-negative brain abscesses is more difficult. In the cancer population, these abscesses usually develop when the patient is terminally ill, so it is difficult to judge the results of antimicrobial treatment. In most instances, the offending organism is not known but can be suspected from the clinical setting and the presence of sepsis with positive blood cultures. The initial treatment should be with high-dose penicillin, 20 million U/24 hours, or ampicillin, 12 g/24 hours, with ceftazidime 2 g every 8 hours. If anaerobic organisms are suspected, metronidazole, 500 mg every 6 hours, may be added.

Brain abscesses can be treated successfully with antibiotics alone, even in immunosuppressed patients. Therefore, when a brain abscess caused by Gram-negative organisms is suspected, begin with antibiotic therapy and follow the patient with MR scans. Stereotactic needle aspiration of abscess contents can both establish a diagnosis and relieve symptoms. Only when antibiotic therapy and stereotactic aspiration have failed is therapeutic excision considered, provided that the patient is in sufficiently good systemic condition. The decision for surgery is based on the patient's clinical response to treatment, not only on the scan; the contrast-enhancing abnormality may persist long after the patient has become asymptomatic and antibiotic therapy has been discontinued.[2834] In a patient with a good clinical response, we discontinue antibiotic treatment after 4 weeks and follow the MR scan. If the lesion is either shrinking or stable, no further therapy is given. If the lesion begins to enlarge or the patient relapses, surgical excision is considered.

FUNGI

In patients with neutrophil deficits, fungal infections usually occur only after prolonged antibiotic treatment for bacterial infection. Thus, fungal infection typically is a nosocomial superinfection, and the particular fungus varies with the hospital environment. Current evidence[49] suggests an increasing incidence of nosocomial systemic fungal infections in both immunocompromised and immunocompetent hosts. In a 25-year experience at Johns Hopkins Hospital,[2736] CNS fungal infections in 57 patients were encountered: 16 *Aspergillus,* 27 *Candida,* and 14 *Cryptococcus.* Patients generally acquired cryptococcosis in the community, while aspergillosis and candidiasis were usually acquired during hospitalization.[2736] Common risk factors were neutropenia, steroid therapy, antibiotic therapy, and prolonged hospitalization.

The fungi usually invade the brain parenchyma, causing abscesses. When meningitis occurs, it is usually caused by *Candida.*[709] The organisms invade blood vessels and thus can cause cerebral infarction from thrombosis or cerebral hemorrhage from disruption of the blood vessel wall.[1609] In most instances, the organisms spread from lung to brain, although in some patients, they may spread from paranasal sinuses and cause rhinocerebral mucormycosis, for example (see the following).[1317,1609] In general, a diagnosis can be made only by biopsy of the involved area. Fungi should be considered a potential cause of CNS infections in any neutropenic patient who fails to respond to appropriate antibiotics. Recent reviews[49,81] address problems of fungal infections and their treatment in the

Table 10–11. **TREATMENT OF COMMON CENTRAL NERVOUS SYSTEM PATHOGENS IN PATIENTS WITH CANCER**

Organism	Recommended Therapy	Alternate Therapy[a]
Listeria monocytogenes	Ampicillin IV, 2 g q4h + gentamicin 1.25 mg/kg q6h	Cotrimoxazole IV 5 mg/kg q6h Vancomycin IV 1 g q12h
Streptococcus pneumoniae	Penicillin IV, 2 × 10^6 U q4h	Ceftriaxone 1–2 g q12h Chloramphenicol IV, 15 mg/kg q6h Vancomycin 1 g q12h
Cryptococcus neoformans	Amphotericin B IV 0.7–1.0 mg/kg per day plus flucytosine po; 75–100 mg/kg per day in 4 divided doses ± intraventricular amphotericin B	Fluconazole po 400 mg qd[b]
Escherichia coli	Ceftazidime 2 g q8h + gentamicin 1.25 mg IV q6h and gentamicin IT 0.1 mg/kg q12–24h	Chloramphenicol IV + gentamicin IV and IT Cotrimoxazole IV 5 mg/kg q6h trimethoprim + gentamicin IV and IT
Klebsiella pneumoniae	A third-generation cephalosporin + gentamicin IV 1.25 mg/kg q6h + gentamicin IT 0.1 mg/kg q12–24h	Chloramphenicol IV 50–100 mg/kg q6h + gentamicin IV and IT[c] Cotrimoxazole IV 5 mg/kg q6h trimethoprim + gentamicin IV and IT
Pseudomonas aeruginosa	Ceftazidime 2g q8h + tobramycin IV 1.25 mg/kg q6h + tobramycin IT 0.1 mg/kg	Imipenem 1g q6h + tobramycin IV and IT
Nocardia asteroides	Sulfadiazine IV 15 mg/kg[d] q6h or 1.5 g orally	Cotrimoxazole as above
Toxoplasma gondii	Sulfadiazine IV 15 mg/kg[d] + pyrimethamine 100 mg po × 1, then 25–50 mg qd	Clindamycin 600–900 mg q6–8h + pyrimethamine
Strongyloides stercoralis	Thiabendazole po 25 mg/kg q12h × 10 days	Ivermectin 200 mg/kg per day Albendazole po 400 mg qd × 10 days
Staphylococcus aureus	Oxacillin IV 2 g q4h[e]	Vancomycin IV 1 g q12h + rifampin 300 mg q12h
Staphylococcus epidermidis	Oxacillin IV 2 g q4h[c]	Vancomycin IV 1 g q12h + rifampin 300 mg q12h
Corynebacterium sp.	Penicillin IV 2 × 10^6 U q4h	Vancomycin 1 g q12h

IT = intrathecal; IV = intravenous; po = oral.

[a] Other semisynthetic penicillins, such as methicillin or nafcillin, may be substitutes for oxacillin; aminoglycosides, such as amikacin or tobramycin, may be substituted for gentamicin; cotrimoxazole is the same preparation as trimethoprim-sulfamethoxazole.

[b] Use only in patients unable to tolerate amphotericin B. This should not be used routinely for induction therapy.

[c] Vancomycin should be used initially; change to oxacillin if the organism is sensitive.

[d] Sulfadiazine IV or PO not commercially available in the United States. For information concerning sulfas, call the Centers for Disease Control, the Division of Parasitic Diseases at (404) 488-4928.

[e] If oxacillin resistance is common, vancomycin should be used initially; change to oxacillin if the organism is sensitive.

Source: Adapted from Armstrong and Polsky,[82] p 169.

immunocompromised host. Newly recognized pathogens include *Fusarium, Curvularia,* and *Trichosporon* genera.[49]

Aspergillus. This fungus causes brain abscess, cerebral infarction, cerebral hemorrhage, or mycotic aneurysms.[11,276,2467] A primary infection is usually present in the lung, and about 10% of pulmonary infections disseminate to the brain. The disease can be isolated to the CNS, usually entering via the respiratory tract and paranasal sinuses. It typically appears in a terminally ill patient who is neutropenic, septic, and treated with multiple antibiotics. Brain involvement is suspected only when the patient becomes delirious or develops seizures or focal signs.[2467] The MR scan usually reveals lesions suggesting infarction in more than one vascular territory; MR angiography or conventional angiography may give evidence of multiple vascular occlusions. The CSF is usually normal except for a slightly elevated protein concentration, and no organisms are isolated. Although pulmonary, sinus,[2698] or skin lesions may be biopsied to suggest the diagnosis, a definitive diagnosis can be made only by a biopsy and isolation of the organism from the brain.

Serologic tests have been helpful in patients with leukemia who were followed prospectively. Radioimmunoassay and enzyme-linked immunosorbent assay tests for antigens also appear promising.

The differential diagnosis usually includes cerebral vascular disease that is due to embolization or cerebral abscess that is due to other organisms. Because most patients are terminally ill when the neurologic symptoms develop, an antemortem diagnosis is rarely made. Amphotericin B should be used empirically in the appropriate clinical situation and has been injected into the abscess cavity.[370] Early diagnosis of systemic or sinus infection may lead to the cure of the infection.[49,344,2056]

Mucorales. Mucormycosis (also called zygomycosis) is a usually fatal fungal infection caused by fungi from the Mucorales order. It occurs in patients with leukemia and lymphoma[1757] with neutropenia, as well as in patients with organ transplants, diabetic ketoacidosis, or metabolic acidosis that is due to renal failure or diarrhea.[49,60] The classic form of CNS mucormycosis is the syndrome of rhinocerebral mucormycosis.[514,720,869,1619] This infection begins in the nasopharynx or pharynx and spreads to involve the paranasal sinuses, the orbit, and then the frontal lobe of the brain. The clinical findings first suggest sinusitis followed by unilateral proptosis, ptosis, and ophthalmoplegia. Decreased vision occurs late. Once the brain is involved, the patient develops seizures, focal neurologic signs, or delirium. Careful examination of the nose, nasopharynx, or palate may reveal a black, necrotic ulcer that, when scraped, will yield the organism. *Aspergillus* hyphae may cause the same clinical symptoms, but the two organisms are easily differentiated: the Mucorales forms are irregular, wide, ribbonlike hyphae that branch at right or nearly right angles, whereas the *Aspergillus,* with uniform caliber and cross septations, branch at acute angles. Successful treatment of rhinocerebral mucormycosis by surgical debridement of infectious tissue, treatment of the underlying condition, and parenteral amphotericin B is now common, but in the cancer population, the disorder is usually fatal.

Mucormycosis also causes brain abscesses by hematogenous dissemination from pulmonary lesions. The single or multiple necrotic mass lesions resemble those caused by aspergillosis. Occasionally, they occlude cerebral vessels and stimulate cerebral infarction.[869] The diagnosis of this particular form of mucormycosis is rarely made antemortem and can only be established by brain biopsy. As with aspergillosis, the CSF is usually normal. In patients suffering from acute cerebral disease, the presence of the organism in skin or in lung is sufficient to warrant treatment.

Candida. The most frequent systemic fungal infections, *Candida albicans* and *C. tropicalis,* in cancer patients[2765] cause meningitis or, more commonly, meningoencephalitis.[709,953] Multiple small abscesses are scattered throughout the cerebral cortex. Vertebral osteomyelitis has also been reported.[2361] *Candida* may also cause vascular occlusions with infarction. The organisms usually disseminate hematogenously from the GI tract, from infected IV catheters, or from other sources of *Candida* sepsis. Unlike aspergillosis and mucormycosis, pleocytosis, elevated protein, and depressed glucose concentrations are often present. CSF cultures may not test positive unless large samples of CSF (20–30 mL) are concentrated and the sediment cultured. If repeated lumbar punctures fail to reveal an organism, cisternal puncture may be positive. In some instances, the organism is never identified in the CSF even when the patient suffers from clinical meningitis.[709] In selected cases, biopsy of the meninges may be helpful. The biopsy specimen should be taken from a symptomatic area,[436] usually at the base of the brain where the infected material tends to concentrate or where enhancement is present on MR scan.[436] In one patient, a hemispheral biopsy failed to reveal the organism even though the patient died of candidal meningitis a few weeks later. The diagnosis of a CNS infection may be helped by the fact that disseminated candidiasis sometimes causes fever, rash, and myalgias from direct infection of muscle.[70] The treatment is amphotericin B and flucytosine.

Splenectomy or B-Cell Abnormalities

Table 10–12 lists the common infections in Hodgkin's disease patients who have undergone a splenectomy and in patients with immunoglobulin deficits (i.e., B-cell abnormalities). The most common infections are bacterial meningitis (most often acute pneumococcal meningitis), usually caused by the encapsulated organisms that cause meningitis in the general population.

BACTERIA

Streptococcus pneumoniae. Pneumococcal meningitis usually occurs in patients with Hodgkin's disease who have undergone splenectomy, after intensive RT and chemotherapy, or in patients with chronic lymphocytic leukemia or multiple myeloma. It may also attack a patient with a CSF fistula following surgery. The splenectomized patient may be in complete remission or cured of the cancer when the meningitis begins, usually with the typically fulminant onset found in the general population. The CSF is purulent, with many hundreds or thousands of neutrophils, but in some patients, WBCs may be absent from the CSF early in the illness, even when the peripheral WBC count is normal. The glucose concentration is typically low, and the protein concentration is high. Organisms are usually visible in Gram's stains; if not, capsular antigen may be demonstrated by counterimmunoelectrophoresis of CSF or urine. The organism tends to cause a vasculitis that often leads to brain infarction with attendant focal neurologic signs.

The drug of choice is penicillin in high doses, and patients should be switched to this drug if they were started on ampicillin before the diagnosis was established. If the diagnosis is made early and effective treatment begun, the patient usually recovers. Permanent sequelae are uncommon. Polyvalent vaccine against pneumococcal polysaccharide is about 80% effective in preventing pneumonia in healthy adults, but almost 40% of bacteremic pneumococcal infections found at MSKCC were caused by nonvaccine serotypes.[82] Because the vaccine is safe, however, it should be given to patients who are at high risk for developing pneumococcal infections, particularly patients who have undergone splenectomy or who have chronic lymphocytic leukemia. The Infec-

Table 10–12. **MENINGITIS IN PATIENTS WITH SPLENECTOMY OR B-CELL ABNORMALITIES (HYPOGAMMAGLOBULINEMIA)**

	Bacteria	Fungi	Parasites	Viruses
Splenectomy	*Streptococcus pneumoniae* *Haemophilus influenzae*—rare *Neisseria meningitidis*—rare	—	—	—
Hypogammaglobulinemia	Same	—	—	Echovirus Coxsackie B

tious Disease Service at MSKCC recommends that high-risk patients receive prophylactic penicillin (penicillin V), 250 mg bid, in addition to the pneumococcal vaccine.

Although *H. influenzae* type B and *N. meningitides* should be common CNS infections in the same population vulnerable to pneumococcal infections, these two organisms rarely cause CNS infections in the cancer population. No instance of either infection in the CNS has been reported at MSKCC.

Cerebrospinal Fluid–Surface Communication

Table 10–13 lists the common infections in cancer patients with a CSF–surface communication caused by either intraventricular shunts or reservoirs or from surgery around the head or spine.

BACTERIA

Staphylococci are the common offenders when a communication develops between the CSF and the surface.[2320] In the patient with cancer and a CSF–surface anatomic connection, *Staphylococcus aureus* usually causes an acute or subacute infection with headache, fever, stiff neck, and abundant WBCs and organisms in the CSF. The diagnosis is suggested on Gram's stain, and the infection can be treated with oxacillin, nafcillin, or methicillin. For occasional resistant strains, vancomycin is the drug of choice.

A more common clinical problem is infection of a ventricular shunt[63,2111] or an Ommaya device[1917] (see Chapter 7). These infections are usually indolent, and the patient may be entirely asymptomatic or suffer only from malaise. The CSF usually, but not always, contains an increased number of WBCs, predominantly mononuclear. The organism may or may not be seen on Gram's stain but grows on culture. In patients with Ommaya devices, pleocytosis and organisms may be identified from ventricular but not lumbar CSF or vice versa. If the clinician suspects CNS infection in this setting, both ventricular and lumbar CSF must be cultured. Because the infection is so indolent and because staphylococci commonly reside on the skin, the positive culture may represent contamination and not a true CNS infection. Thus, unless other clear evidence of CNS infection such as fever, headache, or pleocytosis is noticed, treatment should not be undertaken until cultures have been positive on more than one occasion. These infections are rarely an emergency, and treatment, based on the sensitivity of the organism, should be delivered both parenterally and directly into the shunt or reservoir. It should be continued for 4 to 6 weeks. In some instances, direct treatment of the indwelling device may preserve it,[1169,1584] but often it cannot be sterilized. If it must be removed, a new device may be placed at the time the old one is removed. Parenteral antibiotics prevent the new device from being contaminated by the organism.

Propionibacterium acnes, an anaerobic Gram-positive rod, is present on the skin of healthy individuals and is a common cause of Ommaya device infections. The organism

Table 10–13. **CENTRAL NERVOUS SYSTEM INFECTIONS WITH CEREBROSPINAL FLUID–SURFACE COMMUNICATION**

	Bacteria	Fungi	Parasites	Viruses
Meningitis	Enteric bacilli *Staphylococcus aureus* Coagulase-negative staphylococcus *Propionibacterium acnes*	*Candida*	Trichomonadida	—
Meningoencephalitis	Same	Same	Same	—
Abscess	Same	Same	—	—

causes an indolent infection that may be characterized by only a few cells in the CSF, a feeling of generalized malaise, and a positive culture, but it can also cause a clinically significant meningitis[2631] or brainstem encephalitis.[371] Like coagulase-negative staphylococcus, this organism may contaminate cultures, so that repeatedly positive cultures are necessary to be sure that the CSF is actually infected. Specific treatment depends on sensitivity testing, and as with other infected shunts or reservoirs, drugs should be delivered both parenterally and directly into the reservoir. Drugs successful in treating Ommaya devices have included oxacillin, methicillin, and vancomycin. Daily treatment begins with 25 mg of oxacillin or methicillin and increases to 50 to 100 mg/24 hours. Vancomycin has also been reported to be effective at 75 mg/24 hours. Serious reactions to an oxacillin or methicillin injection are rare. Throbbing headaches may occur as a complication of intraventricular injection of vancomycin. Other drugs such as chloramphenicol have been instilled into the ventricle to treat infections, but I have no experience with these agents. An unusual complication of infected ventriculosystemic shunts is immune-complex–mediated nephritis ("shunt nephritis") caused by coagulase-negative staphylococcus and *P. acnes*.[829]

Anaerobic organisms that occasionally cause meningitis or abscesses in the cancer population include *Fusobacterium, Bacteroides, Clostridium,* and *Actinomyces* species. The infections can occur either with a CSF–surface communication or are seen in severely neutropenic patients. Both CSF and CNS tissues (when available at biopsy) should be cultured for anaerobic as well as aerobic organisms. No special handling of CSF by the clinician is necessary for anaerobic cultures. The treatment depends on the sensitivity of the organisms. Metronidazole, 500 mg qid, may be an effective treatment of many anaerobic organisms causing either meningitis or brain abscess.

PARASITES

Parasites may invade the nervous system via a CSF fistula in patients with cancer. We have encountered one patient with *Trichomonas* meningitis[1702] whose nervous system was invaded via a GI tract-CNS fistula.

Other Infections

Two infections, infectious endocarditis and "malignant" external otitis, also begin outside the brain and secondarily affect the CNS but do not easily fit the classification used in this chapter.

INFECTIOUS ENDOCARDITIS

Bacterial endocarditis in patients with cancer is less common than NBTE, but the increasing use of indwelling venous catheters, with their high rate of infection,[1007] suggests that this disorder will be encountered more commonly in the future. Neurologic complications of infective endocarditis have been reviewed extensively.[1147,1528,2102] These include cerebral emboli causing either symptoms of a diffuse encephalopathy or focal neurologic signs, the same as those in NBTE (see Chapter 9). Because the emboli are infected, they may weaken the blood vessel walls in which they lodge and cause mycotic aneurysms with rupture and subarachnoid hemorrhage,[2686] as well as meningitis, meningoencephalitis, or brain abscess. Seizures are common. The usual infecting organisms are streptococci, but many other bacteria and fungi also can be responsible.[980,2203] The diagnostic clues to the presence of infective endocarditis include conjunctival petechiae, Roth's spots, other retinal hemorrhages, and Osler's nodes. "Splinter" hemorrhages under the nails are nonspecific, as are Roth's spots and retinal hemorrhages, but an Osler's node may establish the diagnosis. All of these changes may also be seen in patients with NBTE.[2194]

"MALIGNANT" EXTERNAL OTITIS

Malignant (also "invasive" or "necrotizing") external otitis is an unusual infection that occurs primarily in elderly diabetic patients,[155,2235] rarely in neutropenic children, and occasionally in young adults. The usual infecting organism is *P. aeruginosa,* but other bacteria (e.g., *S. aureus*) or fungi (an *Aspergillus* species) also cause the disorder. Severe ear pain is often referred to the temporomandibular joint, which impinges on the external ear canal, and sometimes, to the temporal and occipital areas of the head. The pain, often nocturnal, is usually associated with granulation tissue or pus and edema in the external auditory canal. The tympanic membrane is intact. After days to weeks of local discomfort, the patient develops facial nerve paralysis caused by inflammation at the stylomastoid foramen. As the infection invades more centrally, other cranial nerves that exit from the skull base, including glossopharyngeal, vagus, and spinal accessory nerves (jugular foramen syndrome), and the hypoglossal nerve may be affected. Less commonly, mycotic aneurysms, cerebral venous sinus thrombosis, or meningitis complicate the course. Because the disorder is so indolent, it is often mistaken for tumor invasion rather than infection, and the CT scan showing bone destruction may support the incorrect diagnosis. An ear culture confirms the diagnosis, and appropriate antibiotics are the effective treatment,[571] e.g., ceftazidime and tobramycin or ciprofloxacin for *P. aeruginosa.*

CHAPTER 11

METABOLIC AND NUTRITIONAL COMPLICATIONS OF CANCER

Metabolic and nutritional disorders are common in patients with cancer (Table 11–1). Metabolic disorders occur when: (1) The cancer invades vital organs such as liver or kidney, whose normal function is detoxification. The organ damage leads to the accumulation of toxic products that cause neurologic dysfunction.[231,232] (2) The patient may be taking a number of drugs for the treatment of the cancer or its symptoms that interfere with or alter the body's metabolism, or the tumor itself may produce substances that impairthe metabolic function of normal organs or tissues.[2575]

Malnutrition can be caused by the disease itself or by its treatment.[199,555,2575] Taste buds can be affected, leading to a dysgeusia* that sometimes alters total food intake, or specific nutritional disorders may arise even when the patient continues to eat.[632] Several malignancies directly cause weight loss and malnutrition (i.e., cancer cachexia) even in individuals who appear to be eating an adequate and well-balanced diet.[1810]

Metabolic and nutritional disorders frequently affect the CNS. Interference with brain metabolism induces a metabolic encephalopathy with confusion, disorientation, lethargy, and sometimes even stupor or coma, although the brain may be structurally normal. Specific nutritional disturbances may affect particular areas of brain function, such as when a vitamin-B deficiency causes brainstem encephalopathy.[729,1912]

Peripheral nerves are less commonly affected than the brain by metabolic or nutritional disorders, but both diffuse and focal neuropathies can result. For instance, polyneuropathy can be caused by uremia, vitamin-B deficiency, or critical illness.[2806,2902] Cachexia can cause focal peroneal nerve palsy by decushioning the nerve so that it is vulnerable to compression behind the head of the fibula.[2466]

*References 309, 593, 773, 1323, 1514, 1641, 1704, 1957.

Table 11–1. **NERVOUS SYSTEM COMPLICATIONS OF CANCER CAUSED BY METABOLIC AND NUTRITIONAL DISORDERS**

Brain
- Diffuse encephalopathy
  - Lethargic
  - Agitated
- Focal encephalopathy

Spinal cord
- Nutritional myelopathy

Peripheral nerves
- Polyneuropathy
- Focal neuropathy(ies)

Neuromuscular junction and muscle
- Nutritional myopathy

Muscles also may be affected by metabolic or nutritional disorders. Most patients with cancer who lose weight do not develop specific abnormalities of muscle function; although they may complain of "weakness," they usually mean fatigability and are not weak.[329] A few patients develop specific nutritional myopathies that lead to weakness of large proximal muscle groups.[944,1157] Some authorities report that the neuromuscular junction may be adversely affected in malnourished patients, but evidence is not compelling.[1157]

DELIRIUM ASSOCIATED WITH CANCER

Pain is the most common reason for neurologic consultation at Memorial Sloan-Kettering Cancer Center (MSKCC); next is an altered mental state.[461,798] In some, the altered mental state results from focal abnormalities of cognitive function such as aphasia, apraxia, or agnosia and is caused by brain or leptomeningeal metastases. In most, however, the disorder is more diffuse. These patients are delirious; that is, they have clouding of consciousness with reduced capacity to shift focus and sustain attention to environmental stimuli (Table 11–2). Delirium can result from either structural or metabolic brain disease or, in many instances, from both. In an unpublished survey of 100 consecutive admissions to the medical service at MSKCC, careful neurologic evaluation revealed that 15 patients suffered from encephalopathy, presumably of metabolic origin.

Table 11–2. **DIAGNOSTIC CRITERIA FOR DELIRIUM (*DSM-III-R*)***

1. Reduced ability to maintain attention to external stimuli (e.g., questions must be repeated because attention wanders) or to appropriately shift attention to new external stimuli (e.g., perseverates answer to a previous question)
2. Disorganized thinking, as indicated by rambling, irrelevant, or incoherent speech
3. At least two of the following:
   A. Reduced level of consciousness, e.g., difficulty keeping awake during examination
   B. Perceptual disturbance: misinterpretations, illusions, or hallucinations
   C. Disturbance of sleep–wakefulness cycle, with insomnia or daytime sleepiness
   D. Increased or decreased psychomotor activity
   E. Disorientation to time, place, or person
   F. Memory impairment, e.g., inability to learn new material, such as the names of several unrelated objects, after 5 minutes or to remember past events, such as the history of the current episode of illness
4. Clinical features develop over a short period of time (usually hours to days) and tend to fluctuate over the course of a day
5. Either A or B:
   A. Evidence from the history, physical examination, or laboratory tests of a specific organic factor (or factors) judged to be etiologically related to the disturbance
   B. In the absence of such evidence, an etiologic organic factor can be presumed if the disturbance cannot be accounted for by any nonorganic mental disorder, e.g., manic episode accounting for agitation and sleep disturbance

Source: The American Psychiatric Association,[43] p 103, with permission.

These figures are surprisingly close to those reported by Engel and Romano[726] in a similar study conducted on the medical wards of a general hospital. Furthermore, the primary physician and nursing staff were aware that only one-third of their patients were delirious. In a study of 252 consecutive admissions involving 162 patients at the Johns Hopkins Oncology Center, a change in mental status was found in 16% of the patients. In 6%, the cause was believed to be metabolic.[920] In another study of 87 consecutive admissions to Johns Hopkins Oncology Center, approximately 26% of the patients scored in the cognitively impaired range on the Mini-Mental State Examination.[813] Some years later, a 3-day prevalence study of 50 inpatients at the same center found 14% to be cognitively impaired.[813]

In a recent MSKCC study, a single cause of delirium was identified in only about one-third of patients; the other two-thirds suffered multifactorial delirium. When a single cause was identified, structural disease, in the form of multiple brain metastases, bacterial meningitis, or cerebral infarcts accounted for the delirium in half the patients, and metabolic brain disease accounted for the other half (Table 11–3).[2617]

Other series are similar. In one series of 229 elderly patients in a general hospital, 22% were delirious. A single definite cause was identified in only 36% of these, and a single cause was probable in another 20%. The remaining patients each had an average of 2.8 causative factors.[827] Delirious patients had a longer hospital stay and were more likely to die or be institutionalized than nondelirious patients.[827] Among the 67% in whom the cause of the altered mental state was multifactorial, the major contributing factors were more often metabolic than structural; psychoactive drugs and single- or multiple-organ failure were the most common factors contributing (Table 11–4). Structural diseases of the brain leading to delirium are discussed in Chapters 5, 7, 10, and 12. Several reviews address the causes,[77,234,1576] epidemiology,[1546] clinical symptoms and signs,[1548,2559] diagnosis,[1547,2559] and treatment of delirium[1547,1718,2455a] in the general population as well as in the cancer population.[813,2773a]

Table 11–3. **SINGLE CAUSES OF DELIRIUM IN 140 PATIENTS WITH CANCER**

Poor oxygen supply		11
Hypoxia	2	
Hypoperfusion (shock)	6	
Disseminated intravascular coagulation	3	
Organ failure		3
Liver	2	
Kidney	1	
Hyperosmolality		2
Brain metastases		19
Other focal lesions (bacterial meningitis, cerebral infarction)		2
Drugs (steroids, opioids)		6
Total		*43*

Source: Data from Tuma and DeAngelis,[2617] p 288, with permission.

Table 11–4. **MAJOR FACTORS CONTRIBUTING TO DELIRIUM IN 140 PATIENTS WITH CANCER**

Factors	% of Patients
Drugs	59
Organ failure	51
Fluid electrolyte imbalance	45
Infection	45
Hypoxia	35
Brain lesions	21
Environment	21

Source: Data from Tuma and DeAngelis,[2617] p 288, with permission.

METABOLIC BRAIN DISEASE IN PATIENTS WITH CANCER

Metabolic brain disease or metabolic encephalopathy is defined as an abnormality of brain function resulting from interference with brain metabolism by extracerebral factors. The clinical result is often delirium or an acute confusional state. Occasionally, focal signs such as ataxia may predominate, confusing the diagnosis.[1355] Extracerebral disorders that lead to metabolic brain disease (Table

Table 11–5. **CAUSES OF METABOLIC AND NUTRITIONAL ENCEPHALOPATHY IN PATIENTS WITH CANCER**

Drugs*
- Opioids
- Sedatives

Sepsis*
Oxygen deprivation*
- Hypoxia
- Ischemia

Fluid and electrolyte imbalance
- Calcium
- Phosphorus
- Magnesium

Osmolar imbalance
- Hypo-osmolality (hyponatremia)
- Hyperosmolality (hyperglycemia)

Hypoglycemia
Uremia
Hepatic failure
Vitamin deficiencies
- Thiamine (Wernicke's encephalopathy)
- Niacin (pellagra)

Hypercarbia
Endocrine disorders
- Adrenal
- Thyroid

*Particularly common in patients with cancer.

11–5) include deprivation of essential substrates, primarily glucose or oxygen; failure of vital organs; fluid, electrolyte, and acid-base abnormalities; and ingestion of toxic drugs. Because the brain is so sensitive to perturbations of its internal milieu, a bewildering variety of systemic illnesses can cause neurologic dysfunction. These disorders are classified in recent publications[77,231,256,729] that discuss their diagnosis and treatment extensively. In this chapter, those systemic abnormalities that are likely to cause metabolic brain disease in patients with cancer are emphasized. The pathophysiology of metabolic brain disease is discussed in detail elsewhere.[77]

Metabolic encephalopathy is an important neurologic complication of cancer for two reasons:

1. It is common. As indicated previously, delirium is a common symptom in both the cancer and general hospital populations, and in more than 50% of delirious patients, the encephalopathy is metabolic in origin.
2. It can often be treated. If the cause is treated, a patient suffering from a toxic or metabolic disorder can recover normal neurologic function.

Table 11–5 classifies the metabolic encephalopathies; those encountered most frequently in patients with cancer are indicated by an asterisk. The physician must recognize, however, that metabolic brain disease often has no single cause but results from the concurrence of multiple systemic metabolic abnormalities, no one of which alone causes brain dysfunction. A positive consequence of the multiplicity of mild systemic metabolic abnormalities is that, in many instances, if one of the abnormalities can be identified and reversed, the patient often recovers.

Incidence

The exact incidence of metabolic encephalopathy in patients with cancer is not known. The incidence or prevalence of delirium or an acute confusional state is more clearly evaluable. A recent study[1548] of 325 elderly patients admitted to a teaching hospital indicated that at initial evaluation, 10% exhibited symptoms that match the *Diagnostic and Statistical Manual of Mental Disorders,* Third Edition, Revised *(DSM-III-R)* criteria for delirium (see Table 11–2). Furthermore, 31% of the previously normal patients developed delirium during their hospitalization. Although not associated with an increased risk of mortality, delirium was associated with a prolonged hospital stay and an increased risk of institutional placement among community-dwelling patients. Only 4% of the affected patients experienced resolution of all symptoms before hospital discharge, and only 20% had resolved all symptoms by 3 months after discharge. In this population, poor prognostic factors included cognitive impairment on admission, age more than 80 years, cancer on admission, symptomatic infection, male sex, and use of neuroleptics or opioids.

A recent MSKCC study[2617] defined the following risk factors that predispose patients with cancer to metabolic encephalopathy: The cancer is usually disseminated and the patients are older, with a mean age of 64 years. Although old age is a risk factor for the development of delirium (i.e., delirium is more frequent in older patients), the occurrence of delirium in a young person with cancer is a poor prognostic sign for survival, presumably because a more severe systemic insult is required to cause encephalopathy in a younger brain. In addition to younger age, hypoxia and kidney or liver failure are major risk factors for death. Approximately 33% of delirious patients had an altered mental status at the time of hospital admission. Delirium was associated with a 25% mortality rate within 30 days and a 44% mortality rate within 6 months. Nevertheless, two-thirds of the patients were improved by the time of discharge.

An earlier MSKCC study attempted to identify the frequency and causes of metabolic encephalopathy in patients referred for neurologic consultation. In that study of 721 consecutive neurologic consultations during 5 months, 132 patients showed signs of diffuse encephalopathy.[461] Of these, a final diagnosis of metabolic encephalopathy was made in more than 60% (Fig. 11–1); the other 40% suffered from metastatic, vascular, or infectious diseases. These figures undoubtedly underestimate the true frequency of metabolic encephalopathy in hospitalized patients because minor cognitive changes were probably overlooked, as is indicated by our study of consecutive medical admissions, and because when the cause of the encephalopathy was obvious, particularly from drug overdose, hypoxia, and hypercalcemia, the patients were often managed without neurologic consultation. These figures, therefore, can be considered the minimal frequency and probably skew the list of causes toward those most difficult to diagnose. Narcotic drug overdose, hypercalcemia, and hepatic encephalopathy are probably more common causes of encephalopathy than are recognized.

Clinical Signs

Cognitive and behavioral changes characterize all patients with metabolic brain disease. In the beginning, the changes are often so subtle that they escape recognition by the patient's family or physicians. Such patients may have mild difficulty concentrating and be unable to sustain attention. They may appear uninterested or have difficulty understanding explanations of impending medical procedures. Some may appear apathetic, preferring to lie in bed sleeping or staring at the wall rather than reading, watching television, or being active in other ways. If the patients read, they may find themselves spending an unusual amount of

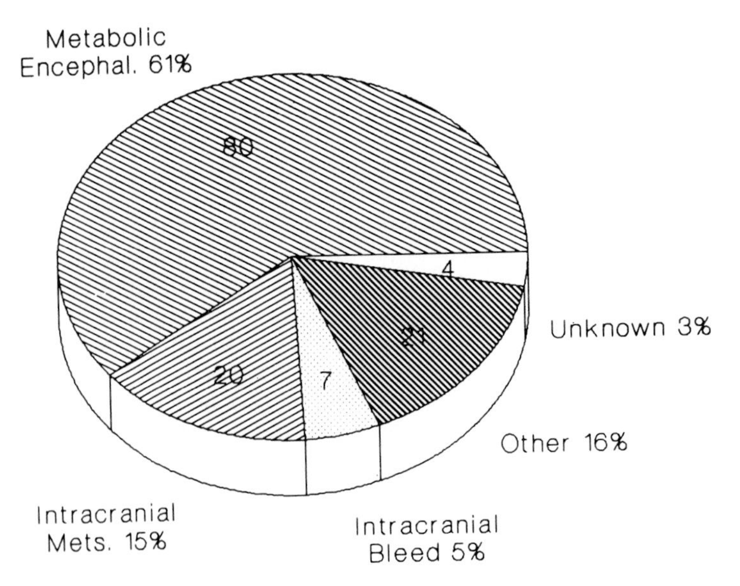

Figure 11–1. Causes of altered mental state in 132 inpatients with cancer in whom neurologic consultation was requested. (From Clouston et al,[461] p 270, with permission.)

time on one paragraph or one page. Often the paragraph must be reread several times before the contents can be related to a questioner. As the illness progresses, behavioral abnormalities become more apparent. Apathy may worsen; patients may become lethargic, drowsy, and unable to attend to external stimuli for an appreciable time. On the other hand, some become restless, develop insomnia, or have vivid nightmares; they may be so distractible that they cannot concentrate or effectively communicate to others. Some patients appear silly or frivolous during the physician's explanation of their illness; conversations in the hall or other noises in the room distract them from the matter at hand. Some become fearful, anxious, and depressed. Patients who retain insight into the problem may express fear of going crazy.

The simplest and best-validated test for abnormalities of cognitive function at the bedside is the Mini-Mental State Examination (Table 11–6). A delirium-symptom interview covering areas similar to the Mini-Mental State Examination, such as orientation, but stressing symptoms, has been reported to yield a sensitivity of .90 and a specificity of .80 when compared with the judgment of a neurologist or psychiatrist. Both examinations can be conducted by lay interviewers.[30,1582]

Table 11–7 categorizes the clinical findings in an MSKCC study of 140 patients with cancer and altered mental state. Nearly half of the patients were alert or hyperalert and

Table 11–6. **MINI-MENTAL STATE EXAMINATION**

Maximum Score	Patient's Score	
		Orientation
5	( )	What is the (year) (season) (date) (day) (month)?
5	( )	Where are we: (state) (county) (town) (hospital) (floor)?
		Registration
3	( )	Name three objects, 1 second to say each, then ask the patient to repeat all three after you have said them. Give 1 point for each correct answer. Continue repeating all three objects until the patient learns all three. Count trials and record.
		Attention and Calculation
5	( )	Serial 7's. One point for each correct response. Stop after five answers. Alternatively, spell *world* backward.
		Recall
3	( )	Ask for the three objects named in *Registration*. Give one point for each correct answer.
		Language
2	( )	Name a pencil and watch.
1	( )	Repeat the following: "No ifs, ands, or buts."
3	( )	Follow a three-stage command: "Take paper in your right hand, fold it in half, and put it on the floor."
1	( )	Read and obey the following: "CLOSE YOUR EYES."
1	( )	Write a sentence.
1	( )	Copy a design.
30	( )	

Assess level of consciousness along a continuum.

Alert Drowsy Stupor Coma

Source: From Folstein et al,[814] pp 196-198, with permission.

Table 11–7. **CLINICAL FINDINGS IN 140 PATIENTS WITH CANCER AND WITH ALTERED MENTAL STATES**

Specific Findings	% of Patients
Consciousness	
Alert	46
Lethargic	52
Comatose	2
Cognition	
Memory poor	91
Inattentive	92
Disoriented	83
Dyscalculia	92
Language impaired	35
Behavior	
Agitated	44
Delusions and/or hallucinations	28
Motor Behavior	
Asterixis	36
Seizures	9
Focal signs	40

Source: Data from Tuma and DeAngelis,[2617] p 288, with permission.

the others were lethargic. Some cognitive abnormalities such as memory impairment, inattention, and dyscalculia were present in more than 90%, but language impairment was identified in only 35%. Over 80% were disoriented and about half displayed motor agitation. Delusions or hallucinations were identified in about one-third of patients; asterixis was present in a similar number. Seizures occurred in about 10%.

Other studies are similar.[1548] A study of 325 elderly patients admitted to a hospital for acute medical problems revealed *DSM-III-R* delirium in 38%. Hyperactive delirium (including hypervigilance, restlessness, fast or loud speech, irritability, and distractibility) occurred in 15%, whereas hypoactive delirium (including decreased alertness, slow speech, lethargy, psychomotor slowness, and apathy) was present in 19%. A mixed picture occurred in 52%, and 14% were neither excessively active nor excessively quiet.[1581] Single signs of delirium such as disorientation or lethargy are often present in elderly patients who do not meet all of the *DSM-III-R* criteria for full-blown delirium.[1546]

Laboratory Tests

Two types of laboratory tests are useful in the diagnosis of metabolic encephalopathy. The first type, which includes MR scan and lumbar puncture, identifies structural lesions of the brain and distinguishes them from metabolic causes of encephalopathy. The second type, which includes biochemical tests of blood and CSF, identifies specific metabolic abnormalities causing delirium.

The MR or CT scan is particularly useful in identifying metastatic brain tumors, abscesses, or subdural effusions. These disorders can affect the brain diffusely and may cause clinical signs and symptoms that mimic those of metabolic brain disease. A lumbar puncture can identify leptomeningeal metastases and infection. Some causes of metabolic brain illness, such as uremia or hypothyroidism, may be associated with an elevated CSF protein concentration; rarely, uremic encephalopathy has been reported to be associated with pleocytosis. The EEG can help to distinguish delirious patients from nondelerious patients (alpha frequency) and those with dementia (theta and delta activity); the EEG also can identify patients with nonconvulsive status epilepticus, whose mental state may mimic delirium.[1265,2873]

Tests of blood and CSF that may be helpful in the diagnosis of metabolic brain disease are listed in Table 11–8. Unless the cause of the encephalopathy is immediately apparent, the physician should err on the side of ordering too many rather than too few laboratory tests because unexpected and sometimes very helpful results may turn up.

Differential Diagnosis

The differential diagnosis of metabolic brain disease has two aspects. The physician must first determine whether the patient suffers from a metabolic or a structural cause of delirium. Having made that determination, the specific metabolic abnormality or abnormalities causing the neurologic dys-

Table 11–8. **LABORATORY EVALUATION OF THE DELIRIOUS PATIENT**

MR scan (gadolinium-enhanced)
  Metastases
  Infection
Lumbar puncture
  Leptomeningeal tumor
  Infection
EEG
Blood cultures
  Sepsis
  Septic emboli
Complete blood count
Blood gases—Po_2, pCO_2, pH
Electrolytes—Na, K, Ca, Mg, Po_4
BUN and creatinine
Lactate
Liver functions including NH_3
Coagulation profile—PT, PTT, FSP, D-dimer
Vitamin B_{12}, folic acid, thiamine
Endocrine tests—T4, cortisol
Glucose
Drug levels: theophylline, digoxin, anticonvulsants, and others

FSP = fibrin split products; PT = prothrombin time; PTT = partial thromboplastin time.

function must be found. Making the first judgment depends on both the clinical and laboratory evaluation. In general, patients should be suspected of suffering from metabolic brain disease if behavioral and cognitive changes represent the earliest or the only signs, if motor signs such as tremor and asterixis are bilateral and symmetric, and if pupillary reactions are preserved even if the patient is comatose. The patient should be suspected of suffering from structural brain disease, either alone or in combination with metabolic brain disease, if focal motor abnormalities (including focal seizures) occur; if specific changes in cognitive function, such as aphasia, acalculia, or agnosia, appear out of proportion to a general overall decrease in mental state; or if the patient is at particular risk for contracting one of the neurologic complications of cancer that may mimic metabolic brain disease, particularly disseminated intravascular coagulation or meningitis. Although clinical signs often are helpful, too much overlap exists to confirm a diagnosis on clinical examination alone. Some patients with hepatic encephalopathy or hypoglycemia may develop hemiparesis or visual field abnormalities strongly suggesting structural brain disease, whereas other patients with multiple brain metastases may show nothing other than a global alteration of cognitive function. Thus, the laboratory tests described previously are essential to exclude structural disease of the nervous system and to ensure that the problem is definitely metabolic brain disease.

Specific Metabolic Causes of Delirium

DRUGS

Certain drugs associated with delirium in patients with cancer are listed in Table 11–9.

Both overdose and withdrawal of the drugs from the tolerant patient can cause delirium. In general, drug overdose causes a passive delirium characterized by drowsiness, inattention, disorientation, and excessive sleeping, whereas the delirium of drug withdrawal is more likely to be characterized by tremulousness, hallucinations, and sometimes seizures.[2807] These distinctions are not absolute. For example, high doses of opioids, particularly meperidine, can cause multifocal myoclonus and seizures, usually phenomena of drug withdrawal.[1318] Sometimes patients with

Table 11–9. **DRUGS ASSOCIATED WITH DELIRIUM IN 140 PATIENTS WITH CANCER**

Classes of Drugs	No. (%) of Patients Taking at Least One Drug
Opioids	75 (53.6)
Benzodiazepines	33 (23.6)
Corticosteroids	30 (21.5)
H_2 blockers	27 (19.3)
Anticholinergics	9 (6.4)
Anticonvulsants	8 (5.7)
Antihistamines	6 (4.3)
Others	12 (8.6)

drug withdrawal become lethargic and withdrawn rather than hyperactive. Furthermore, in many patients, especially those who are elderly, a standard dose—even when the measured blood level is within the "nontoxic" range—of a potentially toxic drug may cause encephalopathy, particularly when other potential causes of metabolic brain disease are also present.[323]

In any patient taking opioids, the drug should be considered as the sole cause or a contributor to a quiet, diffuse encephalopathy. Long-acting opioid agents, such asmethadone and levorphanol (Levo-Dromoran), can accumulate gradually over days, particularly as the dose increases. After days with little pain relief, the patient may suddenly become confused and disoriented, lapsing into stupor or coma. Other characteristic signs are indicated in Table 11–10. This disorder is particularly likely at the time when pain has finally been relieved. Many patients who are wide awake while receiving large doses of opioids that fail to relieve pain may become confused and lethargic on the same dose if pain is alleviated either by the drugs or by other means.

Table 11–10. **CLINICAL FEATURES OF OPIOID INTOXICATION AND WITHDRAWAL**

Intoxication	Withdrawal
Stupor or coma	Anxiety, restlessness
Symmetric, pinpoint, reactive pupils	Insomnia
Hypothermia	Chills, hot flashes
Bradycardia	Myalgias, arthralgias
Hypotension	Nausea, anorexia
Skin cool, moist	Abdominal cramping
Hypoventilation (respiratory slowing, irregular breathing, apnea)	Vomiting, diarrhea
Pulmonary edema	Yawning
Seizures (meperidine, propoxyphene, morphine)	Dilated pupils
Reversal with naloxone	Tachycardia, hypertension (mild)
	Hyperthermia (mild), diaphoresis, lacrimation, rhinorrhea
	Piloerection
	Spontaneous ejaculation

Source: From Benowitz,[185] p 420, with permission.

A stuporous or comatose patient receiving opioids should be given an opioid antagonist such as naloxone. Dilute one ampule (0.4 mg) in 10 mL of saline and inject gradually over several minutes while monitoring the patient's respiratory rate, pupils, and state of consciousness. No more drug than necessary to restore respiration and slightly arouse the patient should be given; in a tolerant patient, larger doses can cause acute withdrawal syndromes and certainly exacerbate pain. Naloxone is a short-acting drug, and many patients who are aroused from stupor relapse into that state if left alone. The relapse can be prevented either by a slow naloxone drip or by careful observation, repeating the naloxone as required.

Opioid withdrawal can also cause delirium, usually in tolerant patients whose pain is successfully relieved by another mechanism. Because these patients are not psychologically dependent on opioids, they stop requesting them once the pain is relieved. The physician must ensure that the drug is tapered rather than abruptly discontinued. The patients, being naive concerning the effects of opioids, generally fail to recognize the premonitory symptoms of withdrawal, such as runny nose, myalgias, yawning, and diarrhea. They frequently tell the doctor that they believe they are getting the flu. If the doctor is as naive as the patient, florid signs of withdrawal (see Table 11–10) may ensue before the cause is recognized and the opioids are restarted at lower doses.

Repetitive doses of meperidine, which is metabolized to normeperidine, can cause delirium, multifocal myoclonus, and seizures, particularly in patients with renal failure.[1318] Consequently, any patient receiving meperidine who becomes tremulous should be carefully observed for seizures and should be switched to another agent. Because of its potential toxicity, meperedine is not preferred to manage acute or chronic cancer pain.

Other drugs, such as benzodiazepines, are rarely the sole cause of delirium in patients with cancer but frequently contribute to it, particularly in patients receiving other drugs. In critically ill patients, even short-acting drugs may accumulate because the patient's ability to detoxify them is impaired. Measurement of blood levels of the drug may assist the physician in determining if a given drug is contributing to the patient's encephalopathy.[1679a]

HYPOXIA-ISCHEMIA-HYPOGLYCEMIA (SUBSTRATE DEPRIVATION)

The average adult brain weighs about 1400 g, about 2% of body weight, but consumes about 20% of the body's oxygen and 65% of glucose production. Cortical gray matter, only 20% of total brain mass, uses about 75% of total brain oxygen. The brain uses no exogenous substrate other than glucose, and 85% of all glucose utilization is aerobic. Consequently, the brain is exceedingly vulnerable to diminution of its supply of either oxygen or glucose. In partial compensation for this vulnerability, the brain can regulate its own blood supply by the process called "autoregulation." If systemic blood pressure falls, cerebral vessels dilate and the blood flow is maintained, at least until the mean pressure falls lower than 50 mm Hg. The brain also protects itself against hypertension by vasoconstricting as blood pressure rises, thus preventing increases in intracranial pressure. In individuals with normal pre-illness blood pressure, cerebral autoregulation maintains normal brain blood flow until blood pressure either falls lower than 50 mm Hg or rises higher than 160 mm Hg. These figures rise for chronically hypertensive persons. In the resting state, the brain and the heart also extract more oxygen from the blood than do other tissues. As its blood supply falls, the brain can extract even more oxygen.

Hypoxemia and hypoperfusion are common metabolic disorders in patients with cancer. Thus, it is not surprising that lack of oxygen or glucose should be important causes of delirium, given the vulnerability of the nervous system to hypoxemia and hypoperfusion (see Table 11–3). These two disorders are also common as associated factors in patients with other metabolic abnormalities.

Hypoxia. The term *hypoxia* implies deprivation of oxygen to the brain when blood flow is maintained. Hypoxia results either from a low partial pressure of oxygen (Po_2) delivered to the brain, such as occurs in pneumonia or other lung disease, or from a low oxygen-carrying capacity of blood, as in severe anemia. The healthy brain can tolerate a Po_2 down to about 40 mm Hg. Levels lower than 40 mm Hg can result in cerebral dysfunction as registered by the EEG and other sensitive tests of brain function, but clinical symptoms are not apparent until the Po_2 falls lower than 30 mm Hg. Nevertheless, even in healthy adults, at high altitudes a steady-state[1203] Po_2 of 30 mm Hg at rest can cause persistent brain dysfunction characterized by abnormalities of motor, intellectual, and psychological function. Oxygen deprivation at higher levels of Po_2 may cause neurologic dysfunction in patients who are already compromised by pre-existing brain disease.

The clinical symptoms of diffuse hypoxia resemble those of other metabolic brain diseases. Patients usually become inattentive to their surroundings and are somewhat drowsy.[799] Hyperactivity and hallucinations are uncommon. Judgment is impaired early. Early-morning headache is a frequent sign of both hypoxia and hypercarbia; tremor, asterixis, and multifocal myoclonus are generally late signs.

Ischemia. *Ischemia* is the term applied when the brain is deprived of blood, either focally or generally. Generalized or global ischemia occurs with cardiac arrest. Focal or multifocal ischemia occurs with occlusion of large vessels supplying the brain, as may occur in nonbacterial thrombotic endocarditis (NBTE), or of multiple small vessels in the brain, as in disseminated intravascular coagulation. In patients with ischemia, the brain is deprived not only of oxygen but also of glucose. Focal ischemia causes focal signs that depend on the part of the brain deprived of substrate. When the focal ischemia involves the right parietal lobe, an agitated delirium without motor or sensory signs is particularly likely.[1807] Patients with elevated cortisol levels associated with focal ischemia are more likely to be delirious.[1033]

Severe global ischemia, as in cardiac arrest, causes coma. In its most severe form, the patient is unconscious and does not respond in any way to painful stimuli. Brainstem reflexes and other motor responses are absent. In a less severe form, brainstem reflexes, including pupillary light responses, may be present, and the patient may develop extensor posturing either spontaneously or in response to noxious stimuli. The prognosis for recovery after cardiorespiratory arrest with global brain ischemia and coma is poor. In the patient with cancer, whose vital organs may already be compromised, the prognosis is even worse.

Multifocal ischemia usually results from either multiple small emboli from NBTE or from disseminated intravascular coagulation (see Chapter 9). Occasionally, it results from a vasculitis.

Hypoglycemia. Approximately two-thirds of the body's glucose consumption in the resting state occurs in the brain. During fasting, plasma glucose levels are maintained by the breakdown of liver glycogen or by new synthesis. Hypoglycemia without ischemia is an uncommon cause of metabolic encephalopathy in the patient with cancer. Fasting hypoglycemia can occur either when glucose synthesis is reduced or when utilization is increased. In patients with cancer, tumor in the liver, either primary hepatoma or metastatic cancer, can decrease glucose synthesis. Metastases to the adrenal glands or the pituitary gland may cause adrenal or growth hormone insufficiency, which may interfere with stimulation of hepatic glucose production. Increases in glucose utilization occur either when large retroperitoneal tumors metabolize large quantities of glucose or when tumors produce insulinlike growth factors that may mimic the biologic actions of insulin.[563] Typically, large retroperitoneal tumors induce repeated episodes of hypoglycemia, causing hunger, confusion, disorientation, and sometimes stupor or coma. Plasma glucose levels during these episodes are low and respond to infusion of glucose. Insulinlike growth factors, insulin, or insulin antibodies can be measured to determine the underlying cause. The disorder is best treated by treating the tumor, but glucagon has also been reported to be successful.[2279,2363]

Insulinomas, tumors of pancreatic beta cells, produce insulin and cause hypoglycemia. Hypoglycemia may also be caused by anti-insulin antibodies spontaneously produced by myeloma cells,[2141] or it may arise in patients with diabetes and cancer who are not eating well; their usual intake of insulin may lead to the disorder. Finally, hypoglycemia may follow the use of drugs such as pentamidine, used in patients with cancer for prophylaxis of *Pneumocystis carinii* pneumonia.

The clinical picture of hypoglycemia can range from a quiet delirium to coma, depending on the level of the glucose and the rapidity with which it has fallen. No clinically distinct characteristics allow the clinician to determine that an encephalopathy is due to hypoglycemia. In a few patients, hypoglycemia causes focal signs, especially hemiplegia, without clinical evidence of diffuse encephalopathy. Such findings can markedly delay the diagnosis, resulting in permanent neurologic disability. Prompt administration of glucose will reverse the focal signs and prevent permanent damage.

One of our patients suffering from a pelvic tumor that had been heavily irradiated developed a vascular occlusion with gangrene of one leg. Although her appetite was poor, she ate and drank. She was found one morning aphasic and hemiplegic. A fingerstick serum glucose level was less than 20 mg/dL; her hemiplegia and aphasia resolved immediately after she received 50 mL of 50% dextrose intravenously; she was then given an infusion of 5% dextrose in water. Later that day, while being observed by the nursing staff, she suddenly became diaphoretic and lethargic, appearing confused and refusing to speak. Right-sided weakness was not present. Again, her glucose level was low, and she responded to immediate IV glucose. Hypoglycemic episodes continued despite glucose infusions but ceased immediately after the gangrenous leg was amputated. The exact cause of the hypoglycemia remains unknown. In this patient, two episodes of hypoglycemia in the same day caused first a focal and then a diffuse encephalopathy. The patient showed no evidence either before or after the hypoglycemia of structural disease of the left hemisphere or any other portion of the brain.

The best treatment of substrate deprivation to the brain is prevention. Patients suffering from disorders that are likely to lead to low Po_2 can be supplemented with oxygen. Those with severe anemia should be given blood, increasing the oxygen-carrying capacity; blood pressure and cardiac output should

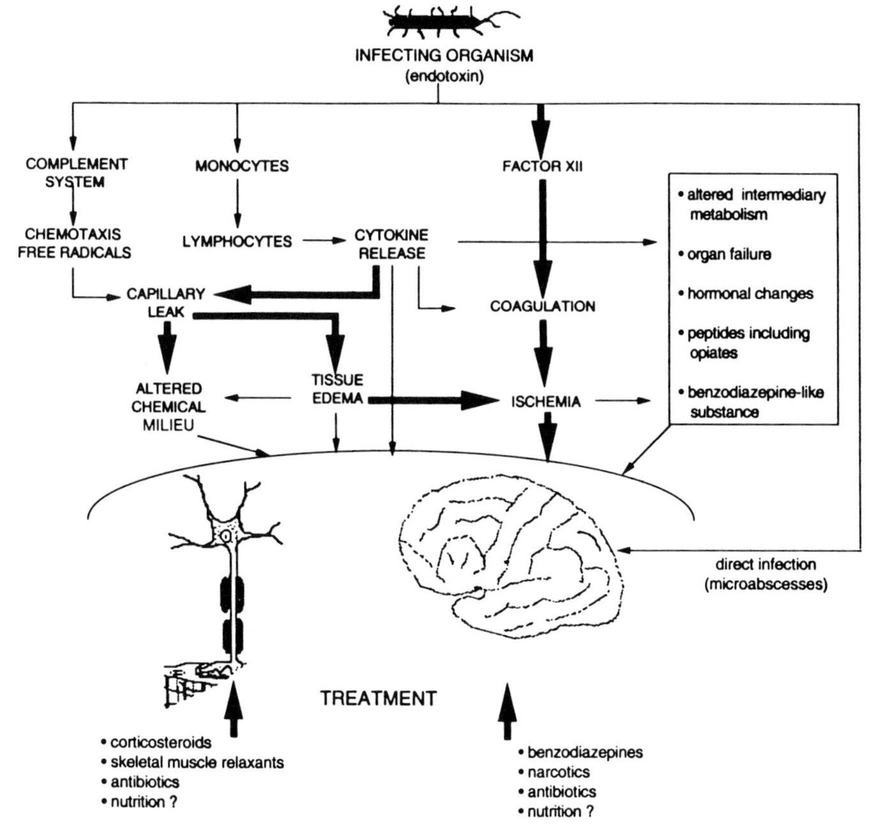

Figure 11–2. The multifactorial pathogenesis of septic encephalopathy. The infecting organism, the immune system, and drugs the patient is receiving all play a role. Mechanisms for septic encephalopathy and critical-illness polyneuropathy are suggested. *Arrows* pointing to the *curved line* indicate mechanisms that may apply to both the central and the peripheral nervous system. The *lower arrows* designate treatments that may affect these systems independently. The *heavy arrows* highlight the most likely mechanisms. These hypotheses are complex but involve the infecting organism's inducing chemical, microvascular, metabolic, or treatment effects that may act independently or in concert. The release of cytokines from macrophages and thence from T lymphocytes may directly affect the brain or act indirectly on the blood–brain barrier and microcirculation. Such vascular effects are abetted by activation of the complement system and factor XII. The encephalopathy may also be due to the failure of other organs or to direct infection of the brain, with the formation of microabscesses. Critical-illness polyneuropathy may be due to disturbances of the microcirculation of peripheral nerve through vascular effects similar to those affecting the brain. Various treatments used in the critical care unit may play an additive role for both the encephalopathy and polyneuropathy. (From Bolton et al,[257] p 96, with permission.)

be maintained. In patients likely to experience hypoglycemia from drugs or disease, glucose should be carefully monitored.

SEPSIS

The cause of septic encephalopathy is unknown. Possible pathogenetic mechanisms are shown in Fig. 11–2.[1787,2808,2872,2874] Blood–brain barrier derangement, permitting entry of otherwise excluded neurotoxic substances, has also been implicated as a potential mechanism.[1286] Regardless of the cause, many patients who become septic, with or without cancer, develop severe delirium.[257,2873] Septic encephalopathy is a relatively frequent sole cause of delirium in patients with cancer and an extremely common cofactor in patients with multifactorial delirium. The symptoms of delirium may precede the onset of fever or be present throughout the course of an afebrile septic episode. Characteristically, affected patients become confused and often agitated, exhibiting tremor, asterixis, and myoclonus.[1099] Many patients develop generalized seizures.[1027] The EEG is usually abnormal even in mildly encephalopathic patients, often before the clinical features become apparent.[2873] Abnormalities include excessive theta activity, slowing of background with prominent delta activity, and, occasionally, triphasic waves. The EEG shows suppression or burst-suppression activity when the encephalopathy becomes severe enough. Encephalopathy is more common with Gram-negative infections but can occur with any form of sepsis. Appropriate antibiotic treatment usually leads to its resolution. Long-term treatment with anticonvulsants is unnecessary even in patients who have had seizures as part of the encephalopathy.

ELECTROLYTE IMBALANCE

Hypercalcemia. Hypercalcemia, a common complication of cancer,[2576] generally is caused either by accelerated bone resorption in patients with widespread bony metastases, or by tumor production of a parathormone-related protein. Less common causes include decreased renal calcium excretion, increased GI calcium absorption, and production by the tumor of vitamin D, cytokines, or parathyroid-like hormone.[2744] Hypercalcemia is an occasional cause of delirium in patients with cancer. Characteristically, such patients become withdrawn and confused and either complain of thirst or develop a markedly increased fluid intake. Constipation is common. As the hypercalcemia worsens, confusion and disorientation develop. Proximal muscle weakness is added to the encephalopathy and reflexes diminish. An occasional patient has an agitated or paranoid delirium, and seizures are a rare complication. The encephalopathy generally resolves when a normal calcium concentration is restored by any one of several treatments.[2744]

Hypocalcemia. This disorder is not a major problem in patients with cancer. However, like hypercalcemia, it can cause encephalopathy and muscle weakness.[645,815]

Hyponatremia. The syndrome of inappropriate antidiuretic hormone (ADH) secretion causing hyponatremia is extremely common in patients with cancer, as it is in the general population of hospitalized patients (about 1%).[75,1433] Hyponatremia was not the sole cause of encephalopathy in any of 140 patients studied at MSKCC,[2617] but it was a contributing cause in a high percentage of those with multifactorial encephalopathy. Hyponatremia, with its associated hypo-osmolality, causes water to shift from the body to the brain, leading to brain edema.[1029] Severe or acute hyponatremia may cause sufficient brain swelling to lead to cerebral herniation and death. The symptoms of less severe hyponatremia depend on the age of the patient and are said to be more severe at higher levels of serum sodium in women than in men.[75] Acute lowering of the serum sodium level to less than 130 mEq/L will cause headaches, nausea, vomiting, and encephalopathy. The rapid lowering of the serum sodium level to 120 mEq/L can cause seizures, coma, and sometimes respiratory arrest. Because the decrease of the serum sodium level is not acute in most patients with cancer, patients with even rather striking hypo-osmolality may be only mildly encephalopathic. My colleagues and I have encountered occasional patients with serum sodium levels as low as 100 mEq/L who had only mild symptoms and recovered without sequelae as osmolality was restored. In patients with concomitant structural brain disease or metabolic derangements, however, relatively mild hyponatremia may contribute significantly to delirium.

Patients who have been severely hyponatremic are susceptible to the development of demyelination in the brain.[2590] A common area to demyelinate is the central pons. The pathogenesis of this central pontine myelinolysis is not completely understood. Most investigators believe it results from rapid correction of hyponatremia and advise that severe hyponatremia should be corrected slowly.[2490] Others believe it results from the edema caused by the hypo-osmolality itself and, thus, offer contrary advice that more rapid correction should be applied.[107] A recent study reports that the only patients who never develop myelinolysis are those whose hyponatremia is treated by water restriction alone, with cessation of diuretics if they are receiving them.[1098]

Treating hyponatremia depends on its

cause and severity. Fluid restriction will often suffice for people with mild, inappropriate ADH secretion. Hypertonic saline may be necessary for people with severe symptoms of hyponatremia. It is probably safe to correct hyponatremia with sodium, 1 to 2 mmol/hr, until symptoms are relieved and then to restrict water. Several formulas have been published for deciding the amount of sodium chloride necessary to restore normal natremia.[1433]

Hypernatremia. Hyperosmolality, usually from hypernatremia, occasionally causes delirium in the cancer population. Hypernatremia can stem from impaired thirst mechanisms from brain disease, from the inability to ingest adequate amounts of fluids, and from excessive fluid losses that are not replaced.[2454] Diabetes insipidus, from the destruction of the pituitary gland by metastases, can cause hypernatremia in patients with breast cancer. Fever causing excessive fluid loss also is a common cause. Patients characteristically have dry mucous membranes, poor skin turgor, and a quiet encephalopathy. Seizures, asterixis, and multifocal myoclonus are uncommon. Rapid correction of hypernatremia may cause symptoms of hyponatremia even at serum sodium levels considered normal. Hypernatremia has been reported to cause a myopathy associated with an elevated serum creatine phosphokinase concentration and electromyographic abnormalities suggesting myopathy. The syndrome reversed when the serum sodium was corrected.[1167a]

Hypomagnesemia. Hypomagnesemia typically develops in patients with cancer who are being treated with *cis*-platinum (see Chapter 12). It rarely causes symptoms, although seizures have been reported. Seizures associated with *cis*-platinum are more likely a result of hypo-osmolality than of hypomagnesemia. Hypermagnesemia rarely occurs in patients with cancer.

Hypophosphatemia. Mild hypophosphatemia, a common abnormality in hospitalized patients with cancer, can result from decreased dietary intake, decreased intestinal absorption, or shifts of phosphorus into cells such as occur with respiratory alkalosis. Rapidly proliferating malignant cells, particularly in leukemia and lymphoma, can absorb phosphorus, causing acute hypophosphatemia. Oncogenic osteomalacia and a paraneoplastic syndrome of prostate or lung cancer[850,2149,2256] can also cause hypophosphatemia. Severe hypophosphatemia has been associated with hyperalimentation (total parenteral nutrition [TPN]) and recovery from severe malnutrition.[77,2424]

Although it rarely occurs now, severe acute hypophosphatemia associated with TPN can cause encephalopathy as well as peripheral neuropathy. Patients develop irritability, apprehension, muscle weakness, numbness, paresthesias, dysarthria, confusion, obtundation, and convulsive seizures that can progress to coma and death. They sometimes have visual hallucinations[145] with or without other aspects of an agitated delirium. A second syndrome, resembling Wernicke's encephalopathy,[2712] occurs with more slowly developing hypophosphatemia. Other patients develop ptosis, amblyopia, paraplegia, and dysphagia. Respiratory weakness leading to hypercarbia, profound muscle weakness, sensory loss, and diminution of deep tendon reflexes may also occur, occasionally mimicking the Guillain-Barré syndrome. Peripheral neuropathy has also been reported.[2424]

Because of careful and effective phosphorus replacement in patients receiving TPN, this disorder does not occur commonly. When it does, it can be effectively treated by replacement of phosphorus.

ENDOCRINE DISORDERS

Neurologic manifestations resulting from abnormalities of both adrenal and thyroid function can affect patients with cancer.[301] Adrenal insufficiency can be caused by metastases to the adrenal gland or hypothalamus[1790,2376] or may follow withdrawal from prolonged corticosteroid therapy. Occasionally, replacement hydrocortisone is inadvertently discontinued in patients with adrenal insufficiency who are begun on dexamethasone, causing florid mineralocorticoid insufficiency. This occurred in the past in patients with breast cancer who had undergone adrenalectomy. These patients were maintained on replacement hydrocortisone, which was changed to dexamethasone when the patients developed CNS metastases. Because dexamethasone has no mineralocorticoid effect, if the cortisol was withdrawn (or rarely even if it was continued), patients developed acute adrenal crisis from inadequate mineralocorticoid. The phenomenon was accompanied by cardiovascular collapse but no encephalopathy.

Adrenal metastases deprive the patient of both glucocorticoids and mineralocorticoids. Symptoms begin with a passive delirium followed by cardiovascular collapse from fluid and electrolyte losses.

Hyperadrenal Corticolism. This abnormality can occur either as a paraneoplastic effect due to increased secretion of adrenocorticotropic hormonelike peptides, usually from lung cancer,[301, 1290, 1521, 2380] or as a result of chronic dexamethasone therapy. In both the paraneoplastic syndrome and chronic steroid ingestion, patients develop metabolic alkalosis. In the paraneoplastic syndrome, compensatory respiratory insufficiency can lead to hypoxia. Respiratory compensation for the metabolic alkalosis of exogenous steroid therapy is unusual. In addition, depression is the common psychological symptom with Cushing's syndrome, whether paraneoplastic or not, whereas mania is more common with exogenous steroid excess (see Chapter 4).

Hyperthyroidism. Transient hyperthyroidism sometimes follows RT to the thyroid gland. It is a rare complication of cancer, unlike hypothyroidism, which is a frequent consequence of RT (see Chapter 13).

Hyperglycemia. Hyperglycemia is common in patients with cancer who have other neurologic complications of cancer. Some hyperglycemic patients are known to be diabetic, but most are not until they begin receiving steroids for a CNS complication of cancer. In a few patients, phenytoin also appears to precipitate hyperglycemia.[1663] As with hypoglycemia, two clinical syndromes are identified. The first is a diffuse encephalopathy generally referred to as *nonketotic hyperosmolar coma.*[76] Its pathogenesis is believed to be cellular dehydration of the brain caused by the very high glucose level and often a moderately elevated adjusted serum sodium level.[564] Patients become lethargic and ultimately comatose, usually without focal signs. They awaken when the hyperglycemia is corrected. Most patients with nonketotic hyperosmolar coma have serum glucose levels greater than 800 mg/dL.

The second syndrome is a focal encephalopathy characterized by recurrent or continuous focal seizures without a change in consciousness.[1138] The seizures do not respond to anticonvulsant medications and generally cease promptly when the hyperglycemia is corrected with insulin and rehydration. Serum glucose levels are usually in the range of 500 to 800 mg/dL, somewhat lower than in patients with nonketotic hyperosmolar coma.

ORGAN FAILURE

Patients with cancer are susceptible to respiratory failure causing hypercarbia, hepatic failure causing hepatic encephalopathy,[1689] and renal failure causing uremia.[256] Hepatic encephalopathy and uremia are occasionally the sole cause of delirium in patients with cancer; more commonly, the conditions are part of a multifactorial delirium. Clinical manifestations resemble those caused by organ failure from other causes.[77,1689] Hyperammonemic coma, similar to hepatic coma, also can occur in the tumor lysis syndrome (see the following), after ureterosigmoidostomy,[2668] and rarely as a manifestation of myeloma.[374]

TUMOR LYSIS SYNDROME

The lysis of tumors can lead to several metabolic disorders that can secondarily affect the brain.[1074] Gross elevations of uric acid, phosphorus, potassium, urea, and ammonia have been reported as part of the syndrome. Uric acid probably has no direct effect on the brain, but it can cause acute uremia as a result of its effect on the kidneys. Hyperammonemia associated with chemotherapy causes a syndrome similar to hepatic encephalopathy.[1784]

LACTIC ACIDOSIS

Its exact cause is unknown, but lactic acidosis may result from tissue hypoxia or hypoperfusion (type A) or it may complicate hematologic malignancy or solid tumor, even when tissue oxygenation is adequate (type B).[2742] Patients with these disorders become confused, but systemic symptoms usually outweigh the neurologic ones.

NUTRITIONAL DISORDERS ASSOCIATED WITH CANCER

Malnutrition and cachexia are frequent complications of advanced cancer.[631,2575] Two general but overlapping categories of malnutrition affect patients with cancer. The first is generalized malnutrition with weight loss, which usually affects the peripheral nervous system and the muscles. The second category involves deprivation of specific nutrients and usually affects the CNS.

Malnutrition and Cachexia

Many studies implicate malnutrition as a cause of neuromuscular disorders in critically ill patients with or without cancer.[2252] Hawley and colleagues,[1118] who studied 71 patients with small-cell lung cancer, report that mononeuropathies from nerve compression occurred in 13%. All patients eventually experienced polyneuropathy, but its severity was less than in patients with chronic alcoholism who had lost a similar amount of weight. These investigators concluded that peripheral neuropathy associated with small-cell lung cancer was a result of weight loss and malnutrition. Hildebrand and Coers[1157] examined biopsy specimens from a number of patients with neuromuscular disorders associated with cancer and found abnormalities at the neuromuscular junction in many. The degree of abnormality was associated with the amount of weight loss. They concluded that the abnormalities were related to cachexia. Histologic changes include axonal degeneration of intramuscular nerve fibers, atrophy of type-I and especially type-II muscle fibers, and the sprouting of nerve endings.[2836] Similar alterations are found in otherwise healthy patients with anorexia nervosa. Of 51 patients with anorexia nervosa, 4 had electrodiagnostic evidence of sensorimotor peripheral neuropathy, compared to none in a matched control group. Three others had an isolated peroneal nerve palsy, presumably from nerve compression with the associated loss of subcutaneous tissue.[1642]

The strength of most cachectic patients with cancer is surprisingly normal. Nonetheless, occasionally the clinician encounters patients with one or both of two clinical syndromes that affect muscle or the neuromuscular junction. The first is probably a nutritional myopathy or perhaps a disorder of neuromuscular transmission in which patients complain of proximal weakness. Like polymyositis or steroid myopathy, the disorder is characterized by difficulty in rising from a low chair or the toilet seat and in climbing stairs. Raising heavy objects over the head or even combing one's hair may also be challenging. Deep tendon reflexes may be preserved. Wasting and weakness of muscles, particularly proximal muscles, also occurs. Myoedema is often apparent when the muscle is struck.[2277] The creatine phosphokinase level is characteristically normal. Electromyograms show little or no abnormality. Patients whose cancer is successfully treated and who gain weight generally recover muscle function. The pathogenesis of this uncommon disorder is not clear. It must be distinguished from paraneoplastic polymyositis and the much more common steroid-induced myopathy.

The second disorder is a sensorimotor peripheral neuropathy (see Chapter 15). Patients complain of numbness and tingling in the toes. Examination frequently reveals distal weakness with absent deep tendon reflexes, particularly ankle jerks and, later, knee jerks.

When the two disorders previously described are combined, they match the diagnostic criteria of Croft and Wilkinson[527] for "neuromyopathy" associated with cancer. Malnutrition may be the major cause of such "paraneoplastic neuromyopathy" (see Chapter 15).

Disorders of Nutrient Deprivation Associated with Cancer

A number of disorders that are due to deprivation of single nutrients have been reported in patients with cancer, including the Wernicke-Korsakoff syndrome from vitamin B_1 deficiency,[729] vitamin B_{12} deficiency,[1377,2383] pellagra associated with carcinoid tumors,[406,1511,1656,2604] and hypophosphatemia in patients receiving TPN.[2424]

WERNICKE-KORSAKOFF SYNDROME

This disorder, also called thiamine-deficiency encephalopathy, is characterized by an acute delirium associated with nystagmus, ocular palsies, and ataxia. Some patients also develop autonomic insufficiency with severe postural hypotension. Unless treated rapidly, patients develop an irreversible amnestic syndrome known as Korsakoff's psychosis. Pathologically, the disorder is characterized by focal, sometimes hemorrhagic, abnormalities in mamillary bodies, thalamus, and brainstem. The disorder can be entirely prevented by thiamine replacement but is sometimes acutely precipitated by the injudicious use of glucose in a thiamine-deprived patient. In one autopsy study of 24 patients with leukemia and lymphoma, 8 had the neuropathologic features of Wernicke's encephalopathy, although in none were clinical symptoms recognized.[579] The syndrome generally occurs when a child or an adult with leukemia or lymphoma is being actively treated. Chemotherapy appears to play no direct role.[326,729,2712] This disorder has also been reported following parenteral nutrition without adequate replacement of thiamine.[2712] The patient may become confused and disoriented, but more characteristically, first develops nystagmus on lateral gaze, followed by lateral-gaze paresis. The ocular motor signs may be accompanied by gait ataxia. This disorder generally begins acutely and, if treated early with thiamine, resolves entirely. Nystagmus may improve within a few minutes after an injection of thiamine. Nevertheless, if treatment is not begun early, the patient may develop a chronic amnestic dementia with severe memory loss but otherwise normal cognitive functions, mimicking the dementia of limbic encephalitis (see Chapter 15). Ataxia may also be permanent, but, unlike the ataxia of paraneoplastic cerebellar degeneration, the patient walks with a stiff-legged, widebased gait and has little or no ataxia of the upper extremities, no nystagmus, and no dysarthria. This clinical difference corresponds to the histopathology of the two syndromes.[2695] In nutritional cerebellar degeneration, destruction of Purkinje cells is limited to the vermis and posterior lobe of the cerebellum. In paraneoplastic cerebellar degeneration, Purkinje cells are lost diffusely. Polyneuropathy or cognitive impairment may be the only signs,[1604a] and some patients present comatose.[2001a] Thiamine deficiency is an unsuspected cause of delirium in some elderly patients admitted to an acute geriatric unit.[1933a]

Any malnourished patient with an encephalopathy and nystagmus should be treated with thiamine. Severely malnourished patients who are going to be given a glucose infusion should also be treated with parenteral thiamine. Only a few milligrams a day are necessary to treat Wernicke's encephalopathy, but larger doses do no harm and ensure replenishment of thiamine stores.

VITAMIN B_{12} DEFICIENCY

Vitamin B_{12} deficiency was found in 10 of 41 patients who underwent radiotherapy for bladder carcinoma.[1377,2714] In 13 patients given full irradiation because of inoperative bladder cancer, 5 had malabsorption of B_{12}. Serum folate levels were normal in all of the patients. Neurologic disturbances were not obvious on examination, but after B_{12} was given, the patients reported that previous weariness and muscular weakness had disappeared. Four patients observed an improvement of numbness and paresthesias in their fingers and toes. The disorder probably represents malabsorption of B_{12} related to high-dose RT that radiated the terminal ilium. Surprisingly, despite the malabsorption, most patients did not have diarrhea or other significant evidence of malabsorption. Vitamin E was not measured in this study, nor was there a careful evaluation of brain function.

Vitamin-B_{12} deficiency can also cause a diffuse encephalopathy, spinal cord signs, and a peripheral neuropathy, all without the well-known hematologic manifestations.

CARCINOID SYNDROME

Carcinoids are interesting neuroendocrine tumors that can secrete several substances causing systemic and neurologic symptoms. The most frequently encountered syndrome is that of flushing and diarrhea. Serotonin appears to play a major role because cyproheptadine substantially reduces the diarrhea,[1793] but histamine, bradykinin, and other vasoactive peptides may also contribute to the syndrome. Serotonin, which requires niacin for its synthesis from tryptophan, also appears to play a role in carcinoid myopathy (see Chapter 15). Pellagra, a disease of niacin deficiency, occurs rarely in patients with a carcinoid syndrome. The disorder appears related to high levels of serotonin produced by the tumor. Under normal circumstances, only 1% of tryptophan is metabolized to serotonin, but in the carcinoid syndrome, as much as 60% of tryptophan may be directed into this pathway. Diversion of tryptophan from its other metabolic pathways impairs both protein synthesis and niacin production and can lead to pellagra.

Pellagra is clinically characterized by a triad of dementia, diarrhea, and dermatitis. The cutaneous eruption appears as an erythematous rash in sun-exposed areas and progresses to produce sharply marginated, symmetrically hyperpigmented and hyperkeratotic lesions, particularly over the dorsum of the hands. The mental symptoms may be those of an agitated delirium; if untreated, the disorder progresses to a stuporous state and eventually to coma and death. Patients respond to replacement of niacin. An alternate explanation for some of the symptomatology may be a tryptophan deficiency in the brain causing low levels of brain serotonin despite the production of serotonin by the tumor.[1656] A review of the mental state of 22 patients with carcinoid syndrome revealed depression in 50%, anxiety in 35%, and altered levels of consciousness in 35%.

An increased production of serotonin and other vasoactive peptides can also cause vasospasm; one case led to ischemic neuropathy of the lower extremities.[1435] Acromegaly[2461] and hypoglycemia have also been associated with carcinoid syndrome.[1791]

CHAPTER 12

SIDE EFFECTS OF CHEMOTHERAPY

Patients with cancer often take several different types of drugs (Table 12–1). Some drugs, including antineoplastic, hormonal, or biologic agents, treat the cancer. Others treat symptoms related to the cancer. In addition, because many patients with cancer are elderly, they may also be taking drugs for illnesses such as hypertension or cardiac disease that are unrelated to the underlying cancer. Some drugs from each category, acting alone or with other agents, are neurotoxic. Experimental antineoplastic agents, the side effects of which are not completely known, may also be neurotoxic. Thus, neurotoxicity caused by medication must be high on the list of potential causes of otherwise unexplained neurologic symptoms. This chapter considers the neurotoxicity of agents used to treat cancer and its complications. Table 12–1 indicates the order in which specific drugs are discussed.

It is surprising that neurotoxicity is a major side effect of antineoplastic agents. Most antineoplastic agents affect rapidly dividing tumor cells, so the clinician expects to see side effects directed at relatively rapidly dividing normal cells such as those in bone marrow and the GI tract. The nervous system consists of cells that either do not divide, such as most neurons (although olfactory neurons do reproduce and are very susceptible to chemotherapeutic agents[912]), or divide slowly, such as glia in the CNS and Schwann cells in the peripheral nervous system. Furthermore, save for a few areas such as the circumventricular organs of the brain and the dorsal root ganglia, the nervous system is protected against easy entry of water-soluble agents. As a result, most chemotherapeutic agents given parenterally achieve much lower concentrations in the nervous system than elsewhere in the body. Despite these theoretic considerations, the nervous system is frequently the site of symptomatic toxicity of antineoplastic agents.

Neurotoxicity can cause significant disability, sometimes appearing or persisting after a patient has been effectively treated or even cured of the cancer. Because regeneration of nervous system structures is poor, once an agent has caused severe damage to nerve cells or supporting structures, recovery is unlikely. Even when regeneration is possible under optimal conditions, as it is in some peripheral neuropathies, the poor nutritional state of many patients precludes useful recovery.

In addition, even minor abnormalities of nervous system function cause symptoms.

Table 12–1. **AGENTS USED TO TREAT PATIENTS WITH CANCER**

Antineoplastic agents
Antineoplastic chemicals (chemotherapeutics)
Hormones and hormone antagonists
Immunotherapeutic agents
Cells
Nonspecific immune enhancers
Cytokines
Adjuvants to radiation or chemotherapy
Radiation enhancers
Radiation protectors (normal tissue)
Chemotherapy rescue drugs
Supportive care agents (see Chapter 4)
Analgesics
Corticosteroids
Anticonvulsants
Anti-emetics
Antibiotics
Anticoagulants
Agents unrelated to cancer therapy
Antihypertensives
Cardiac medication
Others

Toxicity of the liver, lung, or kidney, unless severe, may cause abnormal laboratory tests but usually no symptoms, whereas similarly mild toxicity to the CNS is almost certain to cause at least discernible encephalopathy, and to the peripheral nervous system, distressing paresthesias. Nervous system toxicity often either limits the dose of useful chemotherapeutic agents (e.g., *cis*-platinum and fludarabine) or prevents any use of a new chemotherapeutic agent.

CLINICAL FINDINGS AND DIAGNOSIS

Diagnosing the nature of neurologic abnormalities in patients receiving treatment for cancer is often difficult. A given set of symptoms may result from metastatic or nonmetastatic (e.g., infectious or vascular) complications of the cancer, a paraneoplastic syndrome, or a therapeutic agent. In many instances, because the symptoms and signs are similar (Table 12–2), the diagnosis of a treatment-induced neurologic complication can be established only by clinical inference. The physician is forced to make a diagnosis based on the proximity of the neurologic complication to the treatment and on the knowledge that previous patients have suffered similar complications from these treatments or treatments like these. Recently published reviews* help identify drugs that cause neurotoxic side effects, but new agents, new combinations of agents, and new dosage schedules are often associated with new and different neurologic symptomatology.

In addition, nervous system dysfunction may be caused by either antineoplastic drugs or supportive care agents such as anticonvulsants, corticosteroids, anti-emetics, opioids, and immunosuppressive agents. Furthermore, drugs may act synergistically either with other drugs or with other anticancer treatments, such as radiation therapy (RT), which may cause more serious neurotoxicity in patients who are receiving or have received chemotherapy. Vincristine and corticosteroids together may cause more weakness from combined vincristine neuropathy and corticosteroid myopathy than either alone.

Even when the physician believes that a complication is therapy-related, alternate diagnoses must be considered. In addition, other factors may exacerbate the neurotoxicity of antineoplastic drugs, so that treatment-induced neurotoxicity can be considered the sole cause only after others are excluded. For example, a seizure associated with chemotherapy in a patient with cancer requires a brain image to identify structural disease such as a metastasis, and possibly a CSF evaluation for an infectious cause. If a metastatic or infectious disease is identified, it may not be the sole cause of the neurologic complication. Ample evidence confirms that neurotoxicity from antineoplastic agents is more likely to occur and more likely to be severe in patients with pre-existing nervous system disease, exemplified by the devastating effect of *Vinca* alkaloids on patients with hereditary neuropathies.[1724]

*References 414, 662, 1159, 1633, 2015, 2222, 2420.

Table 12–2. **NEUROTOXIC SIGNS CAUSED BY AGENTS COMMONLY USED IN PATIENTS WITH CANCER**

Acute Encephalopathy (Delirium)
Corticosteroids
Methotrexate (high-dose IV, IT)
Cis-platinum
Vincristine
Asparaginase
Procarbazine
5-Fluorouracil (± levamisole)
Ara-C
Nitrosoureas (high-dose or arterial)
Cyclosporine
Interleukin-2
Ifosfamide/mesna
Interferons
Tamoxifen
VP-16 (high-dose)
PALA

Chronic Encephalopathy (Dementia)
Methotrexate
BCNU
Ara-C
Carmofur
Fludarabine

Visual Loss
Tamoxifen
Gallium nitrate
Nitrosoureas (intra-arterial)
Cis-platinum

Cerebellar Dysfunction/Ataxia
5-Fluorouracil (± levamisole)
Ara-C
Phenytoin
Procarbazine
Hexamethylmelamine
Vincristine
Cyclosporin A

Aseptic Meningitis
Trimethoprim-sulfamethoxazole (Co-trimoxazole)
IVIg
NSAIDs
Levamisole
Monoclonal antibodies
Metrizamide
OKT3
Ara-C
Carbamazepine
Methotrexate (IT)

Headaches without Meningitis
Retinoic acid
Trimethoprim-sulfamethoxazole
Cimetidine
Corticosteroids
Tamoxifen

Seizures
Methotrexate
VP-16 (high-dose)
Cis-platinum
Vincristine
Asparaginase
Nitrogen mustard
BCNU
Dacarbazine (intra-arterial or high-dose)
PALA
mAmsa
Busulfan (high-dose)
Cyclosporine
Mitronidazole
Misonidazole
Beta-lactam antibiotics
Iodinated contrast material (IV or IT)

Myelopathy (Intrathecal Drugs)
Methotrexate
Ara-C
Thiotepa

Peripheral Neuropathy
Vinca alkaloids
Cis-platinum
Hexamethylmelamine
Procarbazine
5-Azacytidine
VP-16
VM-26
Misonidazole
Methyl-G
Ara-C
Taxol
Suramin
Mitotane

Ara-C = cytosine arabinoside or cytarabine; BCNU = carmustine; IV = intravenous; IVIg = intravenous gamma globulin; IT = intrathecal; mAmsa = acridinylaniside or AMSA; NSAIDs = nonsteroidal anti-inflammatory drugs; OKT3 = orthoclone; PALA = *N*-phosphonoacetyl-L-aspartate; VM-26 = teniposide; VP-16 = etoposide.

Peripheral Nervous System

DIFFUSE NEUROPATHY

Diffuse peripheral nervous system neurotoxicity falls into three broad categories:

1. An acute or subacutely developing sensorimotor peripheral neuropathy, often predominantly motor, which resembles the Guillain-Barré syndrome. The drugs probably cause selective demyelination, and the disorder is often reversible when the drug is discontinued. Suramin is the prototypic culprit.
2. A distal sensorimotor neuropathy affecting axons. This disorder begins with paresthesias, but motor weakness soon becomes apparent. Exemplified by vincristine neuropathy, this disorder may reverse with time; even deep tendon reflexes, which usually disappear early, may eventually return.
3. A pure sensory neuropathy, often painful, involving either large fibers or both large and small fibers, probably originating from damage to dorsal root ganglion cells. The patient first complains of numbness and tingling in fingers and toes, but sometimes only fingers. In *cis*-platinum neuropathy, only large fibers are involved, causing loss of proprioception; pin and temperature sensation and motor power are preserved. In Taxol neuropathy, both large and small fibers are lost to an approximately equal degree. Depending on the degree of damage to the dorsal root ganglion cells, the disease may reverse itself if the patient survives in otherwise good health for a year or more after the chemotherapeutic treatment.

FOCAL NEUROPATHY

Neuropathies that affect only one or a few nerves are uncommon but can complicate both vincristine and *cis*-platinum therapy. Focal neuropathy may occur at the site of nerve compression, as in the peroneal nerve palsy from crossed legs, or may be independent of any other focal injury, as in recurrent laryngeal or phrenic nerve paralysis.[1544]

Specific findings in patients with a chemotherapy-induced peripheral neuropathy suggest the offending agent. For example, *cis*-platinum is the only chemotherapeutic agent that causes Lhermitte's sign, electric-shocklike paresthesias in the arms or legs precipitated by neck flexion and indicative of demyelination in the posterior columns of the spinal cord.[2408] Lhermitte's sign may also follow therapeutic irradiation to the spinal cord (see Chapter 13) and rarely occurs in patients who have not received *cis*-platinum or radiation but who have had a bone marrow trasplant.[2793] Muscle cramps also appear to be more common in *cis*-platinum neuropathy[2408] but may be noticed with vincristine therapy.[1056] Cramps may persist more than a year after chemotherapy is discontinued. Paresthesias limited to the fingertips are a more common early sign of vincristine neuropathy. Severe, acute muscle aching, possibly neurogenic, occurs after vincristine injection, steroid withdrawal, and Taxol infusion, but is not a common manifestation of other chemotherapeutic involvement.

Central Nervous System

ACUTE ENCEPHALOPATHY

Acute encephalopathy is characterized by confusion, disorientation, and altered behavior. The patient with a quiet delirium may simply appear depressed and withdrawn; others are agitated and fearful. Most patients develop insomnia. A few suffer florid hallucinations, but they may not report them unless asked. Multifocal myoclonus and generalized seizures often accompany the encephalopathy and give a physical clue to the presence of this condition. Seizures may be the only manifestation of an acute encephalopathy. Encephalopathy induced by chemotherapeutic agents cannot be distinguished clinically from that caused by metabolic disorders (see Chapter 11). Specific chemotherapeutic agents are not usually characterized by specific encephalopathies.

CHRONIC ENCEPHALOPATHY

Chronic encephalopathy is characterized by dementia and sometimes seizures. Those more subacute are often reversible, whereas those that develop more slowly are usually irreversible. Patients are characteristically quiet and withdrawn, often appearing apathetic. They may sleep much of the day or sleep during the daytime and be awake at night. They often sit motionless for long periods and do not spontaneously initiate conversation. They suffer moderate-to-severe memory loss and disorientation, particularly with respect to time. When pressed, however, many patients can (if given sufficient time) answer questions better than the examiner would suspect on the basis of their overall demeanor. These characteristics, often called "subcortical dementia," are caused by several chemotherapeutic agents, especially methotrexate (MTX).

Although severe dementia is rare in adults who have not received RT to the brain, other maladies of cognitive function are relatively common. A recent study evaluated neuropsychologic function in patients with cancer who had widely disseminated metastatic disease and had received chemotherapy. About one third had cognitive defects including memory deficits. Patients who received biologic therapy such as interferon were more likely to have cognitive defects than those who had received antineoplastic chemotherapy.[1760,2416] Long-term survivors of small-cell lung cancer often develop a progressive decline in neurologic function, particularly memory loss. Some patients report gait and coordination abnormalities, which often progress over years. They are more striking in patients who have received a combination of multiagent chemotherapy and RT, but they also occur in others who have received chemotherapy alone. White-matter hyperintensity seen in T_2-weighted images on MR scans often progresses for several years.[1294]

Transient changes in white matter with hyperintensity on MR images are often found in young children who undergo chemotherapy for acute lymphoblastic leukemia. Most of these children also suffer neuropsychological deficits.[2821]

Whether chemotherapy alone, in the absence of radiation, affects long-term cognitive function in children is not fully established. Most survivors of acute lymphoblastic leukemia and small-cell lung cancer have received combined chemotherapy and RT either prophylactically or therapeutically. These patients suffer long-term cognitive defects, particularly with memory and attention.[2232,2717] Pre-irradiation MTX appears to be less toxic to the brain than postirradiation MTX, particularly in young girls. Many investigators believe, however, that patients who undergo intensive systemic chemotherapy, particularly young children and the elderly, are at risk for long-term neuropsychological deficits involving memory and attention, whether or not the brain has been irradiated. These deficits are not as prominent or as severe as those that occur with RT plus chemotherapy, or even with RT alone; they generally do not incapacitate the patient. Animal models may elucidate some of these issues.[2859]

FOCAL DISORDERS

Focal disorders include acute cerebellar syndromes, acute or subacute myelopathy, visual loss, headache, and aseptic meningitis. The cerebellar syndrome caused by 5-fluorouracil (5-FU) and high-dose cytarabine is characterized by truncal and appendicular ataxia. In its mildest form, only gait ataxia is found. Acute cerebellar syndromes are caused by only a few drugs. Sometimes they are reversible, although permanent neurologic deficits characterized pathologically by diffuse loss of Purkinje cells have been reported. A transverse myelopathy following intrathecal therapy can be caused by MTX, cytarabine, or, rarely, thiotepa. Several types of visual loss can complicate chemotherapy: (1) tamoxifen therapy causes reversible retinopathy, (2) gallium nitrate and several other drugs cause an optic neuropathy, and (3) high-dose fludarabine and *cis*-platinum can cause cortical blindness. Isolated headache, seizures, and aseptic meningitis can be caused by several medications (Table 12–2).

SPECIFIC AGENTS

Drugs used to treat cancer include chemotherapeutic agents, hormones, hormone antagonists, biologicals, immunotherapeutic agents, and chemicals that act as adjuvants to RT or chemotherapy (see Table 12–1). Antineoplastic chemotherapeutic agents, gener-

Table 12–3. **CLASSIFICATION OF ANTINEOPLASTIC DRUGS**

Class	Examples
Alkylating agents	*Cis*-platinum Carmustine (BCNU) Cyclophosphamide
Antibiotics	
Anthracyclines	Doxorubicin
Others	Bleomycin
Antimetabolites	Cytarabine 5-Fluorouracil Methotrexate
Plant alkaloids	Vincristine
Miscellaneous	Suramin

ally the most neurotoxic, can be subdivided by their mechanism of action into alkylating agents, antibiotics, antimetabolites, plant alkaloids, and a miscellaneous group (Table 12–3).

Alkylating Agents

Alkylating agents work by covalent bonding of alkyl groups to DNA to form reactive intermediates that attack nucleophilic sites.[414] "Classic" alkylating agents usually contain a chloromethyl group that bifunctionally alkylates macromolecules. "Nonclassic" alkylating agents (e.g., cyclophosphamide) contain an *N*-methyl group and generally must be metabolically activated, usually in the liver, to assume the active form. Individual alkylating agents differ in site and degree of toxicity and in antitumor activity. Drugs such as cyclophosphamide and busulfan cause little or no neurotoxicity, whereas drugs such as *cis*-platinum cause dose-limiting neurotoxicity. The alkylating agents also differ by site of action. The nitrosoureas, such as 1,3-Bis(2-chloroethyl)-1-nitrosourea (BCNU), affect the O_6 position of guanine. Cells that contain guanine O_6 alkyl transferase, as many glial cells do, may be resistant to the nitrosoureas.[2724] Failure of a tumor to be sensitive to one alkylating agent does not predict resistance to other alkylating agents. Table 12–4 lists the commonly used conventional alkylating agents and some experimental ones.

Table 12–4. **ALKYLATING AGENTS**

Platinum-based
Cis-platinum
Carboplatin
Nitrosoureas
Carmustine (BCNU)
Lomustine (CCNU)
Streptozocin
Chlorozotocin
Semustine (methyl CCNU)
ACNU
HECNU
Mustards
Ifosfamide (with mesna)
Cyclophosphamide
Melphalan
Chlorambucil
Mechlorethamine (nitrogen mustard)
Other Alkylating Agents
Busulfan
Dacarbazine (DTIC)
Estramustine
Thiotepa
Procarbazine
Hexamethylmelamine

PLATINUM-BASED AGENTS

Platinum-based chemotherapeutic agents covalently bind to DNA bases and thus disrupt DNA function. Depending on the dose, *cis*-platinum also either augments or suppresses immune function. Whether this mechanism plays a role in its chemotherapeutic action is unknown. These drugs are generally administered intravenously, but the intra-arterial and intracavitary (peritoneal cavity) routes have also been used. Intracarotid platinums have been used to treat tumors of the head, neck, and brain. The platinum drugs are effective against various tumors including ovarian and testicular cancer and some primary brain tumors.

***Cis*-platinum.** This drug binds to plasma proteins (95%) and crosses the blood–brain barrier poorly. The CSF-plasma ratio in experimental animals is less than 0.04.[956] In patients with brain tumors, however, the CSF peak concentration may be as high as 40% of non–protein-bound platinum[596] and is reached about 60 minutes after an IV bolus. Intrathecal injection of more than 20 nmol to rats is toxic.[1938] Although the drug does not easily enter the normal brain or spinal cord, it does enter and accumulate in dorsal root ganglia and peripheral nerves, where concentrations are four to five times the brain concentration.[989] Consequently, as with other heavy-metal compounds, peripheral neuropathy is the most important neurotoxic effect.[264,411,1946] *Cis*-platinum also causes ototoxicity, CNS toxicity, and probably CNS vascular toxicity (Table 12–5).

Peripheral Neuropathy. Peripheral neuropathy occasionally follows cumulative doses of as little as 200 mg/m^2 and is usual after 400 mg/m^2. The degree of peripheral neuropathy correlates both with the total cumulative dose of platinum and with the dose per treatment.[410] Focal lumbosacral plexopathies or mononeuropathies have been reported following infusion of internal or external iliac arteries.[405] Optic neuropathy has followed carotid infusion (see the following).[1653,2389]

The peripheral neuropathy begins with tingling that is occasionally painful in the toes and later the fingers. It then spreads proximally to affect both legs and arms. The deep tendon reflexes disappear (ankle jerks first), and proprioceptive loss (vibration sense first) is sometimes so severe that patients are unable to feed themselves or walk (sensory ataxia). Pin and temperature sensation are spared, and motor power is normal. Autonomic dysfunction is rare.[264,473,2210] Electrical studies reveal decreased conduction velocities in sensory nerves and diminished amplitude of sensory nerve potentials compatible with a sensory axonopathy.[264,2174] In some patients, proprioceptive loss is so severe that patients appear weak when attempting to sustain a muscle contraction not under direct vision. Instructing the patient to look at the limb being tested usually increases strength.

The first neuropathic symptoms may not appear until the *cis*-platinum treatment is completed and then may progress for several months before stabilizing.[1021,2408] If the patient survives the cancer, the neuropathy usually improves and may clear entirely after months or years.[1797] Some patients do not recover.[2657] Pre-existing CNS dysfunction such as myelopathy is a risk factor for *cis*-platinum–induced peripheral neuropathy.[1368] *Cis*-platinum neuropathy is often confused with paraneoplastic sensory neuronopathy (see Chapter 15) but differs from that disorder in that paraneoplastic sensory neuropathy usually affects all sensory modalities equally, does not improve after cessation of chemotherapy, and is often associated with an antineuronal autoantibody in the patient's serum.

Pathologic examination of nerve roots reveals axonal loss with secondary demyelination.[1946,1966,2587,2735] Axonal loss is also found in dorsal but not ventral roots, with secondary degeneration of posterior columns.[2735] Dorsal root ganglion cells are probably the primary site of pathology.[1801] The predominant pathologic abnormality is nuclear.[1946] The degree of histologic change is correlated with platinum levels found in dorsal roots and peripheral nerves.[989]

Once the disorder develops, treatment is ineffective. Protection against the develop-

Table 12–5. NEUROTOXICITY OF *CIS*-PLATINUM

Common
- Peripheral neuropathy (large fiber, sensory)
- Lhermitte's sign
- Hearing loss (high frequency)
- Tinnitus

Uncommon
- Encephalopathy
- Visual loss
  - Retinal toxicity
  - Optic neuropathy
  - Cortical blindness
- Seizures
- Cerebral herniation (hydration related)
- Electrolyte imbalance (Ca^{++}, Mg^{++}, Na^{+}, SIADH)
- Vestibular toxicity
- Autonomic neuropathy

SIADH = syndrome of inappropriate secretion of antidiuretic hormone.

ment of *cis*-platinum neuropathy has been reported with the drug ORG 2766, an adrenocorticotropic hormone 4-9 analog,[2658] and the radioprotective agent WR2721. Nerve growth factor,[66] nimodipine,[402] and reduced glutathione have also been reported effective in clinical and experimental studies.[51,1069] Clinical studies testing some of these agents are under way.

Cranial Neuropathy. Cranial nerve palsies develop in about 6% of patients after common carotid intra-arterial infusion of *cis*-platinum for head and neck cancer. Any or all of the cranial nerves VII through XII[844] can be affected. In one of my patients, sensory loss in the distribution of the ipsilateral superior orbital nerve followed intracarotid infusion. She recovered completely.

Lhermitte's Sign. The appearance of Lhermitte's sign during or shortly after treatment with *cis*-platinum[1083,2408,2737] suggests a transient demyelinating lesion in the posterior columns of the spinal cord. It also can be caused by spinal cord compression and by cervical radiation.[2687] Sensory conduction may be slowed in the spinal cord,[2737] but lesions are not visible on MR scan. In some instances, patients may experience distal paresthesias when they abduct their arms, suggesting that they are stretching a demyelinated brachial plexus.

Muscles. Cramps unrelated to electrolyte imbalance (see the following) are also common but, like Lhermitte's sign, usually resolve spontaneously.[2408]

Hearing and Vestibular Deficits. *Cis*-platinum can cause ototoxicity and vestibulopathy.[1811] Hearing loss results from hair-cell damage.[2850] The hearing loss is often subclinical and affects primarily the high-frequency range (>4000 Hz). When the cumulative *cis*-platinum dose exceeds 300 mg/m^2,[2248] tinnitus may precede hearing loss. Rarely, high-dose *cis*-platinum causes acute deafness. Risk factors for ototoxicity include concomitant ifosfamide,[1759] previous cranial irradiation, young age, and presence of a brain tumor.[2309] If *cis*-platinum is given before radiation, ototoxicity is not increased.[1424,2138] Aminoglycoside antibiotics and diuretics, such as furosemide, may also exacerbate *cis*-platinum ototoxicity.

Vestibular toxicity, characterized by vertigo, oscillopsia, and ataxia, is much less common than hearing loss. It may occur either with or without other symptoms of ototoxicity and may be exacerbated by previous use of aminoglycoside antibiotics.[223,1811]

Visual Loss. Rare, ocular toxicity may include retinopathy (usually after intracarotid infusion[1439]), papilledema,[1955,2735] or retrobulbar neuritis.[1955] Color perception may be disturbed, probably because of retinal cone dysfunction.[2810] Cortical visual loss (homonymous hemianopia and cortical blindness) is sometimes part of the encephalopathy occasionally caused by *cis*-platinum (see the following).[194,472]

Encephalopathy. Characterized by seizures and focal brain dysfunction, particularly cortical blindness, encephalopathy is rare following IV infusion[327,408,955,1155,1737] but more common following intra-arterial infusion.[774,1883] The symptoms are usually reversible. Encephalopathy that is due to the drug must be differentiated from that caused by the hydration preceding *cis*-platinum therapy, that is, water intoxication with herniation,[2727] or by the nephropathy that often follows it; hypocalcemia and hypomagnesemia commonly follow *cis*-platinum treatment and may rarely cause tetany, encephalopathy, or seizures.[178] The syndrome of inappropriate secretion of antidiuretic hormone (SIADH) with hyponatremia and seizures has also been reported,[2176] as has hypozincemia.[2534]

Cis-platinum has been implicated in vascular toxicity (cardiac and cerebral infarction and Raynaud's phenomenon) that sometimes follows multiagent chemotherapy.* Some researchers believe that the late toxicity is caused by the *cis*-platinum, either related to hypomagnesemia or as a direct effect of the drug on endothelial cells[906,1237]; others believe that bleomycin is more likely to be the major culprit.[1888] Other rare complications of *cis*-platinum include irreversible myelopathy, taste disturbances, and a myasthenic syndrome.[1587,2852]

Carboplatin. This drug possesses many of the salutary effects of *cis*-platinum but little neurotoxicity. The drug reaches higher concentrations in CSF than does *cis*-platinum but still crosses the blood–brain barrier poorly.[2166] It has been given to patients and

*References 661, 940, 1240, 1442, 2281, 2706, 2707.

animals intra-arterially with little neurotoxicity other than retinopathy.[2493] One case of carboplatin-induced thrombotic microangiopathy resulted in multiple small cortical infarcts leading to coma and death,[2729] and two patients have developed cortical blindness.[1908] Hypersensitivity reactions with dyspnea, hypotension, anginal pain, and rash have been reported.[2770a]

NITROSOUREAS

The nitrosoureas include lomustine (1-[2-chloroethyl-3-cyclohexyl-l-nitrosourea] [CCNU]), carmustine (BCNU), semustine (methyl CCNU), streptozocin, and chlorozotocin. Investigational drugs include ACNU, widely used in Japan, and HECNU, used in Europe. These drugs are highly lipid-soluble and cross the blood–brain barrier easily. The nitrosoureas, especially BCNU, are frequently used to treat primary brain tumors as well as melanoma and lymphoma. ACNU has been given intrathecally to experimental animals without toxicity.[1397] Bolus injection into the cerebral ventricles, however, fails to provide measurable levels of the drug in lumbar CSF because of its rapid clearance from CSF.[1397] Other drugs such as phenobarbital, phenytoin, and cimetidine increase hepatic microsomal enzyme activity, thus increasing drug metabolism and perhaps decreasing therapeutic activity[1541] of the nitrosoureas.

Nitrosoureas in conventional doses rarely cause neurologic toxicity. Bone marrow suppression appearing 3 to 4 weeks after treatment is the major early side effect. Late side effects include pulmonary fibrosis,[1512] which rarely can occur acutely[1565]; renal failure; hepatotoxicity; myelofibrosis[1728]; or leukemia. Myocardial ischemia has also been reported.[1334]

Patients with CNS tumors who have received previous RT, especially those treated with high-dose IV or intra-arterial BCNU, may develop ocular toxicity[2392] and encephalopathy.[2208] Sudden blindness because of optic neuropathy is a rare complication of oral CCNU combined with brain irradiation.[2826] After intracarotid infusion with BCNU, the first problem is usually visual loss with both retinal and optic nerve damage. The brain disorder is sometimes heralded by seizures and generally characterized by slowly progressive neurologic dysfunction, the exact signs depending on the area infused by the intra-arterial injection. A problem with intra-arterial drug infusion is that laminar flow often prevents uniform perfusion of the entire area supplied by the artery, so that the tumor sometimes receives a smaller dose than normal areas of brain in the same arterial distribution. Rapid or retrograde injection of the drug, by increasing turbulent flow, sometimes prevents this problem. White-matter hypodensity can be seen on CT (hyperintensity on T_2-weighted MR scan), sometimes at a site distant from the tumor (Fig. 12–1) but in the same arterial territory. The affected white matter may calcify, and ipsilateral gyral enhancement has been reported.[1649]

The pathology is necrotizing encephalopathy, which resembles radiation or MTX leukoencephalopathy but is strictly confined to the vascular territories perfused by the BCNU.[345,1388,2208] Both vascular and direct neural damage appear to participate in the pathogenesis of the lesion. Experimental animals receiving intracarotid BCNU develop increased blood–brain-barrier permeability.[1849]

BCNU and other nitrosoureas have also been administered directly to brain tumors by either injection or implanted wafers permeated with a drug. Some of the drugs cause pathologic changes, although their full spectrum has not been reported.

MUSTARDS

This group of highly useful alkylating agents is not particularly neurotoxic; some are prodrugs that cannot become active without first being metabolized by the liver.

Ifosfamide. The most neurotoxic,[1772] ifosfamide requires hydroxylation by microsomal liver enzymes to produce biologically active metabolites. The drug and some of its metabolites cross the blood–brain barrier. It is excreted in the urine and requires the use of a uroprotective agent (mesna) to prevent severe bladder toxicity; mesna itself is probably not neurotoxic. Ifosfamide is reported to be effective in treating pediatric brain tumors.[429] Depending on dose and other factors, 30% of patients receiving high-dose ifosfamide/mesna develop an encephalop-

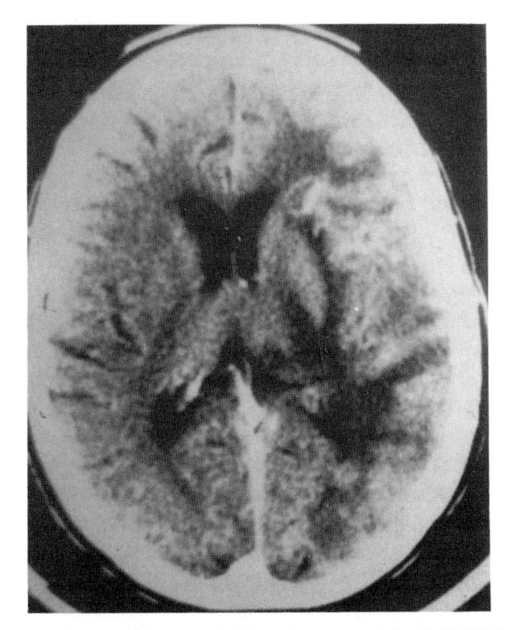

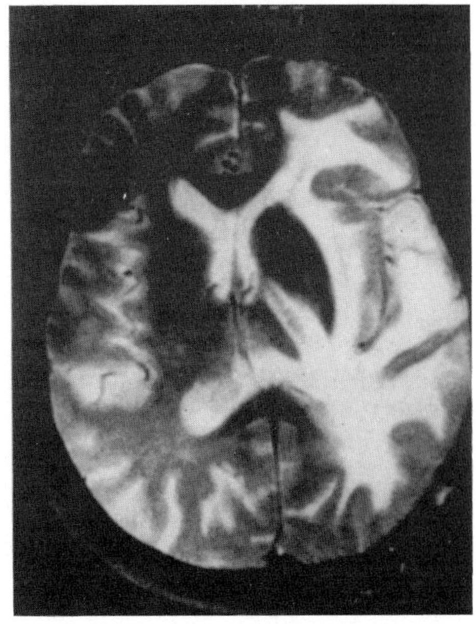

Figure 12–1. Leukoencephalopathy caused by BCNU in a patient who received RT followed by intracarotid administration of BCNU. Hypointensity on the CT scan (*left*) and hyperintensity on the T_2-weighted image (*right*) of the MR scan demonstrate leukoencephalopathy with relative sparing of the gray matter. The entire hemisphere perfused by the BCNU was involved, but the opposite hemisphere, which had received only RT, was less affected. Much of the white matter damage was at a site in the hemisphere remote from the tumor.

athy, usually reversible and characterized by cerebellar dysfunction, extrapyramidal signs,[2088] hallucinations,[644] seizures, quiet or agitated delirium, and sometimes coma. The disorder usually begins within 24 hours of the drug's infusion but may be delayed for 4 to 6 days.[2754] The encephalopathy usually clears in 3 to 4 days (range, 1–12 days) but persistent symptoms or even fatality may occur.[2754] Encephalopathy usually contraindicates further use of the drug at that dose, although some patients have tolerated retreatment without recurrence of the encephalopathy.[2089] Methylene blue may reverse the encephalopathy.[1440] Peripheral neuropathy has also been reported.[1994]

The risk factors for ifosfamide encephalopathy include high dosage, renal impairment, hepatic impairment, low serum albumin level,[540] hypocalcemia, underlying brain disease,[429] phenobarbital,[914] and previous *cis*-platinum therapy.[2088] The EEG during the encephalopathy slows diffusely to 1 to 3 Hz delta waves. The mechanism of the neurotoxicity is unknown[412]; chloroacetaldehyde, a metabolic product with effects similar to acetaldehyde, may be the culprit. If so, drugs such as phenobarbital, which can hasten the metabolic breakdown of ifosfamide, may increase neurotoxicity.[954,2089] Ifosfamide itself may cause the neurotoxicity; rapid infusion appears to be more neurotoxic than slow infusion. Pathologic changes in the nervous system have not been described.

Cyclophosphamide. Cyclophosphamide (Cytoxan) also requires activation by the liver for antitumor activity. Its metabolite, 4-hydroxyperoxycyclophosphamide, has been used experimentally by intrathecal injection to treat leptomeningeal metastases; it appears to be effective and non-neurotoxic except at high doses, which can cause lethargy, seizures, or both.[2035] Vasculitis of superficial arteries has also been observed. Cyclophosphamide intravenously or by mouth has little or no neurotoxicity, although reversible visual blurring,[1357] dizziness, and confusion[2555] have been reported in a few patients receiving high-dose therapy. Hyponatremia[595] has been reported. A rare, peculiar rheumatic disorder with myalgias and arthralgias has been reported to begin 1 to 3 months after completion of adjuvant chemotherapy for breast cancer; cyclophosphamide and 5-FU were given to all such patients.[1601]

Melphalan. This non-neurotoxic drug crosses the blood–brain barrier via the neutral amino acid transporter.[504] As a result, although not much drug enters the brain under normal circumstances, a diet lowering amino acids may promote entry.[1012] At high concentration, melphalan may also open the blood–brain barrier, promoting entry of other molecules. Neuropathologic changes follow intrathecal injection in rats.[69]

Chlorambucil. Although this drug causes encephalopathy and seizures when given in accidental overdose,[244,2674] it is otherwise not neurotoxic. Ocular toxicity, including keratitis, retinal edema, and hemorrhage, is rare.[346]

OTHER ALKYLATING AGENTS

Busulfan. This bifunctional alkylating agent is used to treat chronic myeloid leukemia. The drug easily crosses the blood–brain barrier, with a mean CSF concentration equal to the concentration in blood in children receiving high doses.[2036] With high-dose therapy (e.g., to prepare children for bone marrow transplantation) seizures are common, usually occurring 2 to 4 hours after the dose.[2677] The seizures can be prevented by clonazepam[2677] or phenytoin[1003] and do not occur at conventional doses of busulfan. Isolated case reports indicate that myasthenia gravis,[653] adrenal failure, and Sjögren's syndrome[2402] may complicate chronic busulfan treatment.

Dacarbazine (DTIC; dimethyltraizenyl imidazole carboxamide). Used to treat malignant melanoma, dacarbazine rarely produces neurotoxic side effects, although seizures (in the absence of underlying brain disease), encephalopathy, and occasionally dementia have been reported.[1996]

Estramustine and Nitrogen Mustard (Mechlorethamine). These drugs are not usually neurotoxic, but brain necrosis and necrotizing uveitis following intracarotid infusion of nitrogen mustard have been reported.[78] Both encephalopathy[208] and hearing loss[2352] occur rarely after conventional IV doses.

Diaziquone (aziridinylbenzoquinone). This agent, which crosses the blood–brain barrier and has some activity against primary brain tumors, has no significant neurotoxicity. It has been given intrathecally to treat leptomeningeal tumor, and headache was dose-limiting in a few of these patients.[188]

Procarbazine. This weak monoamine oxidase (MAO) inhibitor rapidly crosses the blood–brain barrier. Because it is an MAO inhibitor, patients are advised to avoid foods containing tyramine, although the importance of this precaution is doubtful. Procarbazine's exact mechanism of action is not known, although it is believed to interfere with DNA synthesis. The drug is given orally because experience with IV administration has revealed unacceptable neurotoxicity. Even with the oral form, however, encephalopathy may occur, ranging from mild drowsiness to stupor. Occasionally, patients develop confusion, agitation, or even psychosis. A reversible peripheral neuropathy with distal paresthesias, decreased deep tendon reflexes, and myalgias[333,2282,2473] has been reported in 10% to 20% of patients. Hypersensitivity reactions, including skin rash, interstitial pneumonitis, and hepatitis may be seen, particularly in patients with glioma.[520]

Mitotane (*o,p*-DDD). This drug is an adrenal cytotoxic agent that acts against adrenal carcinoma. It causes reversible CNS side effects consisting of lethargy and somnolence, dizziness, and vertigo.[1470]

Hexamethylmelamine. This investigational drug, whose mechanism of action is unknown, has some effectiveness against ovarian cancer, lung cancer, and other solid tumors. The drug itself has poor CNS penetration. The CSF concentration is less than 6% of the plasma concentration. Its demethylated metabolites occur in high concentrations and reach CSF-to-plasma ratios close to 1. These metabolites may be concentrated in the brain. Toxicity consists of mood changes including lethargy, depression, agitation, hallucinations, and sometimes coma. Peripheral neuropathy occurs rarely. Dose-limiting vomiting and anorexia may be an effect of the drug on the CNS.

Thiotepa. This drug and its major metabolite, TEPA, cross the blood–brain barrier easily. Systemic administration of thiotepa provides prolonged CSF exposure to TEPA. When the drug is administered intrathecally, as is sometimes done to treat leptomeningeal tumor, concentrations of tepa are not detectable and the rapid clearance of thiotepa results in an uneven neuraxial distribution.[1128] The drug causes marrow suppression but is not neurotoxic even when given systemically in high doses. Myelopathy has been reported[1037] in a few patients after many intrathecal injections.

Antineoplastic Antibiotics

The antineoplastic antibiotics (Table 12–6) consist of the anthracyclines, such as doxorubicin (Adriamycin), and other agents such as mitomycin and bleomycin. All have little or no neurotoxicity in humans.

ANTHRACYCLINES

The anthracycline antibiotics are useful against Hodgkin's disease, non-Hodgkin's lymphoma, acute myelogenous leukemia, and some epithelial tumors including breast cancer. Their mechanism is uncertain but they intercalate into DNA. They also may act by free-radical formation or reaction with topoisomerase type II, leading to DNA cleavage, a nonintercalative mechanism. Except for idarubicin, which has high lipid solubility, anthracyclines do not easily cross the blood–brain barrier.[213] Tumors develop resistance to them by expressing P-glycoprotein, the protein product of the multidrug-resistance gene. P-glycoprotein is present in cell membranes and at the blood–brain barrier. It appears to promote efflux of several chemotherapeutic agents, including doxorubicin and vincristine, from the cell and possibly from the brain.[1817] Thus, metastatic brain tumors could be more resistant to anthracycline therapy than similar tumors elsewhere in the body.

Doxorubicin. This agent causes severe and often fatal myelopathy and encephalopathy after accidental intrathecal injection.[74,1820] Necrosis and hemorrhagic infarcts in the brain sometimes follow intracarotid injection associated with osmotic blood–brain barrier opening.[1875] After systemic administration, cardiac thrombi associated with doxorubicin-induced cardiac toxicity[2305] may lead to transient cerebral ischemia or infarction. Conjunctivitis and excessive lacrimation occur rarely.[2703] One report[170] suggests that the combination of doxorubicin and cyclosporine may increase doxorubicin concentration in the brain and lead to fatal encephalopathy.

The drug does not cause peripheral nerve dysfunction in humans after IV injection, but it damages dorsal root ganglia in experimental animals, causing severe peripheral neuropathy.[1310] Cell loss in dorsal root ganglia also results from retrograde transport after direct injection into a peripheral nerve.[214] The drug affects cardiac and skeletal muscles microscopically[672] and it also accumulates in dorsal root ganglia,[213,2884] where it can be localized intracellularly by its orange fluorescence.

Idarubicin,[193] Epirubicin, and Daunorubicin. Although these anthracycline antibiotics do not appear to be neurotoxic in humans, epirubicin causes neuronal damage to mice after IV injection.[215] Harmless levels of idarubicin have been detected in the CSF of children after systemic therapy.[2150]

Menogaril (NSC-269148). This anthracycline antibiotic is undergoing experimental trial and acts against some solid tumors. Neurotoxicity has not been described.

Mitoxantrone. An analog of the anthracyclines with a similar mechanism of action, mitoxantrone has a narrow spectrum of antitumor activity confined to breast cancer, leukemias, and lymphomas. It is not known to be neurotoxic when given intravenously, but when given intrathecally to treat leukemia,[1667] the drug can cause nerve root damage and myelopathy,[1063] so that intrathecal

Table 12–6. **ANTINEOPLASTIC ANTIBIOTICS**

Anthracyclines
Doxorubicin (Adriamycin)
Daunorubicin
Idarubicin
Epirubicin
Menogaril
Mitoxantrone
Other Antibiotics
Bleomycin
Mitomycin C
Dactinomycin
Plicamycin
Deoxyspergualin
Acivicin

therapy is no longer used. The drug also causes a bluish discoloration of the sclera, fingernails, and urine, as does piroxantrone, a drug that has been used to treat brain tumors.

OTHER ANTIBIOTICS

Bleomycin. This drug is a mixture of peptides containing bleomycinic acid, derived from the fungus *Streptomyces verticillus*. The peptides cleave DNA strands via free radicals. Bleomycin acts against Hodgkin's disease, non-Hodgkin's lymphoma, testicular cancer, and head and neck cancers. The primary toxicity is directed at lung and skin. Raynaud's phenomenon affects 5% to 7% of patients and usually occurs when bleomycin is used in combination with *Vinca* alkaloids, with or without *cis*-platinum.[2817] In most instances, the disorder is mild and not disabling.

More disturbing are delayed effects of bleomycin on the vasculature of the brain and heart, usually when used as part of *cis*-platinum–based chemotherapy. Cerebral and myocardial infarcts have occurred in a very small number of patients apparently cured of testicular or other cancers by the use of bleomycin, *cis*-platinum, and other drugs.[2706] Which of the drugs is at fault is unclear, although bleomycin has been suspected as the main culprit. Strokes and myocardial infarcts are rare but are historically clearly related to the underlying chemotherapy.[277] Hypomagnesemia has been implicated as a risk factor. Recent reviews summarize the vascular toxicity.[663,2289]

Mitomycin C. Originating from *Streptomyces caespitosus*, mitomycin C is useful against several solid cancers, usually without neurotoxicity, although there have been reports of visual blurring in occasional patients and of thrombotic microangiopathy with encephalopathy[2377] similar to that following carboplatin therapy.

Dactinomycin (Actinomycin D). An inhibitor of RNA and protein synthesis, dactinomycin is active against several tumors including choriocarcinoma, Wilm's tumor, and neuroblastoma. Neurotoxicity after IV therapy in humans has not been reported. Intrathecal injection in animals is fatal,[2542] causing a status spongiosus.[2180]

Plicamycin (Mithramycin). This drug has both anticancer and hypocalcemic activity and probably works by inhibiting RNA synthesis. It is rarely used now and has no known neurotoxicity.

Deoxyspergualin (DSG). This investigational antibiotic is effective against some tumors in mice and some human tumors implanted into experimental animals. Neurotoxicity has not been described.

Acivicin. This amino-acid antibiotic appears to have some effect on primary brain tumors[2562]; its neurotoxicity includes a reversible but dose-limiting encephalopathy with somnolence, ataxia, confusion, and hallucinations.[2562,2816] Because acivicin appears to reach the brain via an amino-acid transport system, an adjuvant mixture of amino acids has decreased drug entry into brain and ameliorated encephalopathy in animals without affecting systemic anticancer activity.[2816]

Antimetabolites

The antimetabolites (Table 12–7) can be subdivided into antifolates, cytidine analogs, fluorinated pyrimidines, and purine antimetabolites. Antimetabolites are widely used in cancer therapy and most have some neurotoxicity.

ANTIFOLATES

The antifolates include MTX, trimetrexate, and an investigational compound, edatrexate. The latter has been used experimentally to treat brain tumors because it crosses the blood–brain barrier easily, whereas MTX does not. Antifolates inhibit dihydrofolate reductase, partially depleting reduced folates and causing inhibition of purine and thymidine biosynthesis.

Methotrexate. The most widely used antimetabolite in cancer chemotherapy, MTX has been given orally, intravenously, intraarterially, and intrathecally. The drug is S-phase, cell-cycle–specific and acts primarily against leukemias and lymphomas. MTX crosses the blood–brain barrier poorly; after a continuous IV infusion, the brain-to-blood partition coefficient is 0.1.[2034] MTX levels in the brain can be increased with very high doses intravenously followed by a reversal of the potentially fatal systemic toxicity

Table 12–7. **ANTIMETABOLITES**

Antifolates
Methotrexate
Edatrexate
Trimetrexate
Cytarabine
Hydroxyurea
N-Phosphonoacetyl-L-aspartate (PALA)
Cytidine Analogs
Cytarabine
5-Azacytidine
Fluorinated Pyrimidines
Fluorouracil
Floxuridine
Fotofur
Carmofur
DFUAD
5-Deoxy-5-fluorouridine
FMAU
Purine Analogs
6-Mercaptopurine
6-Thioguanine
Fludarabine
Cladribine (2CdA)
Pentostatin
Chlorodeoxyadenosine
Others
Deoxycoformycin
Tiozofurin
Hydroxyurea

with folinic acid. Folinic acid crosses the blood–brain barrier poorly and thus should not interfere with the CNS effects of MTX, even when it completely prevents systemic toxicity. Intrathecal injection, either by intraventricular injection through an Ommaya device (see Chapter 7) or by lumbar puncture, is used for prophylaxis or treatment of leptomeningeal tumor. Orally administered folinic acid can prevent toxicity from systemic absorption of intrathecal MTX. When injected intrathecally, MTX penetrates the brain variably. In a rabbit study, some drug had reached 40% of the brain 1 hour after intraventricular injection of MTX.[1018] In the larger human brain, penetration is less, so that MTX probably effectively treats only tumor in the leptomeninges, not in the brain.

Acute or chronic neurotoxicity after oral, IV, or intrathecal injection of MTX is a well recognized complication of therapy (Table 12–8).[1159] Risk factors include dose, route of administration, and other concurrent treatments such as RT.[531,2856] Although MTX itself can damage neural tissue, most clinically encountered neurotoxicity results from additive or synergistic effects of cranial irradiation.[141,237,1613,1812] The choroid plexus[248] actively transports MTX out of the nervous system but cytocidal concentrations in CSF are easily achieved after intraventricular injection.[2369]

Aseptic Meningitis. The most common form of acute MTX neurotoxicity is aseptic meningitis, complicating intrathecal administration.[1829] Aseptic meningitis occurs in about 10% of patients who receive intrathecal MTX and is more frequent after lumbar than intraventricular injection. The clinical syndrome is marked by the abrupt onset of headache, stiff neck, nausea, vomiting, lethargy, and fever, usually occurring 2 to 4 hours after MTX instillation and typically lasting for 12 to 72 hours. Examination of the CSF usually reveals a pleocytosis. The disorder may mimic bacterial meningitis, but it occurs too soon after drug instillation to be due to bacterial growth from injection of contaminated material; CSF cultures are negative. The syndrome resolves spontaneously and does not appear to have any long-term sequelae, although one report[266] suggests that such reactions may predispose to later leukoencephalopathy. The reaction may follow either the first or any subsequent injection of MTX, although patients usually do not experience difficulty with continued injections. Risk factors may include higher dose, more frequent instillation, and the presence of leptomeningeal tumor. The pathogenesis is unknown. Some investigators have instilled hydrocortisone with MTX in an attempt to prevent the reaction.[2105]

Encephalomyelopathy. An acute fatal encephalomyelopathy with seizures, paralysis, and coma follows massive overdoses of intrathecal MTX, for example, 650 mg compared to the normal dose of 12 mg.[738] Toxicity from lesser overdoses has been ameliorated by treatment with systemic folinic

Table 12–8. **METHOTREXATE NEUROTOXICITY**

Route of Administration	Dose	Toxic Effect
Oral or intravenous	Conventional	Leukoencephalopathy (if prior brain irradiation)
Intravenous	High-dose	Acute transient encephalopathy
		Chronic leukoencephalopathy
Intra-arterial	Conventional	Hemorrhagic cerebral infarction
Intrathecal	Conventional	Acute aseptic meningitis, paraplegia, seizures
		Chronic leukoencephalopathy, cerebral atrophy, calcification

acid[739] or carboxypeptidase G2,[13] or by CSF exchange.[1272] Rarely, conventional doses of intrathecal MTX cause acute noncardiogenic pulmonary edema,[202,1072] pneumonitis,[1035] an acute tumor lysis syndrome,[2426] or sudden death.[2569]

Transverse Myelopathy. A rare complication of intrathecal MTX, transverse myelopathy usually occurs after several treatments and generally presents within 48 hours of injection, although the onset may be delayed for up to 2 weeks. Graus[970] identified patients whose symptoms began immediately, within 48 hours, or after weeks of delay.[1731] The patient complains of back pain with or without radiation into the legs. The pain is followed by sensory loss,[160,161] paraplegia, and bowel and bladder dysfunction. Recovery varies; some severely affected patients recover fully, others not at all. The exact pathogenesis of MTX myelopathy is unknown but it is believed to be an idiosyncratic drug reaction. Pathologic examination has revealed vacuolar demyelination and necrosis of the spinal cord, sometimes accompanied by brainstem and cerebral hemisphere abnormalities without striking inflammatory or vascular changes.[460] The major site of damage is to areas of the brain and spinal cord closest to the CSF, such as root entry zones, the base of the brain, midbrain, and colliculi. Treatment is ineffective, and the clinician cannot predict which patients will be affected, although the presence of active CNS leukemia or prior spinal irradiation may be predisposing factors. MR scans are usually negative, but at times patchy enhancement can be noted in the spinal cord,[1731] suggesting tumor infiltration. In one of our patients, biopsy did not reveal tumor.

Other symptoms that may rarely follow intrathecal MTX include cranial nerve paresis[263,2865] and transient or permanent hemiparesis.[2865]

Acute Encephalopathy. This disorder sometimes follows the instillation of MTX into the cerebral ventricles, particularly if CSF exit is obstructed.[2365] Encephalopathy has also been reported following inadvertent injection of MTX into the cerebral white matter through a misplaced ventricular cannula.[1522,1963,1965]

High-dose MTX given intravenously can also cause an acute encephalopathy characterized by confusion, disorientation, somnolence, and sometimes seizures (Table 12–9). The onset is within 24 to 48 hours of the treatment and generally resolves without neurologic disability. Prior brain irradiation may be a risk factor.

Subacute Encephalopathy. In a few patients, a subacute encephalopathy follows the administration of weekly IV high-dose MTX (HD MTX). A strokelike syndrome in either adults or children[1697,2725,2860] typically follows the second or third treatment by 5 or 6 days. Patients present with an altered mental status ranging from inappropriate laughter to stupor, usually accompanied by hemiparesis that may fluctuate from one side to the other. Other focal findings include aphasia. Patients generally recover spontaneously within 48 to 72 hours without sequelae and can usually be retreated with HD MTX without recurrence, although a subsequent episode does occur rarely. Serum MTX levels are nontoxic at the time of the syndrome's onset, and the CT scan and CSF are normal. The EEG shows diffuse slowing without epileptiform discharges. The pathogenesis is

Table 12–9. **HIGH-DOSE METHOTREXATE NEUROTOXICITY**

Characteristics	Acute Encephalopathy	Subacute Encephalopathy	Chronic Leukoencephalopathy
Onset	<48 hr	3–10 days	≥3 mo
Symptoms	Confusion, lethargy, headaches, seizures	Multifocal deficits	Spasticity, dementia, seizures
Abnormal CT	No	Rarely	White-matter hypodensity, calcifications
Clinical outcome	Full recovery	Usually full recovery	Persistent neurologic deficits, death

unknown. Brain glucose metabolism decreases following IV infusion with HD MTX, suggesting that derangements in regional glucose metabolism play a role in the clinical presentation.[2033]

HD MTX can cause "dry eyes" with burning and itching,[671] pleuritis,[2637] or osteoporosis with back pain.[2116] Retinal damage can follow intra-arterial MTX after the blood–brain barrier is opened with hyperosmolar agents.[1767] Dizziness, headache, and "fuzzy-headedness," reversible after ceasing treatment, affect as many as 25% of patients receiving weekly low-dose systemic MTX.[2796]

Chronic Encephalopathy. Diffuse leukoencephalopathy is the most devastating form of MTX neurotoxicity. The disorder generally follows repeated doses of IV HD MTX or intrathecal MTX, but it also may occur after standard-dose IV MTX.[2094,2240] Leukoencephalopathy may appear months to years following therapy, beginning either insidiously or abruptly, with personality changes and learning disability.[1920] Children cured of leukemia who have received only IV HD MTX or intrathecal MTX with cranial irradiation show a decrease in IQ after therapy, often by more than 15 points.[1920] Seizures can occur but usually only late in the course. The clinical course varies. Patients may recover slowly over weeks or months, their symptoms may stabilize with a mild-to-moderate dementia, or progress may be relentless with spastic hemiparesis or quadriparesis, severe dementia, and coma, ending in death.

The myelin basic protein concentration may be elevated in CSF, presumably because of myelin breakdown.[881] The CT scan reveals cerebral atrophy, bilateral and diffuse white-matter hypodensities, ventricular dilatation, and sometimes cortical calcifications, findings that are occasionally seen in asymptomatic patients with leukemia.[2023] Focal enhancement may be present in the early stages.[2633] These abnormalities are even more apparent on MR scan.[90,705] Scans may be normal even in patients with diminished intellect,[1418] but usually changes in white matter on the MR scan precede neurologic signs.[1567] Such changes should warn the physician that the patient is at risk for leukoencephalopathy. In patients treated prophylactically, white-matter changes on the MR scan may appear years following treatment with intrathecal and IV MTX, even without RT.[705,1961]

Several different pathologic abnormalities have been reported.* The most common is disseminated foci of white-matter degeneration characterized by demyelination, axonal swelling, and dystrophic mineralization of axonal debris. These necrotizing changes may occasionally be accompanied by fibrinoid necrosis of small blood vessels.[2093] Histologically, leukoencephalopathy from RT cannot easily be distinguished from that of MTX, although axonal swelling is much more characteristic of MTX-induced leukoencephalopathy than of radiation effect.

An unusual pathologic and sometimes radiologic change (now rarely encountered), virtually restricted to children, is mineralizing microangiopathy characterized by noninflammatory fibrosis and calcification of arterial capillaries and venules, particularly in the basal ganglia.[2093]

Pathophysiology. The pathophysiology of MTX neurotoxicity is poorly understood. The depletion of reduced folates in the

*References 307, 2030, 2240, 2386, 2387.

brain, inhibition of cerebral protein or glucose metabolism, injury to cerebral vascular endothelium resulting in increased blood–brain barrier permeability, and inhibition of catecholamine neurotransmitter synthesis have all been implicated but not proved. No effective treatment exists.

Edatrexate. This investigational, lipid-soluble antifolate crosses the blood–brain barrier easily. Used to treat gliomas, its major toxicity at conventional doses is in the skin and GI tract (mucositis). Neurotoxicity has not been reported,[2691] but we have encountered one patient with confusion, gait ataxia, and areas of white matter hyperintensity on MR scan.

Trimetrexate. Possessing many of the properties of MTX, trimetrexate has not been reported to be neurotoxic.

CYTIDINE ANALOGS

Cytosine Arabinoside (Cytarabine, Ara-C). This pyrimidine analog is an S-phase cell-cycle–specific drug that inhibits DNA polymerase α, is incorporated into DNA, and terminates DNA chain elongation. The drug treats leukemia and lymphoma but is not useful for most solid tumors. Although now produced synthetically, arabinose nucleotides were originally isolated from a sponge. Ara-C is given systemically and intrathecally[142,343] in conventional doses and sometimes intravenously in a high-dose regimen. A liposomal ara-C for slow release after intrathecal injection is under clinical trial.[1369] At conventional doses, the drug crosses the blood–brain barrier poorly[558,2348] with blood-to-CSF transport occurring by facilitated diffusion across the choroid plexus. High-dose ara-C yields higher CNS levels; the concentration of ara-C in CSF reaches 6% to 22% of plasma values.[2439] IV ara-C does not cause neurotoxicity at conventional doses but is neurotoxic at high doses.[131] The clinical findings of ara-C toxicity depend on the administration route as well as on patient age, renal function, drug dosage, and the frequency of administration.

Neurotoxicity. Intrathecal ara-C can be neurotoxic. One hour after intrathecal injection of ara-C, more than 67% of the rabbit spinal cord is exposed to the drug,[343] but exposure is certainly much less in humans. Aseptic meningitis and, rarely, myelopathy, both clinically similar to MTX toxicity,[693,2158] can follow intrathecal ara-C. Meningeal irritation causing headache, stiff neck, and pleocytosis has been encountered in approximately 10% of patients given the drug, although no direct relationship between this syndrome and the individual or cumulative dose has been established. The myelopathy begins with back or radicular leg pain. Weakness, sensory alterations, and bowel or bladder dysfunction occur any time from a few days to months following treatment. The clinical picture usually evolves rapidly, sometimes rendering the patient paraplegic. Signs typically persist, but some patients recover.[2276] Examination of the CSF usually reveals an elevated protein level and a modest pleocytosis; an elevated myelin basic protein level has also been reported.[161,460] Pathologically, portions of the spinal cord reveal demyelinization with associated white-matter vacuolization, histologically indistinguishable from MTX-induced myelopathy.[308,460] Forty-eight hours after a single dose of 100 mg of ara-C in conjunction with IV ara-C, *cis*-platinum, and doxorubicin, one patient developed a "locked-in syndrome," in which consciousness was preserved but paralysis prevented communication except by eye movement.[2047] At autopsy, extensive brainstem necrosis was discovered.[1389]

Rarely, intrathecal administration of ara-C is associated with seizures, an acute or subacute encephalopathy, or both.[710,2158] Higher doses and greater frequency of administration increase the risk of intrathecal ara-C neurotoxicity.[2840] The neurotoxic effects of prior radiation or intrathecal MTX treatment may be synergistic with those of intrathecal ara-C,[892] although patients who have suffered MTX neurotoxicity have been successfully treated with intrathecal ara-C without adverse effects.

IV high-dose ara-C, 3 g/m^2 every 12 hours for 8 to 12 doses, may cause several neurologic disorders.[149] Cerebellar dysfunction occurs more frequently in older patients and usually at a cumulative dose of at least 36 g/m^2, but it has been reported after only 3 g/m^2.[183,1234] Patients present with dysarthria, nystagmus, and appendicular and gait ataxia.[698,1149] They may also develop confusion, lethargy, and somnolence. With cessation of the drug, complete resolution of signs and symptoms generally occurs within 2 weeks. Predisposing factors include abnormal renal function, elevated alkaline phosphatase, prior neurologic disorders, age beyond 50 years,[557,957,1107,2234] and perhaps the drug manufacturer.[1302] The EEG may show modest slowing of brain waves. Cerebellar atrophy and reversible white matter abnormalities may be seen on CT or MR scan,[1771] but the CSF is normal.

Although the cerebellar disorder is not fatal, when patients die from their malignancy, neuropathologic changes include widespread loss of Purkinje cells, most pronounced in the deeper portion of the primary and secondary cerebellar sulci. The rest of the CNS appears to be largely unaffected, although white matter demyelination and filamentous degeneration of neurons of brainstem and spinal cord[2705] have also been reported.[1234,2833]

Peripheral neuropathy, either axonal, demyelinating, or both,[270,2081] is a rare complication of ara-C; in most patients, high-dose ara-C was given along with other potentially neurotoxic agents including fludarabine.[1413]

Also reported occasionally are seizures;[710] reversible ocular toxicity,[2177] including blurred vision, photophobia, and burning eye pain[2177]; blindness[1681]; bulbar and pseudobulbar palsy[2374]; Horner's syndrome[1878]; the "painful leg, moving toes syndrome"[1661]; brachial plexus neuropathy[2311]; reversible bilateral lateral rectus palsies[2688]; acute aseptic meningitis (after IV injection)[2589]; and anosmia.[1178] One patient who received a cumulative dose of 72 g developed a parkinsonian syndrome that resolved within 12 weeks.[1621]

The mechanism of ara-C toxicity is unknown. Some investigators believe that ara-C kills neurons by interfering with cytidine-dependent neurotrophic signal transduction. Treatment is unavailable for any of the neurotoxic effects of ara-C, but as indicated previously, many patients recover spontaneously.

5-Azacytidine. A cytidine analog that incorporates into DNA and RNA and prevents DNA methylation, 5-azacytidine has some effect against leukemia. The drug is not usually neurotoxic but is hepatotoxic. Fatal hepatic coma occurred in four patients with extensive hepatic metastases.[177] A neuromuscular syndrome, characterized by muscle tenderness and weakness, may develop after the second or third dose of 200 mg/m^2 per day, as well as encephalopathy, lethargy, and confusion; in one patient, coma was reported.[1532]

FLUORINATED PYRIMIDINES

Fluorinated pyrimidines take advantage of neoplastic cells' absorbing uracil more avidly than nonmalignant cells. These drugs are incorporated into RNA and interfere with its function.

5-Fluorouracil. A pyrimidine analog that binds thymidylate synthase, thereby interfering with DNA synthesis,[2041] 5-FU is useful in GI tumors and breast cancer. In monkeys,[279,1360] it crosses the blood–brain barrier by simple diffusion to achieve a CSF concentration of 11% to 50% that of plasma. In humans, CNS penetration is probably minimal during conventional infusion therapy.[1209,1586] The drug is found in higher concentrations in the cerebellum, especially in granular and Purkinje cell layers, than in the forebrain.[415,1637] In experimental animals, 5-FU may "open" the blood–brain barrier by promoting pinocytotic vesicular transport.[1637]

Neurotoxicity. Neurotoxicity is rare with conventional doses of the drug, except for patients with a congenital abnormality of pyrimidine metabolism who develop ataxia at low doses.[1096,2614] The primary neurotoxicity with higher doses of 5-FU is a cerebellar syndrome, clinically indistinguishable from paraneoplastic or ara-C–induced cerebellar disorders, consisting of truncal and limb ataxia, dysmetria, nystagmus, and dysarthria.[1209,2172] The mechanism of this or other neurotoxicity is unknown. The signs usually reverse within a week after the drug is discontinued but may recur with reintroduction of 5-FU. In experimental animals, 5-FU damages Purkinje cells, granule cells, and neurons of the inferior olive and vestibular nuclei.[2172] If given for several months, 5-FU and some of its derivatives also damage myelin.[1932,1933]

Extraocular muscle abnormalities[222] (particularly vergence disturbances), optic neuropathy,[12] as well as extrapyramidal syndromes[190,1889] have also been reported rarely with the administration of 5-FU. Others have reported encephalopathy with electroencephalographic slowing but without cerebellar symptoms.[988] Ocular toxicity includes blepharitis, conjunctivitis, lacrimal duct stenosis, and excessive lacrimation.[833] Cerebral infarcts have been reported to complicate continuous infusion of the drug.[959] Palmar-plantar erythrodysesthesia, a rare complication, may be confused with a peripheral neuropathy[538] because of painful hands and feet. Acute neurologic symptoms, including somnolence, cerebellar ataxia, and upper motoneuron signs, have been reported following intracarotid arterial infusions. A diffuse encephalopathy occasionally follows conventional IV doses.[1626]

Several modulators have been used to try to enhance the effectiveness of 5-FU or reduce its toxicity in normal tissues. Combining 5-FU with allopurinol, however, can cause acute and subacute cerebellar dysfunction, visual disturbance, dizziness, and, rarely, seizures.[377,1219] The neurotoxicity may be related to reduced 5-FU clearance in the presence of allopurinol. *N*-Phosphonoacetyl-L-aspartate (PALA) inhibits de novo pyrimidine biosynthesis and enhances 5-FU cytotoxicity by increasing its incorporation into RNA. PALA itself may cause ataxia, encephalopathy, and seizures. PALA combined with 5-FU frequently causes cerebellar dysfunction, tremor, memory loss, hallucinations, and seizures.[1832] Thymidine may be neurotoxic when administered in high doses and also appears to enhance the neurotoxicity of 5-FU. Patients develop confusion, disorientation, and lethargy, and a few have experienced nystagmus and dysmetria. When PALA, thymidine, and 5-FU are combined, neurotoxicity is dose-limiting, with dizziness, confusion, ataxia, agitated delirium, and aphasia.[399]

When levamisole is combined with 5-FU,[1792] a few patients develop an inflammatory multifocal leukoencephalopathy.[1197,1371] The disorder usually presents with confusion and focal signs, including ataxia or hemiparesis associated with multiple contrast-enhancing lesions on MR scan, which may be confused with metastases (Fig. 12–2). Levamisole alone may rarely be neurotoxic.[1981]

Floxuridine (5-Fluoro-2′-Deoxyuridine [FUDR]). This drug's mechanism of action, salutary effects, and toxicity are similar to those of 5-FU.

Fotofur. This drug causes encephalopathy, ataxia, and occasionally coma. Because it crosses the blood–brain barrier easily, high concentrations are found in the CSF. Neurotoxicity usually consists of an acute or subacute encephalopathy rather than the cerebellar dysfunction of 5-FU. The neurotoxicity can be dose-limiting.

Carmofur. More widely used in Japan, carmofur causes encephalopathy that sometimes progresses to coma and leaves patients with severe neurologic dysfunction. The CT or MR scan provides evidence of leukoencephalopathy, and the pathologic changes resemble those of MTX leukoencephalopathy.[65,1443,2529]

5′-Deoxy-5-Fluorouridine (DFURD). Effective in breast and colon cancer, DFURD is often neurotoxic, causing dizziness, ataxia, and delirium. Some patients develop a syndrome resembling Wernicke's encephalopathy,[1130] with unsteadiness, weakness, and diplopia.

FMAU. A nucleoside with antiviral and antileukemic activity, this drug has dose-limiting neurotoxicity characterized by extrapyramidal dysfunction that is irreversible at 8 mg/m^2 per day for 5 days. Lower doses may cause transient neurologic dysfunction.[8]

PURINES AND MISCELLANEOUS ANTIMETABOLITES

6-Mercaptopurine and 6-Thioguanine. These agents have little or no neurotoxicity, except for an occasional mild encephalopathy caused by liver toxicity. They do not cross the blood–brain barrier easily.

Deoxycoformycin. This drug is an adenosine deaminase inhibitor that crosses the blood–brain barrier to achieve CSF levels of 10% those of plasma.[1657] In high doses, it causes an encephalopathy characterized by somnolence or agitation and sometimes coma.[1657] The symptoms reverse when the drug is discontinued. Conjunctivitis and complaints of muscle and joint pain[2830] have also been reported.

Tiozofurin. This drug inhibits inosine monophosphate dehydrogenase and causes headache and often severe muscle pains.[2610]

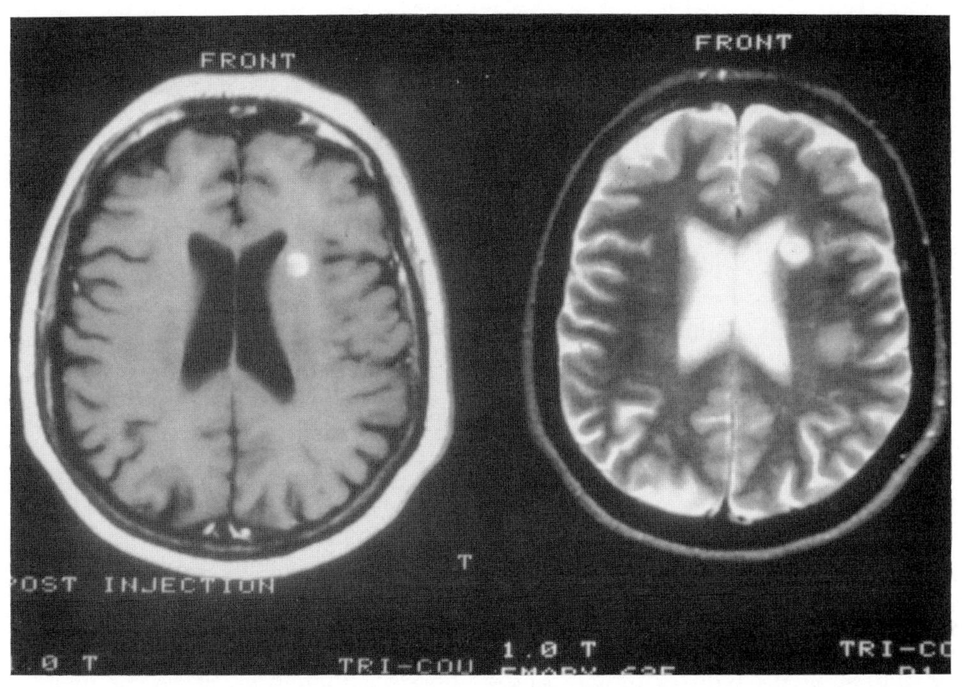

Figure 12–2. Encephalopathy caused by 5-FU-levamisole. This patient with Duke's B colon cancer developed a mild hemiparesis and underwent an MR scan (*left*) that showed a contrast-enhancing lesion in the right hemisphere. Several other lesions did not contrast-enhance but were apparent as hyperintensity on the T_2-weighted image (*right*). After a diagnosis of metastatic tumor, the patient received 3000 cGy to the whole brain. She became demented and bedridden. The needle biopsy specimen of the lesion following the RT revealed the typical demyelination reported as a side effect of 5-FU-levamisole therapy. Metastatic disease was not present.

It may also cause severe encephalopathy with hemiparesis and cortical blindness when given in a prolonged infusion.[2610] The pathogenesis of these disorders is not clear.

Hydroxyurea. An inhibitor of ribonucleotide reductase, an enzyme that catalyzes the rate-limiting step in the de novo synthesis of nucleotide triphosphates required for DNA synthesis, hydroxyurea easily enters CSF[173] to achieve a level of 10% to 25% that of plasma. The drug is widely used to enhance the effect of ionizing radiation and has been used as an adjuvant for radiation of the brain in patients suffering from primary brain tumors. Neurologic toxicity is rare, but when it occurs it includes headache, drowsiness, confusion, and dizziness.

N-Phosphonoacetyl-L-Aspartate (PALA). An inhibitor of aspartate transcarbamoylase, an enzyme catalyzing the second step of de novo pyrimidine biosynthesis, the drug crosses the blood–brain barrier and achieves CSF levels 12% to 40% of plasma levels at 8 hours.[2494] Neurotoxicity includes reversible paresthesias and encephalopathy, sometimes with seizures.[2811] Ataxia occurs when PALA is combined with 5-FU.

Fludarabine. An inhibitor of DNA polymerase and ribonucleotide reductase, fludarabine treats leukemia but can have severe dose-limiting neurotoxicity. In lower doses, the drug causes little neurotoxicity[455] except for transient episodes of somnolence and fatigue[997] or peripheral neuropathy with either paresthesias or weakness.[997] A few patients have reversible focal CNS signs; T_2-weighted MR images show foci of white-matter hyperintensity.[471] At doses greater than 40 mg/m^2 per day, a delayed progressive encephalopathy, characterized by cortical blindness, dementia, coma, and death, can develop.[454,2745] Autopsy shows a diffuse necrotizing leukoencephalopathy most severe in the occipital lobes, medullary pyramids, and posterior columns.[443a,454,2474] Toxicity may increase when fludarabine is combined with cytarabine.[1413] Cladribine(2cdA), a drug also reported useful in patients with multiple sclerosis, causes little neurotoxicity at usual doses. Pentostatin causes dose-related encephalopathy, sometimes with seizures and coma, but at usual doses severe encephalopathy is uncommon.[443a]

Plant Alkaloids

The plant alkaloids all bind to tubulin, the microtubular protein, but the antineoplastic mechanism is different for each group of drugs (Table 12–10). All are highly neurotoxic. They primarily affect the peripheral nervous system but some also have CNS effects.

Table 12–10. **PLANT ALKALOIDS**

Vincas
Vincristine
Vindesine
Vinblastine
Podophyllins
Etoposide (VP-16)
Teniposide (VM-26)
Others
Paclitaxel (Taxol)
Docetaxel (Taxotere)

VINCA ALKALOIDS

The clinically important *Vinca* alkaloids include vincristine, vinblastine, and vindesine. These agents bind to tubulin and prevent microtubule formation, thereby arresting cells in metaphase.[1960] They cross the blood–brain barrier poorly.[1253] Inadvertent intrathecal injection is almost always lethal.[233,860,2815]

Vincristine. The most neurotoxic *Vinca,* vincristine affects primarily the peripheral nerves, although it can also be toxic to the CNS, cranial nerves, and autonomic nervous system (Table 12–11). A dose-limiting sen-

Table 12–11. **SPECTRUM OF VINCRISTINE NEUROTOXICITY**

Toxic Effect	Subacute (1 day–2 wk)	Intermediate (1–4 wk)	Chronic (>4 wk)
Peripheral neuropathy	Depressed Achilles reflex, paresthesias	Other tendon reflexes depressed, paresthesias	Sensory loss, weakness, foot-drop
Myopathy	Muscle pain, tenderness (especially quadriceps); jaw pain		
Autonomic neuropathy	Ileus with abdominal cramping pain	Constipation, urinary hesitancy, impotence, orthostatic hypotension	
Cranial neuropathy (uncommon)			Optic atrophy; ptosis; sixth, seventh, and eighth cranial nerve dysfunction; hoarseness; dysphagia
"Central" toxicity		Seizures, SIADH	

SIADH = syndrome of inappropriate secretion of antidiuretic hormone.
Source: Adapted from Young and Posner,[2870] p 108.

sorimotor neuropathy appears in virtually all patients.[1187] The earliest complaint is tingling and paresthesias of the fingertips and, later, of the toes. Fine movements are often impaired.[583] Loss of ankle jerks is the earliest sign. With continued drug administration, other reflexes also disappear. Muscle cramps, usually diurnal, affect arms and legs and may be the first symptom of neurotoxicity and the last to recover.[1056] Objective sensory loss is uncommon, but weakness, especially of the dorsiflexors of the feet and the wrist extensors, is typical. Foot-drop is either unilateral or bilateral. Unilateral foot-drop is especially common in the superior leg of patients who have lost weight and habitually sit with crossed legs. The weakness seen with vincristine is usually tolerable, but rare patients become bedbound or quadriparetic, particularly if they have a preexisting neuropathy.[433,1724] The sensory symptoms, weakness, and lost reflexes are reversible, although recovery may require several months after the medication is stopped.

Risk factors include age (adults are more severely affected than children), dose, nutritional state, abnormal liver enzymes,[2009] and possibly lymphoma.[2755] Other therapeutic agents such as etoposide,[2573] teniposide,[1002] cyclosporine,[2764] and limb radiation probably also enhance toxicity.[400]

Agents reported to help prevent or relieve vincristine neurotoxicity are gangliosides,[636,1215] glutamic acid,[1255] isaxonine,[1486] prednisone,[2009] pyridoxine,[1255] folinic acid,[1254] and Org 2766.[2667] Transiently occluding the arterial supply to the dominant hand during vincristine infusion is also said to be helpful.[1970] Unfortunately, most treatment is not strikingly effective.[583]

Vincristine occasionally causes unilateral or bilateral focal neuropathies of peripheral or cranial nerves.[1544] Findings include ptosis,[29] ophthalmoplegia,[29] and vocal cord paralysis.[601] The facial nerve,[29] acoustic nerve,[1647] and optic nerve are also occasionally affected.[2287,2568] Night blindness from retinal damage has also been reported.[2175]

Autonomic neuropathy, characterized by colicky abdominal pain and constipation, occurs in as many as 33% of patients. Paralytic ileus is especially frequent in children but is rarely fatal. Amelioration of vincristine-induced ileus with metoclopramide has been reported,[887] but preventing constipation is essential; all patients receiving vincristine should follow a prophylactic bowel regimen of stool softeners and laxatives. This precaution is particularly important when patients are also receiving corticosteroids, because constipation is a major risk factor for steroid-induced bowel perforation (see Chapter 4). Other, infrequent manifestations of autonomic dysfunction include bladder atony, impotence, and postural hypotension.[386]

CNS toxicity of vincristine includes hyponatremia from SIADH.[1910,2182] Encephalopathy[2804] and focal or generalized seizures not due to SIADH[549,1232] have also been reported. Cortical blindness[354,2307] and other focal cerebral signs such as athetosis, ataxia,[388] and parkinsonian symptoms[269] usually reverse after treatment is discontinued.

Diagnosing vincristine neurotoxicity is usually easy, even though the motor weakness typically develops a few weeks following therapy and progresses for several additional weeks. Neurophysiologic studies are usually unnecessary, but when undertaken, they show the features of an axonal neuropathy. These findings have been confirmed by nerve biopsy.[1734]

In experimental animals,[447] vincristine causes focal axonal swellings, primarily in the proximal portion of the peripheral nerves. The swellings result from accumulated maligned neurofilaments with secondary perinodal demyelination. Other changes include a decreased number of microtubules.[2267] In one patient with optic neuropathy, selective loss of β-tubulin from the optic nerve was found.[1836]

Vindesine and Vinblastine. Both these drugs are less neurotoxic than vincristine,[1374] with vindesine being relatively more neurotoxic than vinblastine. The same peripheral and CNS side effects as with vincristine have been reported with both vindesine[804,1145,1919,2768] and vinblastine.[489] The relative cytotoxicity of these *Vinca* alkaloids in cell culture parallels their clinical neurotoxicity.[1374] Vinorelbine, a semisynthetic *Vinca* now in clinical trials, also causes peripheral neuropathy and myalgias.[2195a]

PODOPHYLLINS

Epipodophyllotoxin is an antimitotic agent extracted from the May apple or mandrake plant. The agent binds to tubulin at a different site than the *Vinca* alkaloids. Two synthetic derivatives, etoposide (VP-16) and teniposide (VM-26), are used against many human malignancies including lymphomas, germ-cell tumors, and small-cell lung cancer. These drugs are believed to damage DNA by forming a complex involving the drug, DNA, and topoisomerase type II. Thus, they do not exert their major cytotoxicity through tubulin binding, although this is the mechanism of their peripheral nerve toxicity. They cause an axonal sensory neuropathy or neuronopathy that usually, but not always, reverses after therapy is discontinued.[428] Podophyllotoxins found in herbal medications, particularly those from China, can also cause peripheral neuropathy, as does podophyllin, used topically to treat condyloma acuminatum.* Physicians evaluating a patient with cancer for neurologic symptoms of either peripheral nervous system or CNS origin[1886] must always consider the possibility that the patient is receiving, but not reporting, herbal medicines containing podophyllins or other neurotoxins from an "alternative medicine" practitioner.

Etoposide (VP-16). This drug penetrates CSF poorly, yielding CSF concentrations that are less than 5% of simultaneously measured plasma levels.[2438] It has been given intrathecally to animals without toxicity[2298] but has been reported to occasionally cause a mild and reversible peripheral neuropathy in patients. Intra-arterial injection of etoposide opens the blood–brain barrier.[1922,2472] When combined with other water-soluble agents, it may allow more of those agents to enter the CNS than would enter otherwise. When used in high doses in patients with bone marrow transplantation, etoposide may cause seizures, confusion, and somnolence.[1509]

Teniposide (VM-26). This drug crosses the blood–brain barrier less well than etoposide,[2298] although it is considered to be more effective in treating malignant gliomas. Unlike etoposide, teniposide rarely causes peripheral neuropathy.[1911]

*References 428, 782, 1509, 2298, 2731.

OTHER PLANT ALKALOIDS

Paclitaxel and Docetaxel. Paclitaxel (Taxol[714]) is an agent derived from the Pacific yew tree. Docetaxel (Taxotere) is a partially synthetic Taxol derivative currently used experimentally. Both drugs bind to tubulin but instead of inhibiting polymerization, as do *Vinca* alkaloids, they stabilize and promote microtubular assembly. How this interaction with microtubules causes cytotoxicity is not clear. Both drugs have been useful in treating ovarian and breast cancer. Approximately 60% of patients receiving Taxol at doses of 250 mg/m^2 develop paresthesias of the hands and feet. In most, the symptoms do not progress and may even resolve despite continued therapy.[821,2227] The peripheral neuropathy may be a dose-limiting effect.[432,898a,1578] Itching can be a prominent manifestation of the neuropathy. Arthralgias and myalgias often appear 2 to 5 days after the drug is given. The sensation of light flashing across the visual field has been reported in some patients during Taxol infusion.[2353a]

In some patients, Taxol and Taxotere cause proximal motor weakness that can be disabling. The weakness is probably neuropathic rather than myopathic and may progress or resolve with repeated treatment. The CSF protein may be elevated. Taxol can cause a distal neuropathy that is usually sensory but may be sensorimotor and which, unlike *cis*-platinum neuropathy, affects all sensory modalities. Axonal damage with secondary demyelination probably reflects damage to the cell body.[1880] Taxotere appears to cause a similar sensory neuropathy.[221] Acute arthralgia and myalgia of the legs, curtailing activity and sometimes mistaken for peripheral neuropathy, may occur 2 to 3 days after a course of Taxol and may last for 2 to 4 days. Nerve growth factor prevents Taxol neuropathy in mice and is now in clinical trials.

Miscellaneous Chemotherapeutic Agents

L-ASPARAGINASE

This agent catalyzes the hydrolysis of L-asparagine to aspartic acid and ammonia, depleting asparagine and thus decreasing protein and glycoprotein synthesis. It does not cross the blood–brain barrier but has been given intrathecally.[2165] At high doses, encephalopathy (probably related to liver toxicity) was a problem, but current regimens using lower doses are generally not plagued by this complication.[1526] L-asparaginase interferes with coagulation by inhibiting antithrombin III, possibly leading to thrombosis or hemorrhage. The onset of seizures, headache, or focal neurologic signs should alert the physician to the possibility of sagittal sinus thrombosis with secondary venous infarction.[367,760,2096] Other dural sinuses also may thrombose. Typically, the disorder appears after a few weeks of therapy but sometimes does not until therapy is completed. A definitive diagnosis is made by MR gradient echo sequences, demonstrating clots in the sinus.[1630,1804] An "empty delta sign" seen on a CT scan also suggests the diagnosis.[2898] Treatment is controversial; some investigators recommend anticoagulation but others favor administration of fresh-frozen plasma to replace antithrombin III and depleted fibrinogen. Steroids alleviate the headache; low doses may be necessary for several days to weeks.

AMSACRINE (mAMSA)

This drug[2664] causes muscle aches, cardiac arrhythmias, and (rarely) neurotoxicity that includes transient peripheral neuropathy[2664] and, occasionally, seizures.[1510]

Suramin. A polysulfonated urea and an antihelminthic agent that is useful to treat prostate and some other cancers,[1844] this drug inhibits reverse transcriptase and the binding of several growth factors to their specific receptors.[1777,2558] Suramin serves as a radiation enhancer as well as a cytotoxic agent. Because this drug inhibits cortisol secretion, patients are given hydrocortisone replacement.

Suramin causes a peripheral neuropathy in 40% of patients whose blood levels of the drug reach more than 350 μg/L. The disorder presents as a Guillain-Barré–like syndrome with the rapid onset of a predominantly motor neuropathy with four-extremity paralysis[1447] and sometimes bulbar and respiratory paralysis. Paresthesias in the face and limbs are common prior to the weakness, which often begins proximally. The disorder probably results when demyelination causes a conduction block in the peripheral nerve that can be identified by electromyographic study. The disorder reverses after the drug is discontinued and can be prevented by carefully monitoring blood levels. Suramin-induced neurite growth–inhibition can be overcome by nerve growth factor.[2252a] Whether this is of clinical importance is unclear.

Combined Chemotherapy

Most patients with cancer who are treated with chemotherapeutic agents receive more than one agent because single-agent therapy is rarely curative. Combining chemotherapeutic agents may cause more and sometimes different neurotoxicity than single-agent therapy. For example, a regimen for treating acute lymphoblastic leukemia included vincristine, L-asparaginase, daunorubicin, and prednisone; followed by consolidation with oral MTX and weekly intrathecal injections of MTX, ara-C, and hydrocortisone; and ending the consolidation with IV VP-16 and ara-C. This regimen led to seizures or episodes of transient neurologic dysfunction 10 days after the administration of IV ara-C, VP-16, and triple intrathecal therapy. Discontinuing the intrathecal ara-C did not prevent the neurotoxicity, but giving oral leucovorin 24 to 36 hours after the MTX did.[2831] In another study of multiagent chemotherapy and hormonal therapy for breast cancer, over 1% of patients suffered arterial thromboses, most of which caused cerebral infarcts; 4 of the 9 cerebral infarcts were fatal.[2730] The events occurred while patients received chemotherapy, suggesting that the multiagent chemotherapy was causal. One patient with a urethral cancer developed status epilepticus while being treated with a combination of MTX, vincristine, epirubicin, and *cis*-platinum.[1738] Combination chemotherapy is generally more neurotoxic when administered with cranial RT than it is alone. Complications of RT are discussed in the next chapter.

Antineoplastic Hormones

Both hormone agonists and antagonists have selective antineoplastic activity (Table 12–12). Most are used against breast and

Table 12–12. **TYPES OF ANTINEOPLASTIC HORMONES**

Type	Example
Androgens	Danazol
Antiandrogens	Flutamide
Estrogens	Diethylstilbestrol (DES)
Anti-estrogens	Tamoxifen
Progestins	Megestrol
Adrenocorticosteroids	Dexamethasone
Antiadrenals	Aminogluthamide
Antiprogestins	Mifepristone
Aromatase inhibitors	Aminoglutethimide

prostate carcinomas. The two most widely used, tamoxifen for breast cancer and adrenocorticosteroids (such as dexamethasone and prednisone) for lymphomas and breast cancer, can be neurotoxic. The other hormonal agents have expected endocrine side effects, but neurotoxicity is not a major problem. Steroid side effects are discussed in Chapter 4.

TAMOXIFEN

This synthetic anti-estrogen appears to cross the blood–brain barrier to concentrate both in the brain and brain metastases,[1566] although levels in CSF are low. The most common neurologic side effect is decreased visual acuity with macular edema.[92,1730,1998] In a prospective study of 63 patients on long-term, low-dose tamoxifen, 4 developed either keratitis or retinopathy, both of which were fully reversible when the drug was discontinued. Other rare side effects include priapism,[768] acute reversible encephalopathy characterized by delusions and hallucinations,[2197] depression, irritability, insomnia, headache, poor concentration,[1607] cerebellar dysfunction,[2048] and radiation recall syndrome.[1984] The drug also has been reported to be associated with thromboembolic disease in 1% to 2% of patients.[2289]

DANAZOL AND FLUTAMIDE

When substances having androgenic activity, such as danazol, are used in women, muscle cramps, fatigue, somnolence, headache, and irritability sometimes accompany the androgenic effects of hirsutism and voice deepening, and the anti-estrogenic effects of hot flashes. Luteinizing hormone-releasing hormone agonists used for prostate cancer cause loss of libido, impotence, weight gain, and gynecomastia. Cancer symptoms such as bone pain and spinal cord compression may worsen acutely when the drug is first instituted. This flare can be inhibited by the concurrent use of the antiandrogen flutamide. Side effects of flutamide include gynecomastia, pain, decreased libido, and hot flashes.

OTHER HORMONAL AGENTS

Estrogenic agents such as diethylstilbestrol are used to treat patients with breast and prostate cancer. The drugs sometimes cause dizziness, headache, and depression as well as thromboembolic disease after long-term use. Significant neurologic side effects are rare. Progestational agents such as medroxyprogesterone and megestrol increase appetite and lead to weight gain, so they are often used as supportive care agents as well as antineoplastic agents. Impotence, headache, and insomnia are typical side effects in men. Both men and women sometimes become nervous and develop somnolence or dizziness. Neurologic complications are uncommon. Antiprogestational agents such as mifepristone are said to be useful in treating patients with breast cancer, pituitary tumors, and meningiomas.[1022] Neurologic side effects are not reported. Aromatase inhibitors inhibit production of steroid hormones. The most commonly used one, aminoglutethimide, treats patients with breast carcinoma. It has been reported to cause dizziness, lethargy, and muscle cramps. Because the drug inhibits adrenal secretion, glucocorticoids must be given. Since aminoglutethimide accelerates dexamethasone metabolism, hydrocortisone should be used as adrenal replacement. Additional hormonal agents used less frequently in patients with cancer are listed in Table 12–12.

Biologic Agents

Several biologic approaches may be used to manipulate the immune system to destroy neoplastic cells (Table 12–13). Antibodies

Table 12–13. **TYPES OF ANTINEOPLASTIC BIOLOGICS**

Type	Examples
Antibodies	Epidermal growth factor receptor
Immune cells	Lymphokine-activated killer cells Tumor-infiltrating lymphocytes
Vaccines	Melanoma cells
Immune enhancers	Levamisole
Differentiation agents	Retinoic acid
Cytokines	Interleukin-2, interferon
Immunosuppressants	Immunoglobulins

and either peripheral-blood or tumor-infiltrating lymphocytes (TIL) from the patient, enhanced in vitro[629] (i.e., lymphokine-activated killer [LAK] cells), directly attack the tumor. Tumor vaccines, cytokines, or nonspecific immune-enhancing agents such as levamisole strengthen the patient's intrinsic immunity. Conversely, immunosuppressive drugs may be used to prevent the graft-versus-host reaction[2726] in patients undergoing bone marrow transplantation. Also available are agents that wage a biologic attack on the tumor by differentiating tumor cells or inhibiting tumor angiogenesis.

A few of these agents, to be discussed shortly, cause notable nervous system toxicity (Table 12–14).[629,819,2416,2602] Useful updates on the biologic therapy of cancer are published monthly.[2313]

ANTIBODIES

Monoclonal antibodies raised against various cancers have been used in clinical trials for several years. The antibody itself may be

Table 12–14. **NEUROTOXICITY OF SOME IMMUNOTHERAPEUTIC AGENTS**

	Acute <1 wk	Early-Delayed 1–4 wk	Late-Delayed >1 mo
OTK3 antibody	Aseptic meningitis Seizures Cerebral infarction		
Interleukin-2	Cerebral edema Encephalopathy (frequent) Leukoencephalopathy (rare) Nerve compression (during late vascular syndrome) Brachial plexopathy	Transient focal deficits	
Interferon α	Acute paresthesias Loss of taste/smell Encephalopathy Leukoencephalopathy (intrathecal)	Brachial plexopathy Encephalopathy Headache	Encephalopathy/dementia Parkinsonism Sensory and sensorimotor polyneuropathy Third-nerve palsy Papilledema
Levamisole	Aseptic meningitis		Leukoencephalopathy "MS-like" with 5-FU
Cyclosporine	Seizures Burning feet and hands during infusion	Seizures Tremor Cortical blindness Myelopathy	Myopathy Sensorimotor polyneuropathy Tremor

5-FU = 5-fluorouracil; MS = multiple sclerosis.

cytotoxic or it may be conjugated to a cytotoxic agent such as ricin.[643a] Although most antibodies do not cross the blood–brain barrier, neurotoxicity, especially peripheral neuropathy,[958] has been reported. An antiganglioside monoclonal antibody raised against neuroblastoma, 3F8, reacts with dorsal root ganglion cells to cause severe pain, often necessitating a continuous IV infusion of morphine. No permanent neurotoxicity has been identified. OTK3, an anti–T-cell monoclonal antibody, is sometimes used to suppress the graft-versus-host reaction. This antibody occasionally causes aseptic meningitis[11,2726] or cerebritis with seizures[379] and, rarely, at high doses, cerebral infarction.[2114] Other monoclonal antibodies and immunotoxins have been reported to cause sensorimotor neuropathy[958] or encephalopathy with seizures and coma.[1968]

IMMUNE CELLS

Although lymphocytes, either LAK cells or TIL, seem to have little or no neurotoxicity, interleukin-2 (IL-2) used to activate the lymphocytes is neurotoxic (see the following). Cryopreserved stem cells used for bone marrow rescue have been reported to cause a reversible encephalopathy.[635a]

VACCINES

Vaccines, including those that act against glioma cells, have been injected into patients for many years. At one time, physicians feared that contaminating myelin might cause an immune-mediated encephalomyelitis. The vaccines were not neurotoxic but, unfortunately, were also not very effective.

CYTOKINES

Cytokines used clinically include IL-2, IL-1, tumor necrosis factor, and the interferons.[1081] Colony-stimulating factors (CSF) such as G-CSF and GM-CSF counteract the marrow-suppressive effects of anticancer drugs. Most cross the blood–brain barrier poorly and have little neurotoxicity,[2284] although a case of cerebral arterial thrombosis in a patient receiving G-CSF along with multiagent chemotherapy has been reported.[491]

Interleukin-1 and Interleukin-2. Although IL-2 can cross the blood–brain barrier[1694] and can be safely administered intrathecally, it causes capillaries, including those in the brain, to leak.[2291] After giving patients IL-2, increases in brain water content were inferred from MR scans.[2416] IL-2 can also cause a severe encephalopathy,[1751,2416] but the patients often are so systemically ill that the encephalopathy is not noticed. It is always reversible if the patient recovers from the acute systemic toxicity. Transient focal neurologic signs, such as visual loss, have also been reported,[195] as have occasional transient hypothyroidism,[2771] myalgias, and headache.[2636] Acute brachial plexopathy is a rare effect.[1597] The drug probably alters cerebral vasomotor responses to physiologic stimuli.[723] IL-1 causes encephalopathy and, infrequently, seizures.[1872] IL-4 causes fatigue, anorexia, and headache in some patients[97] and, occasionally, hyponatremia.

Tumor Necrosis Factor. This agent causes asthenia and depression but has no other major side effects.

Interferons. The interferons cause encephalopathy, which may be irreversible.[1749,1761] Milder changes include nightmares, headache, and myalgias. Bilateral brachial plexopathy,[198] oculomotor palsies,[165] hearing loss,[1330] and transient thyrotoxicosis followed by hypothyroidism have been reported.[2297] Meningitis and blood–brain-barrier disruption have been observed in rats.[2110]

IMMUNE ENHANCERS

Nonspecific agents that enhance natural immunity are sometimes used as adjuvants to chemotherapy. The most common of these is levamisole, an antihelminthic agent that enhances immunity.[1636] The drug has been effective when used with fluorouracil in patients with colon cancer. Although it has little neurotoxicity,[1792] levamisole can cause aseptic meningitis with headaches,[1636] stiff neck, fever, and CSF lymphocytic pleocytosis, as well as vertigo[1981] and seizures.[1636] It sometimes alters taste and causes a hyperalert state with anxiety and irritability. When combined with 5-FU, it can cause demyelination of the brain,[1197] characterized by multifocal neurologic symptoms associated with multiple demyelinating lesions of the white matter resembling multiple sclerosis. The lesions may contrast-enhance on a CT or MR scan and can be mistaken for brain metastases, leading to incorrect and probably deleterious treatment with RT (see Fig. 12–2).[2019]

DIFFERENTIATION AGENTS

Retinoic acid, hexamethylene bisacetamide, phenylacetate, and other agents promote the differentiation of tumor cells into their more normal counterparts. All-trans-retinoic acid has proved to be particularly useful in treating promyelocytic leukemia, but like other vitamin A analogs, the drug increases intracranial pressure[2447] and commonly causes diffuse headache. A few cases of papilledema have been reported. The symptoms are rarely disabling but are bothersome to the patient. They always resolve at the end of therapy and can be treated with analgesic agents. Other differentiating agents appear to lack neurotoxic effects.

IMMUNOSUPPRESSIVE AGENTS

Some antineoplastic agents, such as cyclophosphamide and corticosteroids, are also immunosuppressive. Other agents, including cyclosporine, tacrolimus (FK506[2822]), and IV gamma globulin, are sometimes prescribed to prevent graft rejection after transplantation. Cyclosporine is a neurotoxic drug that can cause acute cortical blindness and encephalopathy as well as generalized seizures.[146,170,2143,2233] A reversible demyelinating polyneuropathy has also been reported.[1565a] The incidence of cyclosporine neurotoxicity is 4% to 10%.[2726] The drug damages the vascular endothelium and thus may disrupt the blood–brain barrier and intensify the toxicity of other chemotherapeutic agents.[146] IV immunoglobulin is generally non-neurotoxic, but a few cases[2759] of aseptic meningitis and, more rarely, cerebral infarction[2422] have been reported. The pathogenesis of this infarction is unknown but may be related to hyperviscosity caused by the high-protein load. Tacrolimus sometimes causes an encephalopathy as well as insomnia, headache, and tremor, and has been reported to cause a reversible peripheral neuropathy.[106a]

BONE MARROW TRANSPLANTATION

Most drugs that effectively treat cancer cause dose-limiting bone marrow suppression. Replacing the bone marrow either with the patient's own bone marrow that has been taken and stored before high-dose chemotherapy (autologous bone marrow transplantation or bone marrow rescue) or with the marrow from a human lymphocyte antigen-matched donor (allogeneic transplantation) effectively treats some leukemias and lymphomas. These procedures are also being tested in patients with solid tumors, including breast cancer and brain tumors.[785] Autologous transplants can, when necessary, be purged of tumor cells. After the bone marrow is removed, the next step involves high-dose cytotoxic chemotherapy and sometimes total body irradiation. Supportive drugs, particularly antibiotics and cytokines, are used during the period before the marrow engrafts; immunosuppressive agents are required to prevent rejection of allogeneic transplants.

Frequently, patients undergoing bone marrow transplantation develop neurologic symptoms.* Sometimes it is impossible to identify one particular cause of neurologic signs. It is likely that the neurotoxicity is caused by synergistic effects among agents. Metabolic encephalopathy and seizures are common during the acute phase of marrow transplantation. The seizure is usually a single generalized convulsion and, although most patients are thrombocytopenic at the time, is almost never related to CT-detectable bleeding in the brain. The seizure usually does not recur even if the patient does not receive anticonvulsant drugs, and it does not appear to create a long-term risk for the development of epilepsy. The pathogenesis of the seizure or the metabolic encephalopathy often accompanying it is not generally identifiable, but the symptoms are usually reversible. The few patients who die with metabolic encephalopathy generally have multiple organ failure. Lhermitte's sign as a transient phenomenon[2793] and a Wernicke-like encephalopathy[1655] have also been reported after bone marrow transplantation. Ocular complications include cataracts and,

---

*References 509, 1762, 1973, 1989b, 2452, 2827.

if total body irradiation has been given, dry eyes and conjunctival staining.[297]

Graft-versus-host disease occurring after allogeneic bone marrow transplantation is generally not associated with neurotoxicity, but a polymyositislike illness has been reported in a few patients,[1869] as well as a single case of a subacute panencephalitis with seizures and encephalopathy.[1251]

Adjuvant Agents

Many patients with cancer receive drugs that do not have antineoplastic effects. Instead, they (1) enhance the effects of antineoplastic agents, (2) protect against toxicity, or (3) treat symptoms associated with the cancer or its treatment; that is, they provide supportive care (Table 12–15). Recent reviews describe some in detail.[479,2333] Although neurotoxicity is insignificant in most of these agents, in some it is dose-limiting. Agents used for supportive care are discussed in Chapter 4.

Table 12–15. **ANTINEOPLASTIC AGENT SENSITIZERS AND PROTECTORS**

Sensitizers
Nitromidazoles
Misonidazole
Metronidazole
Etanidazole
Hydrogenated pyrimidines
BuDR
IuDR
Protectors and Rescue Agents
Free-radical scavengers
WR2721
Allopurinol
Mesna
Leucovorin
Uridine
Glutathione depletion
Buthionine sulfoxamine

The nitroimidazole drugs have an oxymimetic effect that sensitizes hypoxic tumor tissue to RT. The drugs also have been used to sensitize tumor tissue to various chemotherapeutic agents. Such radiation sensitivity has not enjoyed striking success. Some drugs, including misonidazole, metronidazole, and etanidazole, cause sensory neuropathy at high doses.[845,1740] This axonal neuropathy begins with numbness and tingling in the lower extremities and sometimes the fingertips, progressing proximally. Once symptoms begin, the drug should be discontinued and the neuropathy, if mild, usually resolves. A small fraction of patients complain of weakness or ototoxicity. CNS toxicity is rare.

Glutathione protects cells against RT and chemotherapy by free-radical scavenging and detoxifying electrophils. Glutathione depletion using buthionine sulfoxamine is being tested as a possible radiation and chemotherapy sensitizer. The drug may cause seizures and hepatotoxicity.

A sulfhydrylradioprotector, WR2721, penetrates the blood–brain barrier poorly and does not appear to protect brain or spinal cord, as it protects other normal tissues, from the damaging effects of RT.[479,2333] It also shields most normal tissues against the cytotoxicity of *cis*-platinum, cyclophosphamide, and some mustards. The drug generally causes mild somnolence, possible hypotension during infusion, and sometimes hypocalcemia that is not usually symptomatic. The pathophysiology of the somnolence is not understood.

Allopurinol has both enhancing and protecting aspects. It prolongs the half-life of 6-mercaptopurine by decreasing the rate of metabolic elimination, thus increasing the cytotoxicity of that drug. It also prevents formation of toxic 5-FU metabolites, however, decreasing the toxicity of that drug. It does not have significant neurotoxicity. Other non-neurotoxic protectors include meprapoethane (mesna), leucovorin, and uridine.

CHAPTER 13

SIDE EFFECTS OF RADIATION THERAPY

Radiation therapy (RT) kills tumor cells. Given a sufficient dose of RT, all neoplasms can be sterilized and the cancer cured. Unfortunately, the curative potential of this therapy is all too often limited by potential damage to normal tissue within the radiation portal. Recent reviews detail RT effects on tumor tissue* and the nervous system.† As Table 13–1 suggests, any part of the nervous system can suffer direct damage from RT, and some areas endure indirect damage. Neoplasms and normal tissue respond differently to RT: (1) Normal cells are better able than tumor cells to repair sublethal radiation damage. (2) Some tumor cells are inherently more sensitive to the direct effects of RT than normal cells. (3) Reproducing cells are more sensitive to RT than cells in the resting phase. This sensitivity of tumor cells, however, may be only slightly greater than that of the normal surrounding tissue. The small differential between gliomas and normal glial tissue, for instance, prohibits doses of external-beam radiation large enough to cure.

* References 1064, 1518, 1825, 2480, 2593, 2835, 2854.
† References 201, 590, 683, 919, 1036, 2222, 2892.

BIOLOGY OF RADIATION DAMAGE

Ionization

X-rays, gamma rays, and atomic particles such as electrons, neutrons, and protons, as well as such elements as helium, cause ionization when they interact with tissue. The average number of ionizations per unit of path length is referred to as the linear energy transfer (LET). Types of radiation with higher LET (e.g., neutron radiation) cause more biologic damage than low-LET radiation (e.g., x-rays). Ionizing radiation causes cellular damage in several ways:

1. It breaks DNA. Single-stranded breaks usually repair themselves, but double-stranded breaks may be repaired either in a mutated form or not at all. The

repair of sublethal damage usually occurs within 6 hours, although some cells in the nervous system may take longer.[1483] Failure to repair sublethal damage leads to either immediate cell death or delayed death at the first or a subsequent attempt of the damaged cell to reproduce. When RT has been directed at the peripheral nervous system or CNS, cell death may occur months or years later because glial and Schwann cells reproduce so slowly.
2. Ionizing radiation may attack RNA, lipids, and proteins, causing cellular damage and probably cell death.
3. Radiation may stimulate apoptosis, programmed cell death,[390,1295,1610] by mechanisms not yet understood but believed to be an important component of radiation and chemotherapy effects on cancer cells.

Fractionation

Therapeutic external RT is usually given in a series of equal-sized fractions, either daily or more than once a day for several weeks. Each fraction kills a similar proportion of tumor cells, resulting in a logarithmic decline in the number of surviving cells as the number of fractions increases. Another result is that smaller tumors are more susceptible than larger tumors to complete sterilization at a given dose. Because of the logarithmic effect of the fractionation schedule, the differential effect on tumor tissue becomes greater with a larger number of fractions. Several techniques attempt to decrease RT toxicity to normal tissue surrounding the tumor. Radiation sensitizers, particularly those that do not cross the normal blood–brain barrier but enter tumors within the CNS, are designed to promote tumor damage relative to normal tissue damage. Radiation protectors are designed to guard normal tissue. Several methods efficient in focusing the radiation beam include using high-energy particles, conformal radiation, radiosurgery, and also brachytherapy, the implantation of the tumor with radioactive sources. Neither radiation sensitizers nor protectors have yet proved effective in treating CNS tumors. High-energy particles have proved particularly effective against pituitary tumors but not against brain tumors. Three-dimensional treatment plans, conformal radiation, stereotactic radiosurgery, and brachytherapy all show promise in treating some CNS tumors by delivering higher doses to the tumor and lower doses to normal tissue.

RT administered in multiple fractions per day is based on the observation that recovery from sublethal damage engendered by RT is accomplished more completely and faster (i.e., in less than 6 hours) in normal cells than in tumor cells.[1067] The repair process may persist beyond 8 hours in some normal tissues, such as the spinal cord, making hyperfractionation less safe than some formulas suggest.[1483] A high total dose of RT is necessary to obtain the same biologic effect in tumor cells, but the lower dose per fraction delivers it with more safety to normal cells. RT administered in multiple doses per fraction has been used to treat primary brain tumors, although clinical evidence that it is more effective than single-dose RT is unavailable.[1067]

Table 13–1. **SITES OF RT-INDUCED INJURY TO THE NERVOUS SYSTEM**

Direct	Indirect
Brain	Cerebral and systemic blood vessels
Spinal cord	
Cranial nerves	Endocrine organs
Peripheral nerves	Secondary tumors

Hypotheses of Damage Mechanisms

Damage to the nervous system from RT depends on many exogenous and endogenous factors (Table 13–2). The mechanism(s) by which the peripheral nervous system and CNS are damaged is controversial. Three hypotheses, not necessarily mutually exclusive, have been proposed. The first is that ionizing radiation directly damages nervous system cells. Because RT-induced nervous system damage predominantly affects white matter more than gray matter, glial cells, par-

Table 13–2. **RISK FACTORS FOR RADIATION DAMAGE TO THE NERVOUS SYSTEM**

Radiation Factors	Host Factors
Doses per fraction	Age[1962,2246,2419,2655a]
Total dose	Sex[2716,2717]
Total duration of therapy	Genetic predisposition
	Pre-existing nervous system disease
Volume of tissue radiated	Infection
Energy of radiation	Systemic diseases (e.g., hypertension, diabetes)
	Chemotherapy

ticularly oligodendroglial, and Schwann cells have been proposed as the most vulnerable. Also, because all but olfactory neurons are postmitotic, they are less susceptible to RT damage, although either apoptosis[1295] or DNA damage, preventing the normal function of critical genes, may lead to neuronal dysfunction or death.

The second proposal is that RT damages vascular endothelium. Hopewell and Wright[1199] postulate that after extensive damage to endothelial cells, a few localized clones survive at irregular locations along the vessel. These multiply, leading to luminal constriction and eventually to vascular occlusion, causing ischemia and necrosis of neural tissue. This hypothesis suffers from the fact that, although vascular occlusions occur in areas of delayed radiation damage, the degree of necrosis is usually greater than can be explained by the degree of vascular damage.

The third hypothesis, proposed by Lampert and colleagues[1461] and Lampert and Davis,[1462] suggests that damaged glial cells release antigens identified as foreign by the immune system. An immune response leads to both the necrosis and vascular changes of a hypersensitivity reaction. Virtually no direct evidence exists for this third hypothesis, although in one patient a focal vasculitis in an irradiated area of brain was associated with circulating immune complexes.[1013] Thus, the exact cause of radiation damage to the peripheral nervous system and CNS is still unknown, although, at least in experimental animals, lower RT doses appear to cause neurotoxicity via the endothelial cells, and higher doses via glial cells.

The Linear-Quadratic Concept

The linear-quadratic concept (Fig. 13–1) posits a double mechanism for cell killing. The first, or linear, component, also called nonrepairable or alpha (α),[1064,1067,2283] results from simultaneous double-stranded DNA breaks by the same electron. The probability of an effect is proportional to the dose (D). The second, or quadratic, component, also called repairable or beta (β), results from two chromosome breaks by different electrons. The probability of an effect is proportional to the square of the dose or D^2. The overall effect is expressed: $E = \alpha D + \beta D^2$. The α/β ratio is the dose at which cell killing by the linear and quadratic components is equal; thus, the ratio measures fractionation sensitivity. For early reactions, such as skin desquamation, α/β is large, approximately 10 Gy,* and, thus, the size of the RT fraction is relatively unimportant. For tissue such as the nervous system, which suffers little early damage but much late damage, the α/β ratio is

*10Gy (gray) = 1000 cGy = 1000 rad.

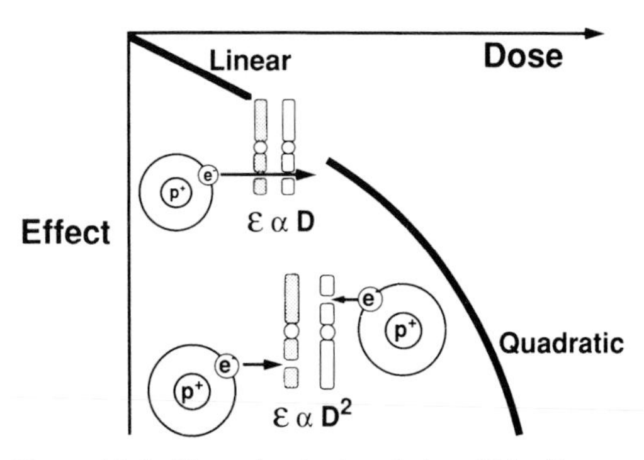

Figure 13–1. Linear-quadratic relation. This diagram shows how breaks in two chromosomes may be caused by a single electron track or by two separate electron tracks. The probability of these events will be proportional to the dose and the square of the dose, respectively. (From Hall,[1064] p 3756, with permission.)

Table 13–3. **FORMULAS TO ESTIMATE NERVOUS SYSTEM TOLERANCE OF RT**

Formulas	TOLERANCE Brain	Spinal Cord	Peripheral	Author/Ref. No.
Linear-Quadratic Formula				
$BED = \frac{E}{\alpha} = Nd\ (1 + \frac{d}{\alpha/\beta})$				Hall[1064]
CNS Formulas				
NSD (ret) $= D \times N^{-.24} \times T^{-.11}$	1700 ret		2000 ret[469]	Ellis[722]
Neuret $= D \times N^{-.41} \times T^{-.03}$	1100 neuret			Sheline et al[2379]
ED ret $= D \times N^{-.377} \times T^{-0.58}$	1250 ret	1000 ret		Wara et al[2740]
BTU $= D \times N^{-.45} \times T^{-.03}$	1050 btu			Pezner and Archambeau[2024]

BED = biologically effective dose (Gy); BTU = brain tolerance unit; D = dose in rad (cGy); d = dose in Gy; E = total effect of radiation; ED = equivalent dose; N = number of fractions; Neuret = ret applied to CNS; NSD = nominal standard dose; Ret = rad equivalent therapy; T = total elapsed time in days.

small, implying that the size of the RT fractions is very important.

The linear-quadratic formula allows the physician to explain the total effect (E) of radiation based on the number of fractions of RT administered (N), the dose per fraction (D), and the α and β factors (Table 13–3). Available evidence[2656] indicates that it is reasonable to use α/β values of 8 to 10 Gy for tissue that suffers early damage, such as rapidly growing tumor, and of 1.5 to 4 Gy for tissue such as the brain, which suffers late damage. Based on these formulas, higher daily doses of radiation, 1.2 cGy bid, can be delivered to the brain with greater biologic effect on the tumor and biologic effect on the normal brain similar to that obtained with conventional daily doses.

Based on a saturable cellular repair mechanism, a newer model[2283] gives results similar to the linear-quadratic model except that they diverge at very low and high doses. This model may predict both early and late radiation damage.

Formulas Predicting Nervous System Toxicity

Several other attempts, rooted in animal experiments and clinical observations, have been made to define a neurologically "safe dose" of RT, using formulas different from the linear-quadratic equation but also based on total dose and fraction size (see Table 13–3). The best-known formula was developed by Ellis[721,722] following experiments on the tolerance of pigskin to radiation. Ellis expressed tolerance in terms of a nominal standard dose (NSD) which he called the "rad equivalent therapy" (ret). The NSD is based on the total dosage in rad or cGy modified by the number of fractions in which the dose is given and the total elapsed time of treatment. The overall treatment time is less relevant in tissues that repair slowly, as do those in the CNS. As shown in Table 13–3, the threshold for brain necrosis is about 1700 to 1800 ret. Wara and colleagues,[2740] using the formula in Table 13–3, estimated the likelihood of spinal cord toxicity as 1% at 1015 ret and 50% at 1480 ret.

Several investigators have modified the Ellis formula, attempting to apply it specifically to neural tissues. These modifications have mostly been based on clinical observations of neural toxicity. Sheline and colleagues[2379] modified the formula with N based on the slope of an isoeffect line below which there is no CNS toxicity in humans and T based on the tolerance of rat spinal cord. He expressed tolerance as "neuret," the neural equivalent of Ellis's ret. In this formula, the threshold tolerance of the nervous system is 1000 to

1100 neuret. The neuret formula better discriminates a threshold dose than does the Ellis formula. Wara and associates[2740] called their modification an "equivalent dose" (ED). Necrosis was not reported in 51 patients with an ED of 1250 or less. With an ED between 1251 and 1330, 2 of 60 patients developed necrosis of the spinal cord; 5 of 28 patients developed spinal necrosis with an ED between 1331 and 1460. Pezner and Archambeau's[2024] modification yielded "brain tolerance units" (BTU). They found a very low risk of brain necrosis at less than 1050 BTU, with a steep rise at greater than 1200 BTU.

All these formulas highlight the importance of the number of doses per fraction as opposed to the time period in which RT is administered for determining nervous tissue tolerance. None clearly identifies a tolerance below which no damage to the nervous system will occur, because individual host factors also determine sensitivity (see Table 13–2). The apparent difference in tolerance between brain and spinal cord may not be real but may instead be an artifact of differences in the volume irradiated (more for the brain), in the underlying disease (parenchymal brain tumor versus extraparenchymal spinal lesions), and in the greater severity of neurologic disability from radiation damage to the spinal cord than to the brain, which prompts more conservative limits for spinal RT.

Although these formulas are not infallible because they cannot estimate all of the risk factors listed in Table 13–2, they are valuable to the clinician who attempts to determine whether neurologic signs developing after RT are related to the RT or are another neurologic complication. A good clinical rule of thumb is that for both brain and spinal cord, 6000 cGy in 200-rad fractions causes a 5% incidence of neurotoxic complications.[2379] With doses given at full tolerance, re-treatment within 2 years carries increased risk of RT damage,[2336,2337] but 2 years after receiving 4400 cGy, the primate spinal cord can tolerate full doses of RT safely.[57] Similar experiments have not been conducted on the brain, but most patients who receive 3000 cGy in 10 fractions (fr) for brain metastases can tolerate re-irradiation at this same dosage if they relapse after a year or more (see Chapter 5).

CLINICAL DIAGNOSIS OF RADIATION-INDUCED NEUROTOXICITY

Clinically diagnosing RT neurotoxicity may be difficult. In any patient with neurologic signs who has previously had RT, the physician should determine:

1. whether the clinical signs correlate with the site previously irradiated,
2. the volume of the nervous system irradiated,
3. the total dose,
4. the dose per fraction, and
5. the time elapsed between RT and the development of neurologic symptomatology.

The physician can then use one of the formulas previously discussed to calculate whether the biologic dose was sufficient to damage the CNS, but it is also important to consider that prior or concomitant chemotherapy may synergize with RT, as may other factors such as the age (either very young or elderly) at which the patient was irradiated. Neurologic disease may also sensitize neural tissue to radiation damage.

In the brain, the differential diagnosis of RT toxicity includes recurrent tumor, brain abscess, or RT necrosis. The diagnosis can be made confidently only with a biopsy. In the spinal cord, the differential diagnosis includes epidural spinal cord compression, intramedullary metastases, or paraneoplastic myelopathy. An MR scan or myelogram easily excludes spinal cord compression, and a high-resolution MR scan with IV contrast identifies intramedullary metastases. It is less important to differentiate radiation myelopathy from paraneoplastic myelopathy because neither is treatable. If the brachial or lumbosacral plexus is involved, the diagnosis is either recurrent tumor or radiation fibrosis. Lack of pain and predominantly motor symptoms suggest radiation fibrosis, whereas severe pain combined with motor and sensory symptoms suggests recurrent tumor. Sometimes only exploration can determine the diagnosis. In a previously radiated patient who complains of neurologic symptoms, the physician should always consider the possibility that symptoms result from an RT-induced vasculopathy causing cerebral infarction or from an endocrinopathy, such as pituitary or thyroid failure.

DIRECT RADIATION DAMAGE TO THE NERVOUS SYSTEM

Brain

Radiation injury can occur at almost any time, from seconds to years, after the therapy is delivered. The side effects of nervous system RT can generally be divided into those that are acute, usually observed within the first few days; early-delayed, seen within 4 weeks to 4 months following RT; or late-delayed, many months to many years after RT is completed. Late-delayed RT-induced brain dysfunction can take several forms (Table 13–4).

ACUTE ENCEPHALOPATHY

The disorder usually follows large fractions (more than 300 cGy) delivered to a large volume of brain in patients with increased intracranial pressure from primary or metastatic brain tumor.[2871] Absence of corticosteroid treatment increases the risk. Immediately or within a few hours following the first treatment, susceptible patients develop headache, nausea, vomiting, somnolence, fever, and worsening of pre-existing neurologic symptoms.[1061,1164,2871] In rare instances, the disorder culminates in cerebral herniation and death. Young and colleagues[2871] report acute complications, usually after the first dose, in 41 of 83 patients given 1500 cGy in 2 fr over 3 days to treat brain metastases. Hindo and coworkers[1164] report four deaths within 48 hours of receiving 1000 cGy in 1 fr. Acute encephalopathy usually follows the first radiation dose and becomes progressively less severe with each ensuing fraction. A mild form of the disorder is common and consists of headache and nausea immediately following radiation. The pathogenesis of acute encephalopathy is probably disruption of the blood–brain barrier by ionizing radiation, causing increased cerebral edema and a rise in intracranial pressure. Evidence indicates that a single dose of 300 cGy to the brain in an experimental animal causes substantial disruption of the blood–brain barrier if measured 2 hours after the radiation. After 24 hours, the barrier reconstitutes itself, but 3000 cGy in 10 doses—a standard treatment regimen for brain metastases—leads to a progressive increase in blood–brain barrier permeability for up to 4 weeks after treatment.[2032] Similar changes in vascular permeability occur in the rat lung and can be ameliorated by dexamethasone.[743] In humans, corticosteroids substantially diminish the disruption of the blood–brain barrier and prevent most clinical symptoms (see Chapter 3). A few investigators have noted an increase in intracranial pressure following a single, high dose of radiation,[2871] but others have failed to document such an increase either in humans or experimental animals, even if clinical symptoms develop.[1061] Most imaging studies[590] in humans do not provide evidence of increased cerebral edema, but such analyses may be insensitive to small, acute changes.

Other experimental animal studies[1775] indicate that even a single, low dose of radiation can affect brain function. A single dose of 50 to 150 cGy alters the late components of visual evoked responses of the brain; the abnormalities peak at about 6 hours after the radiation.

Acute encephalopathy has also been reported in children after the initiation of low-dose cranial RT, often given in conjunction with intrathecal methotrexate (MTX), for prophylaxis of meningeal leukemia. In these patients, the acute disorder was characterized by headache, increased intracranial pressure, ataxia, and depressed state of consciousness, and was ameliorated by corticosteroids.[404,1935,2362]

These observations send two clinical messages. First, patients harboring large brain tumors, particularly tumors causing signs of increased intracranial pressure, should probably be treated with fractions no larger than 200 cGy. In addition, all patients undergoing brain radiation should be protected with corticosteroids such as dexamethasone, 8 mg or 16 mg/24 hr, or more, if increased intra-

Table 13–4. **CEREBRAL RADIATION INJURY**

Designation	Time after RT	Clinical Findings	Pathogenesis	Outcome
Acute	Immediate (min–hr)	Headache, vomiting Neurologic signs	Increased intracranial pressure	Recovery (usually)
Early-delayed	4–16 weeks	Somnolence Increased focal signs Worsening MR scan	Demyelination Possibly cerebral edema	Recovery
Late-delayed	Mo–yr			
Necrosis		Focal signs MR enhancement Memory loss	Brain necrosis Possibly vascular	Responds to steroids Surgical removal
Atrophy		Dementia Gait ataxia Incontinence MR atrophy, ventriculomegaly, leukoencephalopathy	Cellular loss Demyelination Possibly hydrocephalus	Modest response to shunting in some cases
Hemorrhage		Focal signs	Telangiectasia	Partial recovery
Infarction		Focal signs	Cerebral/carotid atherosclerosis	Variable
Encephalopathy		Confusion, disorientation	Hypothyroidism	Recovery
Neoplasm		Focal signs	RT-induced neoplasm	Usually poor

cranial pressure is symptomatic. The drugs should be administered for at least 48 to 72 hours prior to initiating RT.

EARLY-DELAYED ENCEPHALOPATHY

This disorder usually begins 2 weeks to 4 months after RT. The syndrome can take one of several forms depending on the dose, the volume irradiated, and the presence or absence of underlying brain disease.

Neurologic Deterioration. If the patient suffers from a primary or metastatic brain tumor, the symptoms of early-delayed encephalopathy simulate tumor progression. The patient develops headache, lethargy, and worsening or reappearance of the original neurologic symptoms. The disorder usually peaks 2 months after RT and resolves within 6 months.[252,960,1181,2756] Hoffman and colleagues[1181] report such early-delayed symptoms in 7 of 51 patients radiated for glioma. The symptoms suggested tumor progression within 4 months of RT but improved spontaneously over the ensuing 4 months. MR or CT scans reveal an increase in the contrast-enhancing area and surrounding edema. In some instances, new areas of contrast enhancement appear. In some asymptomatic patients, contrast-enhanced lesions are encountered on CT or MR scan at routine follow-up examinations. Both clinical and radiologic changes resolve spontaneously, hastened by corticosteroids. After corticosteroids are discontinued, the patient with radiation encephalopathy remains improved as verified by scans, whereas the patient with tumor relapses. The clinical and scan findings of early-delayed radiation encephalopathy can follow conventional doses of RT to the whole brain or to the tumor alone by either conventional external-beam RT or radiosurgery. The clinical implication is that failure of the patient or the scan to improve, or even worsen within 2 or 3 months of RT, does not mean the therapy has failed. The patient should be supported with corticosteroids, with close follow-up examinations and scanning. A PET scan conducted with glucose helps to resolve these difficult clinical issues. Hypometabolism of the lesion suggests radiation damage, whereas hypermetabolism suggests tumor regrowth.

Several patients have been reported[89] who developed progressive disturbances of cognition with akinesia and tremor within a few months after RT for brain tumors. The clinical symptoms were accompanied by brain atrophy, characterized by ventriculomegaly, attenuation of the white matter, and increased sulcal size on CT scan. In those patients who died, the cortex appeared normal but the white matter was characterized by swelling, loss of myelin sheaths, and reactive astrocytosis.[89] A recent report suggests a decline in long-term memory 1 to 2 months after brain RT, followed by recovery 4 to 8 months later.[80a]

Radiation Somnolence Syndrome. Characterized by somnolence often associated with headache, nausea, vomiting, anorexia, occasional fever, and, rarely, papilledema, the radiation somnolence syndrome[837,1591,1671] appears in patients without tumor, particularly in children, after whole-brain RT. In 1929, Druckmann[687] noted marked somnolence in 3% of children treated with low-dose RT for scalp ringworm. The incidence is 40% to 60% in children administered 1800 to 2400 cGy for prophylaxis of leukemia.[187] The brain's electrical activity slows diffusely,[889] but focal neurologic signs are absent. The MR scan may indicate demyelination.[1013,1786] The syndrome is ameliorated by corticosteroids and may possibly be prevented by giving steroids during RT.[1671] Without treatment, it usually resolves in 3 to 6 weeks. The disorder is sometimes seen in adults following prophylactic RT for small-cell lung cancer, but it is more common in children, especially those younger than 3 years who are treated for leukemia.[1591] Somnolence does not predict late-delayed effects.[1671]

Focal Encephalopathy. A third early-delayed syndrome is a focal encephalopathy that follows high-dose RT to extracranial tumors such as those in an ear or eye when a portion of the brain, especially the brainstem, has been included in the treated field. The symptoms develop 8 to 11 weeks after RT and depend on the portion of the brain radiated. Brainstem signs include ataxia, diplopia, dysarthria, and nystagmus. Transient white matter hyperintensity suggesting demyelination may be found on MR scan. Most patients recover spontaneously within 6 to 8 weeks. Symptoms can progress to stupor, coma, and death.[1461,1462,1800,2169]

The pathogenesis of early-delayed encephalopathy is believed to be demyelination resulting from transient damage to oligodendroglia with the subsequent breakdown of myelin sheaths. The best evidence supporting that hypothesis comes from pathologic studies in patients with early-delayed brainstem encephalopathy in whom confluent areas of demyelination with varying degrees of axonal loss were found in areas receiving the radiation.[1461,1462,2169] Associated are a loss of oligodendrocytes and abnormal, often multinucleated, giant astrocytes. Other pathologic changes include perivenous inflammatory infiltrates. Necrosis and vascular changes are absent.

Experimentally, cerebral metabolic activity is diffusely decreased 2 to 3 weeks after completion of 4000 cGy radiation to the whole brain.[544,1235] Nevertheless, visual, cortical, somatosensory, and brainstem auditory evoked responses usually remain normal after RT to the brainstem delivered for extracranial tumors, suggesting that the focal encephalopathy that occasionally follows brainstem radiation may be idiosyncratic.[1897] Histologic studies of rats subjected to 2000 cGy in 5 fr over 5 days and killed 1 month and 6 months later did not show clear evidence of demyelination but revealed a microglial response and axonal loss in striatal white matter bundles, suggesting vascular insufficiency.[1766] Coincidental with the onset of symptoms in humans, a global decline in cerebral blood flow occurs, as measured by the xenon inhalation method. One case report describes a patient who developed neurologic symptoms 8 weeks after a pituitary adenoma was radiated and who died at 14 weeks; the brain was demyelinated, with loss of oligodendroglia and with abnormal giant astrocytes. Vascularity was not increased and no pathologic changes were found in the vessel wall, suggesting that demyelination was the cause of the neurologic symptoms.[1800] Paradoxically, in the experimental animal, spinal cord doses of 4000 cGy but not 2000 cGy prevent lysolecithin-induced demyelination.[228] Conversely, clinical evidence suggests that, in patients with multiple sclerosis, brain irradiation may enhance the demyelinating process.[2019]

LATE-DELAYED ENCEPHALOPATHY

Late-delayed radiation damage to the brain can be direct or indirect in nature (see Table 13–4), depending on the dose, the volume of tissue irradiated, the radiation portal, and the disease treated.[1687] In patients treated for primary or metastatic brain tumor with focal or whole-brain RT and in some patients treated for extracerebral tumors in whom part of the nervous system is included in the radiation portal, radiation necrosis is the characteristic late-delayed radiation complication.

Radiation Necrosis. Usually beginning 1 to 2 years after RT is completed, radiation necrosis can start as early as 3 months after treatment or be delayed for several years[1687,1813,2223] (Fig.13–2). Approximately 3% to 5% of patients receiving more than 5000 cGy develop radiation necrosis. The longer the patient survives after RT, the greater the risk of RT necrosis.[1687] In patients treated for primary or metastatic brain tumors, the symptoms generally recapitulate those of the brain tumor, leading the physician to suspect tumor recurrence. Rarely, new focal signs indicate a lesion distant from the original lesion.[582] The CT or MR scan may show increased contrast enhancement at the original tumor site or, more rarely, at a remote distance from the original tumor.[2384] Evidence of surrounding cerebral edema increases the clinical suspicion that tumor has recurred. Neither the clinical symptoms nor CT or MR scans distinguish tumor recurrence from necrosis.[91] PET scan measuring glucose consumption shows hypometabolism in areas of necrosis and hypermetabolism in areas containing tumor.[303,604,639,2648] Our experience, however, has been that many patients, particularly those treated for glioma, have a mixture of radiation necrosis and tumor. Radiation necrosis usually occurs near the tumor site, even when the patient has received whole-brain RT, suggesting that tissue damaged either by tumor or by surrounding cerebral edema is more susceptible to radiation damage.

A different clinical picture emerges when normal brain is included in a radiation portal used to treat an extracerebral tumor.[604,2223] Examples include RT of head and neck tumors[2223] such as nasopharyngeal[1495,1502,2846] and pituitary tumors. Radiation necrosis is characterized by new focal neurologic signs, depending on the site radiated. Amnesia, indicating medial temporal lobe destruction, occurs after RT for nasopharyngeal or pituitary tumors. Hemiparesis or personality changes follow RT for eye or maxillary sinus

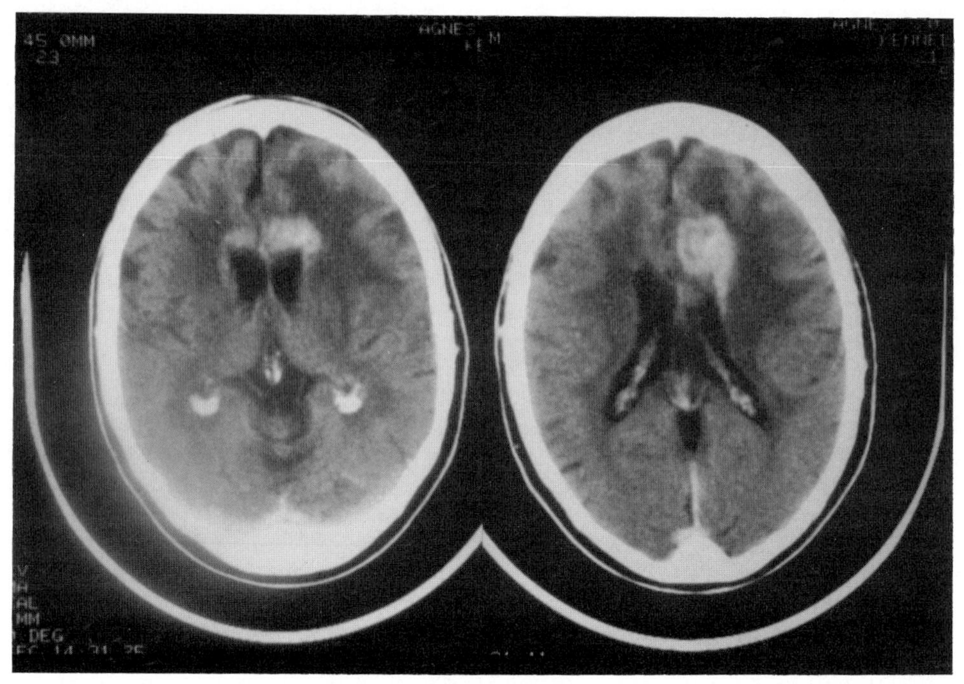

Figure 13–2. CT scans of radiation necrosis following whole-brain RT for metastatic lung cancer. Three years following surgical extirpation of a tumor in the left frontal lobe and whole-brain RT, the patient developed contrast-enhancing lesions in the corpus callosum and the right frontal lobe. The needle biopsy specimen revealed radiation necrosis without evidence of tumor. The patient deteriorated intellectually and eventually became demented and bedridden.

tumors because of damage to frontal or temporal lobes. Symptoms of increased intracranial pressure with headache, lethargy, and papilledema may also be noted.[2223] CT or MR scans show contrast-enhancing mass lesions with surrounding edema (Fig. 13–3). An arteriogram may show an avascular mass containing vessels with beading suggesting a vasculopathy.[2223] The definitive diagnosis can be made only pathologically. PET scans are hypometabolic.[604]

Histologically, the typical radiation necrosis lesion consists of coagulative necrosis in the white matter with relative sparing of the overlying cortex and deep gray matter. Microscopically, striking abnormalities are found in blood vessels, with hyalinized thickening and fibrinoid necrosis often associated with vascular thrombosis, hemorrhage, and accumulated perivascular fibrinoid material.[2223] These pathologic changes cannot be distinguished from the white matter damage caused by MTX (see Chapter 12). In less severely affected areas, demyelination is noted with a loss of oligodendrogliocytes, variable axonal loss, axonal swellings, dystrophic calcifications, fibrillary gliosis, and scattered perivascular infiltrates and mononuclear cells. Telangiectatic vessels also form there and may be responsible for late hemorrhages, particularly in the spinal cord.[38] In experimental animals, disruption of the blood–brain barrier is evident in radionecrotic regions.[2154]

Radiation necrosis is usually treated by surgical resection. Most patients respond transiently to steroids but relapse when steroids are discontinued, although reports have described prolonged responses after steroid therapy without surgery.[2373] A patient at Memorial Sloan-Kettering Cancer Center developed radiation necrosis of the temporal lobe after receiving RT for an ocular tumor. She became aphasic and hemiparetic with a contrast-enhancing mass on MR scan. Both the clinical signs and the necrosis revealed on the scan resolved with corticosteroids. She has remained well 3 years after steroid treatment (Fig. 13–4). A similar patient is well 10 years after surgical resection of the anterior temporal lobe.[604] Other suggested treatments presupposing a vascular

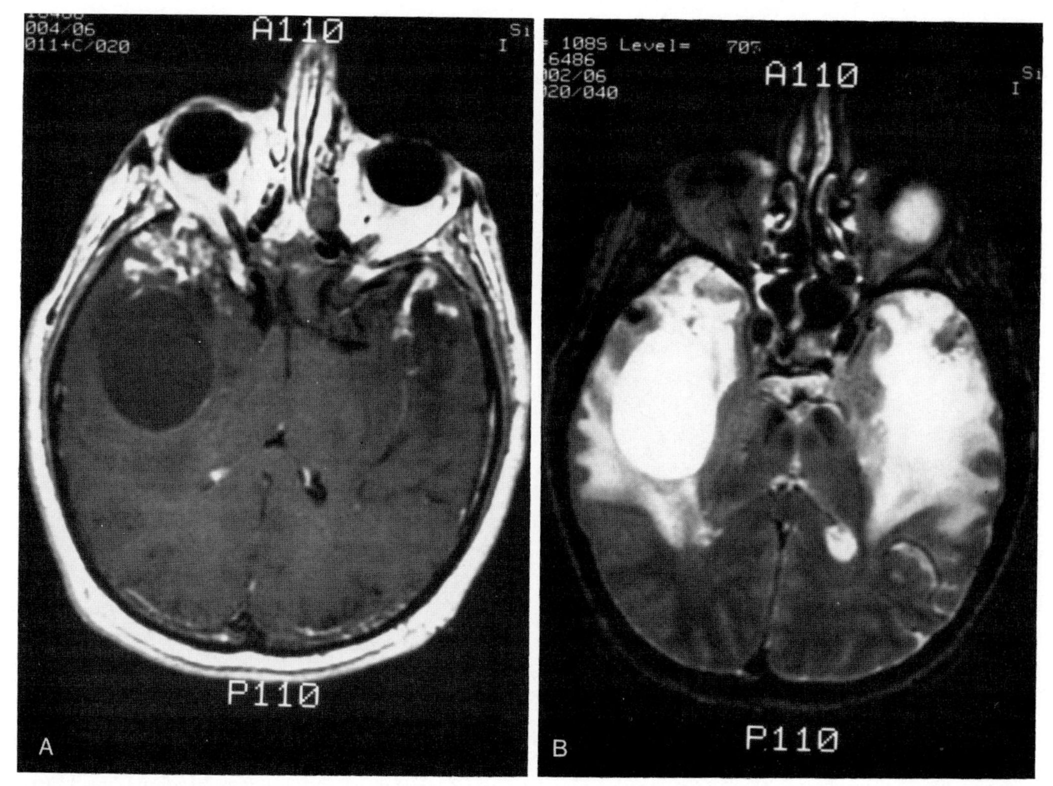

Figure 13–3. Radiation necrosis of the temporal lobes following RT for nasopharyngeal cancer. *A,* The T_1-weighted MR scan shows a cystic mass in the right temporal lobe and a somewhat smaller mass in the left temporal lobe. Contrast enhancement is appreciated anterior to both cysts. *B,* The hyperintensity on the T_2-weighted image suggests fluid surrounded by edema. The patient was demented and aphasic.

mechanism have included aspirin and anticoagulation,[928,2179] but they are not strikingly effective.

Biologic variability from patient to patient and complicating factors such as chemotherapy and patient age make it impossible to calculate exactly the dose that will induce radiation necrosis (see Table 13–3). Depending on the series, 6000 cGy to the whole brain in 30 fr will yield radiation necrosis in 5% to 15% of patients.[1539,1687,2379] The dose-response curve is unfortunately steep; small increments beyond the generally tolerated dose rapidly increase the likelihood of radiation necrosis.

Cerebral Atrophy. A more frequent effect of brain radiation than necrosis is brain atrophy (Fig. 13–5). If substantial volumes of brain tissue are irradiated either for therapy or prophylaxis of leukemia or small-cell lung cancer, most patients develop CT-documented or MR-documented evidence of enlarged cerebral sulci and ventriculomegaly.[1276,1293,1479,1501] MR scans may reveal hyperintensity, most marked in cerebral white matter around the ventricles on the T_2-weighted image; comparatively, hypodensity is noted on the CT scan. These changes, which may worsen over time, almost invariably follow whole-brain RT with 3000 cGy in 10 fr to treat brain metastases or more than 5000 cGy delivered in smaller fractions. The changes documented on the scan are more severe in the very young and the elderly and increase with both dosage and dose per fraction. Concomitant chemotherapy enhances the process.[299] The abnormalities are usually clear-cut by 1 year following RT, but occasionally they may become obvious within 2 or 3 months after RT is completed and persist or progress thereafter.[1045,2486] Prophylactic whole-brain RT doses of 1500 cGy for leukemia, however, do not result in changes on CT in children even after 5 years.[1561]

Long-term alterations in the EEG and visual evoked responses have been reported

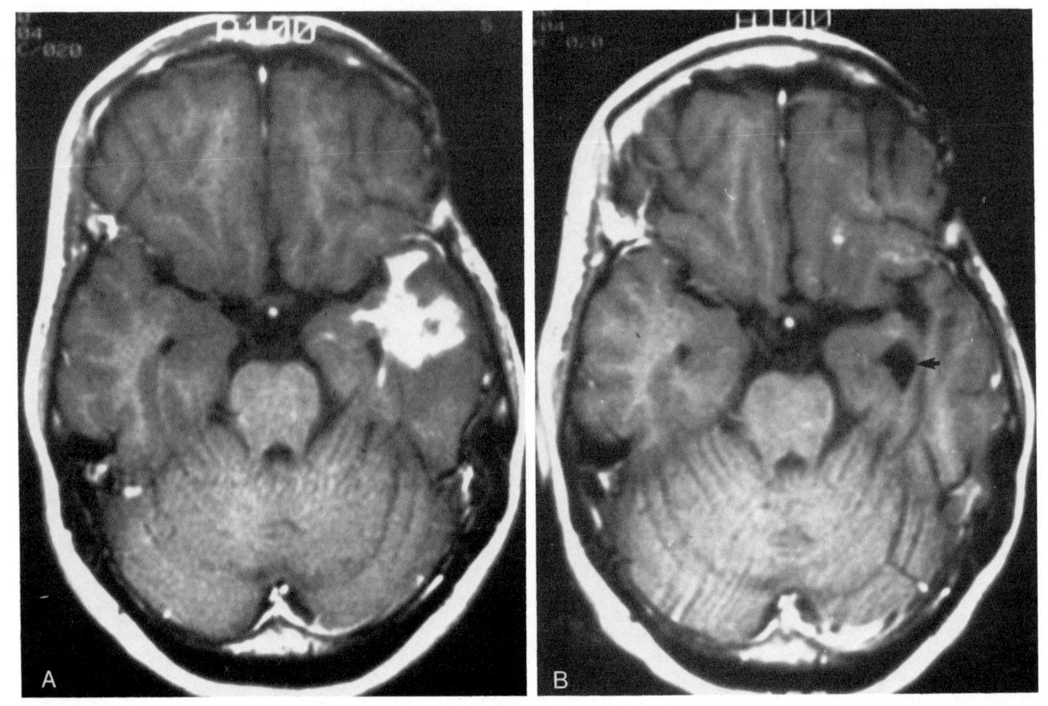

Figure 13–4. Radiation necrosis of the temporal lobe treated by corticosteroids. Three years following exenteration and radiation to the eye for a lacrimal gland tumor, the patient suddenly developed aphasia and a right hemiparesis. *A,* This MR scan revealed a contrast-enhancing lesion with mass effect in the temporal lobe. It was treated with corticosteroids, with amelioration of clinical symptoms. The steroids were then discontinued. The patient has been well for several years. *B,* The temporal lobe now reveals only a dilated ventricle (*arrow*) with no enhancement.

after low-dose (130 cGy) RT to the brains of children to treat tinea capitis,[2855] suggesting that even very low doses of RT may cause mild brain damage in these patients.

The relationship between RT-induced CT-scan or MR-scan abnormalities and clinical symptomatology is uncertain. Many patients with such changes have no symptoms,[1387] but in those who do, the severity of symptoms roughly correlates with scan findings.[1479,1999,2649] Virtually all patients in whom a substantial portion of the brain is radiated to treat primary or metastatic brain tumors complain of memory loss,[528,1833] resembling that experienced by most older people (e.g., forgetting names, telephone numbers, appointments, and recent events but remembering remote events well). The memory loss may even prevent the individual from returning to gainful employment. Recent analysis of long-term survivors of RT for glioma indicate that about 60% were employed at jobs comparable to those they held before receiving RT.[1387] In a minority of patients, perhaps only 10% to 20% who have been treated for brain metastases with 3000 cGy in 10 fr, the memory loss progresses and affects other cognitive functions, leading to a more severe dementia.[582] Some of these patients also have gait abnormalities suggesting gait apraxia and urinary urgency followed by incontinence, a triad suggestive of the syndrome of normal pressure hydrocephalus.[582] If the scan suggests hydrocephalus, that is, if ventricular dilatation is greater than cortical atrophy, the patient may respond at least temporarily to ventricular shunting. These disturbances usually develop 12 to 14 months after RT but occasionally appear earlier or later.

The pathogenesis of the ventricular dilatation and cerebral atrophy is uncertain. In some patients, true communicating hydrocephalus, perhaps from RT-induced arachnoiditis or obliteration of pacchionian granulations, appears to be causal. In others,

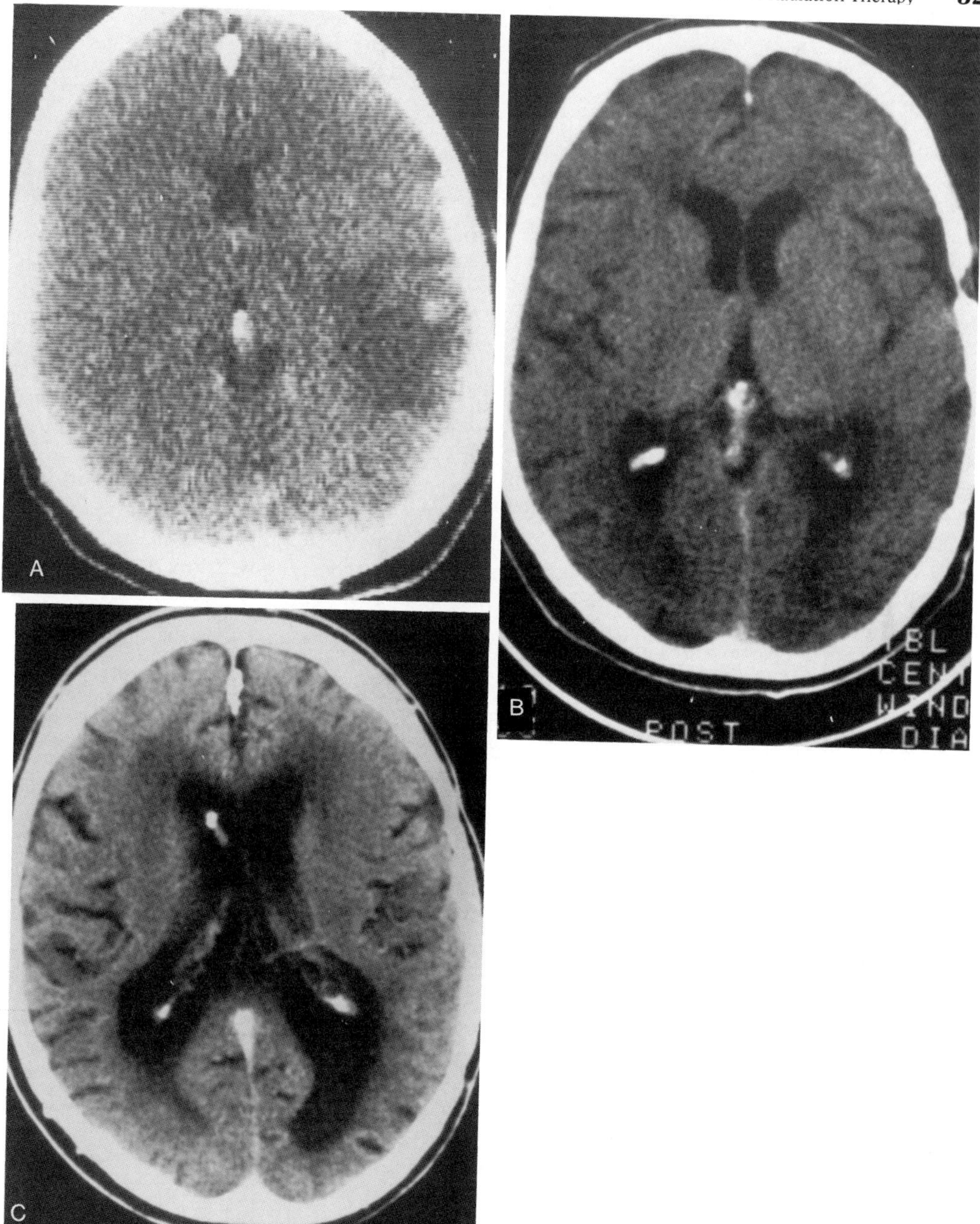

Figure 13–5. CT scans of cerebral atrophy after successful RT for metastatic lung cancer. The patient, whose ventricles were initially small (*A*), developed progressive enlargement of the ventricles several months (*B*) after treatment. Neurologic symptoms after 3 years included dementia, gait ataxia, and incontinence. (*C*) The patient clinically responded transiently to ventriculoperitoneal shunting but eventually became demented and bedridden.

a loss of cerebral substance seems to result from direct radiation damage. Direct damage to neurons is unlikely to be a pathogenetic factor because neurons do not reproduce and ionizing radiation depends on replicating DNA for its effects. Except in those patients who respond to shunting, cerebral atrophy is at present untreatable.

Spinal Cord

ACUTE RADIATION MYELOPATHY

RT to the spinal cord does not cause acute clinical symptoms. Although some physicians are concerned that high doses of RT delivered to the spinal cord to treat epidural spinal cord compression may worsen neurologic symptoms,[943] clinical and experimental evidence refutes this concern. Single fractions of 1000 cGy delivered to the human spinal cord to treat spinal cord compression did not cause acute toxicity.[1768,2567] Likewise, spinal cord dysfunction does not worsen when large fractions are delivered to experimental animals, whether or not the animal is treated with corticosteroids.[2236,2644] Patients with epidural spinal cord compression who suddenly deteriorate during RT are probably suffering from the natural history of the tumor or from sudden hemorrhage into the tumor. Experimental evidence, however, does indicate that spinal cord irradiation acutely increases the blood–to–spinal cord transfer constant for water-soluble agents; that is, it disrupts the blood–spinal cord barrier.[607]

EARLY-DELAYED RADIATION MYELOPATHY

This disorder frequently occurs after radiation is delivered to portals that include[759] the cervical and sometimes the thoracic spinal cord.[1303,2849] It also frequently follows therapeutic RT for Hodgkin's disease as well as for neck and mediastinal tumors; Word and colleagues[2849] estimate its frequency at 15% following mantle RT (i.e., RT to cervical, supraclavicular, infraclavicular, axillary, mediastinal, and hilar lymph nodes in a single portal). Higher doses are more likely to cause the disorder.[2849] This myelopathy is generally characterized by paresthesias or electric shocklike sensations called Lhermitte's sign (Table 13–5), radiating down the spine or into the extremities when the patient flexes the neck. This symptom probably results from demyelination of the spinal posterior columns leading to a spontaneous discharge of sensory axons when the spinal cord is stretched by neck flexion. The patient may not be aware initially that the experience requires neck flexion, but this can easily be demonstrated at the bedside. A tingling paresthesia resembling a mild electric shock, Lhermitte's sign is unpleasant but not painful. It usually begins 12 to 20 weeks after RT has been administered and generally resolves during a few months to 1 year. In occasional patients, it may persist for several years. Prolonged somatosensory-evoked responses (i.e., decreased conduction velocity in the spinal cord) have been reported by some but not all investigators.[669,1492] The demyelination hypothesis is not based on histologic evidence because none exists. Nevertheless, this postradiation symptom resembles the sign that accompanies multiple sclerosis, the timing of its appearance and resolution cor-

Table 13–5. **SPINAL CORD RADIATION INJURY**

Designation	Time after RT	Clinical Findings	Pathogenesis	Outcome
Acute	—	None	—	—
Early-delayed	2–37 wk	Lhermitte's sign	Demyelination	Recovery
Late-delayed	Mo–yr			
Transverse myelopathy		Paraplegia–quadriplegia Brown-Séquard's syndrome Spastic paraparesis	Necrosis	Irreversible
Motor neuron dysfunction		Leg weakness	Possibly neuronal	Irreversible
Hemorrhagic myelopathy		Acute paraparesis	Telangiectasia	Reversible

relates with the turnover of myelin, and histologic evidence in the brain shows that demyelination sometimes follows brain irradiation. The presence of Lhermitte's sign does not predict late-delayed radiation spinal cord injury. In experimental animals, myelin basic protein is transiently increased in the CSF shortly following RT,[444,2247] supporting the demyelination hypothesis for early-delayed myelopathy. The level rises again if a late-delayed myelopathy develops.[444,2247]

LATE-DELAYED RADIATION MYELOPATHY

Late-delayed radiation myelopathy has three forms, a progressive myelopathy, a lower motor neuron syndrome, and hemorrhage in the spinal cord.

Progressive Myelopathy. The most common form is progressive myelopathy. The initial symptoms begin 12 to 50 months after RT and progress during weeks or months to paraparesis or quadriparesis.* Usually, the symptoms progress subacutely, but in some patients they advance slowly over several years, whereas in others they may stabilize, leaving the patient with only mild or moderate paraparesis. The disorder probably never spontaneously resolves. Late-delayed radiation myelopathy is dose-dependent but affects as many as 5% of patients who survive 18 months after receiving 5000 cGy of mediastinal RT for lung tumors. Wara and coworkers[2740] estimate the risk of delayed radiation myelopathy to be 1% at 1015 ret and 50% at 1480 ret. A fraction size of less than 180 cGy appears to lessen the risk of damage. Older age is also a risk factor.[2247]

The first symptom is usually a Brown-Séquard's syndrome with paresthesias and weakness in one leg and a decrease in temperature and pain sensation in the other. Although unusual, pain sometimes occurs first at the lesion site and then radiates into the arm, leg, or trunk. The symptoms begin distally and ascend to reach the irradiated level of the spinal cord. At worst, all motor, sensory, and autonomic functions can be lost below the level of the lesion. Some patients do not develop Brown-Séquard's syndrome but instead exhibit a transverse myelopathy with both legs equally affected by weakness and sensory loss that rise to the level of the radiation portal. I have encountered a few patients with progressive weakness, hyperactive reflexes, and extensor plantar responses associated with sensory loss to position and vibration sense but with sparing of pain and temperature sensation. The progression of the lesion seemed much slower in these patients; several continue to be ambulatory many years after the onset of the syndrome.

Radiation myelopathy must be differentiated from epidural spinal cord compression or intramedullary metastases, which can be excluded by MR scan, and from subacute necrotic myelopathy as a paraneoplastic syndrome (see Chapter 15). The latter is so rare, however, particularly in patients who are known to have cancer, that it is not a major consideration.

The CSF is usually normal but may show an increased protein level. The myelogram is usually normal, but MR scans may be abnormal; in the acute stages, spinal cord swelling may cause a complete block, and the area of damage may contrast-enhance.[1737a,1764,2237] In late stages, the cord appears to be atrophic.[1742] The motor conduction velocity in spinal cord pathways is reduced.[2453] Experimental studies[607] indicate that disruption of the blood–brain barrier precedes the first pathologic changes in the spinal cord. Pathologic abnormalities begin in the posterior column with areas of leukoencephalopathy, which then progress to confluent areas of necrosis with continued predilection for white matter, particularly in the deeper parts of the posterior column and superficial areas of the posterolateral tracts.[607,1038,2659] Vascular changes, including fibrinoid necrosis of vessel walls, hyaline thickening, obliteration of the lumen, telangiectasia, and occasional inflammatory infiltrates,[57,2084,2338] resemble those in the brain but usually are less striking. A recent analysis of the histopathology of human radiation myelopathy suggests that damage to glial cells is the first change in the white matter, followed some months later by vascular damage. These data support the Hopewell hypothesis that vascular and glial damage are independent pathologic changes.[1199,2338]

The pathogenesis of radiation myelopathy is unknown. The lack of early vascular change

*References 648, 649, 823, 935, 2151, 2339.

suggests that the initial damage affects glial cells rather than blood vessels. The early onset of blood–brain barrier disruption suggests that it may participate in causing the disorder. Lipid peroxidation does not appear to be a factor.[1038] Myelin basic protein levels in the spinal cord are decreased,[444] perhaps reflecting the initial demyelination.[2799] Elevated levels of plasminogen activator inhibitor-1 may play a role in the pathogenesis of radiation-induced CNS necrosis.[2302a]

Steroids sometimes delay progression of the lesion,[935] but prevention is the only effective treatment. When radiation portals are designed to spare the spinal cord, radiation myelopathy does not occur.[57a,1436] A recent report suggests that anticoagulation with heparin and warfarin may produce some recovery of function in patients with radiation myelopathy.[928]

The major risk factor for late-delayed radiation myelopathy is the dose. Also important is the dose per fraction[1287] and the oxygenation level.[519] Hemoglobin concentration, which indicates the oxygen availability to tissues, is directly correlated with the incidence of myelopathy[649]; blood pressure is not. In experimental animals, young age hastens the development of radiation myelopathy,[2,908] although human children do not seem to be especially at risk. Additional risk factors include intensive chemotherapy[2121] (intravenously or intrathecally) and perhaps whole-body hyperthermia.[676] Animal experiments, however, suggest that hyperthermia, 1,3-bis-chloro(2-chloroethyl)-1-nitrosurea (BCNU), and aziridinylbenzoquinone chemotherapy do not reduce tolerance of the spinal cord to RT.[58,1879] Vincristine has been reported to do so in humans.[353]

Motor Neuron Syndrome. A second form of late-delayed radiation myelopathy, a lower motor neuron syndrome, characteristically follows pelvic RT for testicular tumors[823,1023,1257,1464] but has also occurred after lumbosacral RT for other tumors[597,1426,1464] or after craniospinal RT for medulloblastoma.[2262] The disorder may occur 3 months to 23 years following RT and is characterized by the subacute onset of a flaccid weakness of the legs[1426] affecting both distal and proximal muscles with atrophy, fasciculations, and areflexia. It is usually bilateral and symmetric but may either begin in or remain restricted to one leg.[1464] Sensory changes are absent, and bowel, bladder, and sexual functions are normal. The CSF may contain an increased protein concentration. The myelogram is normal. Although electromyography reveals varying degrees of denervation, sensory and motor conduction velocities are normal. The deficit usually stabilizes after several months to a few years; often the patient can still walk. One of our patients can walk after 12 years of weakness from abdominal RT. Occasionally, patients become paraplegic.

Impossible to differentiate from a pure motor polyneuropathy or isolated motor neuron loss, it also resembles the paraneoplastic syndrome's subacute motor neuronopathy (see Chapter 15). A single report describes a brachial motor neuron syndrome 3 years following RT that was associated with a cystic hypodense cavity affecting the spinal cord from C-4 to C-6.[1660]

A single pathologic report of a patient with motor neuron syndrome in the lower extremities describes randomly distributed demyelination and axon loss to both sensory and motor roots, with focal areas of complete demyelination. The roots involved were primarily those of the cauda equina; some anterior horn cells (motor neurons) in the lumbar cord exhibited chromatolysis, suggesting secondary damage.[192]

Hemorrhage. Only a few patients have been described with the third form of late-delayed radiation myelopathy, hemorrhage in the spinal cord, which develops many years after RT.[38] Characteristically, 8 to 30 years following RT to the spinal cord, a patient without prior neurologic symptoms suddenly develops back pain and leg weakness. In one of our patients, the syndrome began when the patient was taking a nonsteroidal anti-inflammatory agent (NSAID) for an unrelated disorder. The symptoms may evolve during a few hours to a few days. The MR scan suggests acute or subacute hemorrhage in the spinal cord (Fig. 13–6). The cord may be slightly atrophic, but no other lesions are found. Characteristically, after several days the patient begins to improve and the neurologic symptoms may resolve entirely. A few patients have had recurrent episodes of spinal cord hemorrhage. The pathogenesis is believed to be hemorrhage from telangiectasia caused by RT. A biopsy sample of the spinal

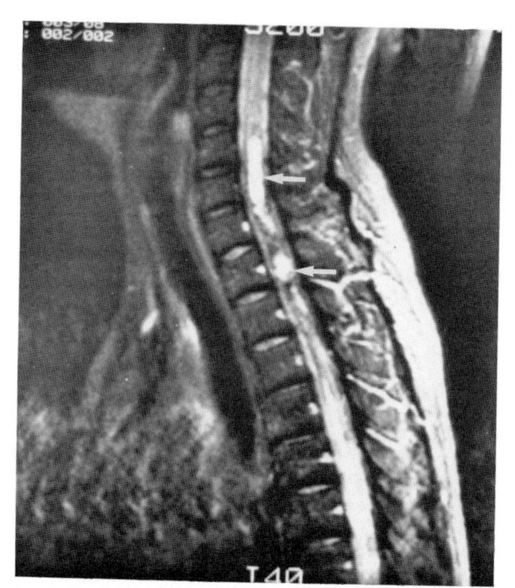

Figure 13–6. Hemorrhage in the spinal cord several years following successful mantle RT for Hodgkin's disease. The patient was taking nonsteroidal anti-inflammatory drugs (NSAIDs) for unrelated pain when she developed sudden back pain associated with weak legs. MR scan revealed an acute hemorrhage in the spinal cord (*arrows*). She subsequently made a full recovery.

cord from one patient was said to show an arteriovenous malformation,[38] but it is more likely that these were telangiectases. Affected patients should be admonished to avoid aspirin and NSAIDs, which might lead to subsequent hemorrhage, but no treatment helps once the hemorrhage has occurred.

Cranial Nerves

RT can damage any of the cranial nerves (Table 13–6).[361,918,1379] Such damage is rare, however, and is usually a late-delayed effect. Apparent exceptions are radiation damage to olfactory and optic nerves, which, strictly speaking, are part of the brain and not truly nerves, and early-delayed conductive hearing loss, which may mimic damage to the acoustic nerve (see the following).

Cranial and other peripheral nerves are susceptible to direct damage. Axonal shrinkage and neurofilament alterations develop before Schwann cell or endothelial capillary damage and substantial fibrosis of surrounding connective tissue. Nevertheless, most late radiation damage to the lower cranial nerves found in the neck probably results from fibrosis of connective tissue causing nerve damage by compression or ischemia. Recent reviews describe cranial nerve damage induced by radiation.[361,918]

OLFACTORY NERVES

The olfactory "nerves" are the only human CNS neurons that reproduce themselves in adults. As a result, they might be expected to be sensitive to radiation. While undergoing head radiation, some patients perceive an odor,[2265] probably because of stimulation of olfactory nerve endings by the radiation. Anosmia is sometimes described,[385,1949] although longitudinal testing of olfactory perception in patients undergoing RT has not been reported. Because many patients confuse taste and smell and because taste is so often affected by RT (see the following), the clinician cannot be certain how frequently olfactory loss occurs after RT.[175]

OPTIC NERVES

The visual system from the cornea to the occipital cortex may be affected by RT.[2400] Visual loss may be caused by an RT-induced dry eye syndrome, glaucoma, cataract,[1986] or, more commonly, by retinopathy[1380,2584] or optic neuropathy.[1041,1634,1986] The only acute effects of RT on the visual system are those resulting from stimulation of retinal photoreceptors by the photons. Patients in a dark room or with closed eyes can perceive visual sensations when the radiation beam is turned on. Late-delayed radiation retinopathy has been reported following RT for nasal carcinoma[2584] or Graves' disease.[1380] The pathogenesis involves direct retinal damage.[621,1884,2584] Late-delayed optic neuropathy, although rare, has followed whole-brain RT for brain metastases, pituitary RT with photons or protons to treat adenomas, and RT for nasopharyngeal tumors.[1634]

Optic neuropathy following whole-brain RT begins 7 to 26 months after RT and is characterized by the painless development of monocular or bilateral blindness. Visual acuity is reduced and is often associated with an altitudinal field defect. The funduscopic examination may show papilledema, telangiectasia, and prepapillary as well as premacular

Table 13–6. **CRANIAL NERVE RADIATION INJURY**

Designation	Time after RT	Clinical Findings	Pathogenesis	Outcome
Acute	During treatment	Smell Lights Paresthesias	Direct stimulation by photons	Benign
Early-delayed	During RT to a few weeks after	Hearing loss	Otitis media	Usually recovers
		Anosmia	Damage to olfactory neurons	Recovers
		Ageusia	Damage to taste buds	Recovers
Late-delayed	Mo–yr	Visual loss	Demyelination, axonal loss	Usually permanent
		Diplopia	Demyelination	Recovers
		Hearing loss	Radiation fibrosis	Permanent
		Hair-cell damage	Radiation fibrosis	Permanent
		Lower cranial-nerve paralysis	Radiation fibrosis	Permanent

hemorrhages. Cotton-wool spots, soft exudates, and retinal arterial narrowing mark damage by RT to the retina. If most of the damage occurs in the retrobulbar area, as with pituitary irradiation, the optic fundus may be normal. MR scans may reveal enhancing lesions of the optic nerve or chiasm that spontaneously resolve.[1041]

Histologic changes include axonal loss, demyelination, gliosis, and thickening and hyalinization of vessel walls. Most affected patients do not recover vision. Steroids are ineffective. More than 2000 ret are probably required to produce optic neuropathy, but pre-existing damage, such as from diabetes, may lower the visual system's tolerance for radiation. The likelihood of visual loss is probably exacerbated with concomitant chemotherapy; visual loss can generally be prevented by shielding the eyes at the time RT is delivered. The optic nerves, however, cannot be shielded completely if whole-brain RT is to be effective. Reversible optic or chiasmal neuropathy has been reported in some patients radiated with protons to treat pituitary adenomas.[1382]

OCULAR MOTOR NERVES

Radiation damage to the motor nerves that move the eye is rarely reported, perhaps because many affected patients suffer a concomitant optic neuropathy that precludes diplopia as a symptom.[2216] Permanent abducens palsies have been reported[1985] following treatment for nasopharyngeal carcinoma, and transient paralysis of ocular motor nerves sometimes follows proton-beam RT to the pituitary. Recovery, either partial or complete, after proton-beam RT suggests that demyelination, not radiation fibrosis, causes these disorders. An unusual ocular complication of RT is neuromyotonia,[1530] characterized by spontaneous spasm of eye muscles secondary to spontaneous discharges of ocular motor nerves. It occurs after RT for sella turcica or cavernous sinus tumors. Affected patients complain of intermittent diplopia, sometimes associated with a feeling of movement of the involved eye. The episodes are painless, can occur as frequently as several times an hour, and last only a few seconds. No electromyographic and pathologic studies are available to determine the pathogenesis of this disorder, although the clinical symptoms suggest the limb myokymia that occurs after radiation of the brachial or lumbosacral plexus[1530] (see pp 330–331).

TRIGEMINAL NERVES

Trigeminal neuropathy has only rarely been reported[189] following RT to the head. A more common cause of trigeminal neuropathy after head and neck tumor therapy is microscopic invasion of the trigeminal nerve by neurotropic tumors (see Chapter 8). Neuromyotonia of the mylohyoid and digastric muscles supplied by the motor branch of the trigeminal nerve has been reported[638] in two patients. Both responded to carbamazepine.

FACIAL NERVES

The motor portion of the facial nerve is rarely, if ever, damaged by RT.[409] If late-delayed facial nerve paralysis occurs, it should be considered to be caused by neurotropic tumor invasion until proved otherwise. Taste perception is a facial-nerve function and susceptible to radiation damage. Taste buds are a rapidly regenerating tissue. Many patients complain of ageusia (loss of taste) during the course of RT,[175,918,1826,1827] and permanent ageusia was reported[918] in 50% of patients who were treated with 5000 to 6000 cGy for head and neck tumors. Dysgeusia, if not permanent, may persist for months after treatment is completed. Confounding factors such as loss of smell and diminished salivary gland output, also from the RT, make it difficult to define the degree of taste loss. Patients with taste loss during RT have greater weight loss than those who do not suffer ageusia.[258] Another problem is that many patients with cancer complain of abnormal taste even before RT[632]; the gustatory loss during RT can occur whether or not the taste buds and facial nerve are included in the radiation portal. Taste aversion is typical in patients being treated with RT or chemotherapy. Experimental animals develop significant RT-induced taste aversion even when low doses are administered to relatively small body areas.[1301]

Just as failure of lacrimal gland secretions can lead to dry eyes and visual loss, decreased salivary gland secretion causes xerostomia and taste abnormalities. If salivary glands are included in the radiation portal, symptoms begin during the first or second week of therapy and persist through the treatment and for months thereafter. Change in the quality and quantity of lacrimal and salivary gland secretions can permanently damage the eyes and mouth.[831] After one or two radiation treatments, a salivary gland in the radiation portal may swell and be acutely painful, reminiscent of viral parotitis (i.e., mumps). Serum amylase levels are also raised, but the swelling, pain, and amylase decrease rapidly without significant sequelae.[366] Experimental evidence indicates that radiation injury to secretory cells is expressed histologically within 24 hours and is associated with an inflammatory infiltrate. Because these cells are normally noncycling, functionally mature cells, cell death is associated not with cell division but with apoptosis.[831] Orally administered pilocarpine has been reported[2647] to be effective in ameliorating the symptoms of post-RT xerostomia.

ACOUSTIC NERVES

Acute radiation damage, probably directly affecting the cochlea, can cause tinnitus and high-frequency hearing loss that are usually reversible but occasionally permanent. An early-delayed hearing loss following RT within a few weeks is due to RT-induced otitis media.[275] Mucosal vasodilatation and eustachian tube edema block exit from the middle ear and lead to serous effusion. Patients complain of decreased hearing and "popping" of their ears; fluid can often be seen behind the tympanic membrane. Although the disorder may resolve spontaneously or in response to nasal vasoconstriction agents, some patients require myringotomy for symptomatic relief. Late-delayed radiation damage occurring months to years after RT probably results from injury to the organ of Corti with secondary acoustic nerve atrophy.[1487,1805] Because of the low dose administered, prophylactic RT for childhood leukemia does not cause sensorineural hearing loss.[2577] Clinically significant damage to the vestibular portion of the eighth nerve is virtually unknown, although labyrinthine damage can be demonstrated histologically.[1721,1824]

LOWER CRANIAL NERVES

The lower cranial nerves (i.e., the glossopharyngeal, vagus, spinal accessory, and hypoglossal nerves) are partially located in the neck and are thus susceptible to radiation damage when RT is directed at head or neck tumors. Large doses, usually greater than 2000 ret, are required. The time of onset varies inversely with the radiation dose. The disorders occur many months to years after RT and are generally associated with obvious fibrosis of cervical soft tissues. The pathogenesis is attributed to radiation fibrosis. The glossopharyngeal nerve has not been reported to be a target of radiation damage but is difficult to assess clinically in isolation. Damage to the vagus nerve leads to unilateral paralysis of the palate and vocal cords.[189] Most patients experiencing such damage who are asked to swallow water during a physical examination are noted to cough just after each swallow, indicating that aspiration is present even if the palate is not obviously paralyzed on examination.[614] Damage to the recurrent laryngeal nerve, a branch of the vagus nerve, paralyzes the vocal cords only, causing hoarseness and often aspiration.[521,2798] Examining the vocal cords identifies the abnormality. Involvement of the spinal accessory nerve leads to shoulder droop and sometimes chronic arm pain. Horner's syndrome may result from radiation damage to sympathetic fibers in the neck; it may be encountered in association with lower cranial nerve dysfunction or in isolation. The hypoglossal nerve is probably the most commonly involved lower cranial nerve. When the radiation dose is greater than 2000 ret, bilateral or unilateral tongue paralysis may occur several years after RT.[158,189,437] Unilateral paralysis is often asymptomatic; at most, affected patients complain of having difficulty with food caught between the teeth and the cheek; dysarthria is uncommon. Bilateral lingual paralysis, however, is extremely disabling and can cause severe dysarthria as well as swallowing difficulty.

Peripheral Nerves

Any peripheral nerve can be damaged by a sufficient dose of RT. The major sites of damage are the brachial plexus after treatment for breast or lung cancer (and occasionally for Hodgkin's disease) and the lumbosacral plexuses after treatment to the pelvis and lower abdomen for a number of cancers (Table 13–7). Radiation injury to peripheral nerves or plexuses is a dose-limiting factor when intraoperative RT is used for pelvic and retroperitoneal tumors.[1378]

BRACHIAL PLEXUS

Peripheral nerves probably do not suffer acute damage from RT, although Haymaker and Lindgren[1123] mention that patients "under the beam" sometimes experience acute paresthesias. Patients with Hodgkin's disease may develop an acute brachial plexus palsy, usually painful but reversible, which is clinically indistinguishable from acute idiopathic brachial neuritis. The disorder begins abruptly a few days to weeks after RT starts.[854,1450] Although its pathogenesis is unknown, the RT can be completed safely. An early-delayed reversible reaction to brachial plexus RT[2278] is characterized by paresthesias in the hand and forearm, sometimes associated with pain and accompanied by weakness and atrophy in a C-6 to T-1 distribution. The disorder begins about 4 months after RT. Nerve conduction velocities reveal segmental slowing; recovery

Table 13–7. **PERIPHERAL NERVE RADIATION INJURY**

Designation	Time after RT	Clinical Findings	Pathogenesis	Outcome
Acute	During treatment	Paresthesias	Direct stimulation	Benign
Early-delayed	2–30 wk	Weakness, paresthesias	Possibly autoimmune Demyelination	Benign Autoimmune
Late-delayed				
Focal	Mo–yrs	Focal neuropathy or plexopathy (painless)	Fibrosis	Permanent
Diffuse	Yrs	Polyneuropathy/myopathy	Hypothyroidism	Reversible
Neoplastic	Yrs	Weakness, pain/tumor mass	RT-induced carcinogenesis	Permanent/sometimes fatal

occurs during a few weeks or months. This disorder affected 14% of patients with breast carcinoma who were radiated in one institution during one 10-year period. The disorder has not been observed since. The pathogenesis of the disorder is not clear, but it does not appear to predispose to late-delayed radiation damage.[2278] A similar reversible disorder of lumbar plexopathy may begin 4 months after wide-field pelvic RT.[725,2316]

Late-Delayed Radiation Plexopathy. This disorder has been reported after RT of either the brachial or lumbosacral plexus, although the former is much more common. It usually occurs a year or more after external-beam RT but often within 4 to 7 months after intraoperative pelvic radiation[1378] if doses are greater than 1700 ret. Brachial plexopathy is characterized by hand and arm paresthesias; loss of sensation in the thumb and index finger; painless weakness of shoulder muscles, biceps, and brachioradialis[125,806,1412,1494,2580]; and, frequently, lymphedema and palpable induration in the supraclavicular fossa. Myokymia detected by an electromyogram affects muscles innervated by the involved nerve trunks and is a useful criterion for differentiating radiation damage from tumor infiltration of the plexus.[27,1494,2219,2809] The disorder often progresses to a panplexopathy that paralyzes the entire arm, usually without severe pain. Sometimes the disorder begins in the lower plexus, affecting the hand muscles before the arm is involved. In one series[1941] of 79 patients radiated for breast cancer, 28 had clinical evidence of brachial plexopathy, 15 of whom had significant disability, and most had panplexopathy. Surgery on the axilla and adjuvant chemotherapy may have been risk factors. In another series[1940] of 161 patients radiated for breast cancer, 5% had late-delayed disabling plexopathy and 9% had mild plexopathy. Cytotoxic therapy, young age, and large RT fractions were risk factors.

The important differential diagnosis in plexus lesions lies between radiation damage and recurrent tumor (see Table 8–3). Pain is the single most important clinical differentiating feature. Severe pain is rare with radiation fibrosis but is almost invariably present if tumor is the culprit. Proximal distribution of the weakness suggests radiation fibrosis but may also be seen with recurrent tumor. The CT or MR scan may identify a discrete tumor mass but often reveals only diffuse, nonspecific loss of tissue planes. Such changes can be seen with either radiation plexopathy or tumor infiltration.[396] Diagnostic certainty may require surgical exploration.[1391] Even this may not exclude tumor if the nerves themselves are infiltrated without perineural tumor. Recurrent tumor may be treated with RT or chemotherapy. No effective treatment exists for radiation plexopathy, although a few reports suggest that surgical neurolysis may help.[1527,1858]

Acute Ischemic Brachial Plexopathy. An acute ischemic brachial plexopathy occurring years after RT to the breast and associated with occlusion of the subclavian artery is a rare late-delayed complication.[905] The plexopathy is painless, acute in onset, and nonprogressive, although not reversible.

LUMBOSACRAL PLEXUS

This disorder causes weakness of one or both legs.[904,931,1378,2579] As with brachial plexopathy, pain is usually absent and, if present, generally mild. The disorder often affects the foot first. Most patients also have sensory loss. The electromyogram frequently reveals myokymic discharges that help differentiate the RT-induced disorder from tumor plexopathy. RT-induced lumbosacral plexopathy often slowly progresses during many years, but it may stabilize while the patient is still functional or it may resolve spontaneously.[725] At times, exploration may be necessary to confirm the diagnosis, but a CT or MR scan can usually exclude recurrent tumor. The pathogenesis of RT damage to the plexus and peripheral nerves may be related to fibrosis that causes compression and ischemia of nerve rather than to direct damage to the nerves.[1378]

SACRAL PLEXUS

Radiation-associated erectile impotence is common following treatment for prostate cancer. In one study, 80% of previously potent patients complained of decreased erectile capacity. Arteriography in some patients revealed bilateral occlusive disease of internal pudendal and penile arteries, suggesting a vascular cause rather than direct damage to sacral nerves.[942]

INDIRECT RADIATION DAMAGE TO THE NERVOUS SYSTEM

Radiogenic Tumors

RT-induced neurogenic tumors,[1683] benign or malignant, include meningioma,[1101,1640] benign or malignant gliomas,[2196,2885] gliosarcoma, and schwannoma.[623,807] Evidence supporting the diagnosis of RT-induced tumor includes the following:

1. the tumor is of a different histologic type than the original neoplasm for which the patient was radiated,
2. the tumor developed within the radiation field, and
3. 10 to 30 years have passed since the initial radiation treatment.[360]

A clinician can never be certain that such a tumor is not a second primary tumor unrelated to the RT, but epidemiologic studies show a higher incidence of certain tumors in irradiated patients than in control subjects and a positive correlation between RT dose and tumor incidence.[2196] The same tumors emerge after low-dose[1117,2196,2903] or high-dose RT.[1629] In addition, identical neoplasms have been experimentally induced in appropriate animal models. Radiation carcinogenesis probably results from radiation damage to DNA with abnormal repair,[1064] although the pathogenesis is not fully established. RT-induced brain tumors occur in patients who have received low-dose brain RT for treatment of tinea capitis as well as in those who have received higher doses for the treatment of brain tumors. In one series of 26 patients with RT-induced nerve sheath tumors, 5 received low-dose radiation for benign illnesses.[623] As with other forms of RT neurotoxicity, biologic variables affect the likelihood that a given patient will develop a tumor. For example, patients with neurofibromatosis are more likely to develop malignant peripheral nerve sheath tumors than are normal subjects receiving the same RT.[807] In experimental animals, genetic factors, sex, age, and hormonal influences appear to play a role.[201]

In a 1988 study,[2196] the relative risk for developing neural tumors of the head and neck following childhood irradiation for tinea capitis was 9.5 for meningioma, 2.6 for glioma, 18.8 for nerve sheath tumors, and 3.4 for other tumors, with a mean latent interval of 17.6 years. With the higher RT doses required to treat childhood malignancies, the increase in brain tumors is sevenfold in those who survive more than 3 years after initial treatment. One of my patients developed a meningioma in the temporal lobe at the site of a low-grade astrocytoma that had been resected and radiated 40 years earlier, when she was an adolescent (Fig. 13–7).

The signs and symptoms of tumors arising in the brain or spinal cord after previous RT do not differ from those of spontaneous tumors. RT-induced tumors can be either malignant or benign and must be examined by biopsy to establish whether the lesion has a different histology from the original tumor irradiated many years before. I have encountered patients with pilocytic astrocytomas recurring as late as 30 years following initial resection and RT.

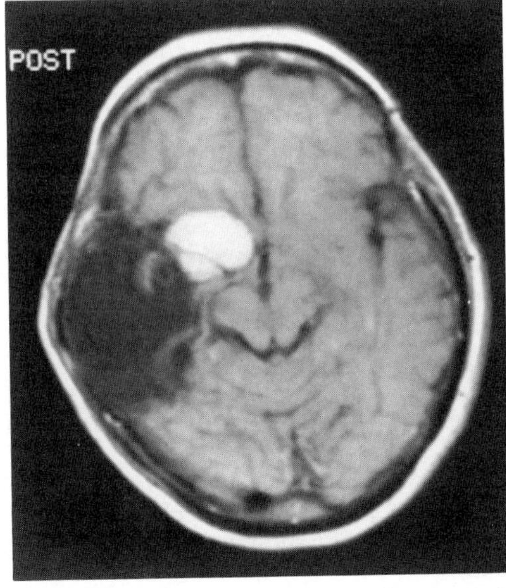

Figure 13–7. Presumed meningioma after successful treatment of a low-grade astrocytoma. This patient, 55 years of age, underwent partial temporal lobe resection for a low-grade astrocytoma at age 15 years. Surgery was followed by RT. She made a noneventful recovery. Forty years later, she underwent a scan of her head for vague dizzy spells that resolved spontaneously. The MR scan revealed a contrast-enhancing lesion within the radiation portal, almost certainly a benign meningioma. The mass has been observed for several years without additional growth.

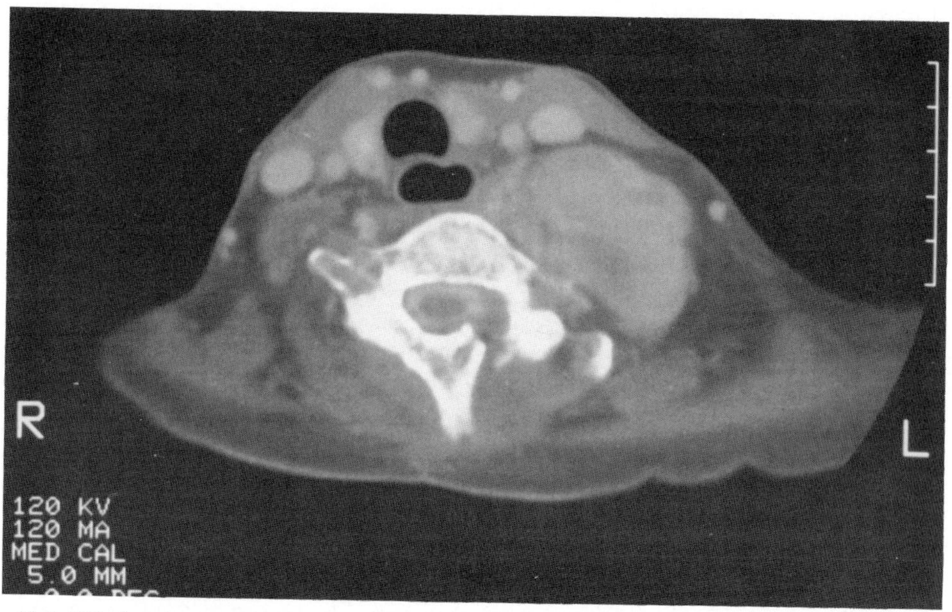

Figure 13–8. RT-induced neurogenic sarcoma of the brachial plexus. This patient, successfully treated for Hodgkin's disease 12 years previously, developed painful weakness of the left upper extremity. A mass was palpated in the supraclavicular fossa that, when biopsied, proved to be a neurogenic sarcoma. The spinal cord was compressed. Continued growth caused the patient's death despite additional RT to the lesion.

Malignant or atypical nerve sheath tumors may follow RT of the brachial, cervical, and lumbar plexuses (Fig. 13–8). It should not be assumed that patients who have been radiated previously for breast, abdominal, or pelvic tumors and who many years later develop painful mass lesions with brachial or lumbosacral plexus dysfunction are experiencing a recurrence of their primary tumor. As mentioned previously, the new lesion should be examined by biopsy or resected before other treatment is initiated. The treatment of nerve sheath tumors is surgical excision where possible and, with malignant tumors, as much external-beam irradiation as the patient can tolerate. Radiosurgery, brachytherapy, and chemotherapy should also be considered if sufficiently large doses of external-beam RT cannot be tolerated because of the prior RT.

Radiation-Induced Large-Vessel Disease

RT can cause late-delayed effects on blood vessels of all sizes. As indicated previously, small-vessel vascular occlusions play an important role in the development of both brain and spinal cord necrosis.[1199] RT-induced telangiectasia can lead to delayed hemorrhage in the brain and spinal cord.[38,731] Late-delayed effects on large vessels can have major secondary effects on CNS function. Lesions of large intracranial or extracranial blood vessels may be apparent 4 months to 20 years after RT. The pathology of large-vessel damage is accelerated atherosclerosis.[1725] The most vulnerable vessel of neurologic interest is the carotid artery.[1841] Several case reports describe carotid occlusion from atherosclerosis leading to transient ischemia or cerebral infarction. The diagnosis of RT-induced carotid occlusion is suggested when a patient's carotid arteries were included in the RT portal. Arteriography often supports the diagnosis by showing that the site of atherosclerotic occlusion in the carotid artery is different from its usual location at the bifurcation in nonirradiated patients. These sites of RT-induced occlusion can be intracranial or extracranial, depending on the RT portal.[98,211,2795] A particularly likely site is the supraclinoid portion of the internal carotid artery in children who have received brain RT. Such occlusions sometimes induce moyamoya disease.[211,1361] Arteriography reveals stenosis or occlusion of the artery within the radiation portal.

The treatment of RT-induced atherosclerosis that is causing neurologic symptoms resembles that of typical atherosclerosis. Experimental evidence indicates that radiation doses insufficient to cause vascular damage in experimental animals may produce significant atheromatous lesions when combined with lipidemia. Thus, lowering serum cholesterol may be helpful in patients. Carotid endarterectomy, when indicated, should be performed, but the surgery may be technically more difficult than usual because periarterial fibrosis may make it difficult to separate the intima from the media.[1596]

Cerebral aneurysms occasionally occur after RT.[111,731] The aneurysms differ from ordinary saccular aneurysms in their location and histologic features. In one patient, the aneurysms followed a combination of external-beam irradiation and intrathecal colloidal radioactive gold. The locations corresponded to areas where the intrathecal gold created a pool around a vessel. Rarely, carotid rupture may complicate the marked periarterial fibrosis that sometimes develops after RT.

Endocrine Dysfunction

RT-induced endocrine dysfunction is relatively common. When severe, abnormal hormonal levels can secondarily affect the nervous system, causing mental changes, sexual dysfunction, and other neurologic disability. Such abnormalities occur after RT that includes the pituitary and hypothalamus, or after RT to the neck when the thyroid and parathyroid glands are within the portal.

RT-induced dysfunction of the hypothalamic-pituitary axis[488,1458,1459,1589] is not rare after treatment for nasopharyngeal carcinoma and pituitary tumors; it also may follow whole-brain irradiation for treatment or prophylaxis. The dose that causes radiation damage to the hypothalamic-pituitary axis is uncertain. Clinical evidence suggests that, in at least some patients, conventional doses and fractionation schedules can cause substantial damage when hormonal levels are measured several years after RT. The radiation damage site in the hypothalamic-pituitary axis differs from patient to patient, depending in part on the fractionation of RT and the portal and in part on the patient's underlying disease. Patients who have had pituitary surgery are more likely to experience pituitary failure, whereas children with acute lymphoblastic leukemia (ALL) tend to suffer hypothalamic failure. Furthermore, each portion of the hypothalamic-pituitary axis has its own intrinsic susceptibility to RT. Growth hormone is most sensitive, thyroid-stimulating hormone the least, with luteinizing hormone/follicle-stimulating hormone and adrenocorticotropic hormone in between.

The most common clinical symptom is growth failure in children. In male adults treated for brain tumors, approximately 67% complain of sexual difficulties, usually decreased libido and impotence, within 2 years of RT. The presumed basis is hypothalamic damage. Adrenal failure and hypothyroidism are rare, but many patients who have received RT to the brain complain of chronically feeling cold, even when thyroid function test results are normal.

Diagnosing hypothalamic-pituitary failure is often difficult. When the condition is florid, standard pituitary hormones are measurably low in the serum, except for the prolactin level, which is usually high because of a failure to secrete dopamine, the prolactin inhibitory factor. However, in a few patients who have symptoms suggesting endocrine dysfunction and low levels of hormone at rest, the results of stimulation study may be normal, making the diagnosis and the identification of the exact site of failure difficult.

In a recent study of 31 adults with nasopharyngeal carcinoma who received approximately 4000 cGy to the hypothalamus and 6000 cGy to the pituitary, more than 50% developed endocrine dysfunction within 5 years of cranial RT. Clinically apparent hypopituitarism was common, following a mean latent interval of 3.8 years.[1459]

Of more neurologic interest is hypothyroidism following neck irradiation. The problem arises particularly in patients who have been treated successfully for Hodgkin's disease. The actuarial risk of developing thyroid disease 20 years after mantle RT is about 52%. Hypothyroidism is the most common complication, although Graves' disease with ophthalmopathy and thyroid cancer also can occur.[1073,1264,1712,1989] Neurologic symptoms involving the peripheral nervous system or CNS, including encephalopathy, ataxia, and peripheral neuropathy, can develop at virtually any time following RT and may occur in the absence of other more obvious symptoms of hypothyroidism. If the spinal-fluid protein is elevated, as it often is in hypothyroidism, the patient with an unrecognized case may undergo extensive and unnecessary neurologic evaluation before recognition that the neurologic disorder is caused by hypothyroidism. Thyroid function studies should be conducted in any neurologic patient who has received prior RT to the neck.

Primary hypothyroidism without symptoms has been described following prophylactic cranial RT for acute lymphoblastic leukemia.[1989]

Hypercalcemic hyperparathyroidism has also been reported to follow RT.[1848,2098]

Combination Radiation and Chemotherapy

As indicated in the previous chapter, the neurotoxicity of chemotherapy is often increased by radiation, and vice versa. Table 13–8 lists chemotherapeutic agents well known to enhance radiation neurotoxicity. Other agents undoubtedly are just as capable of increasing neurotoxicity as those listed, but their interactions are less well established and the pathogenesis of disorders related to their use less well understood. Potential mechanisms by which chemotherapy may increase the neurotoxicity of RT include the following:

1. Chemotherapeutic agents may attack the same cellular structures as does radiation (e.g., some chemotherapeutics stimulate apoptosis, as does RT[390]); thus, their effects are additive.
2. The chemotherapeutic agent may act as a radiosensitizer, increasing the sensitivity of neural tissues to radiation (Fig. 13–9).
3. RT may alter the distribution kinetics of chemotherapeutic agents in the CNS by increasing permeability of the blood–brain barrier,[2505] acting on arachnoid granulations or choroid plexus to decrease clearance of the drug, or interrupting the ependymal barrier to allow drugs in the CSF to leave the ventricles and enter cerebral white matter, particularly after the drug has been injected intrathecally.
4. RT-induced cellular alterations may allow more drug to enter normal cells or may allow less drug to exit.

Table 13–8. **INTERACTIONS BETWEEN CHEMOTHERAPY AND RT**

Agent	Route of Administration	Neurotoxicity
Methotrexate	IV, IT	Leukoencephalopathy Mineralizing microangiopathy Cognitive impairment
Nitrosoureas	IA, high-dose IV	Leukoencephalopathy Cognitive impairment Possibly myelopathy
Cytosine arabinoside	High-dose IV IT	Leukoencephalopathy Possibly cognitive impairment Myelopathy
Multidrug regimens	IV	Cognitive impairment Leukoencephalopathy
Vincristine	IV	Pontine leukoencephalopathy Myelopathy Peripheral neuropathy

IA = intra-arterial; IT = intrathecal; IV = intravenous.
Source: Adapted from DeAngelis and Shapiro,[586] p 362.

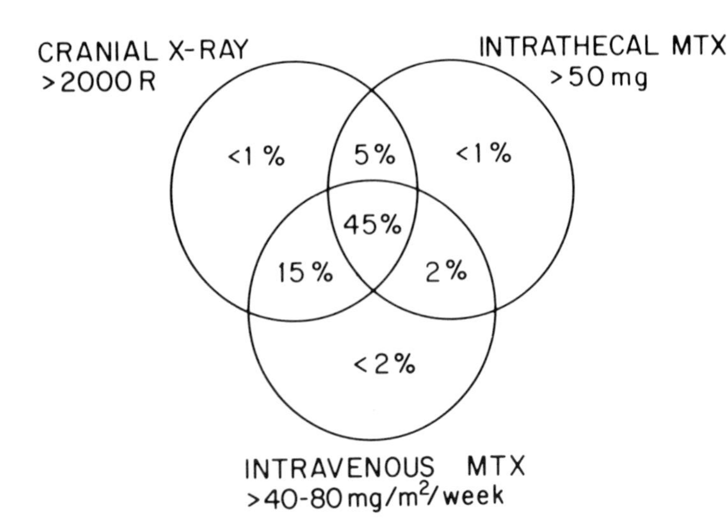

Figure 13–9. A diagram illustrating the relationship among cranial RT, intravenous methotrexate, and intrathecal methotrexate. Of patients who receive all three types of treatment, 45% develop some leukoencephalopathy, whereas less than 2% of patients who receive only one treatment develop the same disorder. (From Bleyer and Griffen,[239] p 171, with permission.)

The relative timing of administering RT and chemotherapy also appears important, at least with respect to MTX. MTX given before RT is less neurotoxic (and may even be protective) than MTX given after or concurrent with RT,[907] perhaps because RT enhances permeability, thus increasing entry of MTX into normal brain.[2505] At least one study, however, suggests no effect of RT on the accumulation of MTX in the brain.[1327] Long-term survivors of childhood acute leukemia who receive prophylactic brain RT and chemotherapy suffer cognitive impairment, with higher doses of radiation causing less impairment than lower doses.[1112a,1275a]

Neurotoxic interactions between MTX and cranial radiation are the most clearly established. Risk factors for neurotoxicity include young age, leptomeningeal disease, the dosages of MTX and cranial radiation, and the timing of chemotherapy. Two disorders, leukoencephalopathy and mineralizing microangiopathy, can be distinguished clinically and by CT scan (Table 13–9). The likelihood of leukoencephalopathy produced by RT is enhanced by the use of MTX following completion of RT. The leukoencephalopathy begins 4 to 12 months following treatment, usually CNS prophylaxis for leukemia. Neurologic signs begin with the insidious onset of dementia, possibly progressive, and may later become associated with ataxia, seizures, and unilateral or bilateral hemiparesis. The disorder may progress to stupor, coma, or death, but most patients survive, albeit with permanent intellectual deficits. CT and MR scans show white matter dysfunction, particularly in the periventricular areas. The pathologic changes are the same whether the disorder is caused by cranial RT alone or by MTX. They include multifocal, coalescing areas of coagulative necrosis in deep white matter, with myelin loss, axonal swelling, fragmentation, and gliosis. The cortical gray matter and the basal ganglia are spared.

Mineralizing microangiopathy occurs only after cranial RT. Restricted to gray matter, it may not be associated with clinical symptoms in children treated for ALL. Previously, it was identified during autopsy examination in 17% of patients with this disease. This disorder can also be identified on CT scan; the mineralization of the walls of small arteries, capillaries, and venules lends a serpentine hyperdensity to the cerebral cortex.

Histopathologically, calcium is deposited in small blood vessels. Some vessels may be occluded and surrounded by mineralized necrotic tissue. Inflammation is absent. The pathogenesis is believed to be related to radiation effects on the microvasculature. Coexistent leukoencephalopathy may or may not be present. The disorder is rarely seen now because it requires more radiation than the 2400 cGy or less that is currently given to children for prophylaxis. A few

Table 13–9. **DELAYED NEUROLOGIC SEQUELAE IN CHILDREN WITH ACUTE LYMPHOBLASTIC LEUKEMIA: LEUKOENCEPHALOPATHY VS. MINERALIZING MICROANGIOPATHY**

Comparative Feature	Leukoencephalopathy	Mineralizing Microangiopathy
Incidence	0–55% (depending on the amount of CNS irradiation, IT MTX, and high-dose IV MTX)	5–50+ %
Lesion sites	White matter (mainly centrum ovale of cerebral hemispheres)	Gray matter (mainly basal ganglia and subcortical zones)
CT scan abnormalities	Periventricular hypodensity, ventricular dilatation, subarachnoid dilatation, subcortical calcifications	Calcifications of basal ganglia and vascular border zones of cerebral cortex
Neurologic dysfunction	Usually severe, progressive, and potentially fatal	Apparently mild, subclinical, or transient
Pathogenesis	Myelin degeneration from combined effects of CNS irradiation and MTX	RT-induced microvascular injury and calcific occlusion
Risk factors	Cranial irradiation <2000 cGy; IT MTX >50 mg; IV MTX >50 mg/m^2 per week	Cranial irradiation >2400 cGy; possibly IV ara-C; possibly IV MTX
Latent period	4–5 mo or longer after RT	About 10 months after RT

IT = intrathecal; IV = intravenous; MTX = methotrexate.
Source: From DeAngelis and Shapiro,[586] p 366, with permission.

patients with this disorder have seizures and poor coordination,[2093] but most are asymptomatic.

Nitrosoureas, including BCNU and CCNU, have been reported[2052] to be more neurotoxic in patients who have received RT, but others have not found such an effect. Similar questions have arisen with respect to the effects of combined BCNU and spinal cord RT. Vincristine has been reported to enhance the neurotoxicity of spinal cord irradiation and peripheral nerve irradiation. Several children have developed a typical vincristine peripheral neuropathy more severe in an irradiated limb than elsewhere.[353,400] The effects of high-dose cytosine arabinoside and intrathecal cytosine arabinoside are probably also enhanced by RT, although the mechanisms are not well established. Various multidrug regimens have been reported to enhance radiation toxicity, especially in elderly patients with small-cell lung cancer who receive prophylactic cranial RT. It is uncertain whether radiation alone causes the dementia or whether the chemotherapy plays a role.

CHAPTER 14

NEUROTOXICITY OF SURGICAL AND DIAGNOSTIC PROCEDURES

In most patients with cancer, iatrogenic neurotoxicity results from either chemotherapy (see Chapter 12) or ionizing radiation (see Chapter 13). In a few, however, tumor surgery, diagnostic tests, and other procedures related to patient care may result in significant neurologic dysfunction. Some of these nervous system abnormalities are described in this chapter.

DISORDERS RESULTING FROM SURGERY OR ANESTHESIA

Neurologic disorders following surgery and anesthesia are uncommon. Nevertheless, neurologic disorders ranging from postoperative delirium to severe and prolonged muscle paralysis in the intensive care unit (Table 14–1) have complicated surgery and anesthesia for patients undergoing treatment for non-neoplastic diseases.[1163,2381] Because surgical procedures in patients with cancer are likely to be more complex and anesthesia more prolonged, complications are more frequent. The type of neurologic disorder depends on the site of the tumor being removed, the patient's position during

Table 14–1. **NEUROTOXICITY OF SURGERY AND ANESTHESIA**

Central Nervous System Injuries
Postoperative delirium
Perioperative stroke
Postanesthetic myelopathy
Cranial and Peripheral Nerve Injuries
Surgical trauma
Compression
Hemorrhage
Vascular Injuries
Hemorrhage
Occlusion
Cerebrospinal Fluid Leak

surgery, and, often, the patient's age and general preoperative condition. Damage to the nervous system may be:

1. a direct result of surgical trauma, for example, section of the intercostal-brachial nerve during mastectomy;
2. an indirect result of metabolic abnormalities that follow the surgery, for example, hypercoagulability and stroke, or delirium;
3. a result of positioning during anesthesia, for example, compression of peripheral nerves; or
4. a result of toxicity of anesthetic agents used, for example, adhesive arachnoiditis following spinal anesthesia.

Central Nervous System Injuries

POSTOPERATIVE DELIRIUM

The incidence of postoperative delirium in patients with cancer is unknown.[1576] Clinically significant delirium that interferes with smooth postoperative care and recovery probably affects less than 1% of patients. When it occurs, it frightens patients, family, and sometimes medical and nursing staff, and it considerably complicates recovery. Although some patients are delirious immediately upon awakening from surgery, a lucid interval of 24 to 48 hours when the patient seems quite normal is more typical. This lucid period is followed by the sudden or gradual onset of confusion, disorientation, and general clouding of consciousness. Most patients are agitated and suffer from delusions, often of persecution, or from visual and auditory hallucinations. The delusions and hallucinations can cause combative behavior; the patient may pull at dressings and tubing and cause extreme difficulty in nursing care. Tachycardia, diaphoresis, and tremor are frequently present even without fever. The disorder may last several days, but the patient virtually always returns to his or her preoperative state.[1753,1847,2429] Persistent delirium may indicate unsuspected pre-existing or concurrent structural brain disease and warrants neuroradiologic investigation with a CT or MR scan. Occult cerebral metastases, compensated hydrocephalus, and cerebrovascular disease are but a few conditions that may manifest only in the postoperative period as a delirium.

The pathogenesis of most postoperative delirium is unknown. No specific metabolic abnormality has been identified, although van der Mast and colleagues[2660] have implicated reduced levels of plasma tryptophan that are due to the patient's metabolic state. In one study,[1819] low serum albumin levels, perhaps a manifestation of premorbid malnutrition, was the only laboratory test result that correlated with delirium. Some patients are hypoxic.[1]

Risk factors for postoperative delirium (Table 14–2) include brain dysfunction prior to surgery[939,2329]; old age; alcoholism; psychological factors, including extreme anxiety in the preoperative period[2429] and the sensory deprivation that can affect patients who are kept in windowless intensive care units[2824] or whose eyes are patched after surgery; and postoperative drugs, particularly opioids and anticholinergics.

A perioperative cerebral infarct, especially if located in the territory of the nondominant or right middle cerebral artery or the left posterior cerebral artery, may also cause a severely agitated delirium with minimal focal signs[624,1807] and should always be considered as a possible cause of postoperative confusion.

The treatment is to try to restore cognition as soon as possible while protecting the patient from self-induced harm. Contributing organic factors should be corrected, and metabolic abnormalities should be reversed. The patient should be in a lighted room, preferably with a relative at the bedside to supply reassurance and assist with orientation. Sedative drugs should be withheld. If the patient's behavior has to be controlled to prevent self-injury, haloperidol rather than benzodiazepines or opioids should be administered. When opioids are necessary for pain relief, they should be closely titrated to avoid excessive sedation. Because restraints increase agitation, they should be used only when absolutely necessary.

ASEPTIC MENINGITIS

Some patients develop a noninfective postcraniotomy meningitis, most often after posterior fossa surgery or when the surgeon

Table 14–2. **ETIOLOGIC FACTORS IN POSTOPERATIVE DELIRIUM**

- Predisposing Factors
  - Age older than 60 years and especially older than 80 years
  - Cerebral disease (dementia, parkinsonism)
  - Chronic illness or disease
  - History of substance abuse
  - Anxiety, depression
- Contributory (Facilitating) Factors
  - Sensory environment of the intensive care unit (sensory deprivation or overload)
  - Sleep deprivation
  - Immobilization
  - Psychological stress
- Precipitating Organic Factors (see Chapter 11)
  - Intoxication with drugs, including agents for premedication (anticholinergics), anesthesia, and analgesics (notably morphine)
  - Metabolic disturbances: hypoxemia, hypercarbia, hypocarbia, dehydration, electrolyte imbalance, acid-base imbalance, hepatic or renal failure
  - Hemodynamic disturbances: hypotension, hypovolemia, cardiac failure
  - Respiratory disorder: hypopnea or apnea, pulmonary embolism
  - Infection: pneumonia, septicemia, bacteremia
  - Acute cerebral disorder: trauma, edema, stroke, fat embolism, metastases
  - Alcohol and/or sedative-hypnotic withdrawal syndrome
  - Malnutrition, vitamin deficiency
  - Seizures
  - Porphyria

Source: Adapted from Lipowski,[1576] p 447.

violates the cerebral ventricular system. Occasionally, the syndrome occurs after spinal operations if the subarachnoid space has been entered. The disorder is caused by blood and blood products in the subarachnoid space (hemogenic meningitis).[384,786] Characteristically, several days after the operation, when the steroid dose is being tapered, the patient complains of headache or backache and develops a low-grade fever. Nuchal rigidity may or may not be present. A few patients become frankly delirious. The CSF pressure is usually high, and the cell count varies from a few hundred to thousands of WBCs, initially dominated by neutrophils that are then replaced by lymphocytes. The protein concentration is raised. The glucose concentration usually remains normal, but sometimes is reduced. Results of CSF cultures are negative. The lumbar puncture may be therapeutic; if not, the aseptic meningitis is treated by increasing the steroid dose and then tapering more slowly. The inflammatory reaction may be severe enough to cause hydrocephalus, although a shunt is rarely required.

Distinguished from bacterial meningitis by its more indolent course and the absence of bacteria in the CSF, this syndrome can also be distinguished from leptomeningeal metastasis, which also may follow posterior fossa craniotomy, by the absence of malignant cells in the CSF.

TENSION PNEUMOCEPHALUS

Operations around the skull-base allow air to enter the intracranial cavity.[945] The air usually resolves but may remain under pressure. Efflux of CSF from the intracranial space during surgery creates a negative pressure that is filled by the entry of air, the "inverted pop bottle" phenomenon (Fig. 14–1).[67] Clinical signs usually appear 2 to 4 days postoperatively. Occasionally, the air appears months to years after the procedure.

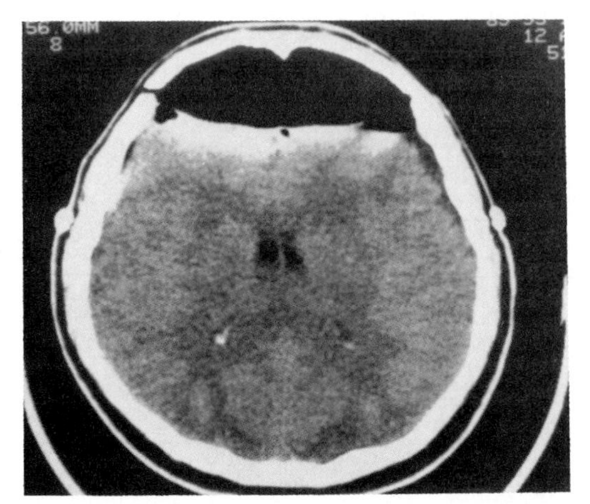

Figure 14–1. CT scan showing a large amount of air entrapped in the frontal region, displacing and compressing the frontal lobes. The frontal horns of the lateral ventricles are deformed and asymmetric. (From Arbit,[67] p 140, with permission.)

Patients complain of headache, may be delirious, and may develop focal neurologic signs dependent on the air site. CT or MR scan clearly identifies the offending agent as air rather than hematoma. Usually the air resolves on its own; at times, it must be aspirated. Occasionally, surgery may be required to repair a skull-base fracture or CSF leak.

Pneumocephalus, not under tension, occurs frequently in the postoperative period. When the amount of air in the intracranial cavity is large, the patient is lethargic and has more headache than expected. Some investigators believe that breathing 100% oxygen may help the patient by replacing the nitrogen component of the intracranial air with oxygen, which is more readily absorbed into the bloodstream.[67]

POSTDECOMPRESSION OPTIC NEUROPATHY

Blindness is a rare but devastating complication of craniotomy performed to remove a brain tumor.[169] Following apparently uncomplicated craniotomies, the disorder occurs in patients with markedly increased intracranial pressure and papilledema. Most patients do not show preoperative evidence of visual field abnormalities, yet the postoperative blindness does not reverse. The pathogenesis of this rare disorder is unknown, but the sudden lowering of intracranial pressure probably alters the vascular supply to the nerves. A similar disorder occasionally follows ventriculostomy for relief of increased intracranial pressure.

Discussed in detail elsewhere[218] are other complications of craniotomy, including intracranial hypertension, hematomas, brain edema, hydrocephalus, cerebral infarction, fluid and electrolyte abnormalities, peripheral venous occlusion, and fevers.

Cranial and Peripheral Nerve Injuries

Nerve injuries during or immediately following surgery can result either from direct damage caused by the surgeon, from postoperative bleeding into nerve beds, or from the patient's position during the course of anesthesia.[574] Pain syndromes related to diagnostic or therapeutic surgical procedures are also an important problem for some patients with cancer.[2061] These acute or chronic syndromes, discussed in the following paragraphs, are summarized in Table 14–3.

HEAD AND NECK SURGERY

Surgery on the neck or head may damage branches of peripheral or cranial nerves (Table 14–4).[2743] For instance, injury to the infraorbital branch of the trigeminal nerve during maxillary sinus surgery leads to a loss of facial sensation lateral to the nose. Another example is damage to the facial nerve during parotid surgery. The marginal mandibular branch of the facial nerve is often damaged during radical neck dissection.[2536] This thin twig descends below the mandible into the upper neck before reascending into the face to innervate the lower lip. The twig is so fine that even if the surgeon identifies the nerve and preserves it anatomically, it often suffers sufficient damage to impair function. Affected patients cannot fully depress the lower lip when grimacing; many women find it diffi-

Table 14–3. **PAIN SYNDROMES FOLLOWING DIAGNOSTIC PROCEDURES OR SURGERY**

Acute Pain
Nociceptive (pain arising from non-neural structures)
Postoperative incisional pain
Venipuncture and infusion
Postural pain
Neuropathic (pain arising from the peripheral nervous system or CNS)
Postoperative from acute nerve injury
Hemorrhage into nerve from venipuncture
Chronic Pain
Nociceptive
Postoperative from nonhealing incision
Neuropathic
Postradical neck dissection
Postmastectomy
Post-thoracotomy
Postamputation

Source: Adapted from Portenoy,[2061] p 1027.

Table 14–4. **INVOLVEMENT OF PERIPHERAL NERVES IN 33 RADICAL NECK DISSECTIONS**

Nerve	No. Involved in Radical Neck Dissection	No. Noted to Be Excised in Operative Report	Percentage Involved
Facial (excluding mandibular, platysmal, and marginal branches)	22	3	67
Glossopharyngeal	3	2	10
Vagus	5	4	15
Spinal accessory	33	33	100
Hypoglossal	13	7	39
Dorsal scapular (rhomboids)	2	0	6
Medial and lateral thoracic nerves (pectorals)	2	0	6
Sympathetic	11	0	33
Cervical plexus and supraclavicular nerves	33	0	100
Suprascapular	2	0	6
Phrenic	3	0	10

Source: Adapted from Swift,[2536] p 695.

cult to apply lipstick to that area. Aside from the mild cosmetic change, the injury has no physiologic consequence.

The vagus nerve runs a long course through the neck and can easily be damaged during neck surgery. Symptomatic damage to branches of the vagus nerve causes palatal and vocal cord paralysis.

Fibers from the cervical sympathetic chain travel with the vagus, as does the glossopharyngeal nerve, which is also vulnerable during neck surgery. Sympathetic damage causes an ipsilateral Horner's syndrome after radical neck dissection. Damage to recurrent laryngeal nerve fibers causes unilateral vocal cord paralysis, a problem that sometimes also follows thyroid surgery.

Florid perspiration of the cheek, jaw, temple, and sometimes neck while eating, known as gustatory sweating, follows aberrant regeneration of surgically damaged autonomic fibers that travel with the glossopharyngeal and vagus nerves. The disorder can follow radical neck dissection.[1845] It is more a nuisance than a disability.

The spinal accessory nerve travels through the neck to innervate the trapezius and sternocleidomastoid muscles. It is often damaged during neck surgery, leading to drooping of the shoulders that can generate chronic arm pain.[950,2230]

The hypoglossal nerve descends into the neck before innervating the ipsilateral half of the tongue; occasional injury during neck surgery causes slurred speech and difficulty in eating.

Sensory branches of supraclavicular and infraclavicular nerves and those of the second and third cervical roots are often sectioned during radical neck dissection.[2536] Sensory loss may affect the anterior chest from below the clavicle, sometimes extending to the nipples; the posterior chest, sometimes to the middle of the scapula; the lateral arm to the lower end of the deltoid; the lateral face anterior to the ear; and the lateral aspect of the jaw (Fig. 14–2). The physician may mistake these last changes for trigeminal nerve involvement, although careful sensory evaluation reveals that the medial portion of the face supplied by the trigeminal nerve, particularly the upper and lower lip, is spared.

The most serious consequence of neck dissection is a rare but extremely painful disorder of the jaw and face, often chronic and disabling. Characteristically, the patient is numb in the C-2 and C-3 distribution over the jaw and lateral face and, within weeks to a few months following surgery, begins to note sharp, lancinating pains in that area, often precipitated by touching the scar. Pa-

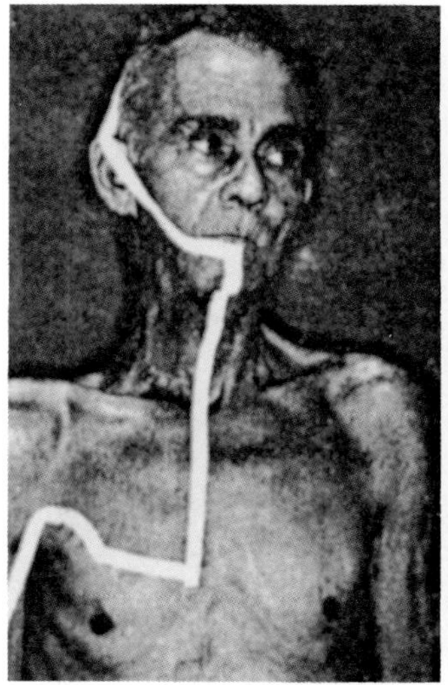
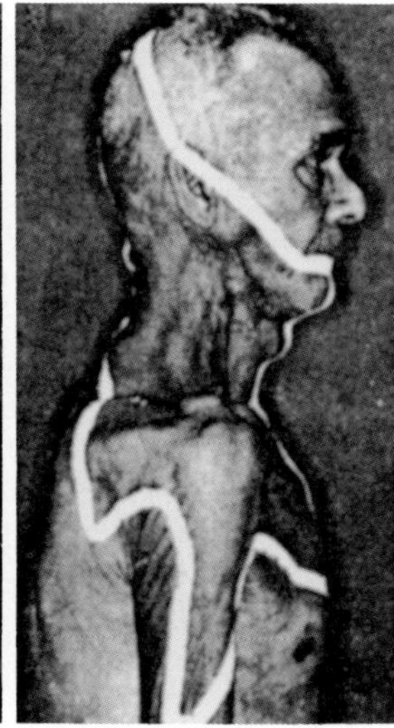
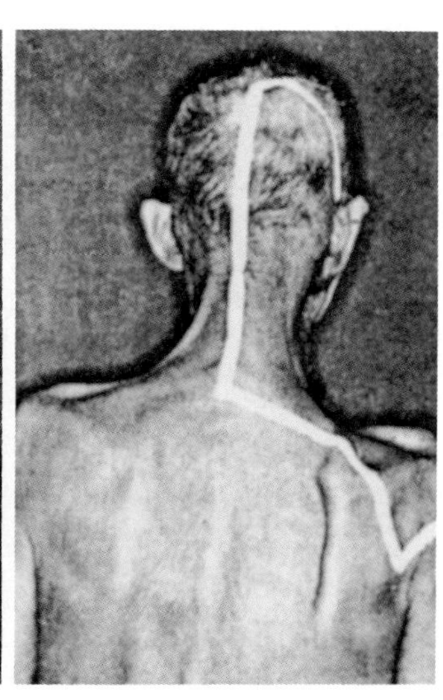

Figure 14–2. The distribution of sensory loss in a patient after radical neck dissection. Note that the sensory loss extends to the cheek and chin and to areas generally thought to be supplied by the trigeminal nerve. Sensory loss also occurs to a variable degree in the anterior and posterior chest and the lateral arm. The spread of sensory loss varies from patient to patient and is always quite extensive. (From Swift,[2536] p 695, with permission.)

tients will generally not allow an examination because touch precipitates lancinating pain. The sharp pains are soon replaced by a chronic dysesthetic pain in the same distribution. The sharp, lancinating pains are often relieved by carbamazepine, but the chronic dysesthetic pain, resembling postherpetic neuralgia, is not relieved by most procedures. Exploration of the scar and removal of neuromas may help, but too often this does not relieve the chronic pain, and many patients never obtain relief.[2061,2682]

Carotid sinus syncope because of tumor involving the carotid sinus nerve (see Chapter 8) usually affects patients who have had a prior neck dissection. The surgery opens the carotid sheath and exposes the sinus to tumor invasion if the tumor recurs.

TRUNK SURGERY

During a mastectomy, the intercostal-brachial nerve is often sacrificed or damaged. Virtually every patient undergoing radical or modified radical mastectomy develops some numbness in the distribution of the intercostal-brachial nerve but may be unaware of it.[1979] About 15% to 20% of these patients complain of a tight, burning sensation in that distribution. The pain may be present immediately after surgery or begin several weeks later[2684] and can be associated with paresthesias in the fingers. The differential diagnosis is outlined in Table 14–5. In a small percentage of patients, the pain may be severe, intractable, and lead to chronic disability. Most patients undergoing mastectomy also recognize a phantom breast that may or may not be painful.[1273,2684]

Damage to intercostal nerves is an inevitable result of thoracotomy. The large overlap of sensory fields of the thoracic roots usually precludes identifiable sensory loss when only one or two nerves have been sectioned, but a few patients develop painful dysesthetic and lancinating sensations in the damaged area. This post-thoracotomy syndrome usually begins within a few weeks after surgery and may persist for many years. It must be distinguished from tumor recurrence invading the chest wall and compressing intercostal nerves or from vertebral body metastasis compressing thoracic roots. The time course and chronicity of the pain usually make the distinction fairly simple.

Damage to lower extremity nerves during abdominal or pelvic surgery is uncommon. Retractor injuries sometimes cause femoral nerve damage that is almost always reversible. Painful postoperative syndromes of the lower extremities are also rare. Autonomic dysfunction on the unoperated side

Table 14–5. **CAUSES OF ARM PAIN FOLLOWING MASTECTOMY**

Postmastectomy Pain (Intercostal-Brachial Neuralgia)
Brachial Plexus Neuropathy
  Tumor infiltration
  Radiofibrosis
  Lymphedema entrapment
  Transient neuritis
Cervical Radiculopathy
  Due to vertebral metastatic compression
  Due to degenerative spine disease
Carpal Tunnel Syndrome
  With lymphedema
  Without lymphedema
Pericapsulitis of Shoulder Joint

Source: Adapted from Vecht et al,[2684] p 172.

after retroperitoneal lymph node dissection has been reported, however. The contralateral leg is cold and sweaty, probably because of compensatory sympathetic hyperfunction.[1129] Painful and nonpainful phantom sensation may follow rectal amputation.[1958]

EXTREMITY SURGERY

When a limb is amputated because of bone or soft-part sarcomas, the patient is left with a phantom sensation[1744] that is painful in about 10% of such patients. Evidence indicates that the patient who has experienced pain prior to the amputation is more likely to have postoperative pain, at least acutely. The phantom pain may be transient or permanent.[1285] With time, the phantom sensation often diminishes; the more distal parts seem to move proximally so that the patient may be left feeling a foreshortened limb with fingers or toes still discernible. A prosthesis is reported to hasten the resolution of the phantom sensation. Painful phantoms are characterized by chronic, unremitting pains often perceived as a cramped, abnormal position of the phantom or as a burning, dysesthetic sensation. The pain does not respond to analgesic agents. Similar phantom sensations may follow nerve injury without amputation, especially when the brachial plexus is affected.

COMPRESSION INJURIES

The patient's position during anesthesia may cause nerve injuries from compression.[574,1982] The most common of these is a brachial plexus palsy that occurs when the arm is abducted above the head during thoracotomy or mastectomy. Abduction to more than 90 degrees causes the head of the humerus to descend into the axilla. The brachial plexus, which passes caudal to the head of the humerus, is stretched and compressed by that structure, especially if the patient remains in that position for several hours. Alternately, a shoulder brace for compressive depression of the shoulder girdle, with the patient in Trendelenburg's position, may also exert pressure on the plexus. Usually, affected patients awaken to find the arm completely paralyzed and numb. Within hours to a few days, the lower portion of the plexus recovers; the patient then is weak in the deltoid and other shoulder muscles, generally with little numbness or sensory loss. The patient usually recovers completely within a few weeks. Permanent loss of neurologic function is uncommon. Idiopathic acute brachial neuritis may follow any surgical procedure.[1659]

Ulnar nerve palsy can result from compression at the elbow by arm boards used to secure the IV line. The patient awakens from surgery with a numb fifth finger; the numbness usually also involves the ulnar aspect of the fourth finger, but the median aspect of the fourth finger, innervated by the median nerve, is spared. The small hand muscles are often weak. Recovery usually occurs in days to weeks, but numbness and weakness may be permanent.

The radial nerve is vulnerable to compression as it winds around the humerus. The nerve can be compressed between the table edge and the humerus or, if the patient is in the lateral decubitus position, between the body and the humerus. Affected patients awaken with a wrist drop and inability to extend the fingers. The brachioradialis muscle is weak, but the triceps muscle is spared because its nerve supply exits the radial nerve above the humeral groove. The patient often complains of a weak grip, suggesting median nerve damage as well, but if the examiner passively extends the wrist, the grip is normal. Sensory loss or paresthesias are usually mild and may not be present at all. If present, they are evident over the dorsum of the median side of the hand and the thumb and index finger. Rarely, a cerebral infarct in its early stages may mimic a radial nerve palsy, but the brachioradialis-triceps muscle disparity is absent.

Compression of the femoral nerve can result from retraction during surgery.[26] The patient suffers weakness when extending the knee and a modest sensory loss in the anterior thigh and medial leg. The patellar reflex is absent. The other thigh and leg muscles are normal, permitting the patient to walk, although the knee may sometimes buckle. Recovery is usually complete after several weeks.

Sciatic neuropathy sometimes follows surgery, particularly if the patient was operated on in the sitting position, for example, to remove a posterior fossa metastasis. Weakness in the leg and foot is evident immediately after surgery, specifically affecting dorsiflexion and plantar flexion of the foot and flexion of the knee. Recovery is usually, but not always, complete.

A peroneal nerve palsy follows compression of that nerve at the fibular head from positioning of the patient or from intraoperative compression boots used to prevent thrombophlebitis.[1452] In contradistinction to sciatic neuropathy, plantar flexion and inversion of the foot remain normal, whereas dorsiflexion and eversion are weak. Sensory loss, if any, is restricted to a small area between the great and second toes. Recovery is usually complete.

Nerve damage may also result from delayed hemorrhage after surgery. Patients usually exhibit normal nerve function when they awaken from surgery, but within the first 24 to 48 hours, they begin to complain of pain and paresthesias in the distribution of affected nerves. The hemorrhage typically is found at such sites as the brachial plexus, where it causes arm paralysis, or at the lumbar plexus, in and around the iliopsoas muscle, where it paralyzes thigh flexion and knee extension. Hematomas in other areas are usually rapidly discovered before nerve compression occurs. CT or MR scan can easily identify an acute hematoma of the brachial or lumbar plexus. When appropriate, draining the hematoma usually relieves neurologic symptoms, although recovery is typical even without drainage.

Vascular Injuries

Vascular injuries can affect either arteries or veins. Disruption of either leads to hemorrhage. Occlusion of an artery leads to infarction of tissues supplied by that vessel; venous occlusion usually increases tissue pressure of the area drained and may cause edema.

ARTERIAL INJURIES

Carotid damage either during or at some time following radical neck dissection, often after RT, may cause bleeding.[1520] When carotid leakage occurs, the artery must be ligated. Many patients tolerate ligation without substantial neurologic injury, but a few may develop cerebral infarction with hemiparesis or hemiplegia. In rare instances, brain swelling, herniation, and death may follow the infarct. The symptoms usually begin immediately after the artery is occluded but can begin at any time within the first several hours. The neurologic damage is usually maximal within a few hours of onset. In patients with cerebral swelling, the symptoms may progress during 24 to 48 hours and then begin to resolve.

Temporary occlusion of the aorta or occlusion during aortic surgery of thoracic branches supplying the spinal cord may lead to spinal cord infarction, characterized clinically either by an acute postoperative transverse myelopathy or Brown-Séquard's syndrome, with paralysis and paresthesias on the ipsilateral side of the body and pain and temperature loss on the contralateral side. Occasionally, the occlusion causes an anterior spinal artery syndrome with bilateral distal paralysis and loss of pain and temperature sensation but preservation of touch, vibration, and position because the posterior columns are spared. Variable, but usually incomplete, recovery occurs after spinal cord ischemia or infarction.

VENOUS INJURIES

Venous occlusion during surgery usually does not lead to neurologic injury. Most patients tolerate the ligation of one or both jugular veins during radical neck surgery. Ligation of one or both jugular veins does increase intracranial pressure, however, and in a few patients may cause the pseudotumor cerebri syndrome characterized by headache, papilledema, and, rarely, blindness.[456,1688] Whether this syndrome results simply from the jugular vein ligation or whether it requires propagation of a clot from the ligated jugular vein into the transverse or sagittal sinus is not certain. In some patients, the venous occlusion leads to hemorrhagic infarction of the brain.[456] Venous occlusion in the trunk or extremities does not cause neurologic injury.

Surgery to the skull-base can fracture it. A carotid-cavernous fistula is possible (but rare) if a bone spicule lacerates the artery in the cavernous sinus. The diversion of blood from the carotid into the cavernous sinus may cause a cerebral infarct on the ipsilateral side in addition to the usual signs of carotid-cavernous fistula, which include proptosis, ocular motor paralysis, and a bruit over the bulging eye (see Fig. 9–9).[1769]

Thrombophlebitis in the postoperative period can complicate virtually any surgery. Patients with cancer, who generally are in a hypercoagulable state, are at greater risk for the development of deep vein thrombosis in the lower extremities followed by pulmonary embolism[2589a] (see Chapter 9) than are patients without cancer. The incidence of thromboembolic complications also appears to be higher in neurosurgical patients than in those undergoing surgery for other neoplasms. Prophylaxis of thromboembolic disorders in the postoperative period includes pneumatic compression boots and low-dose heparin. When the surgery involves nervous system structures, however, particularly the brain, many physicians are reluctant to use low-dose heparin in the immediate postoperative period. Hemorrhagic complications were not noted in a recent study[841] in which patients undergoing neurosurgical procedures were treated with low-dose heparin, 5000 U subcutaneously bid, starting on the morning of the first postoperative day and continuing until they were fully ambulatory. Comparison with historic control subjects indicated that the treatment effectively reduced thromboembolic complications.[841]

Cerebrospinal Fluid Leak

Some patients who undergo head or spinal surgery suffer damage to the dura and arachnoid that leads to a CSF fistula communicating with the nasal passages, the ear, the thoracic or abdominal cavity, or the skin surface of the neck or back. Occasionally, CSF leaks are not immediately evident, such as when CSF empties into chest tubes placed after resection of a thoracic vertebral-body metastasis to alleviate spinal cord compression. These patients are at increased risk for CNS infection from organisms that enter from the skin or nasal passages. CSF leaks also cause intracranial hypotension[1449] (see the following).

Obstruction of the cerebral ventricular system with resulting communicating hydrocephalus often occurs in patients with leptomeningeal tumor (see Chapter 7), as a sequela of bacterial meningitis or subarachnoid hemorrhage. If such patients have related symptoms, shunting the ventricular system will relieve them. In some instances, when the ventricles are decompressed by shunting, fluid accumulates in the subdural space, causing brain compression (Fig. 14–3). Such subdural effusions may resolve spontaneously or may require evacuation.[2675]

DIAGNOSTIC PROCEDURES CAUSING NEUROTOXICITY

Computed Tomographic Scanning

Iodinated contrast material used for diagnostic procedures is generally well tolerated, particularly in patients without previous renal dysfunction. Various adverse reactions may affect systems other than the kidney, however.[216] The agents are epileptogenic, and if a brain lesion such as a metastasis causes blood–brain barrier disruption, a seizure may develop when the intravenously

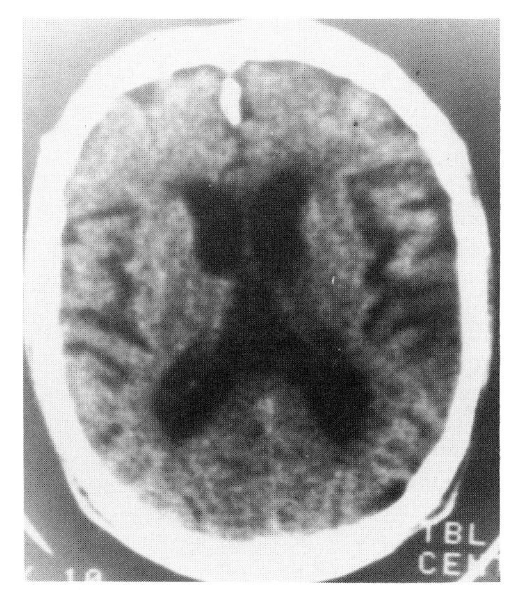

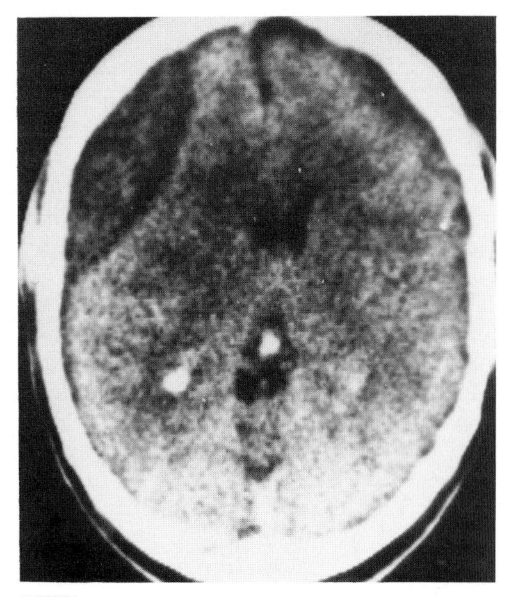

Figure 14–3. Subdural effusion following lumbar puncture. A patient with lung cancer developed slowly progressive dementia. Leptomeningeal metastases were suspected, although the CT scan showed only cerebral atrophy and hydrocephalus ex vacuo. Results of a lumbar puncture were normal. The patient worsened several days after the lumbar puncture. A repeat CT scan showed small ventricles compressed by large subdural effusions.

injected iodinated contrast material leaks across the endothelium. About 15% of patients with brain metastases who undergo CT scanning with contrast suffer a focal or generalized seizure.[1964] If a patient about to undergo CT scanning is suspected of harboring a brain metastasis or other lesion that impairs the blood–brain barrier, administering an oral dose (5 to 10 mg) of diazepam 30 minutes before the procedure considerably lowers the likelihood of an associated seizure. The risk of seizures does not apply to gadolinium contrast enhancement used in MR scanning.

In addition to seizures, other nervous system complications include transient global amnesia, cortical blindness, visual blurring, and worsening of pre-existing myasthenia gravis.[216]

Lumbar Puncture

CEREBRAL HERNIATION

Lumbar puncture, whether used diagnostically or therapeutically, can precipitate neurologic complications. The loss of spinal fluid through myelography or lumbar puncture, or by the CSF leak that often follows them, lowers pressure in the spinal canal, causing a pressure differential between the intracranial and the spinal spaces in those patients in whom cerebral or spinal tumors obstruct free passage of CSF. In patients with large intracranial lesions and increased intracranial pressure, the result may be cerebral herniation and sometimes death.[690] Characteristically, patients who suffer cerebral herniation induced by lumbar puncture are already partially herniated when the lumbar puncture is performed. Lumbar CSF pressure may appear normal because the downwardly displaced brain obstructs the foramen magnum, thereby separating the intracranial and spinal cavities. The patient appears immediately to tolerate the procedure well, but some hours later develops headache, worsening neurologic signs, and then sudden respiratory arrest from tonsillar herniation and brainstem compression. The premonitory signs may evolve rapidly; occasionally, the patient may be found dead the following morning. The apparently normal CSF pressure at the time of the lumbar puncture can give the physician a false sense of security, but it is exactly the apparently normal pressure that increases the risk of herniation. Except for those with suspected bacterial meningitis, lumbar puncture should not be performed in patients suspected of having an intracranial mass until a CT or MR scan of the intracranial contents excludes such lesions. Even in the absence of a mass lesion, lumbar puncture may rarely cause herniation if intracranial pressure is raised by meningitis[1211,2435] or leptomeningeal tumor.

The frequency of cerebral herniation in patients with increased intracranial pressure is unknown but certainly low. Most patients with brain tumor can safely undergo lumbar puncture. Patients whose large lesions are in the posterior fossa or the temporal lobe, or whose scan shows evidence of massive shift and early herniation, are at increased risk of decompressive herniation and lumbar puncture should be avoided. Herniation cannot be prevented by removing a smaller quantity of CSF because the disorder arises mostly from the postpuncture CSF leak through the needle hole. The amount of fluid removed at the time of lumbar puncture probably is irrelevant. Thus, if the needle has already entered the subarachnoid space, the physician should remove as much fluid as is necessary for the appropriate examinations.

Any patient who has elevated intracranial pressure from a mass lesion and who requires lumbar puncture should be started on corticosteroids to decrease the intracranial pressure prior to conducting the lumbar puncture.

INTRACRANIAL HYPOTENSION

The CSF leak from the needle piercing the arachnoid chronically lowers the intracranial pressure and leads to persistent intracranial hypotension.[1974,2120] This leak causes headache in approximately 30% of patients who undergo lumbar puncture. The headache usually begins 24 hours (range, 12 hours to 6 days) after the procedure and persists for 3 or 4 days. If the patient suffers a block to free passage of CSF by an epidural tumor, the headache may appear later, after relief of the epidural block by radiation.[1983] Post–lumbar-puncture headache is usually absent when the patient is recumbent but begins seconds or minutes after the patient assumes an upright position. The pain usually starts in the occipital region and the neck, radiating to the shoulders and then to the forehead. The pain can be mild or severe; severe pain can be associated with autonomic symptoms including pallor, sweating, nausea, and vomiting. The headache usually disappears promptly when the patient returns to the recumbent position. A Valsalva maneuver, a cough, or a sneeze, all of which increase intracranial pressure, may precipitate the headache, even if the patient is in the recumbent position.[2120] Requiring the patient to be flat for several hours after a lumbar puncture does not prevent post–lumbar-puncture headache.

The headache that occurs when the erect position is assumed is believed to result in part from traction on pain-sensitive structures as the brain descends, unbuoyed by the CSF, and in part from compensatory vasodilation, which also results from the decreased volume of CSF. In a few patients, additional symptoms include tinnitus, diplopia from abducens nerve palsy, vertigo, hearing loss,[1993] and visual alterations.[1209a]

Persistent intracranial hypotension can cause subdural effusions that may become large and require surgical evacuation. Patients who suffer persistent intracranial hypotension develop contrast enhancement of the meninges identified on MR and occasionally on CT scan (Fig. 14–4).[1974,2120] Unlike the contrast enhancement of leptomeningeal tumor, which is usually patchy, the contrast enhancement following lumbar puncture is usually diffuse. If a patient with cancer undergoes a lumbar puncture for any reason and then develops headache leading to an MR scan, meningeal enhancement may suggest the diagnosis of leptomeningeal tumor when the headache is only the result of the lumbar-puncture–induced intracranial hypotension. Occasionally, meningeal enhancement can be observed after lumbar puncture in the absence of headache and other signs of intracranial hypotension, further obscuring the diagnosis.

For patients with prolonged postural headache, an epidural blood patch usually relieves the symptoms within a few hours.[1939,2120] Surprisingly, a prophylactic blood patch is be-

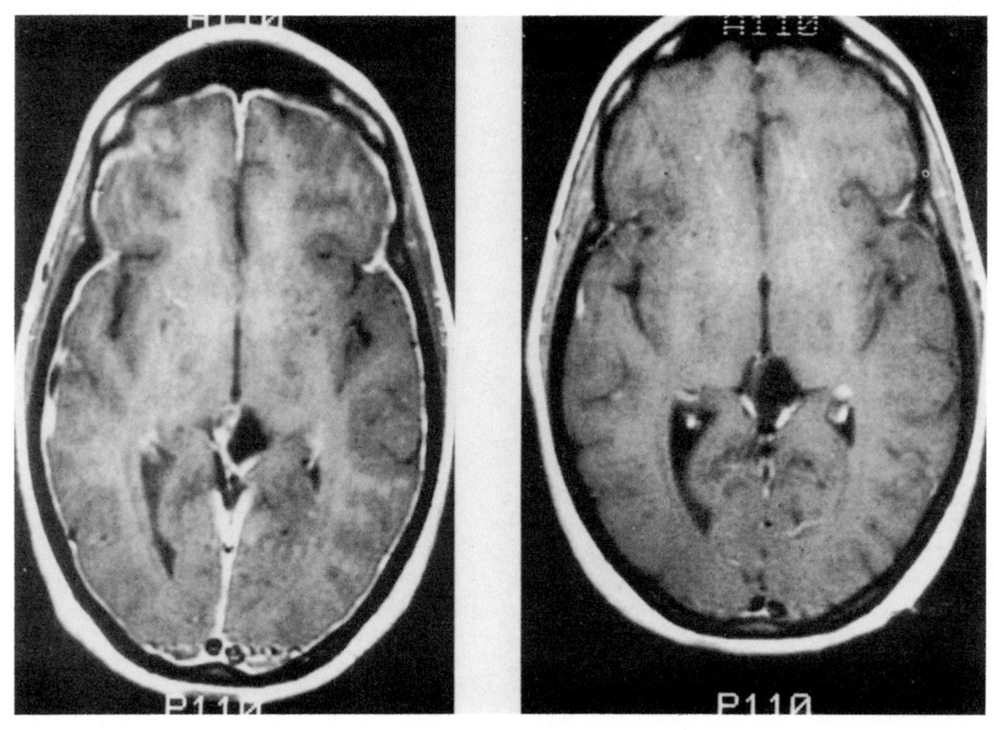

Figure 14–4. MR scans demonstrating intense meningeal enhancement following a lumbar puncture to evaluate possible leptomeningeal metastases in a patient with breast cancer. Persistent postlumbar puncture headache led to an MR scan that showed the intense meningeal enhancement *(left)*. The cerebrospinal fluid was otherwise normal. Several weeks later, after the headaches resolved spontaneously, the MR scan showed no evidence of enhancement. (From Pannullo et al,[1974] p 921, with permission.)

lieved to be ineffective,[203] although one report disagrees.[2603]

SPINAL HERNIATION

In occasional patients with asymptomatic epidural spinal cord compression, the lumbar puncture performed for diagnostic reasons or for spinal anesthesia may cause acute paraplegia, presumably from the sharp reduction of CSF pressure below the level of the epidural compression.[962,1189,1843,2678,2845] Typical is the patient with prostate carcinoma who may have vertebral metastases but shows no evidence of neurologic disability.[1843] The lumbar puncture is performed for spinal anesthesia during prostate surgery. Postoperative numbness from the spinal anesthesia does not resolve, and the patient's condition progresses to paraplegia. A rare situation is paraplegia from upward spinal coning following ventricular shunting to relieve hydrocephalus.[1309]

SPINAL HEMORRHAGE

The third major complication of lumbar puncture is spinal hemorrhage,[227,707] probably resulting from the inadvertent puncture of vessels in the subdural space (Fig. 14–5). The complication particularly affects patients who are thrombocytopenic, with a platelet count lower than 20,000 or lower than 50,000 but dropping rapidly. Patients who are anticoagulated with heparin or warfarin and patients who have a dysfunctional clotting system, such as that caused by liver failure, are also at risk. Most patients with such hemorrhages have suffered multiple attempts to enter the lumbar sac. The CSF may or may not be bloody. The patient characteristically tolerates the procedure well, but within a few hours complains of severe back pain, which may radiate into the legs. The pain is followed by paresthesias, weakness of the legs, urinary retention, and constipation. In some instances, the subdural hematoma

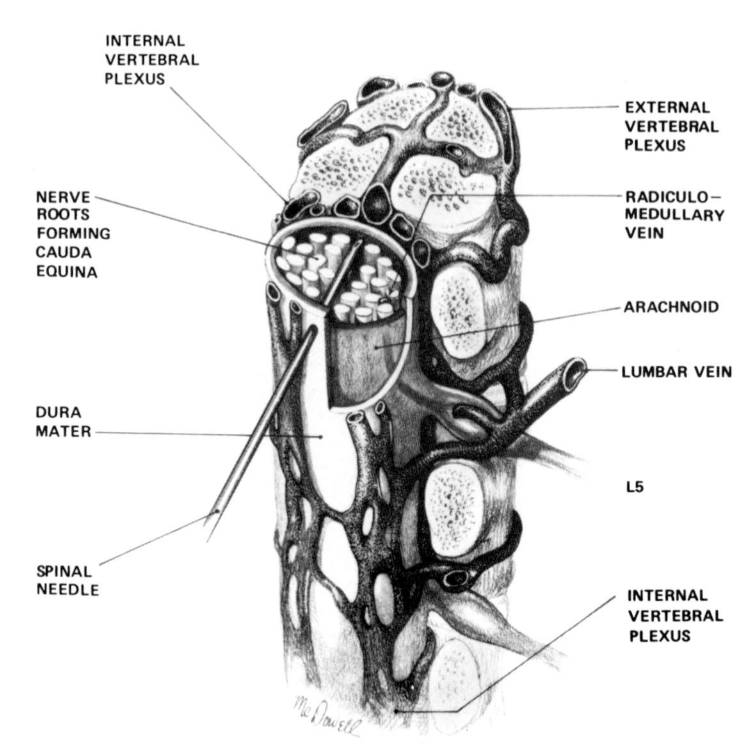

Figure 14–5. Spinal contents at the fourth and fifth lumbar vertebrae, showing the relationship of a lumbar puncture needle to the major vessels at this level. The major radiculomedullary vein, shown accompanying the L-5 nerve root, is situated far laterally to a needle correctly positioned in the dural sac midline. Note the avascular subdural space. (From Edelson et al,[707] p 136, with permission.)

dissects upward, causing paraplegia with sensory and motor levels reaching as high as the upper thoracic area (see Fig. 9–3). Autopsy examination in such instances reveals a large subdural hematoma compressing the spinal cord and cauda equina, probably caused by laceration of radicular vessels by the lumbar puncture needle.[1698] A similar problem occasionally follows lateral cervical puncture, causing quadriparesis and compromising respiratory muscles[5,1678]

Depending on the nature of their coagulopathy, patients who develop such symptoms should receive transfusions of platelets, fresh-frozen plasma, or both. When thrombocytopenic patients require lumbar puncture, the procedure should be done while they receive a platelet transfusion. If the patient complains of back pain at any time during the 24 to 36 hours following the procedure, more platelets should be given. Generally, it is impossible to decompress the subdural hematoma surgically because the coagulopathy precludes surgery. When a lumbar puncture is performed in a patient at risk, the most experienced physician available should do it, using a needle no larger than number 20. Although some patients remain paraplegic, many recover neurologic function spontaneously. A spinal MR or CT scan visualizes the hematoma and establishes the diagnosis (Fig. 14–6).

MENINGITIS

Lumbar puncture almost never causes acute bacterial meningitis, at least in patients older than age 1 year, even when performed in patients with known sepsis.[2566] An exception is the patient harboring a skin or epidural abscess at the site of the needle puncture. Acute aseptic meningitis was rarely reported to follow lumbar puncture in the years that preceded the use of disposable spinal needles.

Myelography

Because a myelogram begins with a lumbar puncture, the complications of lumbar puncture already discussed may also follow myelography. The most serious complication of myelography is spinal herniation when the myelogram is performed to evaluate epidural spinal cord compression. The pathogenic

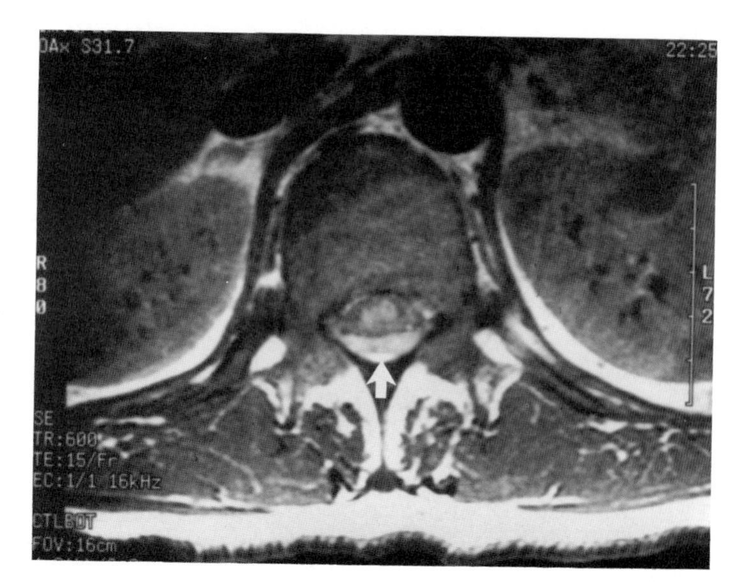

Figure 14–6. MR scan of a 35-year-old man with leukemia who underwent a lumbar puncture 3 days before this scan. Six hours after the lumbar puncture, he began to develop back pain that radiated toward the buttock. He did not develop weakness. The MR scan, however, reveals subdural blood posteriorly from T-12 to L-5. The hyperintense area in the center is the normal conus medullaris.

hypothesis is that the pressure change below the area of compression leads to impaction of the spinal cord against the epidural mass, augmenting compression and causing a transverse myelopathy. The neurologic deterioration after myelography is acute and may occur during the procedure. The incidence of paraplegia after myelography is unknown. One report describes a 15% incidence of neurologic worsening in patients undergoing myelography for the diagnosis of epidural spinal cord compression, but it is unclear from that report or others how much of the neurologic worsening was due to the procedure and how much could be attributed to the natural history of the disease.[1189] In my experience, neurologic worsening after myelography is uncommon, particularly if the physician stops injecting when a patient complains of back pain during the injection of the contrast material. MR scans of the spine should obviate the need for myelography.

CONTRAST MATERIAL

The iodinated contrast material used for myelography can cause aseptic meningitis,[1314,1665] adhesive arachnoiditis, and, in rare instances, encephalopathy, seizures, and cortical blindness.[216,1314] Aseptic meningitis, which is relatively common, is characterized by headache, stiff neck, fever, and pleocytosis following the myelogram. Bacterial meningitis following myelography is rare.[2319] Adhesive arachnoiditis, characterized by pain and progressive neurologic symptoms, is a very rare complication of myelography. In the past at Memorial Sloan-Kettering Cancer Center, myelograms were performed with iodinated, lipid-soluble contrast material, which was left in the canal after the procedure to facilitate reimaging after RT. Arachnoiditis could sometimes be detected by immobility of the dye in the postradiation period, but progressive neurologic symptomatology unrelated to recurrence of spinal cord compression was not seen. Acute transverse myelopathy occurs rarely after myelography with non-ionic, water-soluble contrast media.[127]

VENOUS AND ARTERIAL CATHETERIZATION

Although infection is the most common complication of the placement of indwelling vascular catheters for the infusion of chemotherapy or other agents,[1830] neurologic complications also occur.* Procedures to place subclavian vein catheters may lead to bleeding and compression of the brachial plexus from hematomas. Intrathoracic hemorrhage following laceration of a vertebral artery requiring surgical repair has been reported.[1007] The local anesthesia for internal jugular vein catheterization may cause a transient brachial plexopathy.[2538] A brachial plexopathy also has followed *Aspergillus* infection of a Hickman catheter.[1430] Several cases of stroke temporally associated with subclavian or internal jugular vein catheterization have been reported in patients treated for cancer.[1231,2044,2441] The stroke occurs in the anterior or posterior cerebral circulation and may be caused by paradoxic embolization from a clot on the end of the catheter or by inadvertent arterial damage with subsequent embolization during catheter placement. Brown-Séquard's syndrome that is due to spinal cord infarction has been reported after subclavian vein catheterization.[1400] Similar complications can follow arterial catheterization for the performance of angiograms.

Air embolus from inadvertent disconnection of subclavian catheters has been reported. The negative pressure in the thorax allows air to enter the catheter when it is open to atmospheric pressure.[2044]

Hepatic arterial chemotherapy using an implantable infusion pump sometimes causes neck and shoulder pain referred from diaphragmatic irritation by the pump or by the chemotherapy.[1364] Such shoulder or neck pain should be recognized by the physician as referred pain and not prompt a search for neck or shoulder disease.

*References 572, 594, 832, 853, 883, 1007, 1179, 1205, 2805.

MISCELLANEOUS COMPLICATIONS

Seizures have been reported[2890] following continuous irrigation of the mediastinum with iodine, but their pathogenesis is uncertain.[1110] The serum levels of iodine rise to four orders of magnitude greater than normal levels. One such patient had a previous cerebral infarct, probably compromising blood–brain barrier function and allowing iodine to enter the brain. The mechanism of the seizure disorder probably resembles the mechanism for seizures following a CT scan using iodinated contrast material.

Chewing disorders are common following transtemporal neurosurgical procedures and temporal craniotomies. The limitation in opening the mouth is caused by temporal muscle scarring and shortening and may be relieved by aggressive physical therapy. If not, temporal muscle detachment and coronoidectomy are indicated.[1902]

Occasionally, patients in the intensive care unit who require respiratory support or who receive sedative or paralytic agents, or both, suffer prolonged neurotoxicity. Patients receiving long-term benzodiazepine infusion to maintain sedation during respiratory support frequently remain comatose or stuporous for many days following discontinuation of the drugs, even those with a short half-life. The exact reason is unclear. Also, some may convulse when the benzodiazepine is withdrawn. When long-term treatment with vecuronium is ended, prolonged neuromuscular blockade may cause paralysis for as long as a week or more.[2353] The weakness appears to be dose-related and caused by a polyneuropathy.[1441] Paralysis may also result from a polyneuropathy or myopathy of severe illness often seen in an intensive care unit[2902] (see Chapter 11).

CHAPTER 15

PARANEOPLASTIC SYNDROMES

In patients with cancer, all neurologic abnormalities not caused by the cancer's spread to the nervous system are, by definition, paraneoplastic. Most physicians, however, use this term to refer to a group of disorders, often called "remote effects of cancer on the nervous system,"[293,1144,2070,2074] that are not caused by those nonmetastatic complications of cancer considered in the preceding five chapters. The paraneoplastic disorders differ from other nonmetastatic complications in several respects:

1. The neurologic symptoms of paraneoplastic syndromes usually precede the identification of the cancer, whereas neurologic symptoms of other nonmetastatic disorders usually occur in patients with known cancer.
2. Even when the paraneoplastic-related cancer is identified, it is often small, nonmetastatic, and indolently growing, in contradistinction to the other nonmetastatic complications of cancer, in which the tumors are often large and widely disseminated.
3. The neurologic disability caused by paraneoplastic syndromes is often profound in the absence of any other cancer symptoms. In the other nonmetastatic disorders, systemic disability is usually prominent and often overshadows the neurologic dysfunction.
4. Paraneoplastic syndromes are generally, but not always, irreversible. In other nonmetastatic disorders, treating the cancer often ameliorates the neurologic symptomatology.

These distinctions are not absolute; some disorders initially classified as paraneoplastic syndromes were reclassified once a specific cause was identified. For example, progressive multifocal leukoencephalopathy was once considered a typical remote effect of cancer on the nervous system[293] but is now recognized to be an opportunistic viral infection (see Chapter 10). Other disorders currently classified as paraneoplastic syndromes may eventually be reassigned as having a nutritional or infectious origin.

For the clinician, paraneoplastic syndromes affecting the nervous system can be divided into two large groups. The first group, "classic" paraneoplastic syndromes, is a group of disorders that, when present, strongly suggest an underlying cancer. These disorders include the Lambert-Eaton myasthenic syndrome (LEMS),[1915] opsoclonus/myoclonus found in children,[40] and subacute cerebellar degeneration (Table 15–1). The second group of disorders consists of clinical syndromes sometimes associated with cancer but more often appearing in the absence of a neoplasm. These include polymyositis,[1457] particularly in children and young adults, amyotrophic lateral sclerosis,[1300,2211] and sensorimotor polyneuropathy.[526] Although some of these patients may have an associated cancer, an extensive search for a neoplasm is generally unwarranted.

In this chapter, the term "paraneoplastic syndromes" and the phrase "remote effects of cancer on the nervous system" are used interchangeably to refer to disorders that are associated with an identifiable or occult cancer yet do not result from metastasis to the nervous system or from one of the previously discussed nonmetastatic complications of cancer, such as infection, vascular disorders, nutritional and metabolic disorders, or side effects of cancer therapy.

GENERAL CONSIDERATIONS

Classification

Paraneoplastic syndromes can affect any portion of the nervous system from the cerebral cortex through the brainstem and spinal cord to peripheral nerves, neuromuscular junction, and muscle. Clinical symptomatology can reflect pathologic damage to a single specific structure in the nervous system (e.g., to cerebellar Purkinje cells as in paraneoplastic cerebellar degeneration [PCD] or to the cholinergic synapse as in LEMS) or can reflect damage to multiple areas of the nervous system simultaneously, as in encephalomyelitis associated with cancer.[1142] In some clinically florid paraneoplastic syndromes, such as opsoclonus/myoclonus, the nervous system may be free of any identifiable pathologic change.[52]

Table 15–1. **PARANEOPLASTIC SYNDROMES AFFECTING THE NERVOUS SYSTEM**

Brain and Cranial Nerves
Subacute cerebellar degeneration*
Opsoclonus/myoclonus*
Limbic encephalitis* and other dementias
Brainstem encephalitis
Optic neuritis
Photoreceptor degeneration*
Spinal Cord and Dorsal Root Ganglia
Necrotizing myelopathy
Subacute motor neuronopathy*
Motor neuron disease
Myelitis
Sensory neuronopathy*
Peripheral Nerves
Subacute or chronic sensorimotor peripheral neuropathy
Acute polyradiculoneuropathy (Guillain-Barré syndrome)
Mononeuritis multiplex and microvasculitis of peripheral nerve
Brachial neuritis
Autonomic neuropathy
Peripheral neuropathy with islet-cell tumors
Peripheral neuropathy associated with paraproteinemia
Neuromuscular Junction and Muscle
Lambert-Eaton myasthenic syndrome*
Myasthenia gravis
Dermatomyositis, polymyositis
Acute necrotizing myopathy
Carcinoid myopathies
Myotonia
Cachectic myopathy
Multiple Levels of Central and Peripheral Nervous System or Unknown Site
Encephalomyelitis*
Neuromyopathy
Stiff-man syndrome

*Classic paraneoplastic syndrome.

Frequency

Several studies have addressed the frequency of paraneoplastic syndromes (Table 15–2).[527,733,944,1225,1859] Data from these studies

Table 15–2. **FREQUENCY OF PARANEOPLASTIC SYNDROMES IN SEVERAL STUDIES**

No. of Patients with Cancer Examined	Type of Cancer	Type of Examination	Neurologic Problem Found	% of Patients with Cancer with Neurologic Signs	Reference
1465	Any	Clinical	Neuromyopathy	6.6	527
1465	Any	Clinical	Cerebellar	0.2	527
150	SCLC	Clinical, EMG	LEMS	2.0	733
150	SCLC	Clinical	Weakness	44.0	733
171	Any	Sensory, clinical	Sensory neuropathy	12.0	1579
50	Lung	Postural testing	Cerebellar	26.0	2797
100	Lung	Muscle biopsy	Neuromuscular	33.0	944
641	SCLC	Clinical, EMG	LEMS	0.3	2349
3843	Lung	Clinical	Encephalomyelitis	0.36	1144
3843	Lung	Clinical	Peripheral neuropathy	0.7	1144
908	Ovary	Clinical	Cerebellar degeneration	0.1	1225

EMG = electromyogram; LEMS = Lambert-Eaton myasthenic syndrome; SCLC = small-cell lung cancer.

depend on the definitions of the syndromes, the rigor used to exclude other causes of neurologic dysfunction, and the care with which the neurologic evaluation was performed. For example, typical LEMS occurs in 3% or fewer of patients with small-cell lung cancer (the cancer that, along with ovarian cancer, is believed to have the highest frequency of paraneoplastic disorders), but less well-defined neuromuscular dysfunction, including subjective or objective muscle weakness, affects 44%.[733] Croft and Wilkinson[527] report that 16% of 250 patients with lung cancer had neuromyopathy, a vaguely defined illness characterized by proximal muscular weakness with one or more diminished or absent deep tendon reflexes. Hawley and colleagues,[1118] on the other hand, found that most peripheral neuropathy in patients with small-cell lung cancer could be related to weight loss and nutritional disturbances and thus was not truly paraneoplastic. Croft and Wilkinson[527] found that 6.6% of 1476 patients with any type of cancer had a neuromyopathy as assessed by physical examination; however, Lipton and associates[1579,1580] found abnormalities of peripheral nerve function by quantitative thermal threshold testing in 43% of 29 patients with cancer, and Gomm and colleagues[944] found myopathic changes on muscle biopsy in 33 of 100 patients with lung cancer. Croft and Wilkinson[527] found only 2 instances of cerebellar degeneration in 319 patients with lung cancer and only 3 instances in 1476 patients with any type of cancer. Erlington and coworkers[733] found ataxia or nystagmus in 5 of 150 patients with small-cell lung cancer, whereas Wessel and colleagues[2797] report cerebellar signs by posturographic analysis in 13 of 50 patients with lung cancer.[2797] Although such conflicting figures make it difficult to estimate the incidence of true neurologic paraneoplastic syndromes, my experience indicates that clinically significant paraneoplastic syndromes probably occur in fewer than 1% of patients with cancer.

The low incidence of classic neurologic paraneoplastic syndromes should not lead the physician to believe that patients with cancer do not endure disabling symptoms that *may* be paraneoplastic and *may* be related to nervous system dysfunction. As Table 15–3 indicates, almost half the patients with small-cell lung cancer suffer symptoms that appear to involve the neuromuscular system. Table 15–4 lists various symptoms in 240 unselected patients with cancer. Symptoms such as fatigue, anorexia, drowsiness, and concentration difficulties may very well be neurogenic in origin and possibly are paraneoplastic. Although the symptoms are important, they are usually found in patients being treated for already-identified cancer and are probably

Table 15–3. **NEUROMUSCULAR AND SOMATIC CLINICAL FEATURES OF 150 PATIENTS WITH SMALL-CELL LUNG CANCER**

Clinical Features	% of Total
Symptoms	
Anorexia	53
Weight loss	51
Erectile impotence	44
Dry mouth	41
Weakness	31*
Sphincter disturbance	24
Sweating change	21
Visual change	6
Physical Signs	
Inability to rise from squatting position	21*
Sensory change	16
Brisk reflexes	13
Absent reflexes	10
Diminished reflexes	9
Weakness†	8*
Ataxia or nystagmus	5
Posttetanic potentiation	3

*One or more measures of weakness were present in 44% of subjects.

†Excluding inability to rise from squatting position.

Source: From Erlington et al,[733] p 765, with permission.

Table 15–4. **SYMPTOMS IN PATIENTS WITH CANCER**

Symptom	% Positive
Fatigue	74.2
Worry	70.9
Sadness	66.1
Pain	62.7
Drowsiness	61.0
Dry mouth	56.5
Insomnia	53.7
Poor appetite	45.5
Nausea	44.5
Bloating	39.4
Difficulty in concentration	38.3
Constipation	33.5
Change in taste	36.5
Cough	30.4
Sexual dysfunction	23.9
Incontinence	12.3
Nightmares	11.3

Source: Portenoy R, unpublished data from Memorial Sloan-Kettering Cancer Center, 1992, with permission.

caused by nutritional, metabolic, or toxic effects of cancer or its treatment. By contrast, I describe in this chapter patients with clear, unequivocal involvement of the nervous system usually identified before the cancer and not ascribable to metastases or to the metabolic or toxic effects of cancer and its treatment.

Because of the low incidence of paraneoplastic syndromes in patients with cancer, the oncologist is unlikely to encounter even one patient each year with a paraneoplastic syndrome. Thus, if a patient with cancer complains of neurologic symptomatology, other causes should be assiduously sought. On the other hand, the situation is quite different in a patient without known cancer who develops neurologic symptoms. In this situation, if the cause of the neurologic disability is not immediately obvious and particularly if the patient presents with one of the classic paraneoplastic syndromes (see Table 15–1), the likelihood that the patient has cancer is considerable. Table 15–5 gives estimates of the likelihood that a patient presenting with a specific neurologic symptom has a cancer as the underlying cause. With the exception of LEMS, the data are not well established but represent my own estimates or those of others. Nevertheless, these estimates should encourage the physician to search extensively for cancer in patients with appropriate neurologic syndromes.

Importance

Although neurologic paraneoplastic syndromes are rare, their recognition by the physician is important for several reasons.[1859,2072] First, in about 50% of patients, neurologic symptoms precede and prompt the diagnosis of systemic cancer. Because specific paraneoplastic syndromes are associated with particular cancers, the diagnosis of

Table 15–5. **ESTIMATED LIKELIHOOD THAT A GIVEN NEUROLOGIC DISORDER IS A PARANEOPLASTIC SYNDROME**

Syndrome	% Paraneoplastic
Lambert-Eaton myasthenic syndrome	60
Subacute cerebellar degeneration	50
Subacute sensory neuronopathy	20
Opsoclonus/myoclonus (children)*	50
Opsoclonus/myoclonus	20
Myasthenia gravis	15
Sensorimotor peripheral neuropathy	10
Encephalomyelitis	10
Dermatomyositis	10

*All other percentages refer to adults.

a paraneoplastic syndrome can direct the search for the underlying malignancy to particular organs, such as the lung for LEMS and the ovaries for paraneoplastic cerebellar degeneration (PCD). Second, in patients known to have cancer, paraneoplastic syndromes may be confused with metastatic disease, metabolic or nutritional disorders, or treatment effects; because, with few exceptions, effective treatment is unknown for most paraneoplastic syndromes, other potentially reversible causes of neurologic dysfunction must be carefully excluded before a diagnosis of a paraneoplastic syndrome is made. Third, in many cases, the neurologic syndrome has its onset when the cancer is small and curable. Unfortunately, although the cancer may be relatively easy to control or even to cure, most patients with paraneoplastic syndromes are left with significant neurologic disability. Finally, the recent identification of antibodies associated with several paraneoplastic syndromes gives clues to the underlying etiology of these rare disorders and contributes to our understanding of the interactions of systemic cancers, immunologic mechanisms, and the nervous system.

Pathogenesis

Although the etiology of most neurologic paraneoplastic syndromes is unknown, several potential mechanisms have been proposed (Table 15–6).

1. Oppenheim[1950] in 1888 proposed that some neurologic disorders associated with cancer were caused by a toxic substance released by the tumor. That tumors can secrete substances that interfere with CNS function is now well established. The examples in Table 15–6 are peptide hormones that cause secondary neurologic dysfunction.[1598] Cytokines such as tumor necrosis factor or IL-1 and IL-6, secreted by the tumor or by immune cells reacting to the tumor, may help cause the cachexia,[896] fatigability, asthenia, muscle catabolism,[2571] and general sensation of weakness that can affect as many as 50% of patients with cancer during some stage.[329–331,1611,2570] The role of other cy-

Table 15–6. **POSSIBLE PATHOGENESIS OF PARANEOPLASTIC SYNDROMES**

Hypothesis	Example
Toxin secreted by tumor	ACTH → Cushing's syndrome PTHRP* → hypercalcemia
Competition for essential substrate	Utilization of glucose by large intra-abdominal sarcomas → hypogylcemia Carcinoid tumors compete with brain for tryptophan → pellagralike syndrome
Opportunistic infection	Papovavirus → progressive multifocal leukoencephalopathy
Autoimmune process	Lambert-Eaton myasthenic syndrome

ACTH = adrenocorticotropic hormone; PTHRP = parathyroid hormone-related protein.

tokines in causing nervous system dysfunction remains to be elucidated.[2866]

2. In 1948, Denny-Brown,[612] when describing probably the first cases of anti-Hu–positive subacute sensory neuronopathy, noted a similarity between the dorsal ganglionitis in his patients and that seen in swine deprived of pantothenic acid. He suggested that the malignancy and the nervous system were competing for a vital nutrient. Metastatic carcinoid tumors[406] and large retroperitoneal sarcomas[424] appear to cause neurologic symptoms by such a mechanism, but no evidence is available to show that small and occult cancers, such as those usually encountered in paraneoplastic disorders, deprive the nervous system of any essential substrate.
3. Opportunistic viral infections involving the CNS complicate the clinical course of many patients immunosuppressed by tumor such as lymphomas or by chemotherapy (see Chapter 12). Progressive multifocal leukoencephalopathy (PML), originally classified as a remote effect,[293] is one such infection. Subacute motor neuronopathy (see the following) may be another. Most paraneoplastic syndromes affect patients who are not immunosuppressed, however, making opportunistic infection unlikely unless these patients suffer unrecognized isolated immune dysfunction. The absence of common opportunistic infections such as PML or herpes zoster also indicates that most patients with paraneoplastic syndromes are immunocompetent.
4. Although individual paraneoplastic syndromes such as PCD and LEMS may have different etiologies and a given syndrome such as PCD may have more than one cause, an immune mechanism is now the most attractive hypothesis as the cause of most or, perhaps, all of them. The hypothesis is that antigenic molecules or epitopes known as onconeural antigens are shared between certain tumors and neurons of the peripheral nervous system or CNS.[857] The immune system, recognizing the antigen in the tumor as foreign, directs a response at the tumor but misdirects the same response against the shared antigens or epitopes in the nervous system. This immune response may also be sufficient to retard tumor growth.

The evidence for the autoimmune hypothesis is best for the LEMS.[1555] The presence of autoantibodies in the serum of many patients with CNS paraneoplastic syndromes suggests that immune mechanisms may participate in these disorders as well. For example, in PCD the antibodies react selectively with cerebellar Purkinje cells, those destroyed by the syndrome. CNS synthesis of the antibody is suggested by the higher titer in CSF than in serum. Inflammatory infiltrates found in the CNS of some patients also suggest that immune mechanisms play a role in pathogenesis.[64,552,1142] Similar infiltrates found in the tumor of patients with paraneoplastic syndromes[975,1150,2539] suggest that the immune response is directed against the tumor as well as against the nervous system, perhaps explaining why patients with paraneoplastic syndromes may have more limited and indolent cancers.[40,551] Evidence for an autoimmune mechanism for other paraneoplastic syndromes is presented later in this chapter.

If paraneoplastic syndromes of the CNS are autoimmune, they would represent the end result of a multifactorial process, including the following:

1. Expression of "immunologically privileged" neuronal antigen(s) by tumor cells;
2. The genetically determined propensity to generate self-reactive T- lymphocyte clones;
3. The presence in the major histocompatibility complex of "susceptibility alleles," which allow binding and presentation of the autoantigen(s) to T cells; and
4. Inherited or acquired abnormalities in immunoregulation that lead to activation of self-reactive T cells, deficient suppression of self-reactive T and B cells, and neuronal injury by immune effector elements.[2431]

The relative roles of cellular and humoral immune systems and the actual mechanism of neuronal destruction in these disorders are unknown and may differ from disorder to disorder.

An autoimmune process and opportunistic infections seem to be the most likely causes for most paraneoplastic syndromes.[2072] These two mechanisms could potentially coexist; "molecular mimicry" between viral and CNS proteins could cause an immune response to an opportunistic virus to damage the nervous system.[2431]

Diagnosis

Paraneoplastic syndromes are encountered in three types of patients: those not known to have cancer, the most common situation; those with active cancer; or those in remission after treatment for cancer. When they present in pure form, the classic syndromes are not easily confused with other causes of neurologic disability. Frequently, however, atypical features obscure the diagnosis. In patients with known cancer, other cancer-associated processes need to be excluded before a diagnosis is made (Table 15–7). Depending on the part of the nervous system affected, the workup should include CT or MR scanning to exclude parenchymal or epidural metastasis, CSF examination to exclude leptomeningeal metastasis, measurement of metabolic and endocrine factors, coagulation studies, and electrophysiologic testing. In patients without known cancer, if other causes of nervous system dysfunction have been excluded, an evaluation for systemic cancer needs to be carefully performed. As will be detailed later, certain syndromes associate with particular types of cancer; recognizing these associations helps to focus the search for an underlying neoplasm.

Although the presentation varies, several clinical features suggest a paraneoplastic syndrome:

1. Most are subacute in onset, progress over weeks to months, and then stabilize. Syndromes that begin acutely or are characterized by exacerbations and remissions are less likely to be paraneoplastic.
2. Most cause severe neurologic disability.
3. They often are associated with an inflammatory CSF, including pleocytosis, an elevated protein concentration, and oligoclonal bands.
4. Most patients present with a clinical syndrome that predominantly affects one specific portion of the nervous system, although some show clinical or pathologic evidence of widespread nervous system involvement.
5. Several syndromes present so stereotypically that they become the leading contender for the clinical diagnosis even before testing has excluded alternative diagnoses.

In recent years, diagnosing at least some of the paraneoplastic syndromes has been aided by detecting characteristic autoantibodies (Table 15–8). With the exception of the antibody found in the LEMS, the etiologic significance of most of these autoantibodies is unknown, but their presence helps to confirm the clinical diagnosis and to focus the search for an underlying malignancy.

Table 15–7. **APPROACH TO THE PATIENT WITH A SUSPECTED PARANEOPLASTIC DISORDER**

Known Cancer	No Known Cancer
1. Search for metastases: MR of involved site, CSF cytology	1. Search for cancer: Chest film, pelvic examination, mammograms, examine lymph nodes, serum cancer markers (e.g., CEA)
2. Search for nonmetastatic disorder (see Chapters 9–14)	2. CSF for cells, IgG, oligoclonal bands, cytologic examination
3. CSF for cells and IgG	3. Serum (for autoantibodies) and CSF
4. Serum for autoantibodies and CSF	4. Follow and search again for cancer if numbers 2 and 3 are positive

CEA = carcinoembryonic antigen.

Table 15–8. **SOME WELL-CHARACTERIZED AUTOANTIBODIES ASSOCIATED WITH PARANEOPLASTIC SYNDROMES**

Antibody	Antigen	Syndrome(s)	Tumor(s)
Anti-Yo	34 and 62 kd Purkinje cell cytoplasm	PCD	Ovary Breast
Anti-Hu	37 kd neuronal nuclei	Encephalomyelitis Sensory neuronopathy Limbic encephalitis	Small-cell lung
Anti-Ri	55 and 80 kd neuronal nuclei	Opsoclonus	Breast
Anti-retinal	23, 65, 145, and 205 kd Photoreceptors and ganglion cells	CAR	Small-cell lung
Anti-NMJ	Calcium channel	Lambert-Eaton myasthenic syndrome	Small-cell lung
Anti-NMJ	Acetylcholine receptor	Myasthenia gravis	Thymoma
Hodgkin's	Purkinje cells	Cerebellar degeneration	Hodgkin's

CAR = cancer-associated retinopathy; NMJ = neuromuscular junction; PCD = paraneoplastic cerebellar degeneration.

Treatment

Therapy for the individual paraneoplastic syndromes will be discussed in the following sections. In general, treatment has been unrewarding; most patients are left with severe neurologic disability. Most of the therapies tried have been forms of immunosuppression, particularly in the syndromes that are associated with autoantibodies.[554,2021] With the exception of the LEMS, however, in which plasmapheresis is clearly effective, most patients do not benefit. It is possible that the rapid onset of these syndromes does not allow sufficient time for accurate early diagnosis and for treatment to begin before irreversible neuronal damage has occurred. With earlier diagnosis using specific laboratory tests such as antibodies, therapy may be more successful.[1796]

SPECIFIC SYNDROMES

Paraneoplastic Cerebellar Degeneration

The most common and best characterized of the CNS paraneoplastic syndromes, PCD nevertheless is a rare disorder, with only about 300 cases reported in the literature. It has become increasingly apparent that PCD is a group of related disorders that differ somewhat in their clinical features, prognosis, and types of associated malignancies. Some can be separated on the basis of characteristic antibodies that react to particular tumor-associated antigens. The general characteristics of PCD will be discussed first, followed by the features that identify distinct subclasses of the clinical disorders.

CLINICAL FINDINGS

Although PCD was first described in 1919,[320] the association between PCD and cancer was not recognized until 1938.[321] Its clinical and pathologic features were fully described in 1951,[292] and by 1982, 50 pathologically verified cases had been reported.[1144] PCD can be associated with any cancer, but the most common culprits are lung cancer[462,554] (particularly small-cell lung cancer), ovarian or uterine cancer,[35,2021] and lymphomas, particularly Hodgkin's disease[1070] (Table 15–9). The neurologic symptoms prompt most patients to go to the physician before the cancer is symptomatic. The cancer is usually found within months to a year after the onset of neurologic symptoms, but occasionally the cancer may elude detection for 2 to 4 years or even longer; in some instances, it has been found only at autopsy.

Table 15–9 **MALIGNANCIES ASSOCIATED WITH PARANEOPLASTIC CEREBELLAR DEGENERATION IN 199 PATIENTS**

Malignancy Site/Type	No. of Patients
Ovarian	50
Papillary	3
Serous	3
Unspecified	43
Epithelial	1
Lung	57
Small-cell	36
Squamous	4
Large-cell	4
Adenocarcinoma	5
Unspecified	7
Mixed	1
Uterus	6
Fallopian tube	4
Breast	17
ACA, unknown primary	9
Uterine and colon	1
Ovary and breast	1
Polymorphic sarcoma	1
Lymphoma	32
Hodgkin's	27
NHL	1
Unspecified	1
T-cell	1
Lymphosarcoma	2
Stomach	2
Larynx	1
Prostate	3
Thyroid	1
Rectum	1
Bronchus and rectum	1
Colon	6
Maxillary antrum	1
Tonsil	1
Renal-cell	1
Chondrosarcoma	1
AML	1
Monoclonal gammopathy	1

ACA = adenocarcinoma; AML = acute myelocytic leukemia; NHL = non-Hodgkin's lymphoma.

Typically, the disorder begins with slight incoordination in walking, evolving rapidly over weeks to a few months with progressive gait ataxia; incoordination in arms, legs, and trunk; dysarthria; and often nystagmus associated with oscillopsia (the subjective sensation of oscillation of viewed objects).

Within a few months, the illness reaches its peak and then stabilizes. By this time, most patients cannot walk without support, many cannot sit unsupported, handwriting is impossible, independent eating is difficult, and speech may be understood only with great effort. Patients with cerebellar disease have difficulty coordinating complete closure of air flow when attempting to articulate the stop consonants, P, T, K, B, D, G. For example, when repeating the sequence Pa-Ta-Ka, they usually lose the ability to maintain the voicing distinction and begin to produce the sequence as Ba-Da-Ga. The phenomenon may be present in the absence of any other evidence of dysarthric speech. Oscillopsia may prevent reading or even watching television. The neurologic signs are always bilateral and usually symmetric, although one side is sometimes more affected than the other and the asymmetry is prominent in occasional patients. Diplopia often is an early symptom, although abnormalities of ocular muscles frequently are not detected in a bedside examination.[2021,2069] Vertigo is another common early symptom.[2069]

The signs and symptoms are frequently limited to those of cerebellar or cerebellar pathway dysfunction, but other neurologic abnormalities, usually mild, may be found on careful examination of as many as 50% of patients.[1070,2021] These abnormalities include sensorineural hearing loss, dysphagia, hyperreflexia (with or without extensor plantar responses), extrapyramidal signs, peripheral neuropathy, and dementia and other mental status abnormalities.[292] A recent study using formal cognitive testing found that dementia was not typical when the testing was controlled for motor and speech impairment, however, suggesting that perceived clinical changes in intellectual function may be more apparent than real.[53] Despite this finding, PET scanning of a few patients with PCD has revealed hypometabolism in all areas of the neuraxis, including the cerebral cortex, cerebellum, and brainstem.[53]

Exceptions to these generalizations include occasional patients with more gradual or abrupt onset; some patients progress over a year or more, but one patient became totally disabled by cerebellar signs overnight, having been normal the day before. In some, the disorder may be relatively mild so that the patient can walk, write, and be understood, albeit with some difficulty.

LABORATORY EVALUATION

Early in the course of this disease, CT and MR scans do not reveal an abnormality. If patients are followed for months to a few years, diffuse cerebellar atrophy appears[982] (Fig. 15–1). Occasional patients have hyperintensity found in cerebral and cerebellar white matter on T_2-weighted images.

In most patients who are studied early, the CSF contains an increased number of lymphocytes and slightly elevated protein and IgG concentrations. Oligoclonal bands may be present as well. The pleocytosis usually resolves with time.

A subset of patients (the number of which is unknown) have autoantibodies in serum and CSF that react with Purkinje cells of the cerebellum and with the causal tumor. Some of these antibodies, such as the anti-Yo, the anti-Hu, and the anti-Ri, have been well characterized and appear to be specific for certain clinical syndromes and underlying cancers. Some antibodies react predominantly or exclusively with Purkinje cells, while others have neural reactivity that extends well beyond Purkinje cells of the cerebellum. Anti–Purkinje-cell antibodies also have been reported[561] in patients with nonparaneoplastic subacute cerebellar degeneration, but these are not the same antibodies as previously discussed. The presence or absence of specific antibodies allows the physician to subclassify PCD as indicated in Table 15–10.

PATHOLOGY

The CNS may appear grossly normal when examined at autopsy, but usually the cerebellum is atrophic with abnormally widened sulci and small gyri.

Microscopically, PCD's hallmark is an extensive and often complete loss of Purkinje cells of the cerebellar cortex[292,294,1144] (Fig. 15–2). The degenerating Purkinje cells may have swellings, called torpedoes, along their axons. Other pathologic features sometimes seen include thinning of the molecular and granular layers of the cerebellar cortex, often without marked cell loss, and proliferation of Bergmann's astrocytes. The deep cerebellar nuclei are usually well preserved, although rarefaction of white matter may surround the nuclei, corresponding to the loss of Purkinje cell axons. Basket cells and tangential fibers are usually intact. Lymphocytic infiltrates, if present in the cerebellum, are usually found in the leptomeninges, in the dentate nucleus,

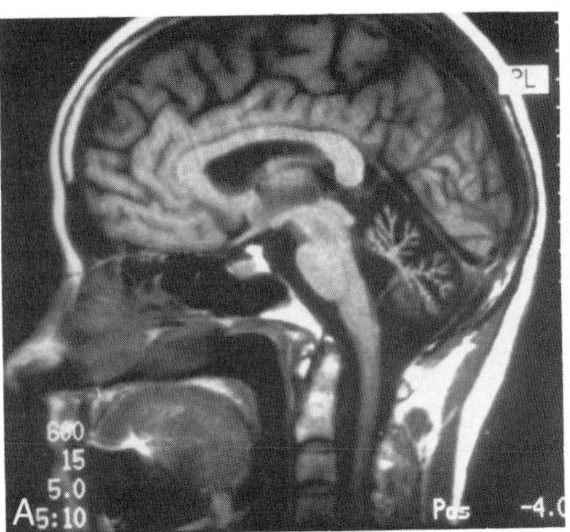

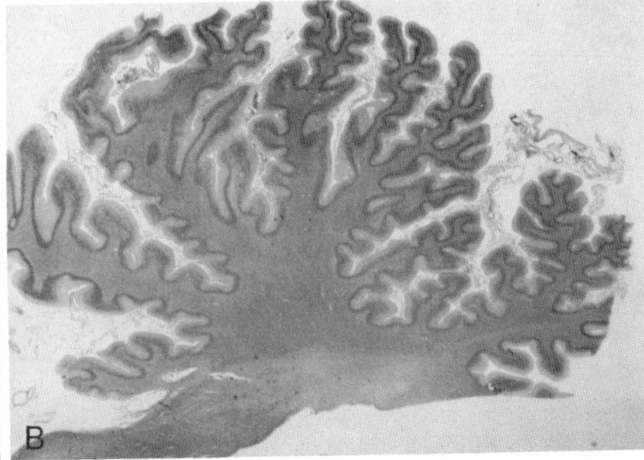

Figure 15–1. *A*, An MR scan of a patient with paraneoplastic cerebellar degeneration (PCD). The scan shows prominent cerebellar sulci and an enlarged fourth ventricle indicating cerebellar atrophy. The cerebral hemispheres are normal. *B*, A mid-sagittal section of cerebellum from a 28-year-old man who died of Hodgkin's disease 6 years after he developed PCD.

Table 15–10. **SUBCLASSES OF PARANEOPLASTIC CEREBELLAR DEGENERATION**

Subclass	Usual Cancer	Sex	Clinical Findings	Onset
Anti-Yo	Ovary	All F	Subacute severe	Before cancer
Anti-Hu	SCLC	F>M	Part of PEM/SN	Before cancer
Hodgkin's	Hodgkin's	M>F	Less severe, may remit	After cancer
PCD and LEMS (Ab neg)	SCLC	M=F	Absent DTRs	Before cancer
Anti-Ri	Breast	F	Opsoclonus/truncal ataxia	Before or after cancer
Miscellaneous	Any	F=M	Variable	Before or after cancer

DTRs = deep tendon reflexes; F = female; LEMS = Lambert-Eaton myasthenic syndrome; M = Male; PCD = paraneoplastic cerebellar degeneration; PEM/SN = paraneoplastic encephalomyelitis/sensory neuronopathy; SCLC = small-cell lung cancer.

and in surrounding white matter, but only rarely in the Purkinje-cell layer.[1144]

In many patients, the disorder is noninflammatory, with all pathologic changes restricted to the Purkinje-cell layer of the cerebellum. Pathologic changes sometimes seen outside the cerebellum differ substantially from patient to patient.[1144] They may include dorsal column and pyramidal tract degeneration of the spinal cord; degeneration of the basal ganglia, specifically the pallidum; loss of peripheral nerve fibers; and inflammatory infiltrates in the brainstem, spinal cord, and cerebral cortex.

The tumors associated with PCD do not differ histologically from similar tumors unassociated with paraneoplastic symptoms. In many patients, however, the tumor is still localized when identified, rather than widely metastatic. Hetzel and colleagues[1150] have reported that the tumors associated with antibody-positive PCD are more likely to contain lymphocytic infiltrates than are tumors of similar histology not associated with PCD.

The diagnosis depends on recognizing the characteristic clinical syndrome while excluding other causes of late-onset cerebellopathy. Cancer-related causes include parenchymal or leptomeningeal metastasis, infections, and toxicity of therapies such as cytarabine (see Chapter 12). Non–cancer-related causes include viral brainstem encephalitis or cerebellitis, demyelinating disease, Creutzfeldt-Jakob disease, infarc-

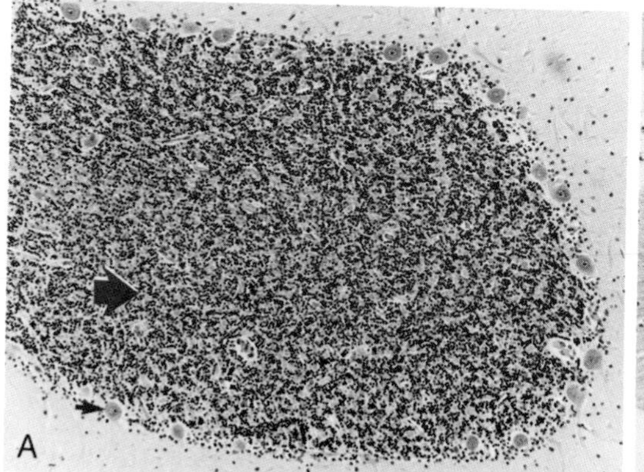

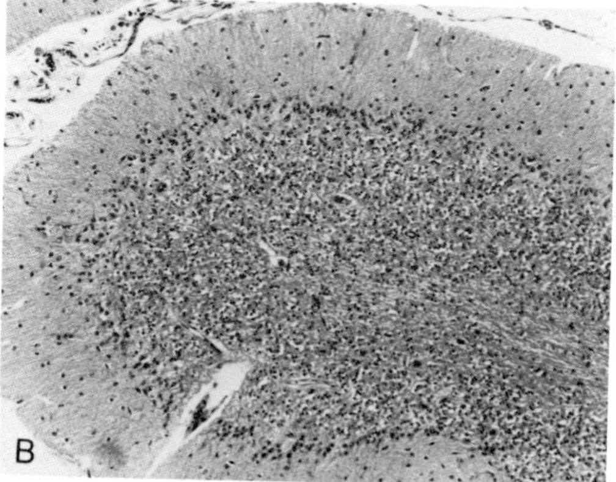

Figure 15–2. *A,* A section of cerebellum taken from a patient who died without neurologic disease. Note the abundant neurons in the granular cell layer (*thick arrow*) and the large number of Purkinje cells (*thin arrow*). *B,* A section of cerebellum taken from a patient with paraneoplastic cerebellar degeneration. Note the absence of Purkinje cells and the thinning of the granular cell layer. (Hematoxylin and eosin stain, magnification × 40.)

tion, hypothyroidism, and alcoholic and hereditary cerebellar degenerations.

The typical clinical picture may be present without a cancer. How often the phenomenon of "subacute cerebellar degeneration" is nonparaneoplastic is not certain. Henson and Urich[1144] estimate that it occurs 50% of the time; others believe that the figure is higher.[2202] Results of autopsy studies of "nonparaneoplastic" subacute cerebellar degeneration are few. Positive antibody studies increase the likelihood that the cerebellar disorder is paraneoplastic, and specific antibodies increase that likelihood to almost 100%. Specific antibodies also indicate specific neoplasms.

Once the disease has reached its peak, it usually does not change, and the patient remains neurologically stable despite treatment and even cure of the underlying cancer. Treatment directed at the cerebellar disorder, including immune suppression with corticosteroids and other drugs and plasmapheresis, usually does not help. Symptomatic improvement in the ataxia occurs in a few patients given clonazepam in doses varying from 0.5 to 1.5 mg/24 hr. On occasion, the disorder may remit spontaneously or coincidentally after treating the tumor[1975] or using thiamine,[1863] plasmapheresis, immunoglobulin, or corticosteroids.[466,1796]

SPECIFIC CATEGORIES OF PARANEOPLASTIC CEREBELLAR DEGENERATION

The discovery of autoantibodies and the increasing number of patients reported with PCD have allowed subcategorization of patients based either on the nature of the underlying tumor or on the presence of a specific autoantibody. Although the clinical and pathologic findings are similar in most cases, small differences have clinical and prognostic significance (see Table 15–10). The following paragraphs attempt to distinguish the categories, emphasizing differences from the general clinical picture.

Anti-Yo–Positive PCD. Anti-Yo is the term first applied by Posner and Furneaux[2074] to designate a polyclonal IgG autoantibody that reacts primarily with Purkinje cell cytoplasm, giving a characteristic granular staining pattern (Fig. 15–3). Immunoelectron mi-

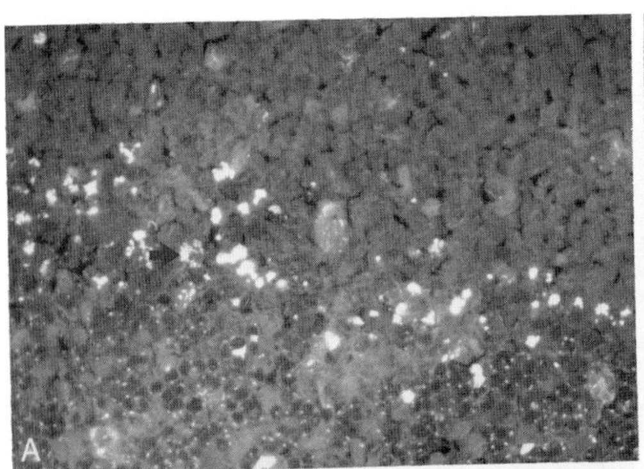

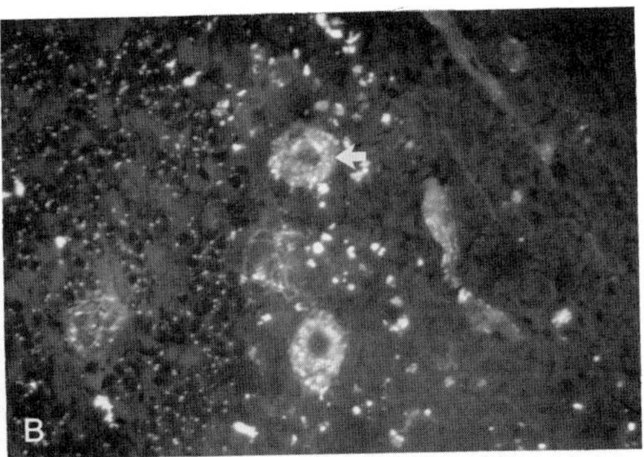

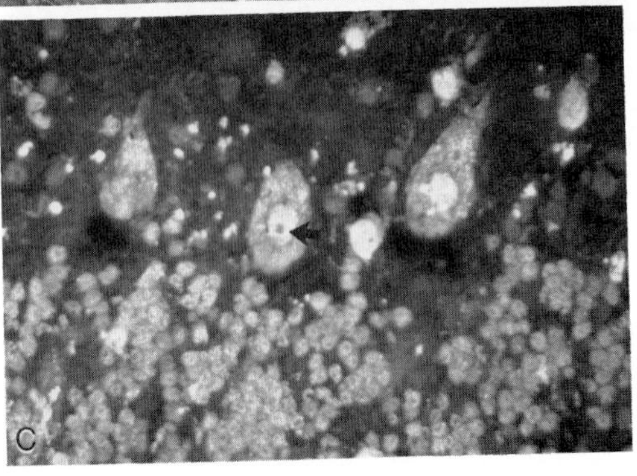

Figure 15–3. Autoantibodies in PCD patients. *A,* A section of the cerebellum reacted with normal human serum. Autofluorescence of lipofuscin is evident in many cells. *B,* Anti-Yo antibody. A section of human cerebellum reacted with serum from a patient with paraneoplastic cerebellar degeneration caused by ovarian cancer. Note the cytoplasmic fluorescence of the Purkinje cells (*arrow*). The nuclei do not react. *C,* Anti-Hu antibody. Section of cerebellum reacted with serum of a patient with subacute sensory neuronopathy-encephalomyelitis associated with small-cell lung cancer. Unlike the anti-Yo antibody that is restricted to Purkinje cells, neurons react with anti-Hu. The reaction is predominantly nuclear, with the nucleoli spared (*arrow*).

croscopy shows the antibody binding to membrane-bound and free ribosomes.[1155a] In one study, there was also binding to the rough endoplasmic reticulum, and the transface of the Golgi complex. Binding to the cell surface has not been unequivocally identified.[2189] The antibody is found at a higher titer relative to total IgG in CSF than in serum, suggesting intrathecal synthesis.[856] The sera also react by Western-blot analysis with extracts of Purkinje cells, identifying at least two bands at approximately 62 and 34 kd (Fig. 15–4). The genes for both 34 and 62 antigens have been cloned, the first by Dropcho and colleagues,[685] the second by Sakai and associates,[2269] and independently by Fathallah-Shaykh and associates.[758] The 34-kd protein is encoded in a single exon consisting of tandem repeats of six amino acids. The mouse gene is somewhat larger than the human gene, but as in the human, amino acids 3, 4, and 6 are always glutamate, aspartate, aspartate, respectively.[434] The function of the protein encoded by this gene is unknown.

Analysis of messenger RNA coding for the 34-kd protein confirms its preferential expression in cerebellum but identifies it to a lesser degree in cerebral cortex and in many tumors and tumor lines from patients who do not have the antibody in their serum and who do not have PCD.[684] Immunohistochemical and Western-blot analyses of ovarian carcinomas reveal that the antigens are expressed in about 20% of tumors of patients without PCD. Antibodies raised against a peptide representing part of the sequence of the 34-kd antigen react to Western-blot and immunohistochemical analyses with both cerebellar Purkinje cells and the tumors of anti-Yo–positive PCD patients.[855] The 34-kd gene has been mapped to the long arm of the X chromosome near the site of the fragile X gene.[2432]

The 62-kd gene encodes for an entirely different protein from the 34-kd gene. The

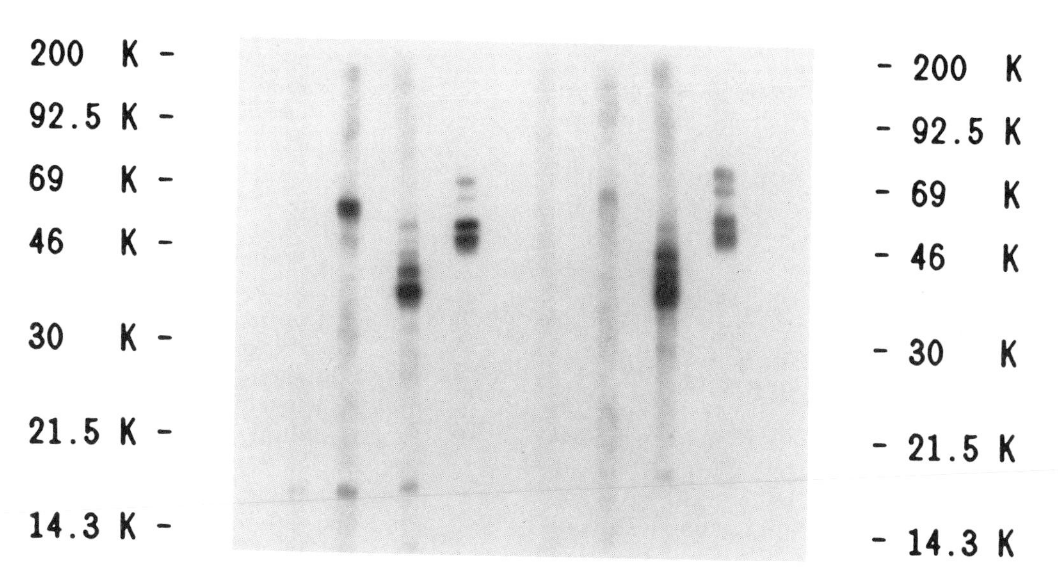

Figure 15–4. A Western-blot of serum of patients with paraneoplastic syndromes. Purkinje cells and cortical neurons are reacted with normal human serum (NHS), serum from a patient with paraneoplastic cerebellar degeneration associated with ovarian cancer (anti-Yo), a patient with encephalomyelitis associated with small-cell lung cancer (anti-Hu), and a patient with opsoclonus associated with breast cancer (anti-Ri). Note that both Purkinje cells and cortical neurons react with anti-Hu and anti-Ri sera. The reaction of the anti-Yo sera with Purkinje cells is much stronger than with cortical neurons.

protein has a leucine zipper as well as a zinc finger motif, suggesting that it may participate in regulating gene expression.[758,2269] The gene has been mapped to chromosome 16. Northern-blot analysis reveals that gene transcript is detected not only in cerebellum and brainstem but also in intestinal mucosa.[2269] A third protein autoantigen has been cloned that appears immunohistologically similar to anti-Yo. This 58-kd "CZF" protein features zinc finger motifs that indicate its possible function as a transcriptional regulatory protein.[2294]

Conclusions from Antibody Studies. Using a fusion protein produced by the cDNA of the gene coding for the 62-kd antigen, the anti-Yo antibody was found by Peterson and colleagues[2021] in 55 patients whose sera, and often CSF, were studied at Memorial Sloan-Kettering Cancer Center. Other investigators, particularly those from the Mayo Clinic, who used immunohistochemical criteria but not Western blotting, have reported a series of patients who probably also have the anti-Yo antibody.[1071] Collectively, more than 100 patients have been reported with either definite or probable anti-Yo antibodies in their serum. From examinations of these patients, certain conclusions are possible:

1. The antibody does not occur in a measurable amount in healthy individuals.
2. With a few exceptions, the antibody does not occur in patients with cancer unless they have PCD. Two exceptions, reported by Brashear and associates,[296] are patients who have ovarian cancer without cerebellar signs and who maintain high titers of antibody in their serum. Because antibody was examined only by immunohistochemical analysis and not by Western-blot, its specificity might be doubted. Our own study of sera from 170 patients with ovarian cancer, but no PCD has found measurable anti-Yo antibody in one patient.
3. All patients harboring the antibody are women, save one male patient with subacute cerebellar degeneration and gynecomastia but no cancer yet discovered, and a man with PCD and non–small-cell lung cancer.
4. The cerebellar disease precedes identification of the cancer in about two thirds of the patients. When identified, the cancer is either breast cancer or cancer of the ovary, fallopian tube, or endometrium. Two exceptions are one woman with lymphoma[2189] and one woman with adenocarcinoma of the lung[2021] who, after 6 years of follow-up, has not developed gynecologic cancer. Whether the antigen was present in those tumors has not been reported.
5. The cancers do not appear histologically different from cancers in the same organ of patients without PCD, but more lymphocytic infiltrates are found in PCD-related tumors than in others.[1150]
6. Although some tumors are quite aggressive and widely metastatic at the time the PCD develops, most are either localized or have spread only to regional nodes. In some instances, the primary tumor is too small to be discovered, and only positive nodes are found. The tumor course after discovery usually appears to be relatively indolent no matter what the treatment.
7. The cerebellar disease is usually subacute in onset, progressing over weeks to months and then stabilizing. At stabilization, virtually all of the patients suffer nystagmus with a downbeating component and many have oscillopsia and diplopia. Dysarthria is usually severe, and truncal and appendicular ataxia are usually disabling. Once stable, the illness usually does not change despite treatment, and the patient, even if cured of the cancer, may remain disabled for years before dying of either cancer recurrence or other disease. Although cerebellar degeneration in and of itself is not lethal, patients may die of the complications associated with being bedridden.
8. The antibody is usually present at a relatively high titer (>1:1000 by immunoperoxidase staining) in the serum with a higher relative specific activity in CSF than in serum.[856] The presence of a higher relative specific activity in CSF suggests intrathecal synthesis of the antibody, presumably from B cells that have invaded the nervous system.

9. When the patients die, usually years to decades after the onset of the disease, the pathology is usually relatively bland, without noticeable inflammation but with a striking loss of Purkinje cells as previously described.
10. Attempts to reproduce the disease in experimental animals have so far been fruitless. Injecting human IgG into the CSF of animals caused antibody to accumulate in Purkinje cells in one study,[972] but Purkinje cells have not been destroyed and neurologic symptomatology has not developed.
11. With a few exceptions, plasmapheresis and immune suppression do not affect the disease course. The failure of immune suppression to affect the disease does not eliminate an autoimmune etiology, however; plasmapheresis with five plasma exchanges was successful in lowering the serum titer of the antibody but did not alter the CSF titer.[856] Furthermore, Purkinje cell destruction probably develops so rapidly that the cells have been destroyed by the time the diagnosis is made and treatment is undertaken. To prove an autoimmune hypothesis, an effective animal model must be developed.
12. Because the anti-Yo antibody is so tightly coupled to breast and gynecologic cancer in patients with cerebellar degeneration, its presence should focus the search for a primary tumor in the pelvis or breasts.[2021] If the initial diagnostic workup of breast and pelvis fails to reveal a mass, then the physician should consider a pelvic examination under anesthesia followed by a dilation and curettage; depending on the findings, a hysterectomy and salpingo-oophorectomy should be performed. In six patients who were approached in this way, the diagnosis of a gynecologic tumor was established in five. The exploration in the sixth patient was negative, but 4 months later the results of the mammogram examination, which had previously been normal, became abnormal and a breast cancer was discovered. Although some believe that immunohistochemistry alone is sufficient to identify the presence of the antibody,[1522a] I believe that unequivocal identification of the anti-Yo antibody requires Western blotting.[544a]
13. The role of the antibody in the pathogenesis of the disease is unknown. It could be pathogenetic or simply a marker, such as anti–striated-muscle antibodies in myasthenia gravis, unrelated to the destruction of Purkinje cells. Autopsy study of two anti-Yo PCD patients showed complete absence of Purkinje cells. In one, inflammatory infiltrates were found in the dorsal medulla but not in the cerebellum.

PCD Associated with Hodgkin's Disease. The first report of an autoantibody in the serum of patients with PCD was that of Trotter and colleagues[2606] in 1976. A subsequent patient was reported by Stefansson and colleagues[2481] in 1981. Hammack and associates[1070] reviewed the clinical and serologic findings in 21 patients with PCD associated with Hodgkin's disease. They also reviewed the literature of previously described cases, reporting a total of 39 patients with PCD associated with Hodgkin's disease. These patients differ from those with anti-Yo and anti-Hu PCD in the following respects: Men outnumber women 6 to 1. The patients tend to be young (age range, 20–40 years) rather than middle-aged or elderly. The diagnosis of PCD was usually made when the patient was known to have Hodgkin's disease and, sometimes, during remission after treatment for that disorder. The biologic meaning of this difference is unclear. It may simply be that Hodgkin's disease, which often presents with palpable nodes in the neck, axilla, and groin, is discovered earlier than asymptomatic lung or gynecologic cancers of the same size. The subacutely evolving onset with a tendency to stabilize and the clinical findings of pancerebellar dysfunction resemble those of the other syndromes. Unlike the others, however, spontaneous or treatment-associated remissions occur in about 15% of patients. The reason for this difference is unknown. In patients with Hodgkin's disease and PCD who are examined at autopsy, the diffuse loss of Purkinje cells is quite similar to the loss seen in PCD associated with other cancers. One of our patients appeared to respond to treatment of the tumor; in another patient, appeared to improve symptoms. These responses were greater than we had seen in patients with anti-Yo or anti-Hu PCD.

Anti–Purkinje-cell antibodies have been identified in a minority of patients with Hodgkin's disease associated with PCD. The antibody that has been identified is usually present at a lower titer than either anti-Hu or anti-Yo. It reacts with cerebellar cytoplasm in a diffuse or small granular pattern sometimes resembling that of anti-Yo but usually sufficiently different to be distinguishable under the microscope. Greenlee and colleagues[987] report a greater reaction with rat than with human Purkinje cells, but we have not identified significant differences. Western-blot analysis of Purkinje-cell extracts has failed to reveal identifiable bands. Because the antibody can only be identified in a minority of patients with PCD associated with Hodgkin's disease, it is difficult to know what relationship, if any, the antibody has to the pathogenesis of the disorder.

Antibody-Negative PCD Associated with Small-Cell Lung Cancer and Lambert-Eaton Myasthenic Syndrome. Some patients with small-cell lung cancer develop PCD without an identifiable antibody. Some of this group also have LEMS.[462] The clinical syndrome is a subacute onset of pancerebellar dysfunction, often associated with weak lower extremities and absent knee and ankle reflexes. The neurologic disorder usually begins before the cancer is identified, and in some patients, no cancer has been identified, either after long follow-up or at autopsy. When cancer is present, it is usually a small-cell lung cancer. Electrophysiologic tests of neuromuscular transmission reveal the typical incrementing pattern associated with the LEMS (see p 382). In some patients, weakness from LEMS dominates. In others, it is subclinical, and the cerebellar disorder predominates. Some patients have antibodies against voltage-gated calcium channels, but others do not.[2212]

Recognizing the syndrome is important so that the physician can identify small-cell lung cancer early and can treat the LEMS by plasmapheresis or immunosuppressive agents. Despite successful treatment of the LEMS, the PCD does not respond and the patient usually remains stable with severe cerebellar disability. The syndrome has been reported in about 30 patients.[462] It has not been established whether the same antibody that causes LEMS can cause Purkinje-cell damage in certain circumstances, nor has the autoimmune nature of the Purkinje-cell portion of the syndrome been established.

Miscellaneous Syndromes. Other PCD patients, some with autoantibodies and some without, have been reported. It is impossible to delineate these disorders clearly without studying a large number of patients possessing a similar autoantibody. The PCD associated with the anti-Hu antibody is discussed in the next section.

Subacute Sensory Neuronopathy/Encephalomyelitis

Henson and coworkers[1142] introduced the term "encephalomyelitis with carcinoma" to describe patients with cancer associated with clinical signs of damage to more than one area of the nervous system[670] and with the postmortem findings of inflammation within the brain, brainstem, spinal cord, dorsal root ganglia,[1142] and nerve roots. Most of these patients had small-cell lung cancer, although similar disorders were found with other cancers. At times, the disorder was clinically and pathologically restricted to the dorsal root ganglion, but many patients presented both clinical and pathologic signs of damage to other areas of the nervous system, either with or without a sensory neuronopathy. The signs included dementia, cerebellar degeneration, brainstem dysfunction, myelopathy, and autonomic neuropathy. It has subsequently been learned that patients in whom this syndrome is caused by small-cell lung cancer usually harbor an antibody in their serum called anti-Hu. The clinical features of the anti-Hu syndrome in 71 patients (Table 15–11) have recently been described by Dalmau and colleagues.[554] The same clinical and pathologic picture can occur in patients without the anti-Hu antibody. At times the syndrome occurs in patients without identifiable cancer even at autopsy.[554,559,1269,1469,2886]

SUBACUTE SENSORY NEURONOPATHY

Sensory neuronopathy (SN) is a rare syndrome that occurs in patients with cancer as well as previously healthy individuals and

Table 15–11. **CLINICAL FINDINGS IN 71 PATIENTS WITH THE ANTI-HU SYNDROME**

	No. of Patients	% of 71 Patients
Unifocal (19 Patients)		
Sensory neuropathy	14	20
Limbic encephalopathy	4	6
Brainstem encephalopathy	1	1
Multifocal (52 Patients)		
Sensory neuropathy	38	54
Limbic encephalopathy	16	22
Cerebellar degeneration	18	25
Brainstem encephalopathy	22	31
Motor neuropathy	32	45
Autonomic dysfunction	20	28
Visual loss	1	1
LEMS	1	1
Myoclonus	1	1
Polymyositis	1	1
Diffuse encephalomyelitis	2	3

LEMS = Lambert-Eaton myasthenic syndrome.
Source: Data from Dalmau et al.[554]

those with a variety of autoimmune conditions, including Sjögren's syndrome[816,1796a]; probably in fewer than 20% is it paraneoplastic. At least 67% of the patients with paraneoplastic SN have small-cell lung cancer.[418,1144] Symptoms typically begin in middle age; men and women are equally affected,[1210] although most anti-Hu patients are women. In the majority, the neurologic syndrome precedes the diagnosis of cancer, and when the cancer is diagnosed, it is usually small and localized. Initial symptoms are dysesthetic pain and numbness, which usually begin in the distal extremities but can begin in the arm(s) or face. The symptoms progress over days to several weeks, eventually affecting all four limbs, the trunk, and sometimes the face, causing a severe sensory ataxia resembling cerebellar degeneration. All sensory modalities are affected, distinguishing this disorder from *cis*-platinum neuropathy, in which pin and temperature sensation are spared. Deep tendon reflexes are lost, but motor function is preserved. The CSF is typically inflammatory. Sensory nerve action potentials have low amplitude or are absent, while motor nerve action potentials are normal and electrical evidence of denervation is absent.[667,1210]

Early pathologic changes are limited mostly to the dorsal root ganglia, which show lymphocytic inflammatory infiltrates and a loss of neurons (Fig. 15–5). As the disease progresses, the inflammatory process may advance to the dorsal roots, posterior columns, and peripheral nerves. About 50% of patients with paraneoplastic SN present with pathologic changes (which may be clinically

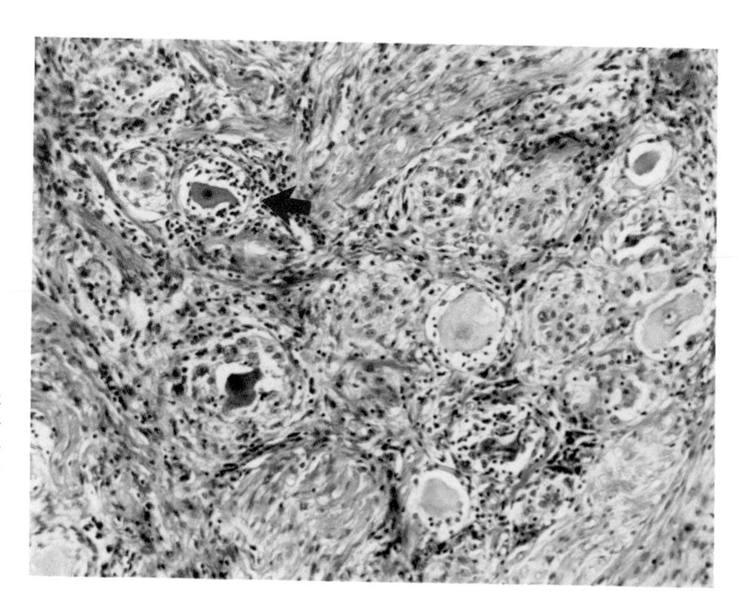

Figure 15–5. A section of dorsal root ganglion from a patient with paraneoplastic encephalomyelitis associated with prostate cancer. Only a few normal neurons can be seen in the section. Lymphocytes can be seen surrounding a few dying neurons (*arrow*).

silent) in other nervous system regions. In most patients, treating the underlying tumor with plasmapheresis or immunosuppressive therapy does not alter the course of the neurologic disease,[979] although one patient with Hodgkin's disease recovered after chemotherapy.[2264] Another with lung cancer had a spontaneous remission.[2650]

LIMBIC ENCEPHALITIS

Paraneoplastic limbic encephalitis is a rare complication of small-cell lung cancer[507] or other cancers.[132,349,2613] A similar clinical syndrome can occur without a neoplasm[310,1269,1469] with an approximately equal incidence in men and women. Typically, personality and mood changes develop over days or weeks, associated with severe impairment of recent memory and sometimes agitation, confusion, hallucinations, and seizures. Limbic encephalitis may occur in isolation or be associated with more diffuse encephalomyelitis or with SN. The diagnosis depends on recognizing the clinical syndrome and excluding other causes of encephalopathy, whether or not they are associated with cancer. The CSF is typically inflammatory, at least early in the disease. The results of CT or MR scans usually appear normal, although abnormalities in one or both medial temporal lobes, some of which contrast enhance, are occasionally seen[349,554,1454] (Fig. 15–6). Hyperintensity of medial temporal lobes seen on a T_2-weighted MR scan has also been reported[647,1496] to follow complex partial status epilepticus in a woman with cancer; her memory loss resolved.

Pathologic changes of paraneoplastic limbic encephalitis are usually restricted to limbic and insular cortex, though other deep gray structures may be involved; in severe

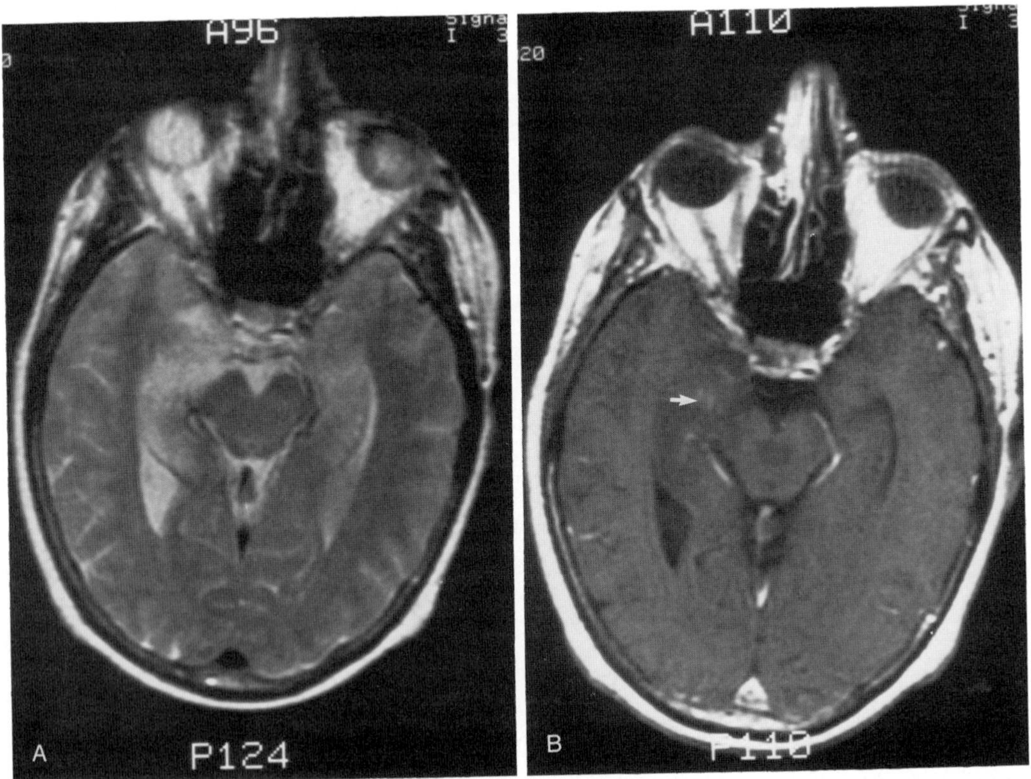

Figure 15–6. An MR scan of an anti-Hu–positive patient with limbic encephalitis as part of paraneoplastic encephalomyelitis associated with small-cell lung cancer. *A,* The T_2-weighted image shows hyperintensity in the medial temporal lobes bilaterally. *B,* The T_1-weighted image with gadolinium shows a modest amount of contrast enhancement in the right medial temporal lobe (*arrow*).

cases, the pathologic abnormalities may affect surrounding white matter. Extensive loss of neurons with reactive gliosis, perivascular lymphocytic cuffing, and microglial proliferation also typify this syndrome.[507,552] No treatment has been routinely beneficial, although several reports relate spontaneous remissions or improvement with treatment of the underlying tumor.*

CEREBELLAR DEGENERATION

The typical clinical findings of PCD may occur as the first or only manifestation of encephalomyelitis.[7,554] The patient with encephalomyelitis is more likely to have evidence of widespread peripheral nervous system and CNS involvement, especially SN, and the pathologic changes are likely to be inflammatory rather than bland.[1144] In one patient with cerebellar signs associated with small-cell lung cancer, infiltrates with T cells were found in the Purkinje-cell layer of the cerebellum despite absent Purkinje cells. Prominent cerebellar signs occur in approximately 15% of patients with the anti-Hu syndrome.[554]

BRAINSTEM ENCEPHALITIS

Paraneoplastic brainstem encephalitis characterized by subacutely developing bulbar, midbrain, or basal ganglia signs usually occurs as part of the more diffuse syndrome of encephalomyelitis, although sometimes it presents clinically as a dominant or isolated finding.[554,1336,2139,2761] Any cranial nerve can be affected.[1030] The syndrome usually affects the lower brainstem, causing diplopia, vertigo, oscillopsia, dysarthria, dysphagia, hypoventilation,[642,2685] hearing loss, and facial numbness. Movement disorders include chorea, dystonia,[32,642,936] bradykinesia,[936] and myoclonus.[667] One of our patients with testicular cancer developed a typical Parkinson's syndrome. The only clinical differences from idiopathic parkinsonism were that the patient was 28 years old and the entire clinical picture evolved during a 3- to 4-week period and then stabilized.

*References 45, 304, 349, 389, 1333, 1685.

MYELITIS

Paraneoplastic non-necrotizing myelitis rarely occurs as an isolated syndrome. More often it is a part of a more diffuse encephalomyelitis. Patients present with progressive weakness, sometimes with lower motor neuron signs including fasciculations, in association with sensory loss and autonomic dysfunction such as incontinence and postural hypotension. In at least one instance, the disorder was episodic and primarily involved posterior column function. Early in its evolution, it may clinically resemble motor neuron disease. The neurologic disorder may precede or follow the diagnosis of cancer. Often upper extremity findings predominate, because of cervical cord involvement; respiratory failure may cause death.[2351] The differential diagnosis includes compressive or intrinsic spinal cord masses, other inflammatory or infectious myelopathies, or radiation injury in patients previously treated for cancer. The CSF typically shows inflammatory changes. Neuroimaging usually shows a normal spinal cord, but hyperintensity occasionally can be identified on a T_2-weighted MR scan, and contrast enhancement may be noted. Effective treatment is not available.

Pathologically, an intense inflammatory reaction and loss of neurons is seen in the anterior and posterior horns, with secondary nerve-root degeneration and neurogenic muscle atrophy. Inflammation and degeneration of white matter tracts also occur.

Paraneoplastic myelitis with small-cell lung cancer is associated with the anti-Hu antibody.[554] Babikian and colleagues[114] also describe a patient with paraneoplastic myelitis associated with small-cell lung cancer and a different serum antibody that reacted with a 52-kd spinal cord antigen and a tumor-associated protein of the same molecular weight.

AUTONOMIC NEUROPATHY

Paraneoplastic autonomic neuropathy is a rare syndrome that occurs alone or with an SN.[554,2417] Usually associated with small-cell lung cancer, it may occur with other cancers[2669,2685] and may present before or after the cancer diagnosis. Patients present with the subacute onset of postural hypotension,[2669] intestinal immotility,[1523,2399] pupillary abnormalities,[1654] and neurogenic bladder. The syndrome is generally progressive but may stabilize or improve with treatment of the underlying tumor. One autonomic symptom may predominate. Lennon and associates[1523] report five patients with small-cell lung cancer and severe constipation from chronic intestinal immotility. In four of these five patients, antibodies were found, probably anti-Hu, that reacted with myenteric and submucosal plexus neurons. Autonomic neuropathy occurring with small-cell lung cancer is usually part of the anti-Hu syndrome. Among patients who had the anti-Hu antibody with paraneoplastic encephalomyelitis and sensory neuronopathy (PEM/SN) as reported by Dalmau and colleagues,[554] 28% had autonomic dysfunction.

ANTI-HU SYNDROME

The term "anti-Hu" was first applied by Graus and associates[971] to an autoantibody found in the serum of two patients with a subacute SN associated with small-cell lung cancer. Anti-Hu may be the same antibody previously reported by Wilkinson and Zeromski[2813] in four patients with SN associated with cancer.[2893] Anti-Hu antibody is a polyclonal, complement-fixing IgG that reacts strongly with the nuclei of virtually all neurons in the peripheral nervous system and CNS, sparing the nucleoli (see Fig. 15–3). It also reacts with the cytoplasm of neurons but much more weakly. Glial cells and other non-neuronal components of the nervous system do not react. Like the anti-Yo antibody, the concentration relative to total IgG is higher in CSF than in serum, suggesting intrathecal synthesis.[856] Unlike anti-Yo, which reacts only with tumor from patients with PCD, the anti-Hu antibody reacts with all small-cell lung cancer tested, whether or not the patient has the antibody in his or her serum or has a paraneoplastic syndrome.[550,971]

By Western-blot analysis of extracts of cortical neurons and small-cell lung cancer, the anti-Hu sera identify several bands between 35 and 40 kd. Western-blot analysis of various tumors and tumor lines indicates that the antigen is present in a percentage of several other tumors, particularly neuroblastomas and other neuroendocrine tumors. The Hu antigen has been cloned and sequenced.[2539] The Hu cDNA predicts a protein of molecular weight of approximately 42 kd with domains suggesting RNA binding sites. The Hu gene has striking homology to a Drosophila protein, Elav, involved in neuronal development.[2539]

Based on a study of 71 patients with high titers of anti-Hu antibody in serum, CSF, or both,[554] the antibody was found to be associated with multifocal neurologic symptoms or signs in most patients. Small-cell lung cancer was the most common underlying malignancy identified (Table 15–12).

About 25% of the patients with the anti-Hu syndrome have a unifocal neurologic disease (see Table 15–11), usually SN. Other patients suffer from limbic or brainstem encephalitis. In the other 75% of patients, dysfunction of the nervous system is widespread, including cerebellar dysfunction in about one-quarter. In a few patients with sensory neuronopathy, the neurologic disease is mild and the course is indolent.[970a]

About 60% of the patients with the anti-Hu syndrome are women. The neurologic disorder usually appears before the cancer is diag-

Table 15–12. **CANCER IN 71 PATIENTS WITH ANTI-HU SYNDROME**

Tumor	No. of Patients
Small-cell lung cancer	55(77.5%)
Small-cell adrenal cancer	1
Adenocarcinoma lung	1
Prostate	2
Neuroblastoma	1
Chondrosarcoma	1
Lung nodule (no biopsy)	1
No tumor	9*
	71

*In two patients who died and were examined at autopsy, no tumor was found.

Source: From Dalmau et al,[554] p 63, with permission.

nosed, and the tumor often is identified only at autopsy. In the majority of patients, death is caused by neurologic dysfunction, usually autonomic failure, and the tumor is found to be restricted to lung and mediastinum.

Neuropathologic changes in patients with the anti-Hu syndrome differ from the changes of anti-Yo in that inflammatory infiltrates are prominent and scattered throughout the CNS[552,1144,2207] (see Fig. 15–5). The lymphocytic infiltrates consist of both B and T cells; they specifically react with the cloned Hu fusion protein.[2539] Similar lymphocytic infiltrates are found in the small-cell lung cancers of patients with the anti-Hu antibody. In several patients with the anti-Hu syndrome, IgG has been found within the nuclei of neurons (Fig. 15–7). When IgG is eluted from those brains, it has a higher relative concentration of anti-Hu than either serum or spinal fluid.[552]

The anti-Hu syndrome also differs from the anti-Yo syndrome in that low but identifiable titers of the anti-Hu antibody can be found in about 15% of patients with small-cell lung cancer who do not have a paraneoplastic syndrome.[551] These patients, similar to those with the higher titers and paraneoplastic syndrome, are predominantly female and tend to have limited rather than extensive disease. Thus, low titers of the anti-Hu antibody are associated with a relatively good prognosis for the small-cell lung cancer.

Opsoclonus/Myoclonus

PARANEOPLASTIC OPSOCLONUS/MYOCLONUS

Opsoclonus, a disorder of saccadic stability, consists of involuntary, arrhythmic, multidirectional, high-amplitude conjugate saccades and is often associated with diffuse or focal myoclonus and truncal titubation, with or without other cerebellar signs. It occurs primarily in children as a self-limited illness and is probably the result of a viral infection in the brainstem. Opsoclonus/myoclonus (OM) also occurs as a paraneoplastic syndrome (POM) said to affect as many as 2% of children suffering from neuroblastoma. First recognized by Solomon and Chutorian[2457] in 1968, other reports indicate that nearly 50% of children with the OM syndrome harbor a neuroblastoma. Given the known tendency of neuroblastoma to differentiate and spontaneously disappear, many of the cases reported as OM without tumor may have truly been paraneoplastic. The age of peak incidence is 18 months; girls are affected more often than boys. Neurologic signs precede identification of the tumor at least 50% of the time, making recognition of the neurologic syndrome an important clue to the presence of neuroblastoma. Ataxia, irritability, vomiting, and dementia may accompany OM. Furthermore, when a neuroblastoma is associated with OM, the incidence of in-

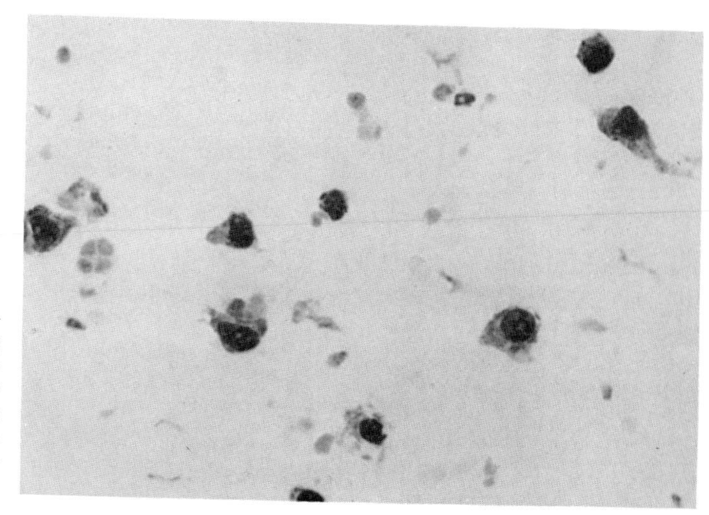

Figure 15–7. A section of hippocampus of a patient with small-cell lung cancer with paraneoplastic encephalomyelitis reacting with an antibody against human IgG. Note that IgG is within the neurons of the hippocampus, specifically within neuronal nuclei, sparing the nucleoli.

trathoracic tumors and of tumors with a benign histology is higher than expected. Independent of these differences, the overall prognosis of the neuroblastoma is better if OM is present than when the neurologic complication is absent, an observation not explained by disease stage or earlier diagnosis as a consequence of neurologic symptoms.[40] One observation[475] suggests that the tumors of children with POM have only one copy of the N-*myc* oncogene, whereas other patients at the same stage of disease but without POM often have multiple copies. A more recent report describes three patients with POM with multiple copies of the N-*myc* gene who had a poor outcome.[1157a] The neurologic disorder responds to corticosteroid-treatment, usually adrenocorticotropic hormone, and to the treatment of the tumor, but 50% of the patients suffer residual neurologic damage. In one study,[1692] only 10 of 26 children with OM but without neuroblastoma recovered fully from their neurologic disorder.

OM occurs less commonly in adults than in children. A recent review[643] of the literature identified 58 adults with OM; 11 cases were believed to be paraneoplastic. The most common tumor was lung cancer, but other cancers also cause the syndrome.[1349] Neurologic symptoms usually preceded the diagnosis of tumor and progressed over several weeks, sometimes faster or slower. Opsoclonus was often associated with truncal ataxia, dysarthria, myoclonus, vertigo, and encephalopathy; some patients appeared to have PCD. The CSF showed a mild pleocytosis in some patients and a mildly elevated protein level. Results of CT and MR scans were usually normal; in a few reports, an abnormality in the brainstem or cerebellum was detected by MR.[1109,2351,2615] POM differs from most other paraneoplastic syndromes of adults in that remissions occur[52] either spontaneously, following treatment of the tumor, or in association with clonazepam or thiamine treatment.

Neuropathologic reports conflict.[52] In some patients, no identifiable neuropathologic abnormalities are found, not even in the omnipause neurons, the putative site of the physiologic lesion in the OM syndrome.[2171] In others, the changes resemble those of PCD, with a loss of Purkinje cells and of cells in the granular layer of the cerebellum and in the inferior olives,[923,2215] and gliosis of the Bergmann astrocytic layer.

Autoantibodies against neurofilaments have been described in the serum of one child with neuroblastoma and POM;[1903] the anti-Hu antibody has been reported in another.[791] We found the anti-Hu antibody in one child with POM but no antibody in several others. Some adult women with POM and carcinoma of the breast or pelvic organs harbor an antibody called anti-Ri (see the following). The characteristics of this and other well-characterized autoantibodies associated with paraneoplastic syndromes can be found in Table 15–8.

ANTI-RI SYNDROME

The anti-Ri antibody has been found[339,1620] in a few patients with eye movement disorders, usually opsoclonus, associated with truncal ataxia and sometimes other cerebellar signs. It is histochemically identical to the anti-Hu antibody but identifies protein bands at 55 kd and 80 kd when cortical neurons are analyzed with the Western-blot method, different from the 35-kd to 40-kd bands identified by anti-Hu. Furthermore, the anti-Ri antibody does not react with neurons of the peripheral nervous system, as does anti-Hu.[977] The gene has been cloned and the protein sequenced.[336] It does not resemble either the Yo or Hu genes. In the 11 patients so far identified with anti-Ri, 5 have breast cancer, 1 a positive axillary lymph node (probably breast), 1 fallopian tube cancer, 1 small-cell lung cancer, and 1 bladder cancer. In the two others, a cancer was not identified, including a patient who was examined at autopsy, although the breasts were not extensively examined. The brain of that patient revealed widespread inflammatory infiltrates, particularly in the dorsal pons and midbrain. Deposits of anti-Ri IgG were found in the dorsal midbrain.[1201]

The clinical syndrome differs from other forms of PCD in that the predominant symptom in most patients is opsoclonus, often precipitated by visual fixation. The opsoclonus is often associated with myoclonus similar to the syndrome that occurs in infants with neuroblastoma. Many patients have ataxia, usually truncal, but sometimes appendicular as well. The prominent opsoclonus and truncal rather than appendicular ataxia distinguish this syndrome from the anti-Yo and anti-Hu PCD. Another difference is that this disorder tends to wax and wane, and some patients have spontaneous resolution, at least of the opsoclonus. The course tends to be independent of the underlying tumor. Because the number of patients is so small, further evaluation will be necessary to define more clearly its clinical and pathologic abnormalities.

Visual Syndromes

RETINAL DEGENERATION

Paraneoplastic retinal degeneration, also called cancer-associated retinopathy (CAR), is a rare syndrome that usually occurs in association with small-cell lung cancer,[1024,2178,2578] melanoma,[37,206,1765] and gynecologic tumors (Table 15–13). The visual symptoms include episodic visual obscurations, night blindness, light-induced glare, photosensitivity, and impaired color vision[1263]; they typically precede the diagnosis of cancer. The symptoms progress to painless visual loss, beginning unilaterally but usually becoming bilateral. Visual testing demonstrates peripheral and ring scotomas and loss of acuity. Funduscopic examination may reveal arteriolar narrowing and abnormal mottling of the retinal pigment epithelium. Results of the electroretinogram are abnormal. The CSF is typically normal, although elevated immunoglobulin concentrations have been reported. Inflammatory cells may be identified in the vitreous by slit-lamp examination. Pathologically, a loss of photoreceptors and ganglion cells with lymphocytic and macrophage infiltration is usually noted. The other parts of the optic pathway are preserved, although a loss of myelin and cellular infiltration of the optic nerve may occur.

Serum antibodies that react immunohistochemically with antigens in retinal photoreceptor and ganglion cells have been found in some patients with CAR, but not in all, and the identified antigens differ from patient to patient.[2178] Retinal deposits of immunoglobulin suggest an immune-mediated mechanism. Some patients produce antibodies that react with a 23-kd calcium-binding protein called recoverin, which regulates the guanylate cyclase resynthesis of cyclic guanylic acid in photoreceptors to allow recovery after light activation.[14,652,2053] Prednisone treatment sometimes reduces antibody titers and stabilizes vision.[1356]

OPTIC NEURITIS

Acute optic neuropathy is much more often a vascular or demyelinating disorder than a paraneoplastic one. When paraneoplastic, it is more likely to be part of a wider encephalomyelitis, not simply isolated blindness.[250] Only a few cases of relatively pure paraneoplastic optic neuritis have been reported.[23,1196,2040,2753] The onset is usually sudden, with painless visual loss, often bilateral, with or without papilledema. More common causes of blindness in patients with cancer are metastatic infiltration of the nerve by tumor, neurotoxicity from chemotherapy or radiotherapy, or anemia.[446,499] None of Dalmau's 71 patients with the anti-Hu antibody and PEM/SN had optic neuritis.[554]

Spinal Cord Syndromes

Paraneoplastic disorders restricted to the spinal cord are rare and much less common than metastatic involvement of the spinal cord. Spinal cord involvement is usually a part of a paraneoplastic encephalomyelitis rather than an isolated spinal disorder.[2006] A few paraneoplastic disorders, discussed in this section, do appear to be restricted to the spinal cord itself.

NECROTIZING MYELOPATHY

This rare syndrome occurs with lymphoma, leukemia, and lung or other cancers.* The syndrome's onset may precede or follow the diagnosis of cancer.[1929,1930,2823] Patients typically present with rapidly ascending flaccid paraplegia; back or radicular pain may precede the onset of neurologic dysfunction, and the process may lead to respiratory failure and death. The CSF is usually inflam-

* References 1005, 1075, 1228, 1531, 1668, 2403, 2823.

Table 15–13. **ELECTROPHYSIOLOGIC AND LABORATORY FINDINGS OF ALL PATIENTS REPORTED WITH PARANEOPLASTIC RETINOPATHY**

Author	Patient No.	Electrophysiology	Tissue Diagnosis	Retinal Immunohistochemistry	Western Blot (kd)
Sawyer	1	Flat/reduced ERG	SCLC	—	—
			PR degeneration		
	2	—	SCLC	—	—
			PR degeneration		
	3	—	SCLC	—	—
			PR degeneration		
Kornguth	4	Flat/reduced ERG	—	Staining of large ganglion cells	20/65
	5	—	SCLC	Nonspecific nuclear staining	—
Keltner	6	Flat ERG	Cervical carcinoma	Diffuse staining	23
			PR degeneration		
Buchanan	7	Flat ERG; normal VEP	PR degeneration	—	—
Klingele	8	Flat ERG	Adenocarcinoma of breast	—	
Grunwald	9	Abnormal VEP	SCLC	Staining of inner retina	145/205
			Ganglion-cell loss		
Thirkill	10	Flat ERG	Non-SCLC	—	23
	11	Flat ERG	SCLC	—	23/48
vanderPol	12	Flat ERG	SCLC	—	—
Nunez	13	Flat ERG; low/reduced VEP	SCLC	—	—
Berson	14	Loss of rod signal on ERG	Melanoma	—	—
Crofts	15	Flat ERG	Endometrial carcinoma	—	50
Thirkill	16	—	SCLC	Diffuse staining of nuclei in all layers	23
Jacobson	17	Almost flat ERG	SCLC	—	23/48
	18	Flat ERG	SCLC	—	23
Rizzo	19	Predominantly rod	SCLC	Selective staining of outer retina	Neg
	20	Flat ERG	SCLC	Selective staining of outer retina	48
Keltner	21	Equal photopic and scotopic effects	SCLC	Photoreceptors	65
				Inner segment	

ERG = electroretinogram; PR = photoreceptor; SCLC = small-cell lung cancer; VEP = visual evoked potential.
Source: Adapted from Rizzo and Gittinger,[2178] p 1293; references can be found in that article.

matory, although malignant cells are absent. The results of an MR scan are usually normal,[1228] but the MR scan may show spinal cord swelling or even contrast enhancement. The absence of an epidural mass or discrete intramedullary enhancement rules out the much more common metastatic myelopathy. Treatment is usually unsuccessful, although one patient was reported[1075] to respond to intrathecal dexamethasone. Pathologically, spinal cord necrosis is widespread, involving all components of the cord, but with some white matter predominance. Inflammatory lesions are not typical. The cause is unknown. A similar disorder also occurs in previously healthy patients without underlying disease.[812]

MOTOR NEURON DISORDERS

Motor Neuron Disease. Motor neuron disease (MND) or amyotrophic lateral sclerosis (ALS), a common neurologic disorder of unknown cause, is rarely paraneoplastic.[2211] Epidemiologic studies of MND or ALS do not show an increased incidence in patients with cancer when compared with the general population,[2211] because the numbers of paraneoplastic patients are so small. Nevertheless, isolated case reports of patients with cancer and clinically typical MND whose neurologic improvement was dramatic after treatment of the underlying tumor suggest that MND can be paraneoplastic.[152,291,741,1782] Paraneoplastic MND may be clinically indistinguishable from the non-neoplastic variety, but its onset and course are usually more rapidly progressive.

The disorder is characterized by weakness with atrophy and fasciculations, usually asymmetric, with a predilection for the small hand or bulbar muscles. Reflex hyperactivity and extensor plantar responses may occur early or they may be absent. In a few of our patients,[822] primary lateral sclerosis, the MND variant, with bilateral corticobulbar or corticospinal signs but without lower motor neuron dysfunction, may have been paraneoplastic.[2097] A patient with small-cell lung cancer from another study developed focal rigidity and myoclonus along with a focal loss of motor neurons.[2198] Bowel and bladder functions are usually spared. The disorder is progressive and usually results in death from respiratory failure. In a few instances, the disease has remitted after treatment of the underlying tumor.

The neuropathologic changes of paraneoplastic MND cannot be distinguished from those of MND or ALS. Although both upper and lower motor neuron findings are evident, either may predominate in an individual patient. Some patients with MND harbor antibodies in their serum and CSF that react with nervous system elements.[635] Younger and colleagues[2877a] describe nine patients with MND and Hodgkin's or non-Hodgkin's lymphoma who had signs of both upper and lower motor neuron dysfunction accompanied by paraproteinemia. In a more recent prospective analysis[2229] of 37 consecutive patients with MND who underwent bone marrow biopsy, 2 were found to have lymphoma. It is not clear whether this disorder, with its combined upper and lower motor neuron signs, is the same disorder that Schold and colleagues[2327] called "subacute motor neuronopathy" (see the following).

The anti-Hu antibody may also be found in patients with paraneoplastic MND. In Dalmau's 71 patients with PEM/SN, 45 had signs of motor neuron dysfunction, and in 20% these were predominant signs, although MND was not an isolated syndrome in any.[554]

Subacute Motor Neuronopathy. Paraneoplastic subacute motor neuronopathy, or spinal muscular atrophy, occurs as a rare complication of Hodgkin's and other lymphomas[2228,2327,2738] and occasionally of other cancers.[2503] The patients develop subacute, progressive, painless, and often patchy lower motor neuron weakness, which usually affects the legs more than the arms. Atrophy is present, but fasciculations are not prominent; the bulbar musculature is spared. Although patients sometimes complain of paresthesias, sensory loss is mild. Weakness is often profound. Motor and sensory nerve conduction velocities are normal or only mildly decreased, but electromyography shows denervation. The CSF is acellular with a mildly elevated protein concentration. The results of the MR scan of the cord are normal. The course is usually benign and independent of the activity of the underlying neoplasm. Unlike MND, the neurologic deficit usually does not incapacitate the patient; it often stabilizes or improves spontaneously, sometimes to full recovery after months or years. Treatment does not hasten recovery.

The main pathologic characteristics are degeneration of neurons in the anterior horns of the spinal cord. Sometimes patchy, mild demyelination is seen in the white matter of the spinal cord, particularly in the dorsal columns. The lateral columns of the spinal cord are typically spared, unlike the findings in MND. Indirect evidence suggests that the disorder may be caused by an opportunistic viral infection of the anterior horn neurons:

1. The disorder is associated with lymphoma, a tumor causing immunosuppression that permits opportunistic viral infections. Of our patients with the disorder, one died of progressive multifocal leukoencephalopathy and another of an opportunistic nocardia infection.
2. The pathologic abnormalities resemble those of burnt-out poliomyelitis. Viral-like particles were identified in the anterior horns of one patient,[2738] but a specific virus has not been isolated.
3. A similar neurologic disorder affecting spinal anterior horn cells in a strain of mice is caused by the murine leukemia virus.[55,885,886]

The relationship between this disorder and the lower motor neuron disorder associated with RT is unclear (see Chapter 13). Some of the subacute motor neuronopathy patients had received prior RT, raising the possibility that the radiation activated a latent virus.

MYELITIS

An inflammatory myelitis sometimes occurs as a part of the encephalomyelitis syndrome. Portions of the nervous system that are not involved clinically sometimes show the typical inflammatory infiltrates of encephalomyelitis on pathologic examination.

Peripheral Nerve Syndromes

The problem of peripheral neuropathy complicating cancer is vexing[817,818,974] (Table 15–14). Peripheral neuropathy is common,

Table 15–14. **PERIPHERAL NEUROPATHY IN PATIENTS WITH CANCER**

Causes	Examples
Metastatic	Spinal cord compression Leptomeningeal metastases Metastases to peripheral nerves
Nonmetastatic, known cause	Metabolic nutritional Side effects of therapy
Paraneoplastic	Subacute or chronic sensorimotor peripheral neuropathy Acute polyradiculoneuropathy (Guillain-Barré syndrome) Mononeuritis multiplex and microvasculitis of peripheral nerve Acute brachial neuritis Autonomic neuropathy Peripheral neuropathy with islet-cell tumors Peripheral neuropathy associated with paraproteinemia
Unrelated to cancer	Diabetes mellitus Vitamin-B_{12} deficiency

and paraneoplastic disorders are rare.[334,1733] Many other nonmetastatic effects of cancer, such as chemotherapy toxicity, cachexia, and malnutrition, probably affect peripheral nerves more commonly in patients with cancer than do paraneoplastic syndromes.[1118] Nevertheless, some surveys indicate that in as many as 10% of patients with a peripheral neuropathy for which the cause (such as diabetes) is not immediately apparent, the neuropathy is paraneoplastic.[903,1222] Surveys of well-nourished patients with cancer using quantitative sensory testing[1579] and electrical testing of nerves[2570] suggest that many patients have subclinical peripheral nerve injuries.

Several different kinds of peripheral nerve injury have been identified as paraneoplastic. The most characteristic is paraneoplastic sensory neuronopathy (discussed previously), which can occur either as an isolated entity or, more commonly, as a fragment of paraneoplastic encephalomyelitis.

The others are discussed in the following paragraphs.[2423a]

SUBACUTE SENSORIMOTOR NEUROPATHY

Subacute sensorimotor neuropathy can be induced by many etiologic mechanisms: diabetes mellitus, nutritional deficiency, alcoholism, chronic illness, vitamin-B_{12} deficiency, toxin exposure, and chemotherapeutic agents, particularly vincristine. A peripheral neuropathy is more likely to be caused by one of these disorders than by a paraneoplastic syndrome, even in the patient with cancer, so the diagnosis of paraneoplastic neuropathy should be made with great caution, only after carefully excluding all other causes. As a true paraneoplastic syndrome, sensorimotor neuropathy is most frequently associated with lung cancer,[526] sometimes preceding the diagnosis of cancer by up to 5 years. The course is variable; a few patients stabilize or remit after treatment of the underlying tumor.

Subacute sensorimotor neuropathy causes a predominantly distal symmetric polyneuropathy, more marked in the lower extremities, with weakness, glove-and-stocking sensory impairment to all modalities, and a loss of tendon reflexes. Although the disorder may pursue the very slow course of idiopathic sensorimotor polyneuropathy, patients with cancer are likely to progress rapidly and develop more disability than patients with diabetes, for example. Accordingly, a rapidly progressive or severe sensorimotor neuropathy should be given greater consideration as a possible paraneoplastic syndrome. Bulbar involvement is exceptional. A few patients with paraneoplastic sensorimotor neuropathy follow a remitting and relapsing course typical of chronic inflammatory demyelinating polyneuropathy. These patients may respond to corticosteroid therapy.

In patients with subacute sensorimotor neuropathy, the CSF is typically acellular, with the protein concentration normal or slightly elevated. Nerve conduction studies are consistent with an axonal neuropathy, with low-amplitude or absent sensory action potentials and normal or decreased motor nerve conduction velocities.[376] A few patients have marked slowing of motor conduction velocities consistent with a demyelinating polyneuropathy.[526]

Pathologically, the nerves usually show axonal degeneration; demyelination is prominent in a few patients.[526] Spinal root demyelination and lymphocytic infiltrates of peripheral nerves have also been reported.

A particular sensorimotor neuropathy is associated with breast cancer. Peterson and colleagues[2020] have described nine patients with a slowly progressive sensorimotor neuropathy (predominantly sensory), sometimes with features that suggest myopathy, such as proximal weakness, or with CNS dysfunction, such as hyperreflexia and extensor plantar responses. The disorder progressed very slowly over many years, was not disabling, and was frequently heralded by itching, muscle cramps, or both. In one patient, itching (initially over the left breast and later diffuse) preceded the identification of the cancer by a year and a half. Most patients remained fully functional, as neither the neuropathy nor the breast cancer was disabling.

Bruera and colleagues,[329] using electrophysiologic tests to examine 61 consecutive patients with advanced breast cancer (compared with control subjects), found diminished muscle strength and increased fatigue that they could not relate to nutritional status or muscle mass.

PERIPHERAL NEUROPATHIES ASSOCIATED WITH PLASMA-CELL DYSCRASIAS

A number of disorders in which clones of B lymphocytes proliferate and produce abnormal amounts of immunoglobulin are associated with peripheral neuropathies.[1308,1351,1735] The plasma-cell dyscrasias associated with peripheral neuropathies are listed in Table 15–15; detailed reviews of these syndromes, beyond the scope of this monograph, are available in other sources.[1351,1735,2478,2700] Only myeloma will be considered in detail here.

In general, patients with neuropathy and paraproteinemia present subacutely with progressive, symmetric, distal sensorimotor and autonomic symptoms. The various disorders do have some distinguishing characteristics, however. For example, benign monoclonal gammopathy is associated with chronic inflammatory demyelinating polyra-

Table 15–15. **PLASMA-CELL DYSCRASIAS AND PERIPHERAL NEUROPATHY**

Benign monoclonal gammopathy
Primary systemic amyloidosis
Multiple myeloma
Osteolytic with amyloidosis
Osteolytic without amyloidosis
Osteosclerotic
Waldenström's macroglobulinemia
Cryoglobulinemia
Gamma heavy-chain disease
Monoclonal gammopathy with solid tumors
Monoclonal gammopathy with benign lymph node hyperplasia
POEMS syndrome

POEMS = polyneuropathy-organomegaly-endocrinopathy-M protein-skin.

diculoneuropathy, with elevated CSF protein, slowing of conduction velocities, and conduction block. The neuropathy of amyloidosis is predominantly sensory, with lancinating pain and burning dysesthesias. Axonal features dominate the electrophysiologic findings.

The most interesting recent development in our understanding of neuropathies associated with plasma-cell dyscrasias is the finding of monoclonal IgM proteins that react with peripheral nerve antigens such as myelin-associated glycoprotein and GM-1 ganglioside.[529,1241,1477,2261] Although direct evidence does not prove that antibodies to these proteins cause neuropathy, intraneural injection of antibody into cat sciatic nerve can cause demyelination.[1124] Patients in whom the titer of antibody in the serum is lowered by plasmapheresis may show clinical improvement.

MULTIPLE MYELOMA

Paraneoplastic peripheral neuropathy (PN) is a rare complication of multiple myeloma (MM), occurring in fewer than 5% of patients.[679] A somewhat higher incidence is observed in prospective studies and when the diagnosis is based on electrophysiologic or histologic criteria rather than clinical ones. Paraneoplastic PN accompanying MM appears in four clinical contexts[1352]:

1. *Associated with Osteolytic Multiple Myeloma without Amyloidosis.* Peripheral neuropathy is rare in osteolytic MM but may be the presenting and dominant clinical feature. These neuropathies resemble the sensorimotor PN associated with carcinoma. The CSF protein concentration is usually normal. The PN is usually slowly progressive, and chemotherapy is not beneficial despite improvement of the MM.
2. *Associated with Osteolytic Multiple Myeloma and Systemic Amyloidosis.* This resembles the PN seen in amyloidosis without MM except that superimposed radicular syndromes may cause a clinical picture resembling mononeuritis multiplex. Treatment of the MM does not improve the PN.
3. *Associated with Osteosclerotic Myeloma.* Patients with osteosclerotic myeloma are usually younger and follow a more indolent clinical course than patients with osteolytic disease.[1352,1353] The bone marrow often is normal, and the concentration of the M protein in serum and urine is low, often detectable only by immunoelectrophoresis.[679] The disorder is especially common among the Japanese. Among patients with MM and a paraneoplastic PN, 50% or more have osteosclerotic lesions, although fewer than 3% of all patients with MM have osteosclerotic disease. Approximately 50% of patients with osteosclerotic myeloma have a PN[1353] and the PN is often the presenting feature. The manifestations are symmetric, distal sensorimotor PN, resembling chronic inflammatory demyelinating polyradiculoneuropathy.[1855] Motor involvement is the dominant feature, and painful dysesthesias and autonomic symptoms are rare. The course is slowly progressive, but most patients eventually are severely disabled. Motor nerve conduction velocity is slowed. The CSF protein concentration is chronically elevated, and the elevation is sometimes associated with papilledema. A detectable IgG or IgA M protein, usually with a λ-light chain, is found in 75% of these patients. All patients have sclerotic bone lesions, either solitary (strictly not *multiple* myeloma) or restricted in number. Osseous lesions

occur in truncal and proximal long bones but spare the skull and distal extremities. Peripheral nerve histology reveals an axonal neuropathy with secondary segmental demyelination and perivascular mononuclear cell infiltration of the epineurium.

4. *POEMS.* Patients with osteosclerotic MM and PN sometimes develop a syndrome of hepatosplenomegaly, lymphadenopathy, endocrinopathy, anasarca, hirsutism, hyperpigmentation, thickening of the skin, and hyperhidrosis, known as the POEMS syndrome: **p**olyneuropathy, **o**rganomegaly, **e**ndocrinopathy, **M** protein, **s**kin.[1672,1778,1855] Of 38 patients with polyneuropathy associated with plasma cell dyscrasia, 31 (82%) had osteosclerotic bone lesions and 5 met all the criteria for the POEMS syndrome.[1778] The male preponderance is striking among patients with this syndrome. A similar constellation of findings is less commonly observed in patients with mixed osteosclerotic and osteolytic MM, osteolytic MM, extramedullary plasmacytoma, and an isolated monoclonal gammopathy.

Excision or RT of solitary osteosclerotic lesions can result in a gradual but often dramatic reversal of the PN and the other clinical manifestations. In patients with multiple bony lesions, chemotherapy may be efficacious.

ACUTE POLYRADICULONEUROPATHY

Paraneoplastic acute polyradiculoneuropathy is usually associated with Hodgkin's disease. The clinical and pathologic features resemble typical Guillain-Barré syndrome.[539,1313,1394,1583] Neurologic symptoms can begin either while the cancer is active or when it is in remission. The clinical course of the neuropathy is independent of that of the lymphoma, and the neuropathy may respond to plasmapheresis.

VASCULITIC NEUROPATHY

Paraneoplastic vasculitic neuropathy has been reported in only a few patients. It usually presents clinically as a mononeuropathy multiplex[1115] with progressive dysfunction of several nerves but not as diffuse as in polyneuropathy. In two of three patients reported by Johnson and colleagues,[1296] an underlying subclinical small-cell lung cancer was detected at autopsy; the third patient had lymphoma. Other investigators have reported an association with renal-cell,[2599] prostate, and endometrial carcinoma.[1924] The pathology is notable for epineural vasculitis, which may be limited to peripheral nerves; in Johnson's patients with small-cell lung cancer, however, it was part of a more diffuse encephalomyelitis. Vincent and associates[2697] report seven patients with sensorimotor polyneuropathy related to cancer who had evidence of both nerve and muscle vasculitis. Among the series reported by Dalmau and coworkers[554] of 71 patients with the anti-Hu antibody and PEM/SN, 2 presented a mononeuritic multiplexlike clinical picture with painful, asymmetric sensory and motor signs.

Immunosuppressive therapy[1924] or plasmapheresis may help, but they are not consistently beneficial. The exact cause of paraneoplastic vasculitic neuropathy multiplex is unknown.

BRACHIAL NEURITIS

The clinical features of brachial neuritis in patients with cancer resemble those in patients without cancer. A causal association has not been established but the disorder appears to occur with increased frequency in patients with Hodgkin's disease.[1450,2025] More common causes of brachial plexopathy that must be excluded in patients with cancer include radiation injury (see Chapter 13), traumatic injury during surgery or anesthesia (see Chapter 14), and ischemic brachial neuritis (see Chapter 8). Brachial neuritis is usually painful at onset, resembling the onset of infiltrating tumor but unlike radiation injury, which is frequently painless.

Neuromuscular Junction Syndromes

MYASTHENIA GRAVIS

Myasthenia gravis occurs in about 30% of patients with thymoma; conversely, 15% of patients with myasthenia are found to have a thymoma. Autoantibodies with specificity for contractile elements of striated muscle are found in 80% to 90% of patients with myasthenia and thymoma.[2814] A few reports indicating that myasthenia complicates lymphoma[284,1907,2814] seem more than just coincidence. The biology and treatment of paraneoplastic myasthenia resemble those of the more common autoimmune but nonparaneoplastic disorder.[2131,2690] The thymomas are usually, but not always, noninvasive and are cured by thymectomy. The myasthenia may also improve.[2690]

LAMBERT-EATON MYASTHENIC SYNDROME

About 60% of patients with LEMS have small-cell lung cancer. A few others have small-cell cancer elsewhere in the body, such as in the prostate or cervix. About 40%, usually women with other evidence of autoimmune dysfunction, do not have cancer.[1915] Patients present with progressive proximal weakness and fatigability, but unlike myasthenia gravis, the symptoms do not significantly affect the bulbar musculature. Respiratory weakness can occur. Power at first increases with effort so that the patient's complaint of weakness may seem greater than the examiner's initial findings. With continued effort, weakness returns. Deep tendon reflexes, especially those in the legs, are diminished or absent but may reappear briefly after exercise. Cholinergic dysautonomia[1365] occurs in more than 50% of the patients, causing dry mouth and impotence. Characteristic abnormalities are found with electrophysiologic testing, including very low compound muscle action potentials (CMAP), which may increase to normal after brief exercise. Repetitive stimulation causes a decrement of the CMAP at low rates of stimulation and an increment at high rates[1460] (Fig. 15–8).

LEMS is believed to result from a reduced release of acetylcholine from presynaptic nerve terminals. In most patients, detectable antibodies react with the voltage-dependent calcium channel at the nerve terminal,[1555,1828a] although a smaller percentage of patients with cancer react than do those without cancer. Evidence that LEMS is actually an autoimmune disease includes its association with other autoimmune diseases, the clinical response to immunosuppression,

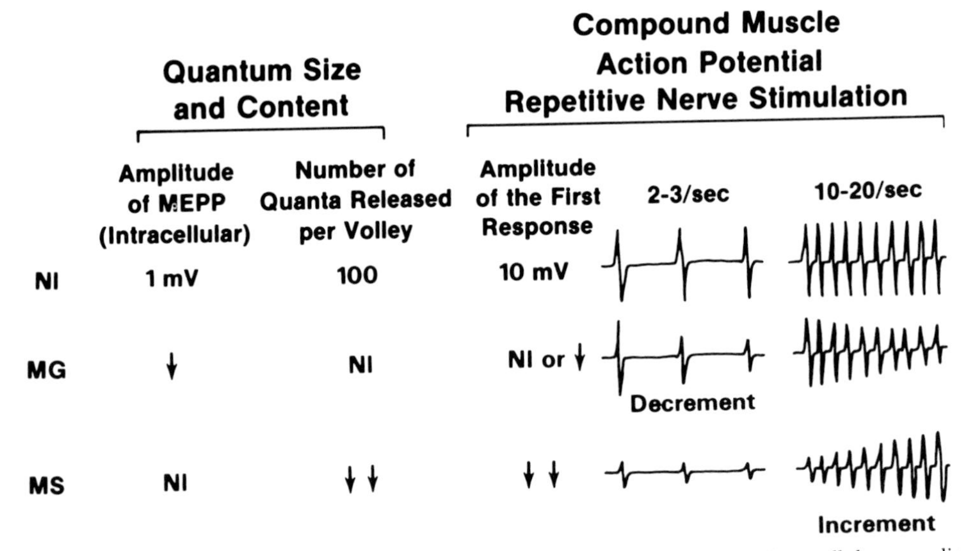

Figure 15–8. Typical changes in quantum size and quantum content as determined by intracellular recordings in myasthenia gravis (MG) and Lambert-Eaton myasthenic syndrome (LEMS) (*left*). Decrement or increment of the compound muscle action potential to repetitive nerve stimulation (*right*). The amplitude of the compound muscle action potential decreases as a result of dropout of individual muscle fibers according to the size of the end-plate potential (EPP), and the amplitude increases with recruitment of additional fibers. (From Kimura,[1372] p 181, with permission.)

and most compellingly, the results of passive transfer experiments in which the disorder has been induced in experimental animals injected with IgG from patients with LEMS.[851,1467] Some patients with small-cell cancer produce IgG antibodies against calcium channel proteins expressed by both the cancer and the neuromuscular junction. These antibodies bind specifically to calcium channels of the presynaptic neuromuscular junction,[1151] causing a disarray visible on electron microscopy.[852] The antibodies cause failure of calcium entry in response to an action potential, leading to diminished acetylcholine release. Using the antibody as a probe, a gene coding for a protein similar in structure to the beta subunit of the calcium channel has been cloned. The protein reacts with antibodies in the sera of about 30% of patients with LEMS.[2212]

Unlike most other paraneoplastic syndromes, LEMS often responds to plasmapheresis or immunosuppressive therapy. Other treatments that increase transmitter release include guanidine hydrochloride, which mobilizes calcium, and 4-aminopyridine, which acts on potassium channels, but both have significant side effects. 3,4-Diaminopyridine also facilitates the release of transmitter but with fewer side effects.[1722] Cholinesterase inhibitors show minimal benefit in most patients. Treatment of the underlying malignancy in some instances improves the neurologic syndrome.[417] In some patients, LEMS may develop in association with other paraneoplastic syndromes, including PCD[462] and PEM/SN.[242,848] One of our patients with small-cell lung cancer developed LEMS associated with POM.

Muscle Syndromes

POLYMYOSITIS/DERMATOMYOSITIS

Polymyositis (PM) and dermatomyositis (DM) are common inflammatory, probably autoimmune, muscle diseases.[547,548,2045] Only a minority of patients suffering from these disorders have an underlying malignancy as the cause.[1670,1699,2335] Some investigators conclude that the incidence of PM or DM is not increased in patients with cancer, but most believe that the disorder, particularly in the older age group, is substantially more common than in the noncancer population.[2167] DM with typical cutaneous changes is more likely to be paraneoplastic than is PM. Women and men are affected in approximately equal numbers. Symptoms of the muscle weakness generally precede identification of the cancer. The tumor may be at any site, but malignancies of breast, lung, ovary, and stomach are the most common. Hodgkin's disease,[2375] prostate cancer,[1980] and colon cancer have also been reported offenders.[2632]

The clinical and laboratory findings in PM/DM associated with malignancy resemble those of the idiopathic disease, although patients with cancer often show more striking abnormalities in muscle biopsy specimens. Patients characteristically present with proximal muscle weakness, elevated serum levels of creatine kinase, and electromyographic evidence suggesting myopathy rather than nerve disease. A muscle biopsy specimen showing an inflammatory myopathy confirms the diagnosis. Although laboratory findings do not distinguish paraneoplastic PM/DM from the nonparaneoplastic variety, autoantibodies are particularly common in PM/DM associated with lung disease[1174] and less common in patients with the paraneoplastic disorder.[1900] No laboratory test is absolutely diagnostic. Normal levels of creatine kinase occasionally found even in patients with profound muscle weakness, with or without malignancy,[1446] indicate a poor prognosis.[847] Toxoplasmosis, an infection common in patients with lymphoma, may be a precipitating factor for the syndrome in some patients. That diagnosis should be considered because at least one patient's muscle disease has responded to treatment of toxoplasmosis.[1091] The disorder has also been reported following bone marrow transplantation for Hodgkin's disease.[2324]

The relationship between the course of the PM/DM and the underlying tumor is inconsistent. Muscle and dermatologic symptoms improve coincident with treatment of the tumor in some patients but not in others. Both paraneoplastic and nonparaneoplastic PM/DM are treated with immunosuppression. Corticosteroids, cyclosporine, and other immunosuppressants have been used successfully.[547] Other reports suggest that high-dose IV gamma globulin is useful in patients unresponsive to other forms of immunosuppression.[1277,2638] Weak respiratory and pharyngeal muscles may contribute to death. The prognosis is poorer for the paraneoplastic disorder than for the nonparaneoplastic disorder.

Abnormalities of both humoral-mediated and cellular-mediated immunity are found in patients with PM/DM; many have autoantibodies. The direct target antigen is not known.[547,1174,2552] Kissel and colleagues[1381] suggest that the disorder is a result of an immune-mediated vasculopathy.

ACUTE NECROTIZING MYOPATHY

Paraneoplastic acute necrotizing myopathy is very rare. In the few patients in which it was described, it was characterized by painful proximal weakness, progressing to respiratory and pharyngeal failure and death.[325,2713,2882] Various associated tumors were described. Usually the onset of neurologic symptoms preceded the diagnosis of cancer. Pathologic changes consisted of widespread necrosis of skeletal muscle with little or no inflammation, distinguishing it from polymyositis. One patient with breast cancer improved after mastectomy, although immunosuppressive therapy was not beneficial. The etiology of this rare disorder is unknown.

CARCINOID MYOPATHY

Carcinoid tumors may be associated with a progressive myopathy that typically begins several years after the carcinoid syndrome.[1493,2533] The symptoms include proximal weakness, fatigability, and sometimes muscle cramps while climbing stairs. The weakness improves when treated with the serotonin blocker cyproheptadine, as does the diarrhea that characterizes the carcinoid syndrome.[1793] These results suggest that the myopathy is related to the increased secretion of serotonin by the tumor. A biopsy specimen reveals type-2 fiber atrophy with little inflammatory change, distinguishing it from PM/DM. Patients with carcinoid should be questioned specifically about muscle weakness and cramps, as this disorder is treatable.

CACHECTIC MYOPATHY

Chronic debilitating diseases, including cancer and anorexia nervosa, which are complicated by cachexia and malnutrition, may be associated with diffuse muscle wasting and with weakness as a later feature.[328,329] Myoedema is also a frequent finding.[1788] Pathologic changes include a predominance of smaller fibers and of grouped atrophy; noninflammatory fiber degeneration and vacuolization of muscles may also be present. The weakness may be reversible if treatment of the underlying illness is successful.

Miscellaneous Disorders

Case reports have described various neurologic disorders as possibly paraneoplastic when they were closely associated with the discovery of a cancer or when treatment of the cancer ameliorated the neurologic disorder. Central pontine myelinolysis[1088] with single or multiple demyelinating plaques of brain or brainstem is an example. The absence of a series of patients with the same neurologic syndrome associated with cancer or of a marker such as an autoantibody suggesting a relationship between cancer and the neurologic disorder raises the question of whether these disorders are, in fact, paraneoplastic.

CARCINOMATOUS NEUROMYOPATHY

Carcinomatous neuromyopathy is a syndrome characterized by the subacute onset of weakness, usually of proximal muscles, appearing before the diagnosis of cancer in patients who are well nourished. It is associated with a decrease or absence of one or more reflexes.[154,1143] During its course, some patients have spontaneous improvement in strength. Pathologic changes are noninflammatory, nonspecific, and minor compared to the degree of clinical weakness. A neurogenic cause has been suggested by the finding of a distal intramuscular axonal neuropathy, but the disorder is not well understood. Some investigators believe that, in most patients, symptoms of neuromyopathy are related to weight loss that either precedes or follows diagnosis of the cancer.[1118,1157]

NEUROMYOTONIA

Muscle cramps are a common complication of cancer[2484]; sometimes they are related to electrolyte imbalances or are induced by chemotherapy (see Chapter 12). A much rarer, but clinically significant paraneoplastic disorder is acquired neuromyotonia,[1062,2733] characterized by progressive aching and stiffness of muscles[2585] associated with spasms or severe rigidity that prevents use of the muscle. Electromyographic studies indicate continuous muscle fiber activity.[884] The muscle spasms and rigidity are sometimes precipitated by activity, forcing patients to become sedentary. The disorder can arise from peripheral nerves or from the CNS, where it may be a part of the encephalomyelitis syndrome.[159,375,2198] Antibodies to voltage-gated potassium channels have been identified in some patients with acquired neuromyotonia.[1101a]

Autoantibodies that react with cerebellum are found in autoimmune, nonparaneoplastic, stiff-man syndrome, as well as in patients with Hodgkin's disease[769] and breast cancer.[811] The stiff-man syndrome has also been associated with lung cancer[2718] and thymoma[884]; it can be distinguished by electromyography[1988,2718] from myoedema, an electrically silent contracture of muscle produced by percussion,[1788] and from pseudomyotonic discharges, a rare manifestation of PM/DM. The disorder often can be treated successfully with phenytoin or diazepam.[1988] Plasmapheresis also has been reported to be successful.[121]

REFERENCES

1. Aakerlund, LP and Rosenberg, J: Postoperative delirium: Treatment with supplementary oxygen. Br J Anaesth 72:286-290, 1994.
2. Abbatucci, JS, Delozier, T, Quint, R, et al: Radiation myelopathy of the cervical spinal cord: Time, dose and volume factors. Int J Radiat Oncol Biol Phys 4:239-248, 1978.

2a. Aavitsland, P, Frohohm, LO, Hoiby, EA, et al: Risk of pneumococcal disease in individuals without a spleen. Lancet 344:1504, 1994.

3. Abdel-Dayem, HM, Oh, YS, and Sil, R: Treated stage IIB Hodgkin's disease complicated by late paraplegia. AJR 132:265-266, 1979.
4. Abello, R, Yeakley, JW, and Goldman, P: Secondary achalasia in a patient with brainstem metastases from lung carcinoma. Letter to the Editor. J Clin Gastroenterol 14:176-178, 1992.
5. Abla, AA, Rothfus, WE, Maroon, JC, et al: Delayed spinal subarachnoid hematoma: A rare complication of C1-C2 cervical myelography. AJNR 7:526-528, 1986.
6. Abramowicz, M (ed): Drugs for pain. Med Lett Drugs Ther 35:1-6, 1993.

6a. Abramowicz, M: Drugs for psychiatric disorders. Med Lett Drugs Ther 36:89-96, 1994.

7. Abrams, HL, Spiro, R, and Goldstein, N: Metastases in carcinoma. Analysis of 1000 autopsied cases. Cancer 3:74-85, 1950.
8. Abruzzese, JL, Schmidt, S, Raber, MN, et al: Phase I trial of 1-(2′deoxy-2′-fluoro-1-beta-D-arabinofuranosyl)-5-methyluracil (FMAU) terminated by severe neurological toxicity. Invest New Drugs 7:195-201, 1989.

8a. Abu-Shakra, M, Kraishi, M, Grosman, H, et al: Primary angiitis of the CNS diagnosed by angiography. QJ Med 87:351-358, 1994.

9. Ackerman, NB and Jacobs, R: The effects of steroidal and nonsteroidal anti-inflammatory agents on uptake of Evans blue in experimental metastasis. Microvasc Res 35:1-7, 1988.
10. Adachi, N: Beta-2-microglobulin levels in the cerebrospinal fluid: Their value as a disease marker. A review of the recent literature. Eur Neurol 31:181-185, 1991.
11. Adair, JC, Woodley, SL, O'Connell, JB, et al: Aseptic meningitis following cardiac transplantation: Clinical characteristics and relationship to immunosuppressive regimen. Neurology 41:249-252, 1991.
12. Adams, JW, Bofenkamp, TM, Kobrin, J, et al: Recurrent acute toxic optic neuropathy secondary to 5-FU. Letter to the Editor. Cancer Treat Rep 68:565-566, 1984.
13. Adamson, PC, Balis, FM, McCully, CL, et al: Rescue of experimental intrathecal methotrexate overdose with carboxypeptidase-G2. J Clin Oncol 9:670-674, 1991.
14. Adamus, G, Guy, J, Schmied, JL, et al: Role of anti-recoverin autoantibodies in cancer-associated retinopathy. Invest Ophthalmol Vis Sci 34:2626-2633, 1993.
15. Aderka, D, Brown, A, Zelikovski, A, et al: Idiopathic deep vein thrombosis in an apparently healthy patient as premonitory sign of occult cancer. Cancer 57:1846-1849, 1986.
16. Adler, JR, Cox, RS, Kaplan, I, et al: Stereotactic radiosurgical treatment of brain metastases. J Neurosurg 76:444-449, 1992.
17. Agamanolis, DP, Tan, JS, and Parker, DL: Immunosuppressive measles encephalitis in a patient with a renal transplant. Arch Neurol 36:686-690, 1979.
18. Ahmad, S, Laidlaw, J, Houghton, GW, et al: Involuntary movements caused by phenytoin intoxication in epileptic patients. J Neurol Neurosurg Psychiatry 38:225-231, 1975.
19. Aichner, F and Schuler, G: Primary leptomeningeal melanoma. Diagnosis by ultrastructural cytology of cerebrospinal fluid and cranial computed tomography. Cancer 50:1751-1756, 1982.
20. Aiken, R, Leavengood, JM, Kim, J-H, et al: Metronidazole in the treatment of metastatic brain tumors. Results of a controlled clinical trial. J Neurooncol 2:105-111, 1984.
21. Aisen, ML, Brown, W, and Rubin, M: Electrophysiologic changes in lumbar spinal cord after cervical cord injury. Neurology 42:623-626, 1992.
22. Aisner, J, Aisner, SC, Ostrow, S, et al: Meningeal carcinomatosis from small cell carcinoma of the lung. Consequence of improved survival. Acta Cytol 23:292-296, 1979.
23. Akihiko, O, Inoue, T, Fukuda, N, et al: A case with paraneoplastic optic neuropathy presenting bitemporal hemianopsia. Neuro-ophthalmology 11:325-328, 1991.
24. Akingbehin, AO: Corticosteroid-induced ocular hypertension. II. An acquired form. Br J Ophthalmol 66:541-545, 1982.
25. Aksamit, AJ, Jr: Nonradioactive in situ hybridization in progressive multifocal leukoencephalopathy. Mayo Clin Proc 68:899-910, 1993.
26. Al-Hakim, M and Katirji, MB: Femoral mononeuropathy induced by the lithotomy position: A report of 5 cases with a review of the literature. Muscle Nerve 16:891-895, 1993.

27. Albers, JW, Allen, AA, II, Bastron, JA, et al: Limb myokymia. Muscle Nerve 4:494-504, 1981.
28. Albert, DM, Rubenstein, RA, and Scheie, HG: Tumor metastasis to the eye. Part I: Incidence in 213 adult patients with generalized malignancy. Am J Ophthalmol 63:723-726, 1967.
29. Albert, DM, Wong, VG, and Henderson, ES: Ocular complications of vincristine therapy. Arch Ophthalmol (Copenh) 78:709-713, 1967.
30. Albert, MS, Levkoff, SE, Reilly, C, et al: The delirium symptom interview: An interview for the detection of delirium symptoms in hospitalized patients. J Geriatr Psychiatry Neurol 5:14-21, 1992.
31. Alberti, E, Hartmann, A, Schutz, HJ, et al: The effect of large doses of dexamethasone on the cerebrospinal fluid pressure in patients with supratentorial tumors. J Neurol 217:173-181, 1978.
32. Albin, RL, Bromberg, MB, Penney, JB, et al: Chorea and dystonia: A remote effect of carcinoma. Mov Disord 3:162-169, 1988.
33. Alcolado, R, Weller, RO, Parrish, EP, et al: The cranial arachnoid and pia mater in man: Anatomical and ultrastructural observations. Neuropathol Appl Neurobiol 14:1-17, 1988.
34. Aldenhovel, HG: The influence of long-term anticonvulsant therapy with diphenylhydantoin and carbamazepine on serum gamma-glutamyltransferase, aspartate aminotransferase, alanine aminotransferase and alkaline phosphatase. Eur Arch Psychiatry Clin Neurosci 237:312-316, 1988.
35. Alessi, D: Lesioni parenchimatose del cervelletto da carcinoma uterino (gliosis carcinotossica): sintomalogia dissinergico-mioclonia. Riv Patol Nerv Ment 55:148-174, 1940.
36. Alexander, JT, Saris, SC, and Oldfield, EH: The effect of interleukin-2 on the blood–brain barrier in the 9L gliosarcoma rat model. J Neurosurg 70:92-96, 1989.
37. Alexander, KR, Fishman, GA, Peachey, NS, et al: "On" response defect in paraneoplastic night blindness with cutaneous malignant melanoma. Optom Vis Sci 33:477-483, 1992.
38. Allen, JC, Miller, DC, Budzilovich, GN, et al: Brain and spinal cord hemorrhage in long-term survivors of malignant pediatric brain tumors: A possible late effect of therapy. Neurology 41:148-150, 1991.
39. Alperin, JB: Coagulopathy caused by vitamin K deficiency in critically ill, hospitalized patients. JAMA 258:1916-1919, 1987.
40. Altman, AJ and Baehner, RL: Favorable prognosis for survival in children with coincident opsomyoclonus and neuroblastoma. Cancer 37:846-852, 1976.
41. Altrocchi, PH and Eckman, PB: Meningeal carcinomatosis and blindness. J Neurol Neurosurg Psychiatry 36:206-210, 1973.
42. Amatruda, TT, Jr, Hurst, MH, and D'Esopo, ND: Certain endocrine and metabolic facets of the steroid withdrawal syndrome. J Clin Endocr 25:1207-1217, 1965.
43. American Psychiatric Association: Diagnostic and Statistical Manual of Mental Disorders, ed 3, rev. (DSM-III-R). American Psychiatric Association, Washington, DC, 1987, pp 100-103.
44. Amico, L, Caplan, LR, and Thomas, C: Cerebrovascular complications of mucinous cancers. Neurology 39:522-526, 1989.
45. Amir, J and Galbraith, RC: Paraneoplastic limbic encephalopathy as a nonmetastatic complication of small cell lung cancer. South Med J 85:1013-1014, 1992.
46. Ampil, FL: Radiotherapy for carcinomatous brachial plexopathy. A clinical study of 23 cases. Cancer 56:2185-2188, 1985.
47. Ampil, FL: Epidural compression from metastatic tumor with resultant paralysis. J Neurooncol 7:129-136, 1989.
48. An-Foraker, SH: Cytodiagnosis of malignant lesions in cerebrospinal fluid. Review and cytohistologic correlation. Acta Cytol 29:286-290, 1985.
49. Anaissie, E: Opportunistic mycoses in the immunocompromised host: Experience at a cancer center and review. Clin Infect Dis 14(Suppl 1):S43-S53, 1992.
50. Andersen, C, Astrup J. and Gyldensted, C: Quantitive MR analysis of glucocorticoid effects on peritumoral edema associated with intracranial meningiomas and metastases. J Comput Assist Tomogr 18:509-518, 1994 .
51. Anderson, ME, Naganuma, A, and Meister, A: Protection against cisplatin toxicity by administration of glutathione ester. FASEB J 4:3251-3255, 1990.
52. Anderson, NE, Budde-Steffen, C, Rosenblum, MK, et al: Opsoclonus, myoclonus, ataxia, and encephalopathy in adults with cancer: A distinct paraneoplastic syndrome. Medicine (Baltimore) 67:100-109, 1988.
53. Anderson, NE, Posner, JB, Sidtis, JJ, et al: The metabolic anatomy of paraneoplastic cerebellar degeneration. Ann Neurol 23:533-540, 1988.
54. Andiman, WA, White-Greenwald, M, and Tinghitella, T: Zoster encephalitis. Isolation of virus and measurement of varicella-zoster-specific antibodies in cerebrospinal fluid. Am J Med 73:769-772, 1982.
55. Andrews, JM and Gardner, MB: Lower motor neuron degeneration associated with type C RNA virus infection in mice: Neuropathological features. J Neuropathol Exp Neurol 33:285-307, 1974.
56. Andrykowski, MA, Schmitt, FA, Gregg, ME, et al: Neuropsychologic impairment in adult bone marrow transplant candidates. Cancer 70:2288-2297, 1992.
57. Ang, KK, Price, RE, Stephens, LC, et al: The tolerance of primate spinal cord to re-irradiation. Int J Radiat Oncol Biol Phys 25:459-464, 1993.
57a. Ang, KK and Stephens, LC: Prevention and management of radiation myelopathy. Oncology 8:71-81, 1994.
58. Ang, KK, van der Kogel, AJ, and van der Schueren, E: Effect of combined AZQ and radiation on the tolerance of the rat spinal cord. J Neurooncol 3:349-352, 1986.
59. Anonymous: Anticonvulsant osteomalacia. Lancet 2:805-806, 1972.

60. Anonymous: Mucormycosis. Ann Intern Med 93:93-108, 1980.
61. Abramowicz, M: Drugs for psychiatric disorders. Med Lett Drugs Ther 36:89-96.
62. Anonymous: Drugs that cause psychiatric symptoms. Table. Med Lett Drugs Ther 35:65-70, 1993.
63. Anonymous: Cerebrospinal fluid shunt infections. Editorial. Lancet 1:1304-1305, 1989.
63a. Antinori, A, DeLuca, A, Ammassari, A, et al: Failure of cytarabine and increased JC virus-DNA burden in the cerebrospinal fluid of patients with AIDS-related progressive multifocal leucoencephalopathy. AIDS 8:1022-1024, 1994.
64. Antoine, JC, Honnorat, J, Vocanson, C, et al: Posterior uveitis, paraneoplastic encephalomyelitis and auto-antibodies reacting with developmental protein of brain and retina. J Neurol Sci 117:215-223, 1993.
65. Aoki, N: Reversible leukoencephalopathy caused by 5-fluorouracil derivatives, presenting as akinetic mutism. Surg Neurol 25:279-282, 1986.
66. Apfel, SC, Arezzo, JC, Lipson, L, et al: Nerve growth factor prevents experimental cisplatin neuropathy. Ann Neurol 31:76-80, 1992.
67. Arbit, E, Shah, J, Bedford, R, et al: Tension pneumocephalus: Treatment with controlled decompression via a closed water-seal drainage system. Case report. J Neurosurg 74:139-142, 1991.
67a. Arbit, E, Wronski, M, Burt, M, et al: The treatment of recurrent brain metastases: A retrospective analysis of 109 patients with non-small cell lung cancer. Neurosurgery. In press, 1995.
68. Archer, BD: Computed tomography before lumbar puncture in acute meningitis: a review of the risks and benefits. Can Med Assoc J 148:961-965, 1993.
69. Archer, GE, Shuster, JM, Fuchs, HE, et al: Neuropathology of multiple versus single dose intrathecal melphalan in rats. Abstract. J Neuropathol Exp Neurol 52:298, 1993.
70. Arena, FP, Perlin, M, Brahman, H, et al: Fever, rash, and myalgias of disseminated candidiasis during antifungal therapy. Case report. Arch Intern Med 141:1233, 1981.
71. Argov, Z and Siegal, T: Leptomeningeal metastases: Peripheral nerve and root involvement—clinical and electrophysiological study. Ann Neurol 17:593-596, 1985.
72. Arguello, F, Baggs, RB, Duerst, RE, et al: Pathogenesis of vertebral metastasis and epidural spinal cord compression. Cancer 65:98-106, 1990.
73. Arguello, F, Baggs, RB, Eskenazi, AE, et al: Vascular anatomy and organ-specific tumor growth as critical factors in the development of metastases and their distribution among organs. Int J Cancer 48:583-590, 1991.
74. Arico, M, Nespoli, L, Porta F, et al: Severe acute encephalopathy following inadvertent intrathecal doxorubicin administration. Med Pediatr Oncol 18:261-263, 1990.
75. Arieff, AI and Ayus, JC: Pathogenesis of hyponatremic encephalopathy: Current concepts. Chest 103:607-610, 1993.
76. Arieff, AI and Carroll, JH: Cerebral edema and depression of sensorium in nonketotic hyperosmolar coma. Diabetes 23:525-531, 1974.
77. Arieff, AI and Griggs, RC (eds): Metabolic Brain Dysfunction in Systemic Disorders. Little, Brown & Company, Boston, 1992.
78. Ariel, IM: Intra-arterial chemotherapy for metastatic cancer to the brain. Am J Surg 102:647-650, 1961.
79. Arita, N, Ushio, Y, Hayakawa, T, et al: Intrathecal ACNU—A new therapeutic approach against malignant leptomeningeal tumors. J Neurooncol 6:221-226, 1988.
80. Ariza, J, Casanova, A, Fernandez Viladrich, P, et al: Etiological agent and primary source of infection in 42 cases of focal intracranial suppuration. J Clin Microbiol 24:899-902, 1986.
80a. Armstrong, C, Mollman, J, Corn, BW, et al: Effects of radiation therapy on adult brain behavior: Evidence for a rebound phenomenon in a phase 1 trial. Neurology 43:1961-1965, 1993.
81. Armstrong, D: Problems in management of opportunistic fungal diseases. Rev Infect Dis 11(Suppl 7):S1591-S1599, 1989.
82. Armstrong, D and Polsky, B: Central nervous system infections in the compromised host. In Rubin, RH and Young, LS (eds): Clinical Approach to Infection in the Compromised Host. Plenum Publishing Corp, 1987, pp 163-194.
83. Armstrong, JG, Fass, DE, Bains, M, et al: Paraspinal tumors: Techniques and results of brachytherapy. Int J Radiat Oncol Biol Phys 20:787-790, 1991.
83a. Armstrong, JG, Wronski, M. Galicich, J, et al: Postoperative radiation for lung cancer metastatic to the brain. J Clin Oncol 12:2340-2344, 1994.
84. Arndt, CA, Colvin, OM, Balis, FM, et al: Intrathecal administration of 4-hydroperoxycyclophosphamide in rhesus monkeys. Cancer Res 47:5932-5934, 1987.
85. Arnold, AC, Hepler, RS, and Foos, RY: Isolated metastasis to the optic nerve. Surv Ophthalmol 26:75-83, 1981.
86. Aroney, RS, Dalley, DN, Chan, WK, et al: Meningeal carcinomatosis in small cell carcinoma of the lung. Am J Med 71:26-32, 1981.
87. Arseni, C and Maretsis, M: Focal epileptic seizures ipsilateral to the tumour. Acta Neurochir 49:47-60, 1979.
88. Arseni, C and Stanciu, M: Particular clinical aspects of chronic subdural haematoma in adults. Eur Neurol 2:109-122, 1969.
89. Asai, A, Matsutani, M, Kohno, T, et al: Subacute brain atrophy after radiation therapy for malignant brain tumor. Cancer 63:1962-1974, 1989.
90. Asato, R, Akiyama, Y, Ito, M, et al: Nuclear magnetic resonance abnormalities of the cerebral white matter in children with acute lymphoblastic leukemia and malignant lymphoma during and after central nervous system prophylactic treatment with intrathecal methotrexate. Cancer 70:1997-2004, 1992.
91. Ashdown, BC, Boyko, OB, Uglietta, JP, et al: Postradiation cerebellar necrosis mimicking tumor: MR appearance. J Comput Assist Tomogr 17:124-126, 1993.
92. Ashford, AR, Doney, I, Tiwari, RP, et al: Reversible ocular toxicity related to tamoxifen therapy. Cancer 61:33-35, 1988.

93. Ashton, N and Morgan, G: Discrete carcinomatous metastases in the extraocular muscles. Br J Ophthalmol 58:112-117, 1974.
94. Askari, A, Vignos, PJ, Jr, and Moskowitz, RW: Steroid myopathy in connective tissue disease. Am J Med 61:485-492, 1976.
95. Assa, J: The intercostobrachial nerve in radical mastectomy. J Surg Oncol 6:123-126, 1974.
96. Athanassiou, A, Begent, RH, Newlands, ES, et al: Central nervous system metastases of choriocarcinoma. 23 years' experience at Charing Cross Hospital. Cancer 52:1728-1735, 1983.
97. Atkins, MB, Vachino, G, Tilg, HJ, et al: Phase I evaluation of thrice-daily intravenous bolus interleukin-4 in patients with refractory malignancy. J Clin Oncol 10:1802-1809, 1992.
98. Atkinson, JL, Sundt, TM, Jr, Dale, AJ, et al: Radiation-associated atheromatous disease of the cervical carotid artery: Report of seven cases and review of the literature. Neurosurgery 24:171-178, 1989.
99. Atkinson, JL, Sundt, TM, Jr, Kazmier, FJ, et al: Heparin-induced thrombocytopenia and thrombosis in ischemic stroke. Mayo Clin Proc 63:353-361, 1988.
100. Atkinson, M: Meniere's famous autopsy and its interpretation. Arch Otolaryngol 42:186-187, 1945.
101. Atlas, SW, Grossman, RI, Gomori, JM, et al: Hemorrhagic intracranial malignant neoplasms: Spin-echo MR imaging. Radiology 164:71-77, 1987.
102. Atweh, GF and Jabbour, N: Intracranial solitary extraskeletal plasmacytoma resembling meningioma. Arch Neurol 39:57-59, 1982.
103. Augsburger, JJ: Differential diagnosis of choroidal neoplasms. Oncology (Huntingt) 5:87-98, 1991.
104. Aurelius, E, Johansson, B, Skoldenberg, B, et al: Rapid diagnosis of herpes simplex encephalitis by nested polymerase chain reaction assay of cerebrospinal fluid. Lancet 337:189-192, 1991.
105. Avvisati, G, ten Cate, JW, Buller, HR, et al: Tranexamic acid for control of haemorrhage in acute promyelocytic leukaemia. Lancet 2:122-124, 1989.
106. Axelrod, L: Glucocorticoid therapy. Medicine (Baltimore) 55:39-65, 1976.
106a. Ayres, RCS, Dousset, B., Wixon, S, et al: Peripheral neurotoxicity with tacrolimus. Lancet 343:862-863, 1994.
107. Ayus, JC and Arieff, AI: Pathogenesis and prevention of hyponatremic encephalopathy. Endocrinal Metab Clin North Am 22:425-446, 1993.
108. Aznavoorian, S, Murphy, AN, Stetler-Stevenson, WG, et al: Molecular aspects of tumor cell invasion and metastasis. Cancer 71:1368-1379, 1993.
109. Azzarelli, B, Itani, A-L, and Catanzaro, PT: Cerebral phlebothrombosis. A complication of lymphoma. Arch Neurol 37:126-127, 1980.
110. Azzarelli, B, Mirkin DL, Goheen, M, et al: The leptomeningeal vein. A site of re-entry of leukemic cells into the systemic circulation. Cancer 54:1333-1343, 1984.
111. Azzarelli, B, Moore, J, Gilmor, R, et al: Multiple fusiform intracranial aneurysms following curative radiation therapy for suprasellar germinoma. Case report. J Neurosurg 61:1141-1145, 1984.
112. Azzarelli, B and Roessmann, U: Pathogenesis of central nervous system infiltration in acute leukemia. Arch Pathol Lab Med 101:203-205, 1977.
113. Baba, T, Chio, C-C, and Black, KL: The effect of 5-lipoxygenase inhibition on blood–brain barrier permeability in experimental brain tumors. J Neurosurg 77:403-406, 1992.
114. Babikian, VL, Stefansson, K, Dieperink, ME, et al: Paraneoplastic myelopathy: Antibodies against protein in normal spinal cord and underlying neoplasm. Letter to the Editor. Lancet 2:49-50, 1985.
115. Babul, N and Darke, AC: Putative role of hydromorphone metabolites in myoclonus. Letter to the Editor. Pain 48-49:260-261, 1992.
116. Bach, F, Agerlin, N, Sorenson, JB, et al: Metastatic spinal cord compression secondary to lung cancer. J Clin Oncol 10:1781-1787, 1992.
117. Bach, F, Larsen, BH, Rohde, K, et al: Metastatic spinal cord compression. Occurrence, symptoms, clinical presentations and prognosis in 398 patients with spinal cord compression. Acta Neurochir 107:37-43, 1990.
118. Bach, F, Soletormos, G, Bach, FW, et al: TPA and CK-BB: New tumor markers in leptomeningeal carcinomatosis secondary to breast cancer. Letter to the Editor. J Natl Cancer Inst 82:320-322, 1990.
119. Bach, F, Soletormos, G, and Dombernowsky, P: Tissue polypeptide antigen activity in cerebrospinal fluid: A marker of central nervous system metastases of breast cancer. J Natl Cancer Inst 83:779-784, 1991.
120. Bach, MC and Davis, KM: *Listeria* rhombencephalitis mimicking tuberculous meningitis. Rev Infect Dis 9:130-133, 1987.
121. Bady, B, Chauplannaz, G, and Vial, C: Autoimmune aetiology for acquired neuromyotonia. Letter to the Editor. Lancet 338:1330, 1991.
122. Baer, MR, Stein, RS, and Dessypris, EN: Chronic lymphocytic leukemia with hyperleukocytosis. The hyperviscosity syndrome. Cancer 56:2865-2869, 1985.
123. Baethge, BA and Lidsky, MD: Intractable hiccups associated with high-dose intravenous methylprednisolone therapy. Ann Intern Med 104:58-59, 1986.
124. Bagenal, FS, Easton, DF, Harris, E, et al: Survival of patients with breast cancer attending Bristol Cancer Help Centre. Lancet 336:606-610, 1990.
125. Bagley, FH, Walsh, JW, Cady, B, et al: Carcinomatous versus radiation-induced brachial plexus neuropathy in breast cancer. Cancer 41:2154-2157, 1978.
126. Baharav, E, Harpaz, D, Mittelman, M, et al: Dexamethasone-induced perineal irritation. N Engl J Med 314:515-516, 1986.
127. Bain, PG, Colchester, AC, and Nadarajah, D: Paraplegia after iopamidol myelography. Letter to the Editor. Lancet 338:252-253, 1991.
128. Bairey, O, Kremer, I, Rakowsky, E, et al: Orbital and adnexal involvement in systemic non-Hodgkin's lymphoma. Cancer 73:2395-2399, 1994.
129. Bakay, L: Olfactory meningiomas. The missed diagnosis. JAMA 251:53-55, 1984.
130. Baker, WF, Jr: Clinical aspects of disseminated

intravascular coagulation: A clinician's point of view. Semin Thromb Hemostas 15:1-57, 1989.
131. Baker, WJ, Royer, GL, Jr, and Weiss, RB: Cytarabine and neurologic toxicity. J Clin Oncol 9:679-693, 1991.
132. Bakheit, AM, Kennedy, PG, and Behan, PO: Paraneoplastic limbic encephalitis: Clinico-pathological correlations. J Neurol Neurosurg Psychiatry 53:1084-1088, 1990.
133. Balch, CM: Surgical management of regional lymph nodes in cutaneous melanoma. J Am Acad Dermatol 3:511-524, 1980.
134. Balducci, L, Little, DD, Khansur, T, et al: Carcinomatous meningitis in small cell lung cancer. Am J Med Sci 287:31-33, 1984.
135. Bale, JF, Jr: Human cytomegalovirus infection and disorders of the nervous system. Arch Neurol 41:310-320, 1984.
136. Balhuizen, JC, Bots, GT, Schaberg, A, et al: Value of cerebrospinal fluid cytology for the diagnosis of malignancies in the central nervous system. J Neurosurg 48:747-753, 1978.
137. Balis, FM, Lester, CM, Chrousos, GP, et al: Differences in cerebrospinal fluid penetration of corticosteroids: Possible relationship to the prevention of meningeal leukemia. J Clin Oncol 5:202-207, 1987.
138. Balis, FM, Lester, CM, and Poplack, DG: Pharmacokinetics of trimetrexate (NSC 352122) in monkeys. Cancer Res 46:169-174, 1986.
139. Balis, FM, Savitch, JL, Bleyer, WA, et al: Remission induction of meningeal leukemia with high-dose intravenous methotrexate. J Clin Oncol 3:485-489, 1985.
140. Balmaceda, CM, Walker, RW, Castro-Malaspina, H, et al: Reversal of amphotericin-B-related encephalopathy. Neurology 44:1183-1184, 1994.
141. Balsom, WR, Bleyer, WA, Robison, LL, et al: Intellectual function in long-term survivors of childhood acute lymphoblastic leukemia: Protective effect of pre-irradiation methotrexate? A Childrens Cancer Study Group study. Med Pediatr Oncol 19:486-492, 1991.
142. Band, PR, Holland, JF, Bernard, J, et al: Treatment of central nervous system leukemia with intrathecal cytosine arabinoside. Cancer 32:744-748, 1973.
143. Bansal S, Brady, LW, Olsen, A, et al: The treatment of metastatic spinal cord tumors. JAMA 202:686-688, 1967.
144. Baram, TZ, van Tassel, P, and Jaffe, NA: Brain metastases in osteosarcoma: Incidence, clinical and neuroradiological findings and management options. J Neurooncol 6:47-52, 1988.
145. Barbe, B, Lejoyeux, M, Bouleau, JH, et al: Visual hallucination related to severe hypophosphataemia. Letter to the Editor. Lancet 338:1083, 1991.
146. Barbui, T, Rambaldi, A, Parenzan, L, et al: Neurological symptoms and coma associated with doxorubicin administration during chronic cyclosporin therapy. Letter to the Editor. Lancet 339:1421, 1992.
147. Barclay, CL, McLean, M, Hagen, N, et al: Severe phenytoin hypersensitivity with myopathy: A case report. Neurology 42:2303, 1992.
148. Barnard, RO and Parsons, M: Carcinoma of the thyroid with leptomeningeal dissemination following the treatment of a toxic goitre with 131-I and methyl thiouracil. Case with a co-existing intracranial dermoid. J Neurol Sci 8:299-306, 1969.
149. Barnett, MJ, Richards, MA, Ganesan, TS, et al: Central nervous system toxicity of high-dose cytosine arabinoside. Semin Oncol 12(2 Suppl 3):227-232, 1985.
150. Barnicoat, MJ, Wierzbicki, AS, and Norman, PM: Cerebral nocardiosis in immunosuppressed patients: Five cases. Q J Med 72:689-698, 1989.
150a. Barohn, RJ, Jackson, CE, Rogers, SJ, et al: Prolonged paralysis due to nondepolarizing neuromuscular blocking agents and corticosteroids. Muscle Nerve 17:647-654, 1994.
151. Barron, KD, Hirano, A, Araski, S, et al: Experiences with metastatic neoplasms involving the spinal cord. Neurology 9:91-106, 1959.
152. Barron, KD and Rodichok, LD: Cancer and disorders of motor neurons. In Rowland, LP (ed): Human Motor Neuron Diseases. Raven Press, New York, 1982, pp 267-272.
153. Barron, KD, Rowland, LP, and Zimmerman, HM: Neuropathy with malignant tumor metastases. J Nerv Ment Dis 131:10-31, 1960.
154. Barron, SA and Heffner, RR, Jr: Weakness in malignancy: Evidence for a remote effect of tumor on distal axons. Ann Neurol 4:268-274, 1978.
155. Barrow, HN and Levenson, MJ: Necrotizing "malignant" external otitis caused by *Staphylococcus epidermidis*. Arch Otolaryngol Head Neck Surg 118:94-96, 1992.
156. Barton, JC, Conrad, ME, and Poon, M-C: Pseudochloroma: Extramedullary hematopoietic nodules in chronic myelogenous leukemia. Ann Intern Med 91:735-738, 1979.
157. Bashe, MA and Popovich, J, Jr: Managing intracranial hypertension to avoid neurologic sequelae. Journal of Critical Illness 6:68-88, 1991.
158. Bataini, JP, Ennuyer, A, Poncet, P, et al: Treatment of supraglottic cancer by radical high dose radiotherapy. Cancer 33:1253-1262, 1974.
159. Bateman, DE, Weller, RO, and Kennedy, P: Stiffman syndrome: A rare paraneoplastic disorder? J Neurol Neurosurg Psychiatry 53:695-696, 1990.
160. Bates, S, McKeever, P, Masur, H, et al: Myelopathy following intrathecal chemotherapy in a patient with extensive Burkitt's lymphoma and altered immune status. Am J Med 78:697-702, 1985.
161. Bates, S, Raphaelson, MI, Price, RA, et al: Ascending myelopathy after chemotherapy for central nervous system acute lymphoblastic leukemia: Correlation with cerebrospinal fluid myelin basic protein. Med Pediatr Oncol 13:4-8, 1985.
162. Bates, T: A review of local radiotherapy in the treatment of bone metastases and cord compression. Int J Radiat Oncol Biol Phys 23:217-221, 1992.
163. Batsakis, JG: Nerves and neurotropic carcinomas. Ann Otol Rhinol Laryngol 94:426-427, 1985.
164. Batson, CV: Function of vertebral veins and their role in spread of metastases. Ann Surg 112:138-149, 1940.

165. Bauherz, G, Soeur, M, and Lustman, F: Oculomotor nerve paralysis induced by alpha II-interferon. Acta Neurol Belg 90:111-114, 1990.
166. Baum, M: New approach for recruitment into randomised controlled trials. Lancet 341:812-813, 1993.
167. Bauman, ML and Price, TR: Intracranial metastatic malignant melanoma: Long-term survival following subtotal resection. South Med J 65:344-346, 1972.
167a. Beal, JE, Olson, R, Laubenstein, L, et al: Dronabinol as a treatment for anorexia associated with weight loss in patients with AIDS. Journal of Pain Symptom Management. In press, 1995.
168. Beamish, NG, Stolinski, C, Thomas, PK, et al: Freeze-fracture observations on normal and abnormal human perineurial tight junctions: Alterations in diabetic polyneuropathy. Acta Neuropathol (Berl) 81:269-279, 1991.
169. Beck, RW and Greenberg, HS: Post-decompression optic neuropathy. J Neurosurg 63:196-199, 1985.
170. Beck, WT and Kuttesch, JF: Neurological symptoms associated with cyclosporin plus doxorubicin. Letter to the Editor. Lancet 340:496, 1992.
171. Becker, DM, Philbrick, JT, and Selby, JB: Inferior vena cava filters. Indications, safety, effectiveness. Arch Intern Med 152:1985-1994, 1992.
172. Becker, JC, Winkler, B, Klingert, S, et al: Antiphospholipid syndrome associated with immunotherapy for patients with melanoma. Cancer 73:1621-1624, 1994.
173. Beckloff, GL, Lerner, HJ, Frost, D, et al: Hydroxyurea (NSC-32065) in biologic fluids: Dose-concentration relationship. Cancer Chemotherapy Reports 48:57-58, 1963.
174. Beggs, JL and Waggener, JD: Transendothelial vesicular transport of protein following compression injury to the spinal cord. Lab Invest 34:428-439, 1976.
175. Beidler, LM and Smith, JC: Effects of radiation therapy and drugs on cell turnover and taste. In Getchell, TV, Doty, RL, Bartoshuk, LM, et al (eds): Smell and Taste in Health and Disease. Raven Press, New York, 1991, pp 753-763.
176. Bell, WR, Starksen, NF, Tong, S, et al: Trousseau's syndrome. Devastating coagulopathy in the absence of heparin. Am J Med 79:423-430, 1985.
177. Bellet, RE, Mastrangelo, MJ, Engstrom, PF, et al: Hepatotoxicity of 5-azacytidine (NSC-102816) (a clinical and pathologic study). Neoplasma 20:303-309, 1973.
178. Bellin, SL, and Selim, M: Cisplatin-induced hypomagnesemia with seizures: A case report and review of the literature. Gynecol Oncol 30:104-113, 1988.
179. Bellur, SN, Chandra, V, and McDonald, LW: Association of meningiomas with extraneural primary malignancy. Neurology 29:1165-1168, 1979.
180. Belt, RJ, Leite, C, Haas, CD, et al: Incidence of hemorrhagic complications in patients with cancer. JAMA 239:2571-2574, 1978.
181. Bender, BL and Mayernik, DG: Hodgkin's disease presenting with isolated craniospinal involvement. Cancer 58:1745-1748, 1986.
182. Bender, CE, Berquist, TH, and Wold, LE: Imaging-assisted percutaneous biopsy of the thoracic spine. Mayo Clin Proc 61:942-950, 1986.
183. Benger, A, Browman, GP, Walker, IR, et al: Clinical evidence of a cumulative effect of high-dose cytarabine on the cerebellum in patients with acute leukemia. A leukemia intergroup report. Cancer Treat Rep 69:240-241, 1985.
184. Benjamin, JC, Moss, T, Moseley, RP, et al: Cerebral distribution of immunoconjugate after treatment for neoplastic meningitis using an intrathecal radiolabeled monoclonal antibody. Neurosurgery 25:253-258, 1989.
185. Benowitz, NL: Central nervous system manifestations of toxic disorders. In Arieff, AI and Griggs, RC (eds): Metabolic Brain Dysfunction in Systemic Disorders. Little, Brown & Company, Boston, 1992, pp 409-436.
186. Benzel, EC: The lateral extracavitary approach to the spine using the three-quarter prone position. J Neurosurg 71:837-841, 1989.
187. Berg, RA, Ch'ien, LT, Lancaster, W, et al: Neuropsychological sequelae of postradiation somnolence syndrome. J Dev Behav Pediatr 4:103-107, 1983.
188. Berg, SL, Balis, FM, Zimm, S, et al: Phase I/II trial and pharmacokinetics of intrathecal diaziquone in refractory meningeal malignancies. J Clin Oncol 10:143-148, 1992.
189. Berger, PS and Bataini, JP: Radiation-induced cranial nerve palsy. Cancer 40:152-155, 1977.
190. Bergevin, PR, Patwardhan, VC, Weissman, J, et al: Neurotoxicity of 5-fluorouracil. Letter to the Editor. Lancet 1:410, 1975.
191. Berlinger, NT, Koutroupas, S, Adams, G, et al: Patterns of involvement of the temporal bone in metastatic and systemic malignancy. Laryngoscope 90:619-627, 1980.
192. Berlit, P and Schwechheimer, K: Neuropathological findings in radiation myelopathy of the lumbosacral cord. Eur Neurol 27:29-34, 1987.
193. Berman, E: Idarubicin. Principles and Practice of Oncology. 6(5):1-10, 1992.
194. Berman, IJ and Mann, MP: Seizures and transient cortical blindness associated with cis-platinum (II) Diamminedichloride (PDD) therapy in a thirty-year-old man. Cancer 45:764-766, 1980.
195. Bernard, JT, Ameriso, S, Kempf, RA, et al: Transient focal neurologic deficits complicating interleukin-2 therapy. Neurology 40:154-155, 1990.
196. Bernat JL, Greenberg, ER, and Barrett, J: Suspected epidural compression of the spinal cord and cauda equina by metastatic carcinoma. Clinical diagnosis and survival. Cancer 51:1953-1957, 1983.
197. Bernat, JL, Sadowsky, CH, Vincent, FM, et al: Sclerosing spinal pachymeningitis. A complication of intrathecal administration of Depo-Medrol for multiple sclerosis. J Neurol Neurosurg Psychiatry 39:1124-1128, 1976.
198. Bernsen, PL, Wong Chung, RE, Vingerhoets, HM, et al: Bilateral neuralgic amyotrophy induced by interferon treatment. Arch Neurol 45:449-451, 1988.
199. Bernstein, IL: Etiology of anorexia in cancer. Cancer 58(Suppl 8):1881-1886, 1986.

200. Bernstein, M and Gutin, PH: Interstitial irradiation of skull base tumours. Can J Neurol Sci 12:366-370, 1985.
201. Bernstein, M and Laperriere, N: Radiation-induced tumors of the nervous system. In Gutin, PH, Leibel, SA, and Sheline, GE (eds): Radiation Injury to the Nervous System. Raven Press, New York, 1991, pp 455-472.
202. Bernstein, ML, Sobel, DB, and Wimmer, RS: Noncardiogenic pulmonary edema following injection of methotrexate into the cerebrospinal fluid. Cancer 50:866-868, 1982.
203. Berrettini, WH, Simmons-Alling, S, and Nurnberger, JI, Jr: Epidural blood patch does not prevent headache after lumbar puncture. Letter to the Editor. Lancet 1:856-857, 1987.
204. Berry, HC, Parker, RG, and Gerdes, AJ: Irradiation of brain metastases. Acta Radiol Ther Phys Biol 13:535-544, 1974.
205. Berry, MP and Jenkin, RD: Parameningeal rhabdomyosarcoma in the young. Cancer 48:281-288, 1981.
206. Berson, EL and Lessell, S: Paraneoplastic night blindness with malignant melanoma. Am J Ophthalmol 106:307-311, 1988.
207. Best, T and Finlayson, M: Two forms of encephalitis in opportunistic toxoplasmosis. Arch Pathol Lab Med 103:693-696, 1979.
208. Bethlenfalvay, NC and Bergin, JJ: Severe cerebral toxicity after intravenous nitrogen mustard therapy. Cancer 29:366-369, 1972.
209. Betz, AL: An overview of the multiple functions of the blood–brain barrier. In Frankenheim, J and Brown, RM (eds): Bioavailability of Drugs to the Brain and the Blood–Brain Barrier. National Institute on Drug Abuse Research Monograph Series, No. 120, United States Department of Health and Human Services, Washington D.C., 1992, pp 54-72.
210. Beuche, W, Thomas, RS, and Felgenhauer, K: Demonstration of zoster virus antibodies in cerebrospinal fluid cells. J Neurol 236:26-28, 1989.
211. Beyer, RA, Paden, P, Sobel, DF, et al: Moyamoya pattern of vascular occlusion after radiotherapy for glioma of the optic chiasm. Neurology 36:1173-1178, 1986.
212. Bick, RL: Coagulation abnormalities in malignancy: A review. Semin Thromb Hemostas 18: 353-372, 1992.
213. Bigotte, L, Arvidson, B, and Olsson, Y: Cytofluorescence localization of adriamycin in the nervous system. I. Distribution of the drug in the central nervous system of normal adult mice after intravenous injection. Acta Neuropathol (Berl) 57:121-129, 1982.
214. Bigotte, L, and Olsson, Y: Degeneration of trigeminal ganglion neurons caused by retrograde axonal transport of doxorubicin. Neurology 37:985-992, 1987.
215. Bigotte, L and Olsson, Y: Distribution and toxic effects of intravenously injected epirubicin on the central nervous system of the mouse. Brain 112:457-469, 1989.
216. Bilazarian, SD, Mittal, S, and Mills, RM, Jr.: Recognizing the extrarenal hazards of intravascular contrast agents. Journal of Critical Illness 6:859-869, 1991.
217. Biller, J, Challa, VR, Toole, JF, et al: Nonbacterial thrombotic endocarditis: A neurologic perspective of clinicipathologic correlations of 99 patients. Arch Neurol 39:95-98, 1982.
218. Bilsky, M and Posner, JB: Intensive and postoperative care of intracranial tumors. In Ropper, A (ed): Neurological and Neurosurgical Intensive Care, ed 3. Raven Press, New York, 1993, pp 309-329.
219. Bindal, RK, Sawaya, R, Leavens, ME, et al: Surgical treatment of multiple brain metastases. J Neurosurg 79:210-216, 1993.
220. Bindoff, LA and Hesteltine, D: Unilateral facial pain in patients with lung cancer: A referred pain via the vagus? Lancet 1:812-815, 1988.
221. Bissett, D, Setanoians, A, Cassidy, J, et al: Phase I and pharmacokinetic study of taxotere (RP 56976) administered as a 24-hour infusion. Cancer Res 53:532-537, 1993.
222. Bixenman, WW, Nicholls, JV, and Warwick, OH: Oculomotor disturbances associated with 5-fluorouracil chemotherapy. Am J Ophthalmol 83:789-793, 1977.
223. Black, FO, Myers, EN, Schramm, VL, et al: Cisplatin vestibular ototoxicity: Preliminary report. Laryngoscope 92:1363-1368, 1982.
224. Black, KL, Hoff, JT, McGillicuddy, JE, et al: Increased leukotriene C4 and vasogenic edema surrounding brain tumors in humans. Ann Neurol 19:592-595, 1986.
225. Black, KL, King, WA, and Ikezaki, K: Selective opening of the blood-tumor barrier by intracarotid infusion of leukotriene C4. Acta Neurochir 51(Suppl): 140-141, 1990.
226. Black, PM, Crowell, RM, and Abbott, WM: External pneumatic calf compression reduces deep venous thrombosis in patients with ruptured intracranial aneurysms. Neurosurgery 18:25-28, 1986.
227. Blade, J, Gaston, F, Montserrat, E, et al: Spinal subarachnoid hematoma after lumbar puncture causing reversible paraplegia in acute leukemia. Case report. J Neurosurg 54:438-439, 1983.
228. Blakemore, WF and Patterson, RC: Suppression of remyelination in the CNS by X-irradiation. Acta Neuropath (Berl) 42:105-113, 1978.
229. Blaney, SM, Balis, FM, and Poplack, DG: Pharmacologic approaches to the treatment of meningeal malignancy. Oncology (Huntingt) 5:107-116, 1991.
230. Blasberg, RG, Groothuis, D, and Molnar, P: A review of hyperosmotic blood-brain-barrier disruption in seven experimental brain tumor models. In Johansson, BB, Owman, CH, and Widner, H (eds): Pathophysiology of the Blood-Brain-Barrier, vol 20. Elsevier Biomedical Division, Amsterdam, The Netherlands, 1990, pp 197-220.
231. Bleck, TP: Metabolic encephalopathy. In Weiner, WJ (ed): Emergent and Urgent Neurology. JB Lippincott, Philadelphia, 1992, pp 27-49.
232. Bleck, TP: Neurologic complications of critical medical illnesses. In Ropper, AH (ed): Neurological and Neurosurgical Intensive Care , ed 3. Raven Press, New York, 1993, pp 193-201.

233. Bleck, TP and Jacobsen, J: Prolonged survival following the inadvertent intrathecal administration of vincristine: Clinical and electrophysiologic analyses. Clin Neuropharmacol 14:457-462, 1991.
234. Bleck, TP, Smith, MC, Pierre-Louis, SJ, et al: Neurologic complications of critical medical illnesses. Crit Care Med 21:98-103, 1993.
235. Bleyer, WA: Clinical pharmacology of intrathecal methotrexate. II. An improved dosage regimen derived from age-related pharmacokinetics. Cancer Treat Rep 61:1419-1425, 1977.
236. Bleyer, WA: Current status of intrathecal chemotherapy for human meningeal neoplasms. Natl Cancer Inst Monogr 46:171-178, 1977.
237. Bleyer, WA: Neurologic sequelae of methotrexate and ionizing radiation: A new classification. Cancer Treat Rep 65(Suppl I):89-98, 1981.
238. Bleyer, WA, Coccia, PF, Sather, HN, et al: Reduction in central nervous system leukemia with a pharmacokinetically derived intrathecal methotrexate dosage regimen. J Clin Oncol 1:317-325, 1983.
239. Bleyer, WA and Griffin, TW: White matter necrosis, mineralizing microangiopathy, and intellectual abilities in survivors of childhood leukemia: Associations with central nervous system irradiation and methotrexate therapy. In Gilbert, HA and Kagan, AR (eds): Radiation Damage to the Nervous System. A Delayed Therapeutic Hazard. Raven Press, New York, 1980, pp 155-174.
240. Bleyer, WA and Poplack, DG: Intraventricular versus intralumbar methotrexate for central-nervous-system leukemia: Prolonged remission with the Ommaya reservoir. Med Pediatr Oncol 6:207-213, 1979.
241. Bleyer, WA and Poplack, DG: Prophylaxis and treatment of leukemia in the central nervous system and other sanctuaries. Semin Oncol 12:131-148, 1985.
242. Blumenfeld, AM, Recht, LD, Chad, DA, et al: Coexistence of Lambert-Eaton myasthenic syndrome and subacute cerebellar degeneration: Differential effects of treatment. Neurology 41:1682-1685, 1991.
243. Blumenreich, MS, Woodcock, TM, Sherrill, EJ, et al: A phase I trial of chlorambucil administered in short pulses in patients with advanced malignancies. Cancer Invest 6:371-375, 1988.
244. Bluming, AZ and Zeegen, PL: Cataracts induced by intermittent Decadron used as an antiemetic. J Clin Oncol 4:221-223, 1986.
245. Boarini, DJ, Beck, DW, and VanGilder, JC: Postoperative prophylactic anticonvulsant therapy in cerebral gliomas. Neurosurgery 16:290-292, 1985.
246. Boccardo, M, Ruelle, A, Mariotti, E, et al: Spinal carcinomatous metastases. Retrospective study of 67 surgically treated cases. J Neurooncol 3:251-257, 1985.
247. Bock, G and Whelan, J (eds): Metastasis. Ciba Foundation Symposium. John Wiley & Sons, New York, 1988.
248. Bode, U, Magrath, IT, Bleyer, WA, et al: Active transport of methotrexate from cerebrospinal fluid in humans. Cancer Res 40:2184-2187, 1980.
249. Bodsch, W, Rommel, T, Ophoff, BG, et al: Factors responsible for the retention of fluid in human tumor edema and the effect of dexamethasone. J Neurosurg 67:250-257, 1987.
250. Boghen, D, Sebag, M, and Michaud, J: Paraneoplastic optic neuritis and encephalomyelitis. Arch Neurol 45:353-356, 1988.
251. Boland, PJ, Lane, JM, and Sundaresan, N: Metastatic disease of the spine. Clin Orthop 169:95-102, 1982.
252. Boldrey, E, and Sheline, G: Delayed transitory clinical manifestations after radiation treatment of intracranial tumors. Acta Radiol 5:5-10, 1966.
253. Boldt, HC and Nerad, JA: Orbital metastases from prostate carcinoma. Arch Ophthalmol 106:1403-1408, 1988.
254. Bolivar, R, Bodey, GP, and Velasquez, WS: Recurrent *Salmonella* meningitis in a compromised host. Cancer 50:2034-2036, 1982.
255. Bollini, P, Riva, R, Albani, F, et al: Decreased phenytoin level during antineoplastic therapy: A case report. Epilepsia 24:75-76, 1983.
256. Bolton, CF and Young, GB: Neurological Complications of Renal Disease. Butterworths, Boston, 1990.
257. Bolton, CF, Young, GB, and Zochodne, DW: The neurological complications of sepsis. Ann Neurol 33:94-100, 1993.
258. Bolze, MS, Fosmire, GJ, Stryker, JA, et al: Taste acuity, plasma zinc levels, and weight loss during radiotherapy: A study of relationships. Radiology 144:163-169, 1982.
259. Bonadio, WA: The cerebrospinal fluid: physiologic aspects and alterations associated with bacterial meningitis. Pediatr Infect Dis J 11:423-431, 1992.
260. Bongers, KM, Willigers, HMM, and Koehler, PJ: Referred facial pain from lung carcinoma. Neurology 42:1841-1842, 1992.
261. Boogerd, W, Dalesio, O, Bais, EM, et al: Response of brain metastases from breast cancer to systemic chemotherapy. Cancer 69:972-980, 1992.
262. Boogerd, W, Hart, AA, van der Sande, JJ, et al: Meningeal carcinomatosis in breast cancer. Prognostic factors and influence of treatment. Cancer 67:1685-1695, 1991.
263. Boogerd, W, Moffie, D, and Smets, LA: Early blindness and coma during intrathecal chemotherapy for meningeal carcinomatosis. Cancer 65:452-457, 1990.
264. Boogerd, W, ten Bokkel Huinink, WW, Dalesio, O, et al: Cisplatin induced neuropathy: Central, peripheral and autonomic nerve involvement. J Neurooncol 9:255-263, 1990.
265. Boogerd, W, van der Sande, JJ, and Kroger, R: Early diagnosis and treatment of spinal epidural metastasis in breast cancer: A prospective study. J Neurol Neurosurg Psychiatry 55:1188-1193, 1992.
266. Boogerd, W, van der Sande, JJ, and Moffie, D: Acute fever and delayed leukoencephalopathy following low dose intraventricular methotrexate. J Neurol Neurosurg Psychiatry 51:1277-1283, 1988.
267. Boogerd, W, Vos, VW, Hart, AAM, et al: Brain metastases in breast cancer; natural history, prognostic factors and outcome. J Neurooncol 15:165-174, 1993.
268. Boogerd, W, Vroom, TM, van Heerde, PV, et al:

CSF cytology versus immunocytochemistry in meningeal carcinomatosis. J Neurol Neurosurg Psychiatry 51:142-145, 1988.
269. Boranic, M and Raci, F: A Parkinson-like syndrome as side effect of chemotherapy with vincristine and adriamycin in a child with acute leukaemia. Biomedicine 31:124-125, 1979.
270. Borgeat, A, DeMuralt, B, and Stalder, M: Peripheral neuropathy associated with high-dose Ara-C therapy. Cancer 58:852-854, 1986.
271. Borgelt, B, Gelber, R, Kramer, S, et al: The palliation of brain metastases: Final results of the first two studies by the Radiation Therapy Oncology Group. Int J Radiat Oncol Biol Phys 6:1-9, 1980.
272. Borgelt, B, Gelber, R, Larson, M, et al: Ultra-rapid high dose irradiation schedules for the palliation of brain metastases: Final results of the first two studies by the Radiation Therapy Oncology Group. Int J Radiat Oncol Biol Phys 7:1633-1638, 1981.
273. Borges, AA, Krasnow, SH, Wadleigh, RG, et al: Nocardiosis after corticosteroid therapy for malignant thymoma. Cancer 71:1746-1750, 1993.
274. Boring, CC, Squires, TS, Tong, T, et al: Cancer statistics, 1994. CA Cancer J Clin 44:7-26, 1994.
275. Borsanyi, SJ and Blanchard, CL: Ionizing radiation and the ear. JAMA 181:958-961, 1962.
276. Bosch, I and Oehmichen, M: Eosinophilic granulocytes in cerebrospinal fluid: Analysis of 94 cerebrospinal fluid specimens and review of the literature. J Neurol 219:93-105, 1978.
277. Bosl, GJ: The late effects of germ cell tumor chemotherapy: More data are needed. J Clin Oncol 10: 1375-1376, 1992.
278. Boston Collaborative Drug Surveillance Program: Acute adverse reactions to prednisone in relation to dosage. Clin Pharmacol Ther 13:694-698, 1972.
279. Bourke, RS, West, CR, Chheda, G, et al: Kinetics of entry and distribution of 5-fluorouracil in cerebrospinal fluid and brain following intravenous injection in a primate. Cancer Res 33:1735-1746, 1973.
280. Bourne, RG: The Costello Memorial Lecture. The spread of squamous carcinoma of the skin via the cranial nerves. Australas Radiol 24:106-114, 1980.
281. Bousser, MG, Chiras, J, Bories, J, et al: Cerebral venous thrombosis: A review of 38 cases. Stroke 16:199-213, 1985.
282. Bovbjerg, D: Psychoneuroimmunology and cancer. In Holland, JC and Rowland, JH (eds): Handbook of Psycho-oncology. Oxford University Press, New York, 1989, pp 727-734.
283. Bowen, BC and Post, JD: Diagnostic imaging of CNS infection and inflammation. In Schlossberg, D (ed): Infections of the Nervous System. Springer-Verlag, New York, 1990, pp 315-380.
284. Bowen, JD and Kidd, P: Myasthenia gravis associated with T helper cell lymphoma. Neurology 37:1405-1408, 1987.
285. Bowyer, SL, LaMothe, MP, and Hollister, JR: Steroid myopathy: Incidence and detection in a population with asthma. J Allergy Clin Med 76(2 Pt 1):234-242, 1985.
286. Boyle, P, Maisonneuve, P, Saracci, R, et al: Is the increased incidence of primary malignant brain tumors in the elderly real? J Natl Cancer Inst 82:1594-1596, 1990.
287. Bozzette, SA, Larsen, RA, Chiu, J, et al: A placebo-controlled trial of maintenance therapy with fluconazole after treatment of cryptococcal meningitis in the acquired immunodeficiency syndrome. California Collaborative Treatment Group. N Engl J Med 324:580-584, 1991.
288. Bradbury, MW: The blood–brain barrier. Transport across the cerebral endothelium. Circ Res 57:213-222, 1985.
289. Bradbury, PG, Levy, IS, and McDonald, WI: Transient uniocular visual loss on deviation of the eye in association with intraorbital tumours. J Neurol Neurosurg Psychiatry 50:615-619, 1987.
290. Braham, J, Sadeh, M, and Sarova-Pinhas, I: Skin wrinkling on immersion of hands. Arch Neurol 36:113-114, 1979.
291. Brain, L, Croft, PB, and Wilkinson, M: Motor neurone disease as a manifestation of neoplasm (with a note on the course of classical motor neuron disease). Brain 88:479-500, 1965.
292. Brain, WR, Daniel, PM, and Greenfield, JG: Subacute cortical cerebellar degeneration and its relation to carcinoma. J Neurol Neurosurg Psychiatry 14:59-75, 1951.
293. Brain, WR and Norris, FH (eds): The Remote Effects of Cancer on the Nervous System. Grune & Stratton, New York, 1965.
294. Brain, WR and Wilkinson, M: Subacute cerebellar degeneration associated with neoplasms. Brain 88:465-478, 1965.
295. Brandes, LJ, Arron, RJ, Bogdanovic, RP, et al: Stimulation of malignant growth in rodents by antidepressant drugs at clinically relevant doses. Cancer Res 52:3796-3800, 1992.
296. Brashear, HR, Greenlee, JE, Jaeckle, KA, et al: Anticerebellar antibodies in neurologically normal patients with ovarian neoplasms. Neurology 39:1605-1609, 1989.
297. Bray, LC, Carey, PJ, Proctor, SJ, et al: Ocular complications of bone marrow transplantation. Br J Ophthalmol 75:611-614, 1991.
298. Brazis, PW, Vogler, JB, and Shaw, KE: The "numb cheek–limp lower lid" syndrome. Neurology 41:327-328, 1991.
299. Brecher, ML, Berger, P, Freeman, AI, et al: Computerized tomography scan findings in children with acute lymphocytic leukemia treated with three different methods of central nervous system prophylaxis. Cancer 56:2430-2433, 1985.
300. Brega, K, Robinson, WA, Winston, K, et al: Surgical treatment of brain metastases in malignant melanoma. Cancer 66:2105-2110, 1990.
301. Breitbart, W: Endocrine-related psychiatric disorders. In Holland, JC and Rowland, JH (eds): Handbook of Psychooncology. Psychological Care of the Patient with Cancer. Oxford University Press, New York, 1989, pp 356-366.
302. Breitbart, W, Stiefel, F, Kornblith, AB, et al: Neuropsychiatric disturbance in cancer patients with epidural spinal cord compression receiving high dose corticosteroids: A prospective comparison study. Psycho-Oncology 2:233-245, 1993.
303. Brennan, KM, Roos, MS, Budinger, TF, et al: A study of radiation necrosis and edema in the

canine brain using positron emission tomography and magnetic resonance imaging. Radiat Res 134:43-53, 1993.

304. Brennan, LV and Craddock, PR: Limbic encephalopathy as a nonmetastatic complication of oat cell lung cancer. Its reversal after treatment of the primary lung lesion. Am J Med 75:518-520, 1983.
305. Brenner, GJ, Felten, SY, Felten, DL, et al: Sympathetic nervous system modulation of tumor metastases and host defense mechanisms. J Neuroimmunol 37:191-202, 1992.
306. Bresalier, RS and Karlin, DA: Meningeal metastasis from rectal carcinoma with elevated cerebrospinal fluid carcinoembryonic antigen. Dis Colon Rectum 22:216-217, 1979.
307. Breuer, AC, Blank, NK, and Schoene, WC: Multifocal pontine lesions in cancer patients treated with chemotherapy and CNS radiotherapy. Cancer 41:2112-2120, 1978.
308. Breuer, AC, Pitman, SW, Dawson, DM, et al: Paraparesis following intrathecal cytosine arabinoside: A case report with neuropathologic findings. Cancer 40:2817-2822, 1977.
309. Brewin, TB: Can a tumour cause the same appetite perversion or taste change as a pregnancy? Lancet 2:907-908, 1980.
310. Brierley, JB, Corsellis, JAN, Hierons, R, et al: Subacute encephalitis of later adult life. Mainly affecting the limbic areas. Brain 83:357-368, 1960.
311. Brightman, MW, Klatzo, I, Olsson, Y, et al: The blood–brain barrier to proteins under normal and pathological conditions. J Neurol Sci 10:215-239, 1970.
312. Brillman, J, Valeriano, J, and Adatepe, MH: The diagnosis of skull base metastases by radionuclide bone scan. Cancer 59:1887-1891, 1987.
313. Brinkley, JR, Jr: Response of a choroidal metastasis to multiple-drug chemotherapy. Cancer 45:1538-1539, 1980.
314. Britton, CB, Romagnoli, M, Sisti, M, et al: Progressive multifocal leukoencephalopathy: Disease progression, stabilization and response to intrathecal ARA-C in 26 patients. Abstract No. ThB1512. Proc VIII Int Conf AIDS/III STD World Cong, Amsterdam, The Netherlands, 1992.
315. Britton, CB, Sisti, MB, Romagnoli, M, et al: Intrathecal cytosine arabinoside treatment of patients with HIV-associated progressive multifocal leukoencephalopathy (PML). Proceeding Neuroscience Conference on HIV Infections: Bask and Clinical Frontiers, Padova, Italy, 1991, p. 23.
316. Broderick, JP and Cascino, TL: Nonconvulsive status epilepticus in a patient with leptomeningeal cancer. Mayo Clin Proc 62:835-837, 1987.
317. Brooks, SM, Werk, EE, Ackerman, SJ, et al: Adverse effects of phenobarbital on corticosteroid metabolism in patients with bronchial asthma. N Engl J Med 286:1125-1128, 1972.
318. Bross, IDG: The role of brain metastases in cascade processes. Implications for research and clinical management. In Weiss, L, Gilbert, HA, and Posner, JB (eds): Brain Metastasis. GK Hall & Co, Boston, 1980, pp 66-80.
319. Brouqui, P, Bollet, C, Delmont, J, et al: Diagnosis of progressive multifocal leucoencephalopathy by PCR detection of JC virus from CSF. Letter to the Editor. Lancet 339:1182, 1992.
320. Brouwer, B: Beitrag zur Kenntnis der chronischen diffusen Kleinhirnerkrankungen. Mendels neurologisches Zentralblblatt 38:674-682, 1919.
321. Brouwer, B and Biemond, A: Les affections parenchymateuses du cervelet et leur signification du point de vue de l'anatomie et la physiologie de cet organe. Journal Belge de Neurologie et Psychiatrie 38:691-757, 1938.
322. Browder, J and Rabiner, AM: Regional swelling of the brain in subdural hematoma. Ann Surg 134:369-375, 1970.
323. Brown, AS and Rosen, J: Lithium-induced delirium with therapeutic serum lithium levels: A case report. J Geriatr Psychiatry Neurol 5:53-55, 1992.
324. Brown, MT, Freidman, HS, Oakes, WJ, et al: Sagittal sinus thrombosis and leptomeningeal medulloblastoma: Resolution without anticoagulation. Neurology 41:455-456, 1991.
325. Brownell, B and Hughes, JT: Degeneration of muscle in association with carcinoma of the bronchus. J Neurol Neurosurg Psychiatry 38:363-370, 1975.
326. Bruck, W, Christen, HJ, Lakomek, H, et al: Wernicke's encephalopathy in a child with acute lymphoblastic leukemia treated with polychemotherapy. Clin Neuropathol 10:134-136, 1991.
327. Bruck, W, Heise, E, and Friede, RL: Leukoencephalopathy after cisplatin therapy. Clin Neuropathol 8:263-265, 1989.
328. Bruera, E: Current pharmacological management of anorexia in cancer patients. Oncology (Huntingt) 6:125-130, 1992.
329. Bruera, E, Brenneis, C, Michaud, M, et al: Muscle electrophysiology in patients with advanced breast cancer. J Natl Cancer Inst 80:282-285, 1988.
330. Bruera, E, Brenneis, C, Michaud, M, et al: Association between asthenia and nutritional status, lean body mass, anemia, psychological status, and tumor mass in patients with advanced breast cancer. Journal of Pain Symptom Management 4:59-63, 1989.
331. Bruera, E and MacDonald, RN: Asthenia in patients with advanced cancer. Issues in symptom control. Journal of Pain Symptom Management 3:9-14, 1988.
332. Bruera, E, Roca, E, Cedaro, L, et al: Action of oral methylprednisolone in terminal cancer patients: A prospective randomized double-blind study. Cancer Treat Rep 69:751-754, 1985.
333. Brunner, KW and Young, CW: A methylhydrazine derivative in Hodgkin's disease and other malignant neoplasms: Therapeutic and toxic effects studied in 51 patients. Ann Intern Med 63:69-86, 1965.
334. Bruyn, RPM: Paraneoplastic polyneuropathy. In Vinken, PJ, Bruyn, GW, Klawans, HL, et al (eds): Neuropathies, Revised Series 7/Handbook of Clinical Neurology, vol 51. Elsevier Science Publishers, Amsterdam, The Netherlands, 1987, pp 465-474.
335. Bryan, CS: Nonbacterial thrombotic endocarditis with malignant tumors. Am J Med 46:787-793, 1969.

336. Buckanovich, RJ, Posner, JB, and Darnell, RB: Nova, a paraneoplastic Ri antigen is homologous to an RNA-binding protein and is specifically expressed in the developing motor system. Neuron 11:1-20, 1993.
337. Buckner, JC: The role of chemotherapy in the treatment of patients with brain metastases from solid tumors. Cancer Metastasis Rev 10:335-341, 1991.
338. Budd, GT, Webster, KD, Reimer, RR, et al: Treatment of advanced ovarian cancer with cisplatin, adriamycin, and cyclophosphamide: Effect of treatment and incidence of intracranial metastases. J Surg Oncol 24:192-195, 1983.
339. Budde-Steffen, C, Anderson, NE, Rosenblum, MK, et al: An anti-neuronal autoantibody in paraneoplastic opsoclonus. Ann Neurol 23:528-531, 1988.
340. Budka, H, Guseo, A, Jellinger, K, et al: Intermittent meningitic reaction with severe basophilia and eosinophilia in CNS leukaemia. J Neurol Sci 28:459-468, 1976.
341. Buerger, LF and Monteleone, PN: Leukemic-lymphomatous infiltration of skeletal muscle. Systematic study of 82 autopsy cases. Cancer 19:1416-1422, 1966.
342. Burch, PA and Grossman, SA: Treatment of epidural cord compressions from Hodgkin's disease with chemotherapy. A report of two cases and a review of the literature. Am J Med 84:555-558, 1988.
343. Burch, PA, Grossman, SA, and Reinhard, CS: Spinal cord penetration of intrathecally administered cytarabine and methotrexate: A quantitative autoradiographic study. J Natl Cancer Inst 80:1211-1216, 1988.
344. Burch, PA, Karp, JE, Merz, WG, et al: Favorable outcome of invasive aspergillosis in patients with acute leukemia. J Clin Oncol 5:1985-1993, 1987.
345. Burger, PC, Kamenar, E, Schold, SC, et al: Encephalomyelopathy following high-dose BCNU therapy. Cancer 48:1318-1327, 1981.
346. Burns, LJ: Ocular toxicities of chemotherapy. Semin Oncol 19:492-500, 1992.
347. Burt, M, Wronski, M, Arbit, E, et al: Resection of brain metastases from non–small-cell lung carcinoma. Results of therapy. Memorial Sloan-Kettering Cancer Center Thoracic Surgical Staff. J Thorac Cardiovasc Surg 103:399-411, 1992.
348. Burt, RK, Sharfman, WH, Karp, BI, et al: Mental neuropathy (numb chin syndrome): A harbinger of tumor progression or relapse. Cancer 70:877-881, 1992.
349. Burton, GV, Bullard, DE, Walther, PJ, et al: Paraneoplastic limbic encephalopathy with testicular carcinoma. A reversible neurologic syndrome. Cancer 62:2248-2251, 1988.
350. Bush, MS, Reid, AR, and Allt, G: Blood–nerve barrier: Distribution of anionic sites on the endothelial plasma membrane and basal lamina of dorsal root ganglia. J Neurocytol 20:759-768, 1991.
351. Buss, DH, Stuart, JJ, and Lipscomb, GE: The incidence of thrombotic and hemorrhagic disorders in association with extreme thrombocytosis: An analysis of 129 cases. Am J Hematol 20:365-372, 1985.
352. Bustamante, CI and Wade, JC: Herpes simplex virus infection in the immunocompromised cancer patient. J Clin Oncol 9:1903-1915, 1991.
353. Byfield, JE: Ionizing radiation and vincristine: Possible neurotoxic synergism. Radiol Clin Biol 41:129-138, 1972.
354. Byrd, RL, Rohrbaugh, TM, Raney, RB, Jr, et al: Transient cortical blindness secondary to vincristine therapy in childhood malignancies. Cancer 47:37-40, 1981.
355. Byrne, P and Clough, C: A case of Pourfour Du Petit syndrome following parotidectomy. Letter to the Editor. J Neurol Neurosurg Psychiatry 53:1014, 1990.
356. Byrne, TN: Spinal cord compression from epidural metastases. N Engl J Med 327:614-619, 1992.
357. Byrne, TN, Cascino, TL, and Posner, JB: Brain metastasis from melanoma. J Neurooncol 1:313-317, 1983.
358. Byrne, TN and Waxman, SG: Spinal Cord Compression. Diagnosis and Principles of Management. FA Davis, Philadelphia, 1990.
359. Bystryn, J-C, Bernstein, P, Liu, P, et al: Immunophenotype of human melanoma cells in different metastases. Cancer Res 45(11 Pt 2):5603-5607, 1985.
359a. Cabantog, AM and Bernstein, M: Complications of first craniotomy for intra–axial brain tumour. Can J Neurol Sci 21:213-218, 1994.
360. Cahan, WG, Woodard, HQ, Higinbotham, NL, et al: Sarcoma arising in irradiated bone. Report of eleven cases. Cancer 1:3-29, 1948.
361. Cairncross, JG: Radiation-induced cranial neuropathy. In Rottenberg, DA (ed): Neurological Complications of Cancer Treatment. Butterworth-Heinemann, Boston, MA, 1991, pp 63-68.
362. Cairncross, JG, Chernik, NL, Kim, J-H, et al: Sterilization of cerebral metastases by radiation therapy. Neurology 29:1195-1202, 1979.
363. Cairncross, JG, Kim, J-H, and Posner, JB: Radiation therapy for brain metastases. Ann Neurol 7:529-541, 1980.
364. Cairncross, JG, Pexman, JHW, Rathbone, MP, et al: Postoperative contrast enhancement in patients with brain tumor. Ann Neurol 17:570-572, 1985.
365. Cairncross, JG and Posner, JB: Neurologic complications of systemic cancer. In Yarbro, JW and Bornstein, RS (eds): Oncologic Emergencies. Grune & Stratton, New York, 1981, pp 73-96.
366. Cairncross, JG, Salmon, J, Kim, J-H, et al: Acute parotitis and hypermylasemia following whole-brain radiation therapy. Ann Neurol 7:385-387, 1980.
367. Cairo, MS, Lazarus, K, Gilmore, RL, et al: Intracranial hemorrhage and focal seizures secondary to use of L-asparaginase during induction of therapy of acute lymphocytic leukemia. J Pediatr 97:829-833, 1980.
368. Callahan, DJ and Noetzel, MJ: Prolonged absence status epilepticus associated with carbamazepine therapy, increased intracranial pressure, and transient MRI abnormalities. Neurology 42:2198-2201, 1992.

369. Calverley, JR and Mohnac, AM: Syndrome of the numb chin. Arch Intern Med 112:819-821, 1963.
370. Camarata, PJ, Dunn, DL, Farney, AC, et al: Continual intracavitary administration of amphotericin B as an adjunct in the treatment of aspergillus brain abscess: Case report and review of the literature. Neurosurgery 31:575-579, 1992.
371. Camarata, PJ, McGeachie, RE, and Haines, SJ: Dorsal midbrain encephalitis caused by *Propionibacterium* acnes. Report of two cases. J Neurosurg 72:654-659, 1990.
372. Camarri, E, Chirone, E, and Benvenuti, C: Double-blind placebo controlled cross-over study on cimetidine-prophylactic effect in patients under steroid treatment. Preliminary data. Int J Clin Pharmacol Ther Toxicol 18:258-260, 1980.
373. Cameron, LB: Neuropsychotropic drugs as adjuncts in the treatment of cancer pain. Oncology (Huntingt) 6:65-77, 1992.
374. Caminal, L, Castellanos, E, Mateos, V, et al: Hyperammonaemic encephalopathy as the presenting feature of IgD multiple myeloma. J Intern Med 233:277-279, 1993.
375. Campbell, AMG and Garland, H: Subacute myoclonic spinal neuronitis. J Neurol Neurosurg Psychiatry 19:268-274, 1956.
376. Campbell, MJ and Paty, DW: Carcinomatous neuromyopathy: 1. Electrophysiological studies. An electrophysiological and immunological study of patients with carcinoma of the lung. J Neurol Neurosurg Psychiatry 37:131-141, 1974.
377. Campbell, TN, Howell, SB, Pfeifle, C, et al: High-dose allopurinol modulation of 5-FU toxicity: Phase I trial of an outpatient dose schedule. Cancer Treat Rep 66:1723-1727, 1982.
378. Cantu, RC: Corticosteroids for spinal metastases. Letter to the Editor. Lancet 2:912, 1968.
379. Capone, PM and Cohen, ME: Seizures and cerebritis associated with administration of OKT3. Pediatr Neurol 7:299-301, 1991.
380. Carey, MP and Burish, TG: Etiology and treatment of the psychological side effects associated with cancer chemotherapy: A critical review and discussion. Psychol Bull 104:307-325, 1988.
381. Carey, RW and Harris, N: Thrombotic microangiopathy in three patients with cured lymphoma. Cancer 63:1393-1397, 1989.
382. Carlin, L, Biller, J, Laster, W, et al: Monocular blindness in nasopharyngeal cancer. Arch Neurol 38:600, 1981.
383. Carlson, J and Wiholm, B-E: Trimethoprim associated aseptic meningitis. Scand J Infect Dis 19:687-691, 1987.
384. Carmel, PW and Greif, LK: The aseptic meningitis syndrome: A complication of posterior fossa surgery. Pediatr Neurosurg 19(5):276-280, 1993.
385. Carmichael, KA, Jennings, AS, and Doty, RL: Reversible anosmia after pituitary irradiation. Ann Intern Med 100:532-533, 1984.
386. Carmichael, SM, Eagleton, L, Ayers, CR, et al: Orthostatic hypotension during vincristine therapy. Arch Intern Med 126:290-293, 1970.
387. Caron, J-L, Souhami, L, and Podgorsak, EB: Dynamic stereotactic radiosurgery in the palliative treatment of cerebral metastatic tumors. J Neurooncol 12:173-179, 1992.
388. Carpentieri, U and Lockhart, LH: Ataxia and athetosis as side effects of chemotherapy with vincristine in non-Hodgkin's lymphoma. Cancer Treat Rep 62:561-562, 1978.
389. Carr, I: The Ophelia syndrome: Memory loss in Hodgkin's disease. Lancet 1:844-845, 1982.
390. Carson, DA and Ribeiro, JM: Apoptosis and disease. Lancet 341:1251-1254, 1993.
391. Carson, JL, Strom, BL, and Schinnar, R: The low risk of upper gastrointestinal bleeding in patients dispensed corticosteroids. Am J Med 91:223-228, 1991.
392. Carson, RE, Zunkeler, B, Blasberg, RG, et al: Quantitative measurement of hyperosmotic blood–brain barrier disruption with ^{82}Rb and PET, Abstract No. 429. J Nucl Med 31:810, 1990.
393. Carter, RL, Tanner, NS, Clifford, P, et al: Perineural spread in squamous cell carcinomas of the head and neck: A clinicopathological study. Clin Otolaryngol 4:271-281, 1979.
394. Carter, SK: Methodology of data reporting in advanced breast cancer trials. Cancer Chemother Pharmacol 3:1-5, 1979.
395. Cascino, TL, Byrne, TN, Deck, MDF, et al: Intra-arterial BCNU in the treatment of metastatic brain tumors. J Neurooncol 1:211-218, 1983.
396. Cascino, TL, Kori, S, Krol, G, et al: CT of the brachial plexus in patients with cancer. Neurology 33:1553-1557, 1983.
397. Cascino, TL, Leavengood, JM, Kemeny, N, et al: Brain metastases from colon cancer. J Neurooncol 1:203-209, 1983.
398. Cash, J, Fehir, KM, and Pollack, SM: Meningeal involvement in early stage chronic lymphocytic leukemia. Cancer 59:798-800, 1987.
399. Casper, ES, Michaelson, RS, Kemeny, N, et al: Phase I evaluation of a biochemically designed combination: PALA, thymidine, and 5-FU. Cancer Treat Rep 68:539-541, 1984.
400. Cassady, JR, Tonnesen, GL, Wolfe, LC, et al: Augmentation of vincristine neurotoxicity by irradiation of peripheral nerves. Cancer Treat Rep 64:963-965, 1980.
401. Cassel, WA, Weidenheim, KM, Campbell, WG, Jr, et al: Malignant melanoma. Inflammatory mononuclear cell infiltrates in cerebral metastases during concurrent therapy with viral oncolysate. Cancer 57:1302-1312, 1986.
402. Cassidy, J: Scottish Gynaecological Cancer Study Group: Pilot study of a novel neuroprotector (nimodipine) in cisplatin-treated ovarian cancer patients. Abstract No. 1334. Progress/Proceedings American Society of Clinical Oncology 33:233, 1992.
403. Cassileth, PA, Lusk, EJ, Torri, S, et al: Antiemetic efficacy of dexamethasone therapy in patients receiving cancer chemotherapy. Arch Intern Med 143:1347-1349, 1983.
404. Casteels-van Daele, M and Van de Casseye, W: Acute encephalopathy after initiation of cranial irradiation for meningeal leukaemia. Letter to the Editor. Lancet 2:834-835, 1978.
405. Castellanos, AM, Glass, JP, and Yung, WKA: Regional nerve injury after intra-arterial chemotherapy. Neurology 37:834-837, 1987.
406. Castiello, RJ and Lynch, PJ: Pellagra and the

carcinoid syndrome. Arch Dermatol 105:574-577, 1972.

406a. Castro, JR, Linstadt, DE, Bahary, JP, et al: Experience in charged particle irradiation of tumors of the skull base. Int J Radiat Oncol Biol Phys 29:647-655, 1994.

406b. Catalona, WJ: Management of cancer of the prostate. N Engl J Med 331:996-1004, 1994.

407. Catane, R, Kaufman, J, West, C, et al: Brain metastasis from prostatic carcinoma. Cancer 38:2583-2587, 1976.

408. Cattaneo, MT, Filipazzi, V, Piazza, E, et al: Transient blindness and seizure associated with cisplatin therapy. J Cancer Res Clin Oncol 114:528-530, 1988.

409. Catterall, M and Errington, RD: The implications of improved treatment of malignant salivary gland tumors by fast neutron radiotherapy. Int J Radiat Oncol Biol Phys 13:1313-1318, 1987.

410. Cavaletti, G, Marzorati, L, Bogliun, G, et al: Cisplatin-induced peripheral neurotoxicity is dependent on total-dose intensity and single-dose intensity. Cancer 69:203-207, 1992.

411. Cavaletti, G, Tredici, G, Marmiroli, P, et al: Morphometric study of the sensory neuron and peripheral nerve changes induced by chronic cisplatin (DDP) administration in rats. Acta Neuropathol (Berl) 84:364-371, 1992.

412. Cerny, T and Kupfer, A: The enigma of ifosfamide encephalopathy. Editorial. Ann Oncol 3:679-681, 1992.

413. Cetto, GL, Iannucci, A, Tummarello, D, et al: Involvement of the central nervous system in non-Hodgkin's lymphoma. Tumori 67:39-44, 1981.

414. Chabner, BA and Collins, JM (eds): Cancer and Chemotherapy: Principles and Practice. JB Lippincott, Philadelphia, 1990.

415. Chadwick, M and Rogers, WI: The physiological disposition of 5-fluorouracil in mice bearing solid L1210 lymphocytic leukemia. Cancer Res 32: 1045-1056, 1972.

416. Chahinian AP, Propert, KJ, Ware, JH, et al: A randomized trial of anticoagulation with warfarin and of alternating chemotherapy in extensive small-cell lung cancer by the Cancer and Leukemia Group B. J Clin Oncol 7:993-1002, 1989.

417. Chalk, CH, Murray, NM, Newsom-Davis, J, et al: Response of the Lambert-Eaton myasthenic syndrome to treatment of associated small-cell lung carcinoma. Neurology 40:1552-1556, 1990.

418. Chalk, CH, Windebank, AJ, Kimmel, DW, et al: The distinctive clinical features of paraneoplastic sensory neuronopathy. Can J Neurol Sci 19:346-351, 1992.

419. Chalk, JB, Ridgeway, K, Tro'r, B, et al: Phenytoin impairs the bioavailability of dexamethasone in neurological and neurosurgical patients. J Neurol Neurosurg Psychiatry 47:1087-1090, 1984.

420. Chamberlain, MC and Corey-Bloom, J: Leptomeningeal metastasis: ^{111}indium-DTPA CSF flow studies. Neurology 41:1765-1769, 1991.

421. Chamberlain, MC, Khatibi, S, Kim, JC, et al: Treatment of leptomeningeal metastasis with intraventricular administration of depot cytarabine (DTC 101). A phase I study. Arch Neurol 50:261-264, 1993.

422. Champagne, MA and Silver, HKB: Intrathecal decarbazine treatment of leptomeningeal malignant melanoma. J Natl Cancer Inst 84:1203-1204, 1992.

423. Chan, PH and Fishman, RA: The role of arachidonic acid in vasogenic brain edema. Fed Proc 43:210-213, 1984.

424. Chandalia, HB and Boshell, BR: Hypoglycemia associated with extrapancreatic tumors. Report of two cases with studies on its pathogenesis. Arch Intern Med 129:447-456, 1972.

425. Chandler, JR: Malignant external otitis: Further considerations. Ann Otol Rhinol Laryngol 86:417-428, 1977.

426. Chang, D-B, Yang, P-C, Luh, K-T, et al: Late survival of non-small cell lung cancer patients with brain metastases. Influence of treatment. Chest 101:1293-1297, 1992.

427. Chang, M-H, Liao, K-K, Wu, Z-A, et al: Reversible myeloneuropathy resulting from podophyllin intoxication: An electrophysiological follow up. Letter to the Editor. J Neurol Neurosurg Psychiatry 55:235-236, 1992.

428. Chang, M-H, Lin, K-P, Wu, Z-A, et al: Acute ataxic sensory neuronopathy resulting from podophyllin intoxication. Letter to the Editor. Muscle Nerve 15:513-514, 1992.

429. Chastagner, P, Sommelet-Olive, D, Kalifa, C, et al: Phase II study of ifosfamide in childhood brain tumors: A report by the French Society of Pediatric Oncology (SFOP). Med Pediatr Oncol 21:49-53, 1993.

430. Chatani, M, Teshima, T, Hata, K, et al: Whole brain irradiation for metastases from lung carcinoma. A clinical investigation. Acta Radiologica: Oncology, Radiation, Physics, Biology (Stockholm) 24:311-314, 1985.

431. Chatani, M, Teshima, T, Inoue, T, et al: Radiation therapy for nasopharyngeal carcinoma. Retrospective review of 105 patients based on a survey of Kansai Cancer Therapist Group. Cancer 57:2267-2271, 1986.

431a. Chaturvedi, S, Ansell, J and Recht, L: Should cerebral ischemic events in cancer patients be considered a manifestation of hypercoagulability? Stroke 25:1215-1218, 1994.

432. Chaudhry, V, Rowinsky, EK, Sartorius, SE, et al: Peripheral neuropathy from Taxol and cisplatin combination chemotherapy: Clinical and electrophysiological studies. Ann Neurol 35:304-311, 1994.

433. Chauncey, TR, Showel, JL, and Fox, JH: Vincristine neurotoxicity. Letter to the Editor. JAMA 254:507, 1985.

434. Chen, Y-T, Rettig, WJ, Yenamandra, AK, et al: Cerebellar degeneration-related antigen: A highly conserved neuroectodermal marker mapped to chromosomes X in human and mouse. Proc Natl Acad Sci USA 87:3077-3081, 1990.

435. Cheng, CL, Greenberg, J, and Hoover, LA: Prostatic adenocarcinoma metastatic to chronic subdural hematoma membranes. Case report. J Neurosurg 68:642-644, 1988.

436. Cheng, TM, O'Neill, BP, Scheithauer, BW, et al: Chronic meningitis: The role of meningeal or cortical biopsy. Neurosurgery 34:590-596, 1994.
437. Cheng, VST and Schultz, MD: Unilateral hypoglossal nerve atrophy as a late complication of radiation therapy of head and neck carcinoma: A report of four cases and a review of the literature on peripheral and cranial nerve damages after radiation therapy. Cancer 35:1537-1544, 1975.
438. Chernik, NL, Armstrong, D, and Posner, JB: Central nervous system infections in patients with cancer. Medicine (Baltimore) 52:563-581, 1973.
439. Chernik, NL, Armstrong, D, and Posner, JB: Central nervous system infections in patients with cancer. Changing patterns. Cancer 40:268-274, 1977.
440. Chernik, NL, Loewenson, RB, Posner, JB, et al: Cerebral atherosclerosis and stroke in cancer patients. Abstract. Neurology 28:350, 1978.
441. Cherny, NI and Portenoy, RK: Practical issues in the management of cancer pain. In Wall, PD and Melzack, R (eds): Textbook of Pain, ed 3. Churchill Livingstone, Edinburgh, 1994, pp 1437-1467.
442. Cherubin, CE, Marr, JS, Sierra, MF, et al: *Listeria* and gram-negative bacillary meningitis in New York City, 1972-1979. Am J Med 71:199-209, 1981.
443. Cheruku, R, Tapazoglou, E, Ensley, J, et al: The incidence and significance of thromboembolic complications in patients with high-grade gliomas. Cancer 68:2621-2624, 1991.
443a. Cheson, BD, Vena, DA, Foss, FM. et al: Neurotoxicity of purine analogs: A review. J Clin Oncol 12:2216-2228, 1994.
444. Chiang, CS, Mason, KA, Withers, HR, et al: Alteration in myelin-associated proteins following spinal cord irradiation in guinea pigs. Int J Radiat Oncol Biol Phys 24:929-937, 1992.
445. Chio, C-C, Baba, T, and Black, KL: Selective blood–tumor barrier disruption in leukotrienes. J Neurosurg 77:407-410, 1992.
446. Chisholm, IA: Optic neuropathy of recurrent blood loss. Br J Ophthalmol 53:289-295, 1969.
447. Cho, E-S, Lowndes, HE, and Goldstein, BD: Neurotoxicology of vincristine in the cat. Morphological study. Arch Toxicol 52:83-90, 1983.
448. Cho, KG, Hoshino, T, Pitts, LH, et al: Proliferative potential of brain metastases. Cancer 62:512-515, 1988.
449. Choi, KN, Withers, HR, and Rotman, M: Intracranial metastases from melanoma. Clinical features and treatment by accelerated fractionation. Cancer 56:1-9, 1985.
450. Chou, M-Y, Brown, AE, Blevins, A, et al: Severe pneumococcal infection in patients with neoplastic disease. Cancer 51:1546-1550, 1983.
451. Choucair, AK: Myelopathies in the cancer patient: Incidence, presentation, diagnosis and management. Oncology (Huntingt) 5:25-37, 1991.
452. Christy, WC and Powell, DL: Knee pain exacerbated by recumbency: An unusual manifestation of spinal cord involvement by diffuse histiocytic lymphoma. Arthritis Rheum 27(3):341-343, 1984.
453. Chromiak, JA and Vandenburgh, HH: Glucocorticoid-induced skeletal muscle atrophy in vitro is attenuated by mechanical stimulation. Am J Physiol 262:C1471-C1477, 1992.
454. Chun, HG, Leyland-Jones, B, Caryk, SM, et al: Central nervous system toxicity of fludarabine phosphate. Cancer Treat Rep 70:1225-1228, 1986.
455. Chun, HG, Leyland-Jones, B, and Cheson, BD: Fludarabine phosphate: A synthetic purine antimetabolite with significant activity against lymphoid malignancies. J Clin Oncol 9:175-188, 1991.
456. Chutkow, JG, Sharbrough, FW, and Riley, FC, Jr: Blindness following simultaneous bilateral neck dissection. Mayo Clin Proc 48:713-717, 1973.
457. Cibas, ES, Malkin, MG, Posner, JB, et al: Detection of DNA abnormalities by flow cytometry in cells from cerebrospinal fluid. Am J Clin Pathol 88:570-577, 1987.
458. Cieplinski, W, Ciesielski, TE, Haine, C, et al: Choroid metastases from transitional cell carcinoma of the bladder: A case report and a review of the literature. Cancer 50:1596-1600, 1982.
459. Clamon, G and Doebbeling, B: Meningeal carcinomatosis from breast cancer: Spinal cord vs brain involvement. Breast Cancer Res Treat 9:213-217, 1987.
460. Clark, AW, Cohen, SR, Nissenblatt, MJ, et al: Paraplegia following intrathecal chemotherapy: Neuropathologic findings and elevation of myelin basic protein. Cancer 50:42-47, 1982.
460a. Clark, J and Rubin, RN: A practical approach to managing disseminated intravascular coagulation. Journal of Critical Illness 9:265-280, 1994.
461. Clouston, PD, DeAngelis, LM, and Posner, JB: The spectrum of neurologic disease in patients with systemic cancer. Ann Neurol 31:268-273, 1992.
462. Clouston, PD, Saper, CB, Arbizu, T, et al: Paraneoplastic cerebellar degeneration. III. Cerebellar degeneration, cancer and the Lambert-Eaton myasthenic syndrome. Neurology 42:1944-1950, 1992.
463. Clouston, PD, Sharpe, DM, Corbett, AJ, et al: Perineural spread of cutaneous head and neck cancer. Arch Neurol 47:73-77, 1990.
464. Coakham, HB, Garson, JA, Brownell, B, et al: Use of monoclonal antibody panel to identify malignant cells in cerebrospinal fluid. Lancet 1:1095-1098, 1984.
465. Cobb, CA, III, Leavens, ME, and Eckles N: Indications for nonoperative treatment of spinal cord compression due to breast cancer. J Neurosurg 47:653-658, 1977.
466. Cocconi, G, Ceci, G, and Juvarra, G: Successful treatment of subacute cerebellar degeneration in ovarian carcinoma with plasmapheresis. A case report. Cancer 56:2318-2320, 1985.
467. Cocconi, G, Lottici, R, Bisagni, G, et al: Combination therapy with platinum and etoposide of brain metastases from breast carcinoma. Cancer Invest 8:327-334, 1990.
468. Coffey, RJ, Flickinger, JC, Bissonette, DJ, et al: Radiosurgery for solitary brain metastases using the cobalt-60 gamma unit: Methods and results in 24 patients. Int J Radiat Oncol Biol Phys 20:1287-1295, 1991.
469. Cohen, L and Svensson, H: Cell population kinetics and dose-time relationships for post-

irradiation injury of the brachial plexus in man. Acta Radiol Oncol Radiat Phys Biol 17:161-166, 1978.

470. Cohen, N, Strauss, G, Lew, R, et al: Should prophylactic anticonvulsants be administered to patients with newly diagnosed cerebral metastases? A retrospective analysis. J Clin Oncol 6:1621-1624, 1988.
471. Cohen, RB, Abdallah, JM, Gray, JR, et al: Reversible neurologic toxicity in patients treated with standard-dose fludarabine phosphate for mycosis fungoides and chronic lymphocytic leukemia. Ann Intern Med 118:114-116, 1993.
472. Cohen, RJ, Cuneo, RA, Cruciger, MP, et al: Transient left homonymous hemianopsia and encephalopathy following treatment of testicular carcinoma with cisplatinum, vinblastine, and bleomycin. J Clin Oncol 1:392-393, 1983.
473. Cohen, SC and Mollman, JE: Cisplatin-induced gastric paresis. J Neurooncol 5:237-240, 1987.
474. Cohn, KH, et al: Association of nm23-H1 allelic deletions with distant metastases in colorectal carcinoma. Lancet 338:722-724, 1991.
474a. Cohn, SL, Hamre, M, Kletzel, M, et al: Intraspinal Wilms' tumor metastases. Cancer 73:2444-2449, 1994.
475. Cohn, SL, Salwen, H, Herst, CV, et al: Single copies of the N-*myc* oncogene in neuroblastomas from children presenting with the syndrome of opsoclonus-myoclonus. Cancer 62:723-726, 1988.
476. Coia, LR: The role of radiation therapy in the treatment of brain metastases. Int J Radiat Oncol Biol Phys 23:229-238, 1992.
477. Cold, GE and Felding, M: Even small doses of morphine might provoke "luxury perfusion" in the postoperative period after craniotomy. Letter to the Editor. Neurosurgery 32(2):327, 1993.
478. Cole, K and Kohn, E: Calcium-mediated signal transduction: Biology, biochemistry, and therapy. Cancer Metastasis Review 13:31-44, 1994.
479. Coleman, CN, Glover, DJ, and Turrisi, AT: Radiation and chemotherapy sensitizers and protectors. In Chabner, BA and Collins, JM (eds): Cancer Chemotherapy: Principles and Practice. JB Lippincott, Philadelphia, 1990, pp 424-448.
480. Colice, GL: How to ventilate patients when ICP elevation is a risk: Monitor pressure, consider hyperventilation therapy. Journal of Critical Illness 8:1003-1020, 1993.
481. Collier, J: The false localising signs of intracranial tumour. Brain 27:490-508, 1904.
482. Collins, RC, Al-Mondhiry, H, Chernik, NL, et al: Neurologic manifestations of intravascular coagulation in patients with cancer. A clinicopathologic analysis of 12 cases. Neurology 25:795-806, 1975.
483. Colman, RW and Rubin, RN: Disseminated intravascular coagulation due to malignancy. Semin Oncol 17:172-186, 1990.
484. Colucci, M, Delaini, F. de Bellis Viti, G, et al: Warfarin inhibits both procoagulant activity and metastatic capacity of Lewis lung carcinoma cells. Role of vitamin K deficiency. Biochem Pharmacol 32:1689-1691, 1983.
485. Comaish, S: A case of hypersensitivity to corticosteroids. Br J Dermatol 81:919-925, 1969.
486. Coman, D and DeLong, RP: The role of the vertebral venous system in the metastasis of cancer to the spinal column. Cancer 4:610-618, 1951.
487. Conley, FK: Metastatic brain tumor model in mice that mimics the neoplastic cascade in humans. Neurosurgery 14:187-192, 1984.
488. Constine, LS, Wolff, PD, Cann, D, et al: Hypothalamic-pituitary dysfunction after radiation for brain tumors. N Engl J Med 328:87-94, 1993.
489. Conter, V, Rabbone, ML, Jankovic, M, et al: Overdose of vinblastine in a child with Langerhans' cell histiocytosis: Toxicity and salvage therapy. Pediatr Hematol Oncol 8:165-169, 1991.
490. Conti, DJ and Rubin, RH: Infection of the central nervous system in organ transplant recipients. Neurol Clin 6:241-260, 1988.
491. Conti, JA and Scher, HI: Acute arterial thrombosis after escalated-dose methotrexate, vinblastine, doxorubicin, and cisplatin chemotherapy with recombinant granulocyte colony-stimulating factor. A possible new recombinant granulocyte colony: Stimulating factor toxicity. Cancer 80: 2699-2702, 1992.
492. Coomes, EN: The rate of recovery of reversible myopathies and the effects of anabolic agents in steroid myopathy. Neurology 15:523-530, 1965.
493. Cooper, DL, Sandler, AB, Wilson, LD, et al: Disseminated intravascular coagulation and excessive fibrinolysis in a patient with metastatic prostate cancer. Response to epsilon-aminocaproic acid. Cancer 70:656-658, 1992.
494. Cooper, JS and Carella, R: Radiotherapy of intracerebral metastatic malignant melanoma. Radiology 134:735-738, 1980.
495. Cooper, JS, Steinfeld, AD, and Lerch, IA: Cerebral metastases: Value of reirradiation in selected patients. Radiology 174(3 Pt 1):883-885, 1990.
496. Cooper, K, Bajorin, D, Shapiro, W, et al: Decompression of epidural metastases from germ cell tumors with chemotherapy. J Neurooncol 8:275-280, 1990.
497. Cooper, PR, Errico, TJ, Martin, R, et al: A systematic approach to spinal reconstruction after anterior decompression for neoplastic disease of the thoracic and lumbar spine. Neurosurgery 32:1-8, 1993.
498. Cooper, WH, Ringel, SP, Treihaft, MM, et al: Calf enlargement from S-1 radiculopathy. Report of two cases. J Neurosurg 62:442-444, 1985.
499. Coppeto, JR, Monteiro, M, and Cannarozzi, DB: Optic neuropathy associated with chronic lymphomatous meningitis. Journal of Clinical Neuro-Ophthalmology 8:39-45, 1988.
500. Corbett, JJ and Mehta, MP: Cerebrospinal fluid pressure in normal obese subjects and patients with pseudotumor cerebri. Neurology 33:1386-1388, 1983.
501. Cordon-Cardo, C, Fuks, Z, Drobnjak, M, et al: Expression of HLA-A,B,C antigens on primary and metastatic tumor cell populations of human carcinomas. Cancer Res 51:6372-6380, 1991.
502. Cordon-Cardo, C, O'Brien, JP, Casals, D, et al: Multidrug-resistance gene (P-glycoprotein) is expressed by endothelial cells at blood–brain barrier sites. Proc Natl Acad Sci U S A 86:695-698, 1989.

503. Cordonnier, C, Vernant, JP, Brun, B, et al: Acute promyelocytic leukemia in 57 previously untreated patients. Cancer 55:18-25, 1985.
504. Cornford, EM, Young, D, Paxton, JW, et al: Melphalan penetration of the blood–brain barrier via the neutral amino acid transporter in tumor-bearing brain. Cancer Res 52:138-143, 1992.
505. Cornuz, J, Bogousslavsky, J, Schapira, M, et al: Ischemic stroke as the presenting manifestation of localized systemic cancer. Schweiz Arch Neurol Psychiatr 139(2):5-11, 1988.
506. Correale, J, Monteverde, DA, Bueri, JA, et al: Peripheral nervous system and spinal cord involvement in lymphoma. Acta Neurol Scand 83:45-51, 1991.
507. Corsellis, JA, Goldberg, GJ, and Norton, AR: "Limbic encephalitis" and its association with carcinoma. Brain 91:481-496, 1968.
508. Cosgrove, GR, Bertrand, G, Fontaine, S, et al: Cavernous angiomas of the spinal cord. J Neurosurg 68:31-36, 1988.
509. Coskuncan, NM, Jabs, DA, Dunn, JP, et al: The eye in bone marrow transplantation. VI. Retinal complications. Arch Ophthalmol 112:372-379, 1994.
510. Cosolo, WC, Martinello, P, Louis, WJ, et al: Blood–brain barrier disruption using mannitol: Time course and electron microscopy studies. Am J Physiol 256:R443-R447, 1989.
511. Costans, JP, de Divitiis, E, Donzelli, R, et al: Spinal metastases with neurological manifestations. Review of 600 cases. J Neurosurg 59:111-118, 1983.
512. Costello, P and Del Maestro, R: Human cerebral endothelium: Isolation and characterization of cells derived from microvessels of non-neoplastic and malignant glial tissue. J Neurooncol 8:231-243, 1990.
513. Costigan, DA and Winkelman, MD: Intramedullary spinal cord metastasis. A clinicopathological study of 13 cases. J Neurosurg 62:227-233, 1985.
514. Couch, L, Theilen, F, and Mader, JT: Rhinocerebral mucormycosis with cerebral extension successfully treated with adjunctive hyperbaric oxygen therapy. Arch Otolaryngol Head Neck Surg 114:791-794, 1988.
515. Coulam, CM, Seshul, M, and Donaldson, J: Intracranial ring lesions: Can we differentiate by computed tomography? Invest Radiol 15:103-112, 1980.
516. Couldwell, WT, Chandrasoma, PT, and Weiss, MH: Pituitary gland metastasis from adenocarcinoma of the prostate. J Neurosurg 71:138-140, 1989.
517. Coventry, MB and Mitchell, WC: Osteitis pubis. Observations based on a study of 45 patients. JAMA 178:130-137, 1961.
518. Cox, JD, Stanley, K, Petrovich, Z, et al: Cranial irradiation in cancer of the lung of all cell types. JAMA 245:469-472, 1981.
519. Coy, P and Dolman, CL: Radiation myelopathy in relation to oxygen level. Br J Radiol 44:705-707, 1971.
520. Coyle, T, Bushunow, P, Winfield, J, et al: Hypersensitivity reactions to procarbazine with mechlorethamine, vincristine, and procarbazine chemotherapy in the treatment of glioma. Cancer 69:2532-2540, 1992.
521. Craswell, PW: Vocal cord paresis following radioactive iodine therapy. Br J Clin Pract 26:571-572, 1972.
522. Craven, W and Donofrio, P: Sensory and autonomic polyneuropathy associated with trimethoprim-sulfamethoxazole. Abstract. Ann Neurol 32:281-282, 1992.
523. Creutzig, U, Ritter, J, Budde, M, et al: Early deaths due to hemorrhage and leukostasis in childhood acute myelogenous leukemia. Associations with hyperleukocytosis and acute monocytic leukemia. Cancer 60:3071-3079, 1987.
524. Crevel, HV: Absence of papilloedema in cerebral tumours. J Neurol Neurosurg Psychiatry 38:931-933, 1975.
525. Criscuolo, GR, Merrill, MJ, and Oldfield, EH: Further characterization of malignant glioma-derived vascular permeability factor. J Neurosurg 69:254-262, 1988.
526. Croft, PB, Urich, H, and Wilkinson, M: Peripheral neuropathy of sensorimotor type associated with malignant disease. Brain 90:31-66, 1967.
527. Croft, PB and Wilkinson, M: The incidence of carcinomatous neuromyopathy in patients with various types of carcinomas. Brain 88:427-434, 1965.
528. Crossen, JR, Garwood, D, Glatstein, E, et al: Neurobehavioral sequelae of cranial irradiation in adults: A review of radiation-induced encephalopathy. J Clin Oncol 12:627-642, 1994.
529. Cruz, M, Jiang, Y-P, Ernerudh, J, et al: Antibodies to myelin-associated glycoprotein are found in cerebrospinal fluid in polyneuropathy associated with monoclonal serum IgM. Arch Neurol 48:66-70, 1991.
530. Cruz, T, Reboucas, G, and Rocha, H: Fatal strongyloidiasis in patients receiving corticosteroids. N Engl J Med 275:1093-1096, 1966.
531. Cruz-Sanchez, FF, Artigas, J, Cervos-Navarro, J, et al: Brain lesions following combined treatment with methotrexate and craniospinal irradiation. J Neurooncol 10:165-171, 1991.
532. Cserr, HF, Harling-Berg, CJ, and Knopf, PM: Drainage of brain extracellular fluid into blood and deep cervical lymph and its immunological significance. Brain Pathol 2:269-276, 1992.
533. Cserr, HF and Knopf, PM: Cervical lymphatics, the blood-brain barrier and the immunoreactivity of the brain: A new view. Immunol Today 13:507-512, 1992.
534. Cubeddu, LX: Mechanisms by which cancer chemotherapeutic drugs induce emesis. Semin Oncol 19:2-13, 1992.
535. Cullis, PA and Cushing, R: Vidarabine encephalopathy. J Neurol Neurosurg Psychiatry 47:1351-1354, 1984.
536. Culpepper-Morgan, JA, Inturrisi, CE, Portenoy, RK, et al: Treatment of opioid-induced constipation with oral naloxone: A pilot study. Clin Pharmacol Ther 52:90-95, 1992.
537. Cuneo, RA, Caronna, JJ, Pitts, L, et al: Upward transtentorial herniation: Seven cases and a literature review. Arch Neurol 36:618-623, 1979.
538. Curran, CF and Luce, JK: Fluorouracil and palmar-plantar erythrodysesthesia. Letter to the Editor. Ann Intern Med 111:858, 1989.

539. Currie, S, Henson, RA, Morgan, HG, et al: The incidence of the non-metastatic neurological syndromes of obscure origin in the reticuloses. Brain 93:629-640, 1970.
540. Curtin, JP, Koonings, PP, Gutierrez, M, et al: Ifosfamide-induced neurotoxicity. Gynecol Oncol 42:193-196, 1991.
541. Cushing, H: Anosmia and sellar distension as misleading signs in the localization of a cerebral tumor. J Nerv Ment Dis 44:415-419, 1916.
542. Czerwinski, AW, Czerwinski, AB, Whitsett, TL, et al: Effects of a single, large intravenous injection of dexamethasone. Clin Pharmacol Ther 13:638-642, 1972.
543. D'Angio, GJ, French, LA, Stadlan, EM, et al: Intrathecal radioisotopes for the treatment of brain tumors. Clin Neurosurg 15:288-299, 1968.
544. d'Avella, D, Cicciarello, R, Albiero, F, et al: Effect of whole brain radiation on local cerebral glucose utilization in the rat. Neurosurgery 28:491-495, 1991.
545. D'Elia, F, Bonucci, I, Biti, GP, et al: Different fractionation schedules in radiation treatment of cerebral metastases. Acta Radiol Oncol 25:181-184, 1986.
546. Dakhil, S, Ensminger, W, Kindt, G, et al: Implanted system for intraventricular drug infusion in central nervous system tumors. Cancer Treat Rep 65:401-411, 1981.
547. Dalakas, MC: Polymyositis, dermatomyositis, and inclusion-body myositis. N Engl J Med 325:1487-1498, 1991.
548. Dalakas, MC (ed): Polymyositis and Dermatomyositis. Butterworths, Boston, 1988.
549. Dallera, F, Gamoletti, R, and Costa, P: Unilateral seizures following vincristine intravenous injection. Tumori 70:243-244, 1984.
550. Dalmau, J, Furneaux, HM, Cordon-Cardo, C, et al: The expression of the Hu (paraneoplastic encephalomyelitis/sensory neuronopathy) antigen in human normal and tumor tissues. Am J Pathol 141:881-886, 1992.
551. Dalmau, J, Furneaux, HM, Gralla, RJ, et al: Detection of the anti-Hu antibody in the serum of patients with small cell lung cancer—A quantitative western blot analysis. Ann Neurol 27:544-552, 1990.
552. Dalmau, J, Furneaux, HM, Rosenblum, MK, et al: Detection of the anti-Hu antibody in specific regions of the nervous system and tumor from patients with paraneoplastic encephalomyelitis/sensory neuronopathy. Neurology 41:1757-1764, 1991.
553. Dalmau, J, Graus, F, and Marco, M: "Hot and dry foot" as initial manifestation of neoplastic lumbosacral plexopathy. Neurology 39:871-872, 1989.
554. Dalmau, J, Graus, F, Rosenblum, MK, et al: Anti-Hu-associated paraneoplastic encephalomyelitis/sensory neuronopathy. A clinical study of 71 patients. Medicine (Baltimore) 71:59-72, 1992.
554a. Dalmau, J and Posner, JB: Neurologic paraneoplastic antibodies (anti-Yo; anti-Hu; anti-Ri): The case for a nomenclature based on antibody and antigen specificity. Neurology 44:2241-2246, 1994.
555. Daly, JM and Torosian, MH: Nutritional support. In DeVita, VT, Jr, Hellman, S, and Rosenberg, SA (eds): Cancer. Principles & Practice of Oncology, ed 4. JB Lippincott, Philadelphia, 1993, pp 2480-2501.
556. Damasio, AR and Benton, AL: Impairment of hand movements under visual guidance. Neurology 29:170-174, 1979.
556a. Dameron, KM, Volpert, OV, Tainsky, MA, et al: Control of angiogenesis in fibroblasts by p53 regulation of thrombospondin-1. Science 265:1582-1584, 1994.
557. Damon, LE, Mass, R, and Linker, CA: The association between high-dose cytarabine neurotoxicity and renal insufficiency. J Clin Oncol 7:1563-1568, 1989.
558. Damon, LE, Plunkett, W, and Linker, CA: Plasma and cerebrospinal fluid pharmacokinetics of 1-β-D-arabinofuranosylcytosine and 1-β-D-arabinofuranosyluracil following the repeated intravenous administration of high- and intermediate-dose 1-β-D-arabinofuranosylcytosine. Cancer Res 51:4141-4145, 1991.
559. Daniel, SE, Love, S, Scaravilli, F, et al: Encephalomyeloneuropathy in the absence of a detectable neoplasm. Clinical and postmortem findings in three cases. Acta Neuropathol (Berl) 66:311-317, 1985.
560. Danziger, J, Wallace, S, Handel, SF, et al: Metastatic osteogenic sarcoma to the brain. Cancer 43:707-710, 1979.
561. Darnell, RB, Furneaux, HM, and Posner, JB: Antiserum from a patient with cerebellar degeneration identifies a novel protein in Purkinje cells, cortical neurons and neuroectodermal tumors. J Neurosci 11:1224-1230, 1991.
562. Darouiche, RO, Hamill, RJ, Greenberg, SB, et al: Bacterial spinal epidural abscess. Review of 43 cases and literature survey. Medicine (Baltimore) 71:369-385, 1992.
563. Daughaday, WH, Emanuele, MA, Brooks, MH, et al: Synthesis and secretion of insulin-like growth factor II by a leiomyosarcoma with associated hypoglycemia. N Engl J Med 319:1434-1440, 1988.
564. Daugirdas, JT, Kronfol, NO, Tzamaloukas, AH, et al: Hyperosmolar coma: Cellular dehydration and the serum sodium concentration. Ann Intern Med 110:855-857, 1989.
565. Dauplat, J, Nieberg, RK, and Hacker, NF: Central nervous system metastases in epithelial ovarian carcinoma. Cancer 60:2559-2562, 1987.
566. Davey, P and O'Brien, P: Disposition of cerebral metastases from malignant melanoma: Implications for radiosurgery. Neurosurgery 28:8-15, 1991.
567. Davids, D, Henslee, PJ, and Markesbery, WR: Fatal adenovirus meningoencephalitis in a bone marrow transplant patient. Ann Neurol 23:385-389, 1988.
568. Davidson, JE, Willms, DC, and Hoffman, MS: Effect of intermittent pneumatic leg compression on intracranial pressure in brain-injured patients. Crit Care Med 21:224-227, 1993.
568a. Davies, SWV: Intravenous fluids and parageustia. Lancet 343:1432, 1994.

569. Davis, CL, Springmeyer, S, and Gmerek, BJ: Central nervous system side effects of ganciclovir. Letter to the Editor. N Engl J Med 322:933-934, 1990.
570. Davis, DL, et al: Is brain cancer mortality increasing in industrial countries? Am J Ind Med 19:421-431, 1991.
571. Davis, JC, Gates, GA, Lerner, C, et al: Adjuvant hyperbaric oxygen in malignant external otitis. Arch Otolaryngol Head Neck Surg 118:89-93, 1992.
572. Davis, P and Watson, D: Horner's syndrome and vocal cord paralysis as a complication of percutaneous internal jugular vein catherisation in adults. Case report. Anaesthesia 37:587-588, 1982.
573. Davis, PC, Hudgins, PA, Peterman, SB, et al: Diagnosis of cerebral metastases: Double-dose delayed CT vs contrast-enhanced MR imaging. AJNR 12:293-300, 1991.
574. Dawson, DM and Krarup, C: Perioperative nerve lesions. Arch Neurol 46:1355-1360, 1989.
575. Dawson, TM, Lavi, E, Raps, EC, et al: Thrombotic microangiopathy isolated to the central nervous system. Ann Neurol 30:843-846, 1991.
576. Dayes, LA, Rouhe, SA, and Barnes, RW: Excision of multiple intracranial metastatic hypernephroma. Report of a case with a 7-year survival. J Neurosurg 46:533-535, 1977.
577. De Angelis, LM: Primary central nervous system lymphoma: A new clinical challenge. Neurology 41:619-621, 1991.
578. de Divitiis, E, Spaziante, R, Stella, L, et al: Le syndrome pseudo-vasculaire des metastases intracraniennes. Neurochirurgie 24:235-238, 1978.
579. De Reuck, J, Sieben, G, De Coster, W, et al: Prospective neuropathologic study on the occurrence of Wernicke's encephalopathy in patients with tumors of the lymphoid-hemopoietic systems. Acta Neuropathol (Berl) Suppl 7:356-358, 1981.
580. DeAngelis, LM: Primary CNS lymphoma. A new clinical challenge. Neurology 41:619-621, 1991.
581. DeAngelis, LM, Currie, VE, Kim, J-H, et al: The combined use of radiation therapy and lonidamine in the treatment of brain metastases. J Neurooncol 7:241-247, 1989.
582. DeAngelis, LM, Delattre, J-Y, and Posner, JB: Radiation-induced dementia in patients cured of brain metastases. Neurology 39:789-796, 1989.
583. DeAngelis, LM, Gnecco, C, Taylor, L, et al: Evolution of neuropathy and myopathy during intensive vincristine/corticosteroid chemotherapy for non-Hodgkin's lymphoma. Cancer 67:2241-2246, 1991.
584. DeAngelis, LM, Mandell, LR, Thaler, HT, et al: The role of post-operative radiotherapy after resection of single brain metastases. Neurosurgery 24:798-865, 1989.
585. DeAngelis, LM and Payne, R: Lymphomatous meningitis presenting as atypical cluster headache. Pain 30:211-216, 1987.
586. DeAngelis, LM and Shapiro, WR: Drug/radiation interactions and central nervous system injury. In Gutin, PH, Leibel, SA, and Sheline, GE (eds): Radiation Injury to the Nervous System. Raven Press, New York, 1991, pp 361-382.
586a. DeAngelis, LM, Weaver, S, Rosenblum, M: Herpes varicella zoster (HVZ) encephalitis in immunocompromised patients. Abstract: Neurology 44:A332, 1994.
587. DeAngelis, LM, Yahalom, J, Rosenblum, M, et al: Primary CNS lymphoma: Managing patients with spontaneous and AIDS-related disease. Oncology (Huntingt) 1:52-59, 1987.
588. DeCarvalho, C, Shuttleworth, E, Knox, D, et al: Bilateral gaze paralysis with positive computerized tomography findings. A clinicoanatomic correlation. Arch Neurol 37:184-186, 1980.
589. Deck, JH and Lee, MA: Mucin embolism to cerebral arteries: A fatal complication of carcinoma of the breast. Can J Neurol Sci 5:327-330, 1978.
590. Deck, MD: Imaging techniques in the diagnosis of radiation damage to the central nervous system. In Gilbert, HA and Kagan, AR (eds): Radiation Damage to the Nervous System. Raven Press, New York, 1980, pp 107-127.
591. Decker, DA, Decker, VL, Herskovic, A, et al: Brain metastases in patients with renal cell carcinoma: Prognosis and treatment. J Clin Oncol 2:169-173, 1984.
592. Dee, RR and Lorber, B: Brain abscess due to *Listeria monocytogenes*: Case report and literature review. Rev Infect Dis 8:968-977, 1986.
593. Deems, DA, Doty, RL, Settle, RG, et al: Smell and taste disorders, a study of 750 patients from the University of Pennsylvania Smell and Taste Center. Arch Otolaryngol Head Neck Surg 117:519-528, 1991.
594. Defalque, RJ and Fletcher, MV: Neurological complications of central venous cannulation. JPEN 12:406-409, 1988.
595. DeFronzo, RA, Braine, H, Colvin, OM, et al: Water intoxication in man after cyclophosphamide therapy. Time course and relation to drug activation. Ann Intern Med 78:861-869, 1973.
596. DeGregorio, M, Wilbur, B, King, O, et al: Peak cerebrospinal fluid platinum levels in a patient with ependymoma: Evaluation of two different methods of cisplatin administration. Cancer Treat Rep 70:1437-1438, 1986.
597. DeGreve, JLP, Bruyland, M, DeKeyser, J, et al: Lower motor neuron disease in a patient with Hodgkin's disease treated with radiotherapy. Clin Neurol Neurosurg 86-1:43-46, 1984.
598. Dekker, AW, Elderson, A, Punt, K, et al: Meningeal involvement in patients with acute nonlymphocytic leukemia. Incidence, management, and predictive factors. Cancer 56:2078-2082, 1985.
599. Del Maestro, RF, Megyesi, JF, and Farrell, CL: Mechanisms of tumor-associated edema: A review. Can J Neurol Sci 17:177-183, 1990.
600. del Regato, JA: Pathways of metastatic spread of malignant tumors. Semin Oncol 4:33-38, 1977.
601. Delaney, P: Vincristine-induced laryngeal nerve paralysis. Neurology 32:1285-1288, 1982.
602. Delarive, J, and de Tribolet, N: Metastases cerebrales. Etude d'un collectif chirurgical de 81 cas. Neurochirurgie 38:89-97, 1992.
603. Delattre, J-Y, Arbit, E, Thaler, HT, et al: A dose-

response study of dexamethasone in a model of spinal cord compression caused by epidural tumor. J Neurosurg 70:920-925, 1989.

604. Delattre J-Y, et al: Cerebral necrosis following neutron radiation of an extracranial tumor. J Neurooncol 6:113-117, 1988.
605. Delattre, J-Y, Krol, G, Thaler, HT, et al: Distribution of brain metastases. Arch Neurol 45:741-744, 1988.
606. Delattre, J-Y, and Posner, JB: The blood–brain barrier: Morphology, physiology and its change in cancer patients. In Hildebrand, J (ed): Neurological Adverse Reactions to Anticancer Drugs, European School of Oncology Monographs (Veronesi, U, series ed), Springer-Verlag, Berlin, 1990, pp 3-24.
607. Delattre, J-Y, Rosenblum, MK, Thaler, HT, et al: A model of radiation myelopathy in the rat. Pathology, regional capillary permeability changes and treatment with dexamethasone. Brain 111:1319-1336, 1988.
608. Delattre, J-Y, Safai, B, and Posner, JB: Erythema multiforme and Stevens-Johnson syndrome in patients receiving cranial irradiation and phenytoin. Neurology 38:194-198, 1988.
609. Delattre, J-Y, Shapiro, WR, and Posner, JB: Acute effects of low-dose cranial irradiation on regional capillary permeability in experimental brain tumors. J Neurol Sci 90:147-153, 1989.
610. Della Cuna, GR, Pellegrini, A, and Piazzi, M: Effect of methylprednisolone sodium succinate on quality of life in preterminal cancer patients: A placebo-controlled, multicenter study. The Methylprednisolone Preterminal Cancer Study Group. Eur J Cancer Clin Oncol 25:1817-1821, 1989.
611. Demirer, T, Dail, DH, and Aboulafia, DM: Four varied cases of intravascular lymphomatosis and a literature review. Cancer 73:1738-1745, 1994.
612. Denny-Brown, D: Primary sensory neuropathy with muscular changes associated with carcinoma. J Neurol Neurosurg Psychiatry 11:73-87, 1948.
613. Denny-Brown, D and Yanagisawa, N: The function of the descending root of the fifth nerve. Brain 96:783-814, 1973.
614. DePippo, KL, Holas, MA, and Reding, MJ: Validation of the 3-oz water swallow test for aspiration following stroke. Arch Neurol 49:1259-1261, 1992.
615. Deppisch, LM and Fayemi, AO: Non-bacterial thrombotic endocarditis: Clinicopathologic correlations. Am Heart J 92:723-729, 1976.
616. Derby, BM and Guiang, RL: Spectrum of symptomatic brain-stem metastasis. J Neurol Neurosurg Psychiatry 38:888-895, 1975.
617. Deuel, TF: Polypeptide growth factors: Roles in normal and abnormal cell growth. Annu Rev Cell Biol 3:443-492, 1987.
618. Deutsch, AD, Levin, BE, Nathanson, DC, et al: Temporary reversal of cord compression with hyperosmolar glucose. Letter. Neurology 42:2220, 1992.
619. Devereaux, MW, Brust, JC, and Keane, JR: Internuclear ophthalmoplegia caused by subdural hematoma. Neurology 29:251-255, 1979.
620. Devesa, SS and Fears, T: Non-Hodgkin's lymphoma time trends: United States and international data. Cancer Res 52(Suppl 19):5432S-5440S, 1992.
621. Devi, SK, Burns, CA, Riley, EF, et al: Visual function responses of patients receiving X- or 60Co gamma-radiation therapy in the region of head and neck. Int J Radiat Biol Rel Std Phys Chem Med 19:379-392, 1971.
622. Devine, JW, Mendenhall, WM, Million, RR, et al: Carcinoma of the superior pulmonary sulcus treated with surgery and/or radiation therapy. Cancer 57:941-943, 1986.
623. Devinsky, O: Radiation-induced tumors of the central and peripheral nervous system. In Rottenberg, DA (ed): Neurological Complications of Cancer Treatment. Butterworth-Heineman, Boston, MA, 1991, pp 79-94.
624. Devinsky, O, Bear, D, and Volpe, BT: Confusional states following posterior cerebral artery infarction. Arch Neurol 45:160-163, 1988.
625. Devinsky, O, Cho, E-S, Petito, CK, et al: Herpes zoster myelitis. Brain 114(Pt 3):1181-1196, 1991.
626. Devinsky, O, Lemann, W, Evans, AC, et al: Akinetic mutism in a bone marrow transplant recipient following total-body irradiation and amphotericin B chemoprophylaxis. A positron emission tomographic and neuropathologic study. Arch Neurol 44:414-417, 1987.
627. DeVita, VT and Canellos, GP: Hypoglycorrhachia in meningeal carcinomatosis. Cancer 19:691-694, 1966.
628. DeVita, VT, Jr: The problem of resistance. In DeVita, VT, Jr, Hellman, S, and Rosenberg, SA (eds): Cancer. Principles & Practice of Oncology, ed 4. JB Lippincott, Philadelphia, 1990, pp 1-12.
629. DeVita, VT, Jr, Hellman, S, and Rosenberg, SA (eds): Biologic Therapy of Cancer. JB Lippincott, Philadelphia, 1991.
630. Devor, M, Govrin-Lippmann, R, and Raber, P: Corticosteroids suppress ectopic neural discharge originating in experimental neuromas. Pain 22:127-137, 1985.
631. Dewys, WD, Begg, C, Lavin, PT, et al: Prognostic effect of weight loss prior to chemotherapy in cancer patients. Eastern Cooperative Oncology Group. Am J Med 69:491-497, 1980.
632. Dewys, WD and Walters, K: Abnormalities of taste sensation in cancer patients. Cancer 36:1888-1896, 1975.
633. Dexter, DD, Jr, Westmoreland, BF, and Cascino, TL: Complex partial status epilepticus in a patient with leptomeningeal carcinomatosis. Neurology 40:858-859, 1990.
634. Dexter, DL and Leith, JT: Tumor heterogeneity and drug resistance. J Clin Oncol 4:244-257, 1986.
635. Dhib-Jalbut, S and Liwnicz, BH: Immunocytochemical binding of serum IgG from a patient with oat cell tumor and paraneoplastic motoneuron disease to normal human cortex and molecular layer of the cerebellum. Acta Neuropathol (Berl) 69:96-102, 1986.
635a. Dhodapkar, M, Goldberg, SL, Tefferi, A, et al: Reversible encephalopathy after cryopreserved peripheral blood stem cell infusion. Am J Hematol 45:187-188, 1994.

636. Di Gregorio, F, Favaro, G, Panozzo, C, et al: Efficacy of ganglioside treatment in reducing functional alterations induced by vincristine in rabbit peripheral nerves. Cancer Chemother Pharmacol 26:31-36, 1990.
637. Di Napoli, RP and Thomas, JE: Neurologic aspects of malignant external otitis: Report of three cases. Mayo Clin Proc 46:339-344, 1971.
638. Diaz, JM, Urban, ES, Schiffman, JS, et al: Post-irradiation neuromyotonia affecting trigeminal nerve distribution: An unusual presentation. Neurology 42:1102-1104, 1992.
639. DiChiro, G, Oldfield, E, Wright, DC, et al: Cerebral necrosis after radiotherapy and/or intracranial chemotherapy for brain tumors: PET and neuropathologic studies. AJR 150:189-197, 1988.
640. Dickenman, RC and Chason, JL: Alterations in the dorsal root ganglia and adjacent nerves in the leukemias, the lymphomas and multiple myeloma. Am J Pathol 34:349-357, 1958.
641. Dieckert, JP and Berger, BB: Prostatic carcinoma metastatic to choroid. Br J Ophthalmol 66:234-239, 1982.
642. Dietl, HW, Pulst, SM, Engelhardt, P, et al: Paraneoplastic brainstem encephalitis with acute dystonia and central hypoventilation. J Neurol 227:229-238, 1982.
643. Digre, KB: Opsoclonus in adults. Report of three cases and review of the literature. Arch Neurol 43:1165-1175, 1986.
643a. Dillman, RO: Antibodies as cytotoxic therapy. J Clin Oncol 12:1497-1515, 1994.
644. DiMaggio, JR, Brown, R, Baile, WF, et al: Hallucinations and ifosfamide-induced neurotoxicity. Cancer 73:1509-1514, 1994.
645. Dimich, A, Bedrossian, PB, and Wallach, S: Hypoparathyroidism. Clinical observations in 34 patients. Arch Intern Med 120:449-458, 1967.
646. DiResta, GR, Lee, J, Larson, SM, et al: Characterization of neuroblastoma xenograft in rat flank: I. Growth, interstitial fluid pressure, and interstitial fluid velocity distribution profiles. Microvas Res 46:158-177, 1993.
647. Dirr, LY, Elster, AD, Donofrio, PD, et al: Evolution of brain MRI abnormalities in limbic encephalitis. Neurology 40:1304-1306, 1990.
648. Dische, S, Martin, WM, and Anderson, P: Radiation myelopathy in patients treated for carcinoma of bronchus using a six fraction regimen of radiotherapy. Br J Radiol 54:29-35, 1981.
649. Dische, S, Warburton, MF, and Saunders, MI: Radiation myelitis and survival in the radiotherapy of lung cancer. Int J Radiat Oncol Biol Phys 15:75-81, 1988.
650. DiTullio, M, Sacco, RL, Gopal, A, et al: Patent foramen ovale as a risk factor for cryptogenic stroke. Ann Intern Med 117:461-465, 1992.
651. Dixon, RA, and Christy, NP: On the various forms of corticosteroid withdrawal syndrome. Am J Med 68:224-230, 1980.
652. Dizhoor, AM, Ray, S, Kumar, S, et al: Recoverin: A calcium sensitive activator of retinal rod guanylate cyclase. Science 251:915-918, 1991.
653. Djaldetti, M, Pinkhas, J, Vries, AD, et al: Myasthenia gravis in a patient with chronic myeloid leukemia treated by busulfan. Blood 32:336-340, 1968.
654. Doblin, RE and Kleiman, MA: Marijuana as antiemetic medicine: A survey of oncologists' experiences and attitudes. J Clin Oncol 9:1314-1319, 1991.
655. Dodge, HW, Svien, HJ, Camp, JD, et al: Tumors of the spinal cord without neurologic manifestations, producing low back and sciatic pain. Mayo Clin Proc 26:88-96, 1951.
656. Dodi, G, Farini, R, Pedrazzoli, S, et al: Effect of cimetidine on steroid experimental peptic ulcers. Acta Hepato-Gastroenterologica (Stuttgart) 25:395-397, 1978.
657. Dodson, WE, DeLorenzo, RJ, Pedley, TA, et al: Treatment of convulsive status epilepticus. Recommendations of the Epilepsy Foundation of America's Working Group on Status Epilepticus. JAMA 270:854-859, 1993.
658. Dofferhoff, AS, Berendsen, HH, Naalt, VD, et al: Decreased phenytoin level after carboplatin treatment. Am J Med 89:247-248, 1990.
659. Doge, H and Hliscs, R: Intrathecal therapy with ^{198}Au-colloid for meningosis prophylaxis. Eur J Nucl Med 9:125-128, 1984.
660. Doig, RG, Olver, IN, Jeal, PN, et al: Symptomatic choroidal metastases in breast cancer. Aust N Z J Med 22:349-352, 1992.
661. Doll, DC, List, AF, Greco, FA, et al: Acute vascular ischemic events after cisplatin-based combination chemotherapy for germ-cell tumors of the testis. Ann Intern Med 105:48-51, 1986.
662. Doll, DC, Ringenberg, QS, and Yarbro, JW: Vascular toxicity associated with antineoplastic agents. J Clin Oncol 4:1405-1417, 1986.
663. Doll, DC and Yarbro, JW: Vascular toxicity associated with antineoplastic agents. Semin Oncol 19:580-596, 1992.
664. Dolman, CL, Sweeney, VP, and Magil, A: Neoplastic angioendotheliosis. The case of the missed primary? Arch Neurol 36:5-7, 1979.
665. Dommasch, D, Przuntek, H, Gruninger, W, et al: Intrathecal cytostatic chemotherapy of meningitis carcinomatosa. Clinical manifestation and cerebrospinal fluid cytology in a case of metastatic carcinoma of the breast. Eur Neurol 14:178-191, 1976.
666. Donato, T, Shapria, Y, Artru, A, et al: Effect of mannitol on cerebrospinal fluid dynamics and brain tissue edema. Anesth Analg 78:58-66, 1994.
667. Donofrio, PD, Alessi, AG, Alberts, JW, et al: Electrodiagnostic evolution of carcinomatous sensory neuronopathy. Muscle Nerve 12:508-513, 1989.
668. Doppman, JL: The mechanism of ischemia in anteroposterior compression of the spinal cord. Invest Radiol 10:543-551, 1975.
669. Dorfman, LJ, Donaldson, SS, Gupta, PR, et al: Electrophysiologic evidence of subclinical injury to the posterior columns of the human spinal cord after therapeutic radiation. Cancer 50:2815-2819, 1982.
670. Dorfman, LJ and Forno, LS: Paraneoplastic encephalomyelitis. Acta Neurol Scand 48:556-574, 1972.
671. Doroshow, JH, Locker, GY, Gaasterland, DE, et al:

Ocular irritation from high-dose methotrexate therapy: Pharmacokinetics of drug in the tear film. Cancer 48:2158-2162, 1981.

672. Doroshow, JH, Tallent, C, and Schechter, JE: Ultrastructural features of Adriamycin-induced skeletal and cardiac muscle toxicity. Am J Pathol 118:288-297, 1985.

673. Doshi, HM, Schochet, SS, Jr, Gold, M, et al: Granulocytic sarcoma presenting as an epidural mass with acute paraparesis in a leukemic patient. Am J Clin Pathol 95:228-232, 1991.

674. Doshi, R and Fowler, T: Proximal myopathy due to discrete carcinomatous metastases in muscle. J Neurol Neurosurg Psychiatry 46:358-360, 1983.

675. Dosoretz, DE, Blitzer, PH, Russell, AH, et al: Management of solitary metastasis to the brain: The role of elective brain irradiation following complete surgical resection. Int J Radiat Oncol Biol Phys 6:1727-1730, 1980.

676. Douglas, MA, Parks, LC, and Bebin, J: Sudden myelopathy secondary to therapeutic total-body hyperthermia after spinal cord irradiation. N Engl J Med 304:583-585, 1981.

677. Dresel, SHJ, Mackey, JK, Lufkin, RB, et al: Meckel cave lesions: Percutaneous fine-needle-aspiration biopsy cytology. Radiology 179:579-582, 1991.

678. Drew, WL: Nonpulmonary manifestations of cytomegalovirus infection in immunocompromised patients. Clin Microbiol Rev 5:204-210, 1992.

679. Driedger, H and Pruzanski, W: Plasma cell neoplasia with peripheral polyneuropathy: A study of five cases and a review of the literature. Medicine (Baltimore) 59:301-310, 1980.

680. Dritschilo, A, Bruckman, JE, Cassady, JR, et al: Tolerance of brain to multiple courses of radiation therapy. I. Clinical experiences. Br J Radiol 54:782-786, 1981.

681. Drlicek, M, Grisold, W, Liszka, U, et al: Angiotropic lymphoma (malignant angioendotheliomatosis) presenting with rapidly progressive dementia. Acta Neuropathol (Berl) 82:533-535, 1992.

682. Drobyski, WR, Knox, KK, Majewski, D, et al: Brief report: Fatal encephalitis due to variant B human herpesvirus-6 infection in a bone marrow-transplant recipient. N Engl J Med 330:1356-1360, 1994.

683. Dropcho, EJ: Central nervous system injury by therapeutic irradiation. Neurol Clin 9:969-988, 1991.

684. Dropcho, EJ: Expression of the "onconeural" CDR34 gene in human carcinomas. Abstract. Neurology 41(Suppl 1) 1:238, 1991.

685. Dropcho, EJ, Chen, Y-T, Posner, JB, et al: Cloning of a brain protein identified by autoantibodies from a patient with paraneoplastic cerebellar degeneration. Proc Natl Acad Sci U S A 84:4552-4556, 1987.

686. Dropcho, EJ and Soong, S-J: Steroid-induced weakness in patients with primary brain tumors. Neurology 41:1235-1239, 1991.

687. Druckmann, A: Schlafsucht als Folge der Rontegenbestrahlung. Beitrag zur Strahlenempfindlichkeit des Gehirns. Strahlentherapie 33:382-384, 1929.

688. Dubuisson, AS, Kline, DG, and Weinshel, SS: Posterior subscapular approach to the brachial plexus. Report of 102 patients. J Neurosurg 79:319-330, 1993.

689. Dueland, AN, Devlin, M, Martin, JR, et al: Fatal varicella-zoster virus meningoradiculitis without skin involvement. Ann Neurol 29:569-572, 1991.

690. Duffy, GP: Lumbar puncture in the presence of raised intracranial pressure. BMJ 1:407-409, 1969.

691. Duncan, JS, Shorvon, SD, and Trimble, MR: Effects of removal of phenytoin, carbamazepine, and valproate on cognitive function. Epilepsia 31(5):584-591, 1990.

692. Dunn, DW, Daum, RS, Weisberg, L, et al: Ischemic cerebrovascular complications of *Haemophilus influenzae* meningitis. The value of computed tomography. Arch Neurol 39:650-652, 1982.

693. Dunton, SF, Nitschke, R, Spruce, WE, et al: Progressive ascending paralysis following administration of intrathecal and intravenous cytosine arabinoside. A Pediatric Oncology Group study. Cancer 57:1083-1088, 1986.

694. Durand, ML, Calderwood, SB, Weber, DJ, et al: Acute bacterial meningitis in adults. A review of 493 episodes. N Engl J Med 328:21-28, 1993.

695. Dutcher, JP, Marcus, SL, Tanowitz, HB, et al: Disseminated strongyloidiasis with central nervous system involvement diagnosed antemortem in a patient with acquired immunodeficiency syndrome and Burkitts lymphoma. Cancer 66:2417-2420, 1990.

696. Dux, R, Kindler-Rohrborn, A, Annas, M, et al: A standardized protocol for flow cytometric analysis of cells isolated from cerebrospinal fluid. J Neurol Sci 121:74-78, 1994.

697. Dvorak, HF: Thrombosis and cancer. Hum Pathol 18:275-284, 1987.

698. Dworkin, LA, Goldman, RD, Zivin, LS, et al: Cerebellar toxicity following high-dose cytosine arabinoside. J Clin Oncol 3:613-616, 1985.

699. Dyck, P: Lumbar reservoir for intrathecal chemotherapy. Cancer 55:2771-2773, 1985.

700. Eapen, L, Vachet, M, Catton, G, et al: Brain metastases with an unknown primary: A clinical perspective. J Neurooncol 6:31-35, 1988.

701. Easton, HG: Zoster sine herpete causing acute trigeminal neuralgia. Lancet 2:1065-1066, 1970.

702. Ebb, DH, Kerasidis, H, Vezina, G, et al: Spinal cord compression in widely metastatic Wilms' tumor. Paraplegia in two children with anaplastic Wilms' tumor. Cancer 69:2726-2730, 1992.

703. Ebels, EJ and van der Meulen, JDM: Cerebral metastasis without known primary tumour—A retrospective study. Clin Neurol Neurosurg 80(3):195-197, 1978.

704. Eberth, CJ: Zur Entwickelung des Epithelioms (Cholesteatoms) der Pia und der Lunge. Virchows Arch 49:51-63, 1870.

705. Ebner, F, Ranner, G, Slavc, J, et al: MR findings in methotrexate-induced CNS abnormalities. AJNR 10:959-964, 1989.

706. Eby, NL, Grufferman, S, Flannelly, CM, et al: Increasing incidence of primary brain lymphoma in the US. Cancer 62:2461-2465, 1988.

707. Edelson, RN, Chernik, NL, and Posner, JB: Spinal subdural hematomas complicating lumbar puncture. Arch Neurol 31:134-137, 1974.

708. Edelson, RN, Deck, MD, and Posner, JB: In-

tramedullary spinal cord metastases. Clinical and radiographic findings in nine cases. Neurology 22:1222-1231, 1972.
709. Edelson, RN, McNatt, EN, and Porro, RS: *Candida* meningitis with cerebral arteritis. New York State Journal of Medicine 75:900-904, 1975.
710. Eden, OB, Goldie, W, Wood, T, et al: Seizures following intrathecal cytosine arabinoside in young children with acute lymphoblastic leukemias. Cancer 42:53-58, 1978.
711. Ehrenkranz, JRL and Posner, JB: Adrenocorticosteroid hormones. In Weiss, L, Gilbert, HA, and Posner, JB (eds). Brain Metastasis. GK Hall & Co, Boston, 1980, pp 340-363.
712. Eidelberg, D, Sotrel, A, Horoupian, S, et al: Thrombotic cerebral vasculopathy associated with herpes zoster. Ann Neurol 19:7-14, 1986.
713. Einhaupl, KM, Villringer, A, Meister, W, et al: Heparin treatment in sinus venous thrombosis. Lancet 338:597-600, 1991.
714. Einzig, AI, Wiernik, PH, Sasloff, J, et al: Phase II study and long-term follow-up of patients treated with taxol for advanced ovarian adenocarcinoma. J Clin Oncol 10:1748-1753, 1992.
715. Eisenberg, L: The social imperatives of medical research. Impeding medical research, no less than performing it, has ethical consequences. Not to act is to act. Science 198:1105-1110, 1977.
716. Ekbom, K, Hornsten, G, and Johansson, T: Posterior cranial fossa tumors. Headaches, oculostatic disorders and scintillation camera findings. Headache 14:119-132, 1974.
717. Elerding, SC, Fernandez, RN, Grotta, JC, et al: Carotid artery disease following external cervical irradiation. Ann Surg 194:609-615, 1981.
718. Elkington, JSC: Metastatic tumors of the brain. Proceedings of the Royal Society of Medicine 28:1080-1096, 1935.
719. Elkon, KB, Hughes, GR, Catovsky, D, et al: Hairy-cell leukaemia with polyarteritis nodosa. Lancet 2:280-282, 1979.
720. Ellis, CJK, Daniel, SE, Kennedy, PG, et al: Rhino-orbital zygomycosis. J Neurol Neurosurg Psychiatry 48:455-458, 1985.
721. Ellis, F: Dose, time and fractionation: A clinical hypothesis. Clin Radiol 20:1-7, 1969.
722. Ellis, F: Nominal standard dose of the ret. Br J Radiol 44:101-108, 1971.
723. Ellison, MD, Krieg, RJ, and Merchant, RE: Cerebral vasomotor responses after recombinant interleukin 2 infusion. Cancer Res 50:4377-4381, 1990.
724. Elster, AD and DiPersio, DA: Cranial postoperative site: Assessment with contrast-enhanced MR imaging. Radiology 174:93-98, 1990.
725. Enevoldson, TP, Scadding, JW, Rustin, GJ, et al: Spontaneous resolution of a postirradiation lumbosacral plexopathy. Neurology 42:2224-2225, 1992.
726. Engel, GL and Romano, J: Delirium, a syndrome of cerebral insufficiency. J Chronic Dis 9:260-277, 1959.
727. Engel, IA, Straus, DJ, Lacher, M, et al: Osteonecrosis in patients with malignant lymphoma. A review of 25 cases. Cancer 48:1245-1250, 1981.
728. Engel, J: Seizures and Epilepsy. FA Davis Company, Philadelphia, 1989.
729. Engel, PA, Grunnet, M, and Jacobs, B: Wernicke-Korsakoff syndrome complicating T-cell lymphoma: Unusual or unrecognized? South Med J 84:253-256, 1991.
730. Epelbaum, R, Haim, N, Ben-Shahar, M, et al: Non-Hodgkin's lymphoma presenting with spinal epidural involvement. Cancer 58:2120-2124, 1986.
731. Epstein, MA, Packer, RJ, Rorke, LB, et al: Vascular malformation with radiation vasculopathy after treatment of chiasmatic/hypothalamic glioma. Cancer 70:887-893, 1992.
732. Epstein, N, Hood, DC, and Ransohoff, J: Gastrointestinal bleeding in patients with spinal cord trauma. Effects of steroids, cimetidine, and minidose heparin. J Neurosurg 54:16-20, 1981.
733. Erlington, GM, Murray, NM, Spiro, SG, et al: Neurological paraneoplastic syndromes in patients with small cell lung cancer. A prospective survey of 150 patients. J Neurol Neurosurg Psychiatry 54:764-767, 1991.
734. Ersboll, J, Schultz, HB, Thomsen, BL, et al: Meningeal involvement in non-Hodgkin's lymphoma: Symptoms, incidence, risk factors and treatment. Scand J Haematol 35:487-496, 1985.
735. Espana, P, Chang, P, and Wiernik, PH: Increased incidence of brain metastases in sarcoma patients. Cancer 45:377-380, 1980.
736. Estevez, CM and Corya, BC: Serial echocardiographic abnormalities in nonbacterial thrombotic endocarditis of the mitral valve. Chest 69:801-804, 1976.
737. Ethelberg, S and Jensen, VA: Obscurations and further time-related paroxysmal disorders in intracranial tumors: Syndrome of initial herniation of parts of the brain through the tentorial incisure. J Neurol Psychiatry 68:130-149, 1952.
738. Ettinger, LJ: Pharmacokinetics and biochemical effects of a fatal intrathecal methotrexate overdose. Cancer 50:444-450, 1982.
739. Ettinger, LJ, Freeman, AI, and Creaven, PJ: Intrathecal methotrexate overdose without neurotoxicity: Case report and literature review. Cancer 41:1270-1273, 1978.
740. Etzioni, A, Levy, J, Lichtig, C, et al: Brain mass as a manifestation of very late relapse in nonendemic Burkitt's lymphoma. Cancer 55:861-863, 1985.
741. Evans, BK, Fagan, C, Arnold, T, et al: Paraneoplastic motor neuron disease and renal cell carcinoma: Improvement after nephrectomy. Neurology 40:960-962, 1990.
742. Evans, CH, Westfall, V, and Atuk, NO: Astrocytoma mimicking the features of pheochromocytoma. N Engl J Med 286:1397-1399, 1972.
743. Evans, ML, Graham, MM, Mahler, PA, et al: Use of steroids to suppress vascular response to radiation. Int J Radiat Oncol Biol Phys 13:563-567, 1987.
744. Ewing, J: Metastasis. In Ewing, J (ed): Neoplastic Diseases: A Treatise on Tumours, ed 4. WB Saunders, Philadelphia, 1940, pp 62-74.
745. Ey, FS and Goodnight, SH: Bleeding disorders in cancer. Semin Oncol 17:187-197, 1990.
746. Eyre, HJ, Ohlsen, JD, Frank, J, et al: Randomized trial of radiotherapy versus radiotherapy plus metronidazole for the treatment of metastatic cancer

to brain. A Southwest Oncology Group study. J Neurooncol 2:325-330, 1984.
747. Ezrin-Waters, C, Klein, M, Deck, J, et al: Diagnostic importance of immunological markers in lymphoma involving the central nervous system. Ann Neurol 16:668-672, 1984.
748. Fadul, C, Misulis, KE, and Wiley, RG: Cerebellar metastases: Diagnostic and management considerations. J Clin Oncol 5:1107-1115, 1987.
749. Fadul, CE, Lemann, W, Thaler, HT, et al: Perforation of the gastrointestinal tract in patients receiving steroids for neurological disease. Neurology 38:348-352, 1988.
750. Fagius, J and Westerberg, C-E: Pseudoclaudication syndrome caused by a tumour of the cauda equina. J Neurol Neurosurg Psychiatry 42:187-189, 1979.
751. Fain, JS, Naeim, F, Becker, DP, et al: Chronic lymphocytic leukemia presenting as a pituitary mass lesion. Can J Neurol Sci 19:239-242, 1992.
752. Falk, WE, Mahnke, MW, and Poskanger, DC: Lithium prophylaxis of corticotropin-induced psychosis. JAMA 241:1011-1012, 1979.
753. Farcet, J-P, Weschsler, J, Wirquin, V, et al: Vasculitis in hairy-cell leukemia. Arch Intern Med 147:660-664, 1987.
754. Farmer, L, Echlin, FA, Loughlin, WC, et al: Pachymeningitis apparently due to penicillin hypersensitivity. Ann Intern Med 52:910-914, 1960.
755. Farrar, WB: Clinical trials. Access and reimbursement. Cancer 67(Suppl 6):1779-1782, 1991.
756. Farrell, CL and Shivers, RR: Capillary junctions of the rat are not affected by osmotic opening of the blood–brain barrier. Acta Neuropathol (Berl) 63:179-189, 1984.
757. Fast, A, Alon, M, Weiss, S, et al: Avascular necrosis of bone following short-term dexamethasone therapy for brain edema. J Neurosurg 61:983-985, 1984.
758. Fathallah-Shaykh, H, Wolf, S, Wong, E, et al: Cloning of a leucine-zipper protein recognized by the sera of patients with antibody-associated paraneoplastic cerebellar degeneration. Proc Natl Acad Sci U S A 88:3451-3454, 1991.
759. Fein, DA, Marcus, RB, Jr, Parsons, JT, et al: Lhermitte's sign: Incidence and treatment variables influencing risk after irradiation of the cervical spinal cord. Int J Radiat Oncol Biol Phys 27:1029-1033, 1994.
760. Feinberg, WM and Swenson, MR: Cerebrovascular complications of L-asparaginase therapy. Neurology 38:127-133, 1988.
761. Feldenzer, JA, McKeever, PE, Schaberg, DR, et al: The pathogenesis of spinal epidural abscess: Microangiographic studies in an experimental model. J Neurosurg 69:110-114, 1988.
762. Feldman, M and Eisenbach, L: What makes a tumor cell metastatic? Sci Am 259:60-65, 68, 85, 1988.
763. Feldman, S, Hughes, WT, and Daniel, CB: Varicella in children with cancer: Seventy-seven cases. Pediatrics 56:388-397, 1975.
764. Feldmann, E, Gandy, SE, Becker, R, et al: MRI demonstrates descending transtentorial herniation. Neurology 38:697-701, 1988.
765. Feldmann, E and Posner, JB: Episodic neurologic dysfunction in patients with Hodgkin's disease. Arch Neurol 43:1227-1233, 1986.
766. Felsen, DT and Anderson, JJ: A cross-study evaluation of association between steroid dose and bolus steroids and avascular necrosis of bone. Lancet 1:902-905, 1987.
767. Fenstermacher, JD: Pharmacology of the blood–brain barrier. In Neuwelt, EA (ed): Implications of the Blood–Brain Barrier and Its Manipulation, vol 1, Basic Science Aspects, Plenum Medical Book Company, New York, 1989, pp 137-155.
768. Fernando, IN and Tobias, JS: Priapism in patient on tamoxifen. Letter to the Editor. Lancet 1:436, 1989.
769. Ferrari, P, Federico, M, Grimaldi, LM, et al: Stiff-man syndrome in a patient with Hodgkin's disease. An unusual paraneoplastic syndrome. Hematologica (Pavia) 75:570-572, 1990.
770. Ferrigno, D and Buccheri, G: Lumbar muscle metastasis from lung cancer—report of a case. Letter to the Editor. Acta Oncol 31:680-681, 1992.
771. Ferry, AP and Font, RL: Carcinoma metastatic to the eye and orbit. I. A clinicopathologic study of 227 cases. Arch Ophthalmol 92:276-286, 1974.
772. Fessler, RG, Dietze, DD, Jr, Millan, M, et al: Lateral parascapular extrapleural approach to the upper thoracic spine. J Neurosurg 75:349-355, 1991.
773. Fetting, JH, Wilcox, PM, Sheidler, VR, et al: Tastes associated with parenteral chemotherapy for breast cancer. Cancer Treat Rep 69:1249-1251, 1985.
774. Feun, LG, Wallace, S, Stewart, DJ, et al: Intracarotid infusion of cis-diamminedichloroplatinum in the treatment of recurrent malignant brain tumors. Cancer 54:794-799, 1984.
775. Fidler, IJ: Critical factors in the biology of human cancer metastasis: Twenty-eighth G.H.A. Clowes memorial award lecture. Cancer Res 50:6130-6138, 1990.
776. Fidler, IJ: 7th Jan Waldenstrom Lecture. The biology of human cancer metastasis. Acta Oncol 30:668-675, 1991.
777. Fidler, IJ and Lieber, S: Quantitative analysis of the mechanism of glucocorticoid enhancement of experimental metastasis. Res Commun Chem Pathol Pharmacol 4:607-613, 1972.
778. Fidler, IJ and Poste, G: The cellular heterogeneity of malignant neoplasms: Implications for adjuvant chemotherapy. Semin Oncol 12:207-221, 1985.
779. Fidler, IJ and Radinsky, R: Genetic control of cancer metastasis. Editorial. J Natl Cancer Inst 82:166-168, 1990.
779a. Fidler, IJ, Wilmanns, C, Staroselsky, A, et al: Modulation of tumor cell response to chemotherapy by the organ environment. Cancer Metastasis Rev 13:209-222, 1994.
780. Figlin, RA, Piantadosi, S, Feld, R, et al: Intracranial recurrence of carcinoma after complete surgical resection of stage I, II, and III non-small cell lung cancer. N Engl J Med 318:1300-1305, 1988.
781. Filler, AG, Howe, FA, Hayes, CE, et al: Magnetic resonance neurography. Lancet 341:659-661, 1993.
782. Filley, CM, Graff-Richard, NR, Lacy, JR, et al:

Neurologic manifestations of podophyllin toxicity. Neurology 32:308-311, 1982.
783. Findlay, GF: Adverse effects of the management of malignant spinal cord compression. J Neurol Neurosurg Psychiatry 47:761-768, 1984.
784. Findlay, GF: The role of vertebral body collapse in the management of malignant spinal cord compression. J Neurol Neurosurg Psychiatry 50:151-154, 1987.
785. Finlay, JL: High-dose chemotherapy followed by bone marrow "rescue" for recurrent brain tumors. In Bleyer, A and Packer, R (eds): Pediatric Neurooncology: New Trends in Clinical Research. Harwood Academic Publishers, New York, 1992, pp 278-297.
786. Finlayson, AI and Penfield, W: Acute postoperative aseptic leptomeningitis: Review of cases and discussion of pathogenesis. Archives of Neurology and Psychiatry 46:250-276, 1941.
787. Fisher, CM: Transient paralytic attacks of obscure nature: The question of non-convulsive seizure paralysis. Can J Neurol Sci 5:267-273, 1978.
788. Fisher, CM: Late-life migraine accompaniments as a cause of unexplained transient ischemic attacks. Can J Neurol Sci 7:9-17, 1980.
789. Fisher, CM: Hydrocephalus as a cause of disturbances of gait in the elderly. Neurology 32:1358-1363, 1982.
790. Fisher, MS: Lumbar spine metastasis in cervical carcinoma: A characteristic pattern. Radiology 134:631-634, 1980.
791. Fisher, PG, Wechsler, DS, and Singer, HS: Anti-Hu antineuronal antibody in neuroblastoma-associated paraneoplastic syndrome. Pediatr Neurol 10: 309-312, 1994.
792. Fishman, RA: Studies of the transport of sugars between blood and cerebrospinal fluid in normal states and in meningeal carcinomatosis. Trans Am Neurol Assoc 88:114-118, 1963.
793. Fishman, RA: Carrier transport and the concentration of glucose in cerebrospinal fluid in meningeal diseases. Editorial. Ann Intern Med 63:153-155, 1965.
794. Fishman, RA: Is there a therapeutic role for osmotic breaching of the blood–brain barrier? Editorial. Ann Neurol 22:298-299, 1987.
795. Fishman, RA: Cerebrospinal Fluid in Diseases of the Nervous System, ed 2. WB Saunders, Philadelphia, 1992.
796. Fishman, RA, Sligar, K, and Hake, RB: Effects of leukocytes on brain metabolism in granulocytic brain edema. Ann Neurol 2:89-94, 1977.
797. Flavin, DK, Frederickson, PA, Richardson, JW, et al: Corticosteroid abuse—an unusual manifestation of drug dependence. Mayo Clin Proc 58:764-766, 1983.
798. Fleishman, S and Lesko, LM: Delirium and dementia. In Holland, JC and Rowland, JH (eds): Handbook of Psychooncology: Psychological Care of the Patient with Cancer. Oxford University Press, New York, 1989, pp 342-355.
799. Flenly, DC: Clinical hypoxia: Causes, consequences and correction. Lancet 1:542-546, 1978.
800. Flickinger, JC, Kondziolka, D, Lunsford, LD, et al: A multi-institutional experience with stereotactic radiosurgery for solitary brain metastasis. Int J Radiat Oncol Biol Phys 28:797-802, 1994.
801. Flickinger, JC, Loeffler, JS, and Larson, DA: Stereotactic radiosurgery for intracranial malignancies. Oncology 8:81-86, 1994.
802. Floeter, MK, So, YT, Ross, DA, et al: Miliary metastasis to the brain: Clinical and radiologic features. Neurology (NY) 37:1817-1818, 1987.
803. Flowers, A and Levin, VA: Management of brain metastases from breast carcinoma. Oncology (Huntingt) 7:21-34, 1993.
804. Focan, C, Olivier, R, Le Hung, S, et al: Neurological toxicity of vindesine used in combination chemotherapy of 51 human solid tumors. Cancer Chemother Pharmacol 6:175-181, 1981.
805. Fogelholm, R, Uutela, T, and Murros, K: Epidemiology of central nervous system neoplasms. A regional survey in Central Finland. Acta Neurol Scand 69:129-136, 1984.
806. Foley, KM: Brachial plexopathy in patients with breast cancer. In Harris, JR, Hellman, S, Henderson, IC, et al (eds): Breast Diseases ed 2. JB Lippincott, Philadelphia, 1990, pp 722-729.
807. Foley, KM, Woodruff, JM, Ellis, FT, et al: Radiation-induced malignant and atypical peripheral nerve sheath tumors. Ann Neurol 7:311-318, 1980.
808. Folkman, J: How is blood vessel growth regulated in normal and neoplastic tissue? G.H.A. Clower Memorial Award Lecture. Cancer Res 46:467-473, 1986.
809. Folkman, J: What is the evidence that tumors are angiogenesis dependent? J Natl Cancer Inst 82:4-6, 1990.
810. Folkman, J, Langer, R, Linhardt, RJ, et al: Angiogenesis inhibition and tumor regression caused by heparin or a heparin fragment in the presence of cortisone. Science 221:719-725, 1983.
811. Folli, F, Solimena, M, Cofiell, R, et al: Autoantibodies to a 128-kd synaptic protein in three women with the stiff-man syndrome and breast cancer. N Engl J Med 328:546-551, 1993.
812. Folliss, AG and Netsky, MG: Progressive necrotic myelopathy. In Vinken, PJ and Bruyn, GW (eds): Handbook of Clinical Neurology, vol 9, Multiple Sclerosis and Other Demyelinating Diseases. North-Holland, Amsterdam, 1970, pp 452-468.
812a. Folpe, A, Lapham, LW, and Smith, HC: Herpes simplex myelitis as a cause of acute necrotizing myelitis syndrome. Neurology 44:1955-1957, 1994.
813. Folstein, MF, Fetting, JH, Lobo, A, et al: Cognitive assessment of cancer patients. Cancer 53(Suppl 10):2250-2257, 1984.
814. Folstein, MF, Folstein, SE, and McHugh, PR: "Mini-mental state." A practical method for grading the cognitive state of patients for the clinician. J Psychiatr Res 12:189-198, 1975.
815. Fonseca, OA and Claverley, JR: Neurological manifestations of hypoparathyroidism. Arch Intern Med 120:202-206, 1967.
816. Font, J, Valls, J, Cervera, R, et al: Pure sensory neuropathy in patients with primary Sjögren's syndrome: Clinical, immunological, and electromyographic findings. Ann Rheum Dis 49:775-778, 1990.
817. Forman, A: Peripheral neuropathy in cancer

patients: Incidence, features, and pathophysiology. Part 1. Oncology 4:57-62, 1990.
818. Forman, A: Peripheral neuropathy in cancer patients: Clinical types, etiology, and presentation. Part 2. Oncology 4:85-89, 1990.
819. Forman, AD: Neurologic complications of cytokine therapy. Oncology 8:105-110, 1994.
820. Fornasier, VL and Horne, JG: Metastases to the vertebral column. Cancer 36:590-594, 1975.
821. Forsyth, PA, Balmaceda, C, Peterson, K, et al: Prospective study of taxol-induced peripheral neuropathy (PN) with quantitative sensory testing (QST). Abstract. Neurology 43:A397, 1993.
822. Forsyth, PA, Dalmau, J, Graus, F, et al: Paraneoplastic motor neuron disease. Ann Neurol 34:277, 1993.
822a. Forsyth, PA and Posner, JB: Headaches in patients with brain tumors: A study of 111 patients. Neurology 43:1678-1683, 1993.
823. Fossa, SD, Aass, N, and Kaalhus, O: Long-term morbidity after infradiaphragmatic radiotherapy in young men with testicular cancer. Cancer 64:404-408, 1969.
824. Foster, O, Crockard, HA, and Powell, MP: Syrinx associated with intramedullary metastasis. J Neurol Neurosurg Psychiatry 50:1067-1070, 1987.
825. Fox, MW and Onofrio, BM: The natural history and management of symptomatic and asymptomatic vertebral hemangiomas. J Neurosurg 78:36-45, 1993.
826. Foy, PM, Chadwick, DW, Rajgopalan, N, et al: Do prophylactic anticonvulsant drugs alter the pattern of seizures after craniotomy? J Neurol Neurosurg Psychiatry 55:753-757, 1992.
827. Francis, J, Martin, D, and Kapoor, WN: A prospective study of delirium in hospitalized elderly. JAMA 263:1097-1101, 1990.
828. Frank, JA, Girton, M, Dwyer, AJ, et al: Meningeal carcinomatosis in the VX2 rabbit tumor model: Detection with Gd-DTPA-enhanced MR imaging. Radiology 167:825-829, 1988.
829. Frank, JA, Jr, Friedman, HS, Davidson, DM, et al: *Propionibacterium* shunt nephritis in two adolescents with medulloblastoma. Cancer 52:330-333, 1983.
830. Frankenheim, J and Brown, RM (eds): Bioavailability of Drugs to the Brain and the Blood–Brain Barrier. National Institute on Drug Abuse Research Monograph Series, No. 120, United States Department of Health and Human Services, Washington, D.C., 1992.
831. Franzen, L, Funegard, U, Ericson, T, et al: Parotid gland function during and following radiotherapy of malignancies in the head and neck. A consecutive study of salivary flow and patient discomfort. Eur J Cancer 28:457-462, 1992.
832. Frasquet, FJ and Belda, FJ: Permanent paralysis of C-5 after cannulation of the internal jugular vein. Letter to the Editor. Anesthesiology 54:528, 1981.
833. Fraunfelder, FT and Meyer, SM: Ocular toxicity of antineoplastic agents. Ophthalmology 90:1-3, 1983.
834. Freedman, LS, Parkinson, MC, Jones, WG, et al: Histopathology in the prediction of relapse of patients with stage I testicular teratoma treated by orchiectomy alone. Lancet 2:294-298, 1987.
835. Freedman, MD, Schocket, AL, Chapel, N, et al: Anaphylaxis after intravenous methylprednisolone administration. JAMA 245:607-608, 1981.
836. Freedman, MI and Folk, JC: Metastatic tumors to the eye and orbit. Patient survival and clinical characteristics. Arch Ophthalmol 105:1215-1219, 1987.
837. Freeman, JE, Johnston, PG, and Voke, JM: Somnolence after prophylactic cranial irradiation in children with acute lymphoblastic leukaemia. BMJ 4:523-525, 1973.
837a. Freilich, RJ, Krol, G, and DeAngelis, LM: Neuroimaging and cerebrospinal fluid cytology in the diagnosis of leptomeningeal metastasis. Abstract. Ann Neurol 36:394, 1994.
838. Friden, PM, Walus, LR, Watson, P, et al: Blood–brain barrier penetration and in vivo activity of an NGF confugate. Science 259:373-377, 1993.
838a. Friedman, HS, Archer, GE, McLendon, RE, et al: Intrathecal melphalan therapy of human neoplastic meningitis in athymic nude rats. Cancer Res 54:4710-4714, 1994.
839. Friedman, JH: Hemifacial gustatory sweating due to Pancoast's tumor. Am J Med 82:1269-1272, 1987.
840. Friedman, WA, Sceats, DJ, Jr, Nestok, BR, et al: The incidence of unexpected pathological findings in an image-guided biopsy series: A review of 100 consecutive cases. Neurosurgery 25:180-184, 1989.
841. Frim, DM, Barker, FG, II, Poletti, CE, et al: Postoperative low-dose heparin decreases thromboembolic complications in neurosurgical patients. Neurosurgery 30:830-833, 1992.
842. Front, D, Even-Sapir, E, Iosilevsky, G, et al: Monitoring of 57Co-bleomycin delivery to brain metastases and their tumors of origin. J Neurosurg 67:506-510, 1987.
843. Froula, PD, Bartley, GB, Garrity, JA, et al: The differential diagnosis of orbital calcification as detected on computed tomographic scans. Mayo Clin Proc 68:256-261, 1993.
844. Frustaci, S, Barzan, L, Comoretto, R, et al: Local neurotoxicity after intra-arterial cisplatin in head and neck cancer. Cancer Treat Rep 71:257-259, 1987.
845. Frytak, S, Moertel, CH, and Childs, DS: Neurologic toxicity associated with high-dose metronidazole therapy. Ann Intern Med 88:361-362, 1978.
846. Fuchs, HE, Archer, GE, Colvin, OM, et al: Activity of intrathecal 4-hydroperoxycyclophosphamide in a nude rat model of human neoplastic meningitis. Cancer Res 50:1954-1959, 1990.
847. Fudman, EJ, and Schnitzer, TJ: Dermatomyositis without creatinine kinase elevation. A poor prognostic sign. Am J Med 80:329-332, 1986.
848. Fueyo, J, Gomez-Manzano, C, Pascual, J, et al: Paraneoplastic syndromes. Letter to the Editor. Neurology 43:236, 1993.
849. Fujita, NK, Reynard, M, Sapico, FL, et al: Cryptococcal intracerebral mass lesions: The role of computed tomography and nonsurgical management. Ann Intern Med 94:382-388, 1981.
850. Fukumoto, Y, Tarui, S, Tsukiyama, K, et al: Tumor-induced vitamin D–resistant hypophosphatemic osteomalacia associated with proximal renal tubu-

lar dysfunction and 1,25-dihydroxyvitamin D deficiency. J Clin Endocrinol Metab 49:873-878, 1979.

851. Fukunaga, H, Engel, AG, Lang, B, et al: Passive transfer of Lambert-Eaton myasthenic syndrome with IgG from man to mouse depletes the presynaptic membrane active zones. Proc Natl Acad Sci U S A 80:7636-7640, 1983.
852. Fukuoka, T, Engel, AG, Lang, B, et al: Lambert-Eaton myasthenic syndrome: I. Early morphological effects of IgG on the presynaptic membrane active zones. Ann Neurol 22:193-199, 1987.
853. Fuller, GN, Dick, JP, and Colquhoun, IR: Brachial plexus compression by hematoma following jugular puncture. Neurology 44:775-776, 1994.
854. Fulton, DS: Brachial plexopathy in patients with breast cancer. Developments in Oncology 51:249-257, 1987.
855. Furneaux, HM, Dropcho, EJ, Barbut, D, et al: Characterization of a cDNA encoding a 34-kd Purkinje neuron protein recognized by sera from patients with paraneoplastic cerebellar degeneration. Proc Natl Acad Sci U S A 86:2873-2877, 1989.
856. Furneaux, HM, Reich, L, and Posner, JB: Autoantibody synthesis in the central nervous system of patients with paraneoplastic syndromes. Neurology 40:1085-1091, 1990.
857. Furneaux, HM, Rosenblum, MK, Dalmau, J, et al: Selective expression of Purkinje-cell antigens in tumor tissue from patients with paraneoplastic cerebellar degeneration. N Engl J Med 322:1844-1851, 1990.
858. Furukawa, T: Numb chin syndrome in the elderly. Letter to the Editor. J Neurol Neurosurg Psychiatry 53:173, 1990.
859. Gaffey, CM, Chun, B, Harvey, JC, et al: Phenytoin-induced systemic granulomatous vasculitis. Arch Pathol Lab Med 110:131-135, 1986.
860. Gaidys, WG, Dickerman, JD, Walters, CL, et al: Intrathecal vincristine Report of a fatal case despite CNS washout. Cancer 52:799-801, 1983.
861. Gaillard, J-L, Abadie, V, Cheron, G, et al: Concentrations of ceftriaxone in cerebrospinal fluid of children with meningitis receiving dexamethasone therapy. Antimicrob Agents Chemother 38:1209-1210, 1994.
862. Galandiuk, S and Fazio, VW: Pneumatosis cystoides intestinalis. A review of the literature. Dis Colon Rectum 29:358-363, 1986.
863. Galasko, CS: Spinal instability secondary to metastatic cancer. J Bone Joint Surg [Br] 73:104-108, 1991.
864. Galasko, CS and Sylvester, BS: Back pain in patients treated for malignant tumours. Clin Oncol 4:273-283, 1978.
865. Galasko, CSB: The anatomy and pathways of skeletal metastases. In Weiss, L and Gilbert, HA (eds): Bone Metastasis. GK Hall & Co, Boston, 1981, pp 49-63.
866. Gale, GB, O'Connor, DM, Chu, JY, et al: Successful chemotherapeutic decompression of epidural malignant germ cell tumor. Med Pediatr Oncol 14:97-99, 1986.
867. Galer, BS and Portenoy, RK: Acute herpetic and postherpetic neuralgia: Clinical features and management. Mt Sinai J Med 58:257-266, 1991.
868. Galetta, SL, Sergott, RC, Wells, GB, et al: Spontaneous remission of a third-nerve palsy in meningeal lymphoma. Ann Neurol 32:100-102, 1992.
869. Galetta, SL, Wulc, AE, Goldberg, HI, et al: Rhinocerebral mucormycosis: Management and survival after carotid occlusion. Ann Neurol 28:103-107, 1990.
870. Galicich, JH and French, LA: Use of dexamethasone in the treatment of cerebral edema resulting from brain tumors and brain surgery. American Practitioner and Digest of Treatment 12:169-174, 1961.
871. Galicich, JH and Guido, LJ: Ommaya device in carcinomatous and leukemic meningitis. Surgical experience in 45 cases. Surg Clin North Am 54:915-922, 1974.
872. Galicich, JH, Sundaresan, N, Arbit, E, et al: Surgical treatment of single brain metastasis: Factors associated with survival. Cancer 45:381-386, 1980.
873. Gallie, BL, Graham, JE, and Hunter, WS: Clinicopathologic case reports: Optic nerve head metastasis. Arch Ophthalmol 93:983-986, 1975.
874. Galluzzi, S and Payne, PM: Brain metastases from primary bronchial carcinoma: A statistical study of 741 necropsies. Br J Cancer 10:408-414, 1956.
875. Gamache, DA and Ellis, EF: Effect of dexamethasone, indomethacin, ibuprofen, and probenecid on carrageenan-induced brain inflammation. J Neurosurg 65:686-692, 1986.
876. Gamache, DA, Povlishock, JT, and Ellis, EF: Carrageenan-induced brain inflammation. Characterization of the model. J Neurosurg 65:679-685, 1986.
877. Gamache, FW, Jr, Galicich, JH, and Posner, JB: Treatment of brain metastases by surgical extirpation. In Weiss, L, Gilbert, HA, and Posner, JB (eds): Brain Metastasis. GK Hall & Co, Boston, 1980, pp 394-414.
878. Ganapathi, R, Hercbergs, A, Grabowski, D, et al: Selective enhancement of vincristine cytotoxicity in multidrug-resistant tumor cells by Dilantin (phenytoin). Cancer Res 53:3262-3265, 1993.
879. Ganel, A, Engel, J, Sela, M, et al: Nerve entrapments associated with postmastectomy lymphedema. Cancer 44:2254-2259, 1979.
880. Gangji, D: Treatment of leptomeningeal metastases. In Hildebrand, J (ed): Management in Neuro-oncology, European School of Oncology Monographs. Springer-Verlag, Berlin, 1992, pp 41-62.
881. Gangji, D, Reaman, GH, Cohen, SR, et al: Leukoencephalopathy and elevated levels of myelin basic protein in the cerebrospinal fluid of patients with acute lymphoblastic leukemia. N Engl J Med 303:19-21, 1980.
882. Garcia, CA, Weisberg, LA, and Lacorte, WS: Cryptoccal intracerebral mass lesions: CT-pathologic considerations. Neurology 35:731-734, 1985.
883. Garcia, EG, Wijdicks, EF, and Younge, BR: Neurologic complications associated with internal jugular vein cannulation in critically ill patients: A prospective study. Neurology 44:951-952, 1994.
884. Garcia-Merino, A, Cabello, A, Mora, JS, et al: Continuous muscle fiber activity, peripheral neu-

ropathy, and thymoma. Ann Neurol 29: 215-218, 1991.

885. Gardner, MB: Retroviral spongiform polioencephalomyelopathy. Rev Infect Dis 7:99-110, 1985.
886. Gardner, MB: Retroviral leukemia and lower motor neuron disease in wild mice: Natural history, pathogenesis and genetic resistance. In Rowland, LP (ed): Advances in Neurology, vol 56. Raven Press, New York, 1991, pp 473-480.
887. Garewal, HS and Dalton, WS: Metaclopramide in vincristine-induced ileus. Cancer Treat Rep 69:1309-1311, 1985.
888. Garson, JA, Coakham, HB, Kemshead, JT, et al: The role of monoclonal antibodies in brain tumour diagnosis and cerebrospinal fluid (CSF) cytology. J Neurooncol 3:165-171, 1985.
889. Garwicz, S, Aronson, S, Elmqvist, D, et al: Postirradiation syndrome and EEG findings in children with acute lymphoblastic leukaemia. Acta Paediatr Scand 64:399-403, 1975.
890. Gasecki, AP, Bashir, RM, and Foley, J: Leptomeningeal carcinomatosis: A report of 3 cases and review of the literature. Eur Neurol 32:74-78, 1992.
891. Gassel, MM: False localizing signs. Arch Neurol 4:526-554, 1961.
892. Gay, CT, Bodensteiner, JB, Nitschke, R, et al: Reversible treatment-related leukoencephalopathy. J Child Neurol 4:208-213, 1989.
893. Gay, PC, Litchy, WJ, and Cascino, TL: Brain metastasis in hypernephroma. J Neurooncol 5:51-56, 1987.
894. Gelber, C, Plaksin, D, Vadai, E, et al: Abolishment of metastasis formation by murine tumor cells transfected with "foreign" H-2K genes. Cancer Res 49:2366-2373, 1989.
895. Gelber, RD, Larson, M, Borgelt, BB, et al: Equivalence of radiation schedules for the palliative treatment of brain metastases in patients with favorable prognosis. Cancer 48:1749-1753, 1981.
896. Gelin, J and Lundholm, K: Cancer cachexia, what are the mediators? Topics in Supportive Care in Oncology 3:4-5, 1991.
897. Gellert, GA, Maxwell, RM, and Siegel, BS: Survival of breast cancer patients receiving adjunctive psychosocial support therapy. A 10-year follow-up study. J Clin Oncol 11:66-69, 1993.
898. Gellin, BG and Broome, CV: Listeriosis. JAMA 261:1313-1320, 1989.
898a. Gelman, K: The taxoids: paclitaxel and docetaxel. Lancet 344:1267-1272, 1994.
899. Genta, RM, Miles, P, and Fields, K: Opportunistic *Strongyloides stercoralis* infection in lymphoma patients. Report of a case and review of the literature. Cancer 63:1407-1411, 1989.
900. Gentili, F, Lougheed, WM, Yamashiro, K, et al: Monitoring of sensory evoked potentials during surgery of skull base tumours. Can J Neurol Sci 12:336-340, 1985.
901. Geny, C, Yulis, J, Azoulay, A, et al: Thalamic infarction following lingual herpes zoster. Case report. Neurology 41:1846, 1991.
902. Geopfert, H, Dichtel, WJ, Medina, JE, et al: Perineural invasion in squamous cell skin carcinoma of the head and neck. Am J Surg 148:542-547, 1984.
903. George, J and Twomey, JA: Causes of polyneuropathy in the elderly. Age Ageing 15:247-249, 1986.
904. Georgiou, A, Grigsby, PW, and Perez, CA: Radiation induced lumbosacral plexopathy in gynecologic tumors: Clinical findings and dosimetric analysis. Int J Radiat Oncol Biol Phys 26:479-482, 1993.
905. Gerard, JM, Franck, N, Moussa, Z, et al: Acute ischemic brachial plexus neuropathy following radiation therapy. Neurology 39:450-451, 1989.
905a. Gerl, A, Clemm, C, Koh., P, et al: Central nervous system as sanctuary site of relapse in patients treated with chemotherapy for metastatic testicular cancer. Clin Exp Metastasis 12:226-230, 1994.
906. Gerl, A, Clemm, C, and Wilmanns, W: Acute and late vascular complications following chemotherapy for germ cell tumors. Onkologie 16:88-92, 1993.
907. Geyer, JR, Taylor, EM, Milstein, JM, et al: Radiation, methotrexate, and white matter necrosis: Laboratory evidence for neural radioprotection with preirradiation methotrexate. Int J Radiat Oncol Biol Phys 15:373-375, 1989.
908. Geyer, JR, Taylor, EM, Milstein, JM, et al: The effect of age on the latency of radiation myelopathy. J Neurooncol 10:145-151, 1991.
909. Ghatak, NR: Pathology of cerebral embolization caused by nonthrombotic agents. Hum Pathol 6:599-610, 1975.
910. Ghatak, NR and Sawyer, DR: A morphologic study of opportunistic cerebral toxoplasmosis. Acta Neuropathol (Berl) 42:217-221, 1978.
911. Gherardi, R, Gaulard, P, Prost, C, et al: T-cell lymphoma revealed by a peripheral neuropathy. Cancer 58:2710-2716, 1986.
912. Ghobrial, M and Struble, R: Antineoplastic therapy and the olfactory bulb. Abstract. J Neuropathol Exp Neurol 52:298, 1993.
913. Ghosh, C, Lazarus, HM, Hewlett, JS, et al: Fluctuation of serum phenytoin concentrations during autologous bone marrow transplant for primary central nervous system tumors. J Neurooncol 12:25-32, 1992.
914. Ghosn, M, Carde, P, Leclerq, B, et al: Ifosfamide/mesna related encephalopathy: A case report with a possible role of phenobarbital in enhancing neurotoxicity. Bull Cancer (Paris) 75:391-392, 1988.
915. Giannone, L, Greco, FA, and Hainsworth, JD: Combination intraventricular chemotherapy for meningeal neoplasia. J Clin Oncol 4:68-73, 1986.
916. Giannone, L, Johnson, DH, Hande, KR, et al: Favorable prognosis of brain metastases in small cell lung cancer. Ann Intern Med 106:386-389, 1987.
917. Gibson, WC: The cost of not doing medical research. JAMA 244:1817-1819, 1980.
917a. Gidal, B, Spencer, N, Maly, M, et al: Valproate-mediated disturbances of hemostasis: Relationship to dose and plasma concentration. Neurology 44:1418-1422, 1994.
918. Giese, WL and Kinsella, TJ: Radiation injury to peripheral and cranial nerves. In Gutin, PH, Leibel, SA, and Sheline, GE (eds): Radiation Injury to the Nervous System. Raven Press, New York, 1991, pp 383-403.

919. Gilbert, HA and Kagan, AR (eds): Radiation Damage to the Nervous System: A Delayed Therapeutic Hazard. Raven Press, New York, 1980.
920. Gilbert, MR and Grossman, SA: Incidence and nature of neurologic problems in patients with solid tumors. Am J Med 81:951-954, 1986.
921. Gilbert, RW, Kim, J-H, and Posner, JB: Epidural spinal cord compression from metastatic tumor: Diagnosis and treatment. Ann Neurol 3:40-51, 1978.
921a. Gilden, DH, Wright, RR, Schneck, SA, et al: Zoster sine herpete, a clinical variant. Ann Neurol 35:530-533, 1994.
921b. Gilden, DH, Beinlich, BR, Rubenstein, EM, et al: Varicella-zoster virus myelitis: An expanding spectrum. Neurology 44:1818-1823, 1994.
922. Giles, CL and Henderson, JW: Horner's syndrome: Analysis of 216 cases. Am J Ophthalmol 46:289-296, 1958.
923. Giordana, MT, Sofietti, R, and Schiffer, D: Paraneoplastic opsoclonus: A neuropathologic study of two cases. Clin Neuropathol 8:295-300, 1989.
924. Giraldi, T, Perissin, L, Zorzet, S. et al: Metastasis and neuroendocrine system in stressed mice. Int J Neurosci 74:265-278, 1994.
925. Girgis, NI, Farid, Z, Mikhail, IA, et al: Dexamethasone treatment for bacterial meningitis in children and adults. Pediatr Infect Dis J 8:848-851, 1989.
926. Girmenia, C, Iori, AP, Arcese, W, et al: Fatal *Listeria* meningitis in immunosuppressed patient. Letter to the Editor. Lancet 1:794, 1989.
927. Giulian, D, Woodward, J, Young, DG, et al: Interleukin-1 injected into mammalian brain stimulates astrogliosis and neovascularization. J Neurosci 8:2485-2490, 1988.
928. Glantz, MJ, Burger, PC, Friedman, AH, et al: Treatment of radiation-induced nervous system injury with heparin and warfarin. Neurology 44:2020-2027, 1994.
928a. Glantz, M, Friedberg, M, Cole, B, et al: Double-blind, randomized, plecebo-controlled trial of anticonvulsant prophylaxis in adults with newly diagnozed brain metastases. Abstract. Program/Proceedings American Society of Clinical Oncology 13:176, 1994.
929. Glass, J, Hochberg, FH, and Miller, DC: Intravascular lymphamatosis. A systemic disease with neurologic manifestations. Cancer 71:3156-3164, 1993.
930. Glass, JP, Melamed, M, Chernik, NL, et al: Malignant cells in cerebrospinal fluid (CSF): The meaning of a positive CSF cytology. Neurology 29:1369-1375, 1979.
931. Glass, JP, Pettigrew, LC, and Maor, M: Plexopathy induced by radiation therapy. Letter to the Editor. Neurology 35:1261, 1985.
932. Glaves, D: Correlation between circulating cancer cells and incidence of metastasis. Br J Cancer 48:665-673, 1983.
933. Gledhill, RF, Harrison, BM, and McDonald, WI: Demyelination and remyelination after acute spinal cord compression. Exp Neurol 38:472-487, 1973.
934. Goday, A, Lozano, F, Santamaria, J, et al: Transient immunologic defect in a case of *Listeria* rhombencephalitis. Arch Neurol 44:666-667, 1987.
935. Godwin-Austen, RB, Howell, DA, and Worthington, B: Observations on radiation myelopathy. Brain 98:557-568, 1975.
936. Golbe, LI, Miller, DC, and Duvoisin, RC: Paraneoplastic degeneration of the substantia nigra with dystonia and parkinsonism. Mov Disord 4:147-152, 1989.
937. Goldberg, LD and Ditchek, NT: Thyroid carcinoma with spinal cord compression. JAMA 245:953-954, 1981.
938. Goldberg, RI, Rams, H, Stone, B, et al: Dysphagia as the presenting symptom of recurrent breast carcinoma. Cancer 60:1085-1088, 1987.
939. Golden, WE, Lavender, RC, and Metzer, WS: Acute postoperative confusion and hallucinations in Parkinson disease. Ann Intern Med 111:218-222, 1989.
940. Goldhirsch, A, Joss, R, Markwalder, TC, et al: Acute cerebrovascular accident after treatment with *cis*-platinum and methylprednisolone. Oncology 40:344-345, 1983.
941. Goldstein, GW and Betz, AL: The blood–brain barrier. Sci Am 255:74-83, 1986.
942. Goldstein, I, Feldman, MI, Deckers, PJ, et al: Radiation-associated impotence. JAMA 251:903-910, 1984.
943. Goldwein, JW: Radiation myelopathy: A review. Med Pediatr Oncol 15:89-95, 1987.
944. Gomm, SA, Thatcher, N, Barber, PV, et al: A clinicopathological study of the paraneoplastic neuromuscular syndromes associated with lung cancer. Q J Med 278:577-595, 1990.
945. Gonzalez Moles, D and Mezzadri, JJ: Postoperative fourth ventricle tension pneumocephalus. Letter to the Editor. J Neurol Neurosurg Psychiatry 55:511-512, 1992.
946. Gonzalez-Vitale, JC and Garcia-Bunuel, R: Meningeal carcinomatosis. Cancer 37:2906-2911, 1976.
947. Goodkin, R, Carr, BI, and Perrin, RG: Herniated lumbar disc disease in patients with malignancy. J Clin Oncol 5:667-671, 1987.
948. Goodman, A, Ramos, R, Petrelli, M, et al: Gingival biopsy in thrombotic thrombocytopenic purpura. Ann Intern Med 89:501-504, 1978.
949. Goodpasture, HC, Hershberger, RE, Barnett, AM, et al: Treatment of central nervous system fungal infection with ketoconazole. Arch Intern Med 145:879-880, 1985.
950. Gordon, SL, Graham, WP, III, Black, JT, et al: Accessory nerve function after surgical procedures in the posterior triangle. Arch Surg 112:264-268, 1977.
951. Gore, JM, Appelbaum, JS, Greene, HL, et al: Occult cancer in patients with acute pulmonary embolism. Ann Intern Med 96:556-560, 1982.
952. Gorelik, E, Fogel, M, Feldman, M, et al: Differences in resistance of metastatic tumor cells and cells from local tumor growth to cytotoxicity of natural killer cells. J Natl Cancer Inst 63:1397-1404, 1979.
953. Gorell, JM, Palutke, WA, and Chason, JL: *Candida* pachymeningitis with multiple cranial nerve pareses. Arch Neurol 36:719-720, 1979.

954. Goren, MP, Wright, RK, Pratt, CB, et al: Dechloroethylation of ifosfamide and neurotoxicity. Letter to the Editor. Lancet 2:1219-1220, 1986.
955. Gorman, DJ, Kefford, R, and Stuart-Harris, R: Focal encephalopathy after cisplatin therapy. Med J Aust 150:399-401, 1989.
956. Gormley, PE, Gangji, D, Wood, JH, et al: Pharmacokinetic study of cerebrospinal fluid penetration of cis-diamminedichloroplatinum II. Cancer Chemother Pharmacol 5:257-260, 1981.
957. Gottlieb, D, Bradstock, K, Koutts, J, et al: The neurotoxicity of high-dose cytosine arabinoside is age-related. Cancer 60:1439-1441, 1987.
958. Gould, BJ, Borowitz, MJ, Groves, ES, et al: Phase I study of an anti–breast cancer immunotoxin by continuous infusion: Report of a targeted toxic effect not predicted by animal studies. J Natl Cancer Inst 81:775-781, 1989.
959. Gradishar, WJ, Vokes, EE, Schilsky, RL, et al: Catastrophic vascular events in patients receiving 5-fluorouracil (5-FU) based chemotherapy. Abstract. Proceedings American Association for Cancer Research 31:A1128, 1990.
960. Graeb, DA, Steinbok, P, and Robertson, WD: Transient early computed tomographic changes mimicking tumor progression after brain tumor irradiation. Radiology 144:813-817, 1982.
961. Graham, BS and Tucker, WS, Jr: Opportunistic infections in endogenous Cushing's syndrome. Ann Intern Med 101:334-338, 1984.
962. Graham, GP, Dent, CM, and Mathews, P: Paraplegia following spinal anaesthesia in a patient with prostatic metastases. Br J Urol 70:445, 1992.
963. Grain, GO and Karr, JP: Diffuse leptomeningeal carcinomatosis. Clinical and pathologic characteristics. Neurology 5:706-722, 1955.
964. Gralnick, HR, Bagley, J, and Abrell, E: Heparin treatment for the hemorrhagic diathesis of acute promyelocytic leukemia. Am J Med 52:167-174, 1972.
965. Gram, L and Bentsen, KD: Valproate: An updated review. Acta Neurol Scand 72:129-139, 1985.
966. Granberg-Ohman, IF, Andersson, BI, Gupta, SK, et al: Chromosome analysis in meningeal carcinomatosis. Acta Neurol Scand 60:255-259, 1979.
967. Grant, R, Naylor, B, Greenberg, HS, et al: Clinical outcome in aggressively treated meningeal carcinomatosis. Arch Neurol 51:457-461, 1994.
968. Grant, R, Naylor, B, Junck, L, et al: Clinical outcome in aggressively treated meningeal gliomatosis. Neurology 42:252-254, 1992.
969. Grant, R, Papadopoulos, SM, and Greenberg, HS: Metastatic epidural spinal cord compression. Neurol Clin 9:825-841, 1991.
970. Graus, F: Acute meningospinal syndromes: Acute myelopathy and radiculopathy. In Hildebrand, J (ed): Neurological Adverse Reactions to Anticancer Drugs, European School of Oncology Monographs (Veronesi, U, series ed). Springer-Verlag, Berlin, 1990, pp 87-92.
970a. Graus, F, Bonaventura, I, Uchuya, M, et al: Indolent anti-Hu-associated paraneoplastic sensory neuropathy, Neurology 44:2258-2261, 1994.
971. Graus, F, Elkon, KB, Cordon-Cardo, C, et al: Sensory neuronopathy and small cell lung cancer. Antineuronal antibody that also reacts with the tumor. Am J Med 80:45-52, 1986.
972. Graus, F, Illa, I, Agusti, M, et al: Effect of intraventricular injection of an anti-Purkinje cell antibody (anti-Yo) in a guinea pig model. J Neurol Sci 106:82-87, 1991.
973. Graus, F, Krol, G, and Foley, KM: Early diagnosis of spinal epidural metastasis (SEM): Correlation with clinical and radiological findings. Abstract No. C-1047, Program/Proceedings American Society of Clinical Oncology 4:269, 1985.
974. Graus, F and Rene, R: Paraneoplastic neuropathies. Eur Neurol 33:279-286, 1993.
975. Graus, F, Ribalta, T, Campo, E, et al: Immunohistochemical analysis of the immune reaction in the nervous system in paraneoplastic encephalomyelitis. Neurology 40:219-222, 1990.
976. Graus, F, Rogers, LR, and Posner, JB: Cerebrovascular complications in patients with cancer. Medicine (Baltimore) 64:16-35, 1985.
977. Graus, F, Rowe, G, Fueyo, J, et al: The neuronal nuclear antigen recognized by the human anti-Ri autoantibody is expressed in central but not peripheral nervous system neurons. Neurosci Lett 150:212-214, 1993.
978. Graus, F and Slatkin, NE: Papilledema in the metastatic jugular foramen syndrome. Arch Neurol 40:816-818, 1983.
979. Graus, F, Vega, F, Delattre, J-Y, et al: Plasmapheresis and antineoplastic treatment in CNS paraneoplastic syndromes with antineuronal autoantibodies. Neurology 42:536-540, 1992.
979a. Gray, F, Belec, L, Lescs, MC, et al: Varicella-zoster virus infection of the central nervous system in the acquired immune deficiency syndrome. Brain 117:987-999, 1994.
980. Gray, JR: Rational approaches to the treatment of culture-negative infective endocarditis. Drugs 41:729-736, 1991.
981. Green, D, Lee, MY, Lim, AC, et al: Prevention of thromboembolism after spinal cord injury using low-molecular-weight heparin. Ann Intern Med 113:571-574, 1990.
982. Greenberg, HS: Paraneoplastic cerebellar degeneration: A clinical and CT study. J Neurooncol 2:377-382, 1984.
983. Greenberg, HS, Deck, MD, Vikram, B, et al: Metastasis to the base of the skull: Clinical findings in 43 patients. Neurology 31:530-537, 1981.
984. Greenberg, HS, Kim, J-H, and Posner, JB: Epidural spinal cord compression from metastatic tumor: Results with a new treatment protocol. Ann Neurol 8:361-366, 1980.
985. Greene, GM, Hart, MN, Poor, MM, Jr, et al: Carcinoma metastatic to a cerebellar vascular malformation: Case report. Neurosurgery 26: 1054-1057, 1990.
986. Greenlee, JE: Cerebrospinal fluid in central nervous system infections. In Scheld, WM, Whitley, RJ, and Durack, DT (eds): Infections of the Central Nervous System. Raven Press, New York, 1991, pp 861-886.
987. Greenlee, JE, Brashear, HR, and Herndon, RM: Immunoperoxidase labeling of rat brain sections with sera from patients with paraneoplastic cerebellar degeneration and systemic neoplasia. J Neuropathol Exp Neurol 47:561-571, 1988.
988. Greenwald, ES: Organic mental changes with

fluorouracil therapy. Letter to the Editor. JAMA 235:248-249, 1976.

989. Gregg, RW, Molepo, JM, Monpetit, VJ, et al: Cisplatin neurotoxicity: The relationship between dosage, time, and platinum concentration in neurologic tissues, and morphologic evidence of toxicity. J Clin Oncol 10:795-803, 1992.
990. Gregorius, FK, Johnson, BL, Jr, Stern, WE, et al: Pathogenesis of hematogenous bacterial meningitis in rabbits. J Neurosurg 45:561-567, 1976.
991. Gregory, RE, Grossman, S, and Sheidler, VR: Grand mal seizures associated with high-dose intravenous morphine infusions: Incidence and possible etiology. Pain 51:255-258, 1992.
992. Greig, NH: Chemotherapy of brain metastases: Current status. Cancer Treat Rev 11:157-186, 1984.
993. Greig, NH: Drug delivery to the brain by blood–brain barrier circumvention and drug modification. In Neuwel, EA (ed): Implications of the Blood–Brain Barrier and Its Manipulation, vol 1, Basic Science Aspects. Plenum Medical Book Company, New York, 1989, pp 311-367.
994. Greig, NH, Ries, LG, Yancik, R, et al: Increasing annual incidence of primary malignant brain tumors in the elderly. J Natl Cancer Inst 82:1621-1624, 1990.
995. Grem, JL, Burgess, J, and Trump, DL: Clinical features and natural history of intramedullary spinal cord metastasis. Cancer 56:2305-2314, 1985.
996. Grem, JL, Neville, AJ, Smith, SC, et al: Massive skeletal muscle invasion by lymphoma. Arch Intern Med 145:1818-1820, 1985.
997. Grever, MR, Kopecky, KJ, Coltman, CA, et al: Fludarabine monophosphate: A potentially useful agent in chronic lymphocytic leukemia. Nouv Rev Fr Hematol 30:457-459, 1988.
998. Greydanus, DE, Burgert, EO, Jr, and Gilchrist, GS: Hypothalamic syndrome in children with acute lymphocytic leukemia. Mayo Clin Proc 53:217-220, 1978.
999. Griffeth, LK, Rich, KM, Dehashti, F, et al: Brain metastases from non-central nervous system tumors: Evaluation with PET. Radiology 186:37-44, 1993.
1000. Griffin, BR, Livingston, RB, Stewart, GR, et al: Prophylactic cranial irradiation for limited non-small cell lung cancer. Cancer 62:36-39, 1988.
1001. Griffin, MR, Stanson, AW, Brown, ML, et al: Deep venous thrombosis and pulmonary embolism. Risk of subsequent malignant neoplasms. Arch Intern Med 147:1907-1911, 1987.
1002. Griffiths, JD, Stark, RJ, Ding, JC, et al: Vincristine neurotoxicity enhanced in combination chemotherapy including both teniposide and vincristine. Cancer Treat Rep 70:519-521, 1986.
1003. Grigg, AP, Shepherd, JD, and Phillips, GL: Busulphan and phenytoin. Letter to the Editor. Ann Intern Med 111:1049-1050, 1989.
1004. Grines, C, Plouffe, JF, Baird, IM, et al: Toxoplasma meningoencephalitis with hypoglycorrhachia. Arch Intern Med 141:935, 1981.
1005. Grisold, W, Lutz, D, and Wolf, D: Necrotizing myelopathy associated with acute lymphoblastic leukemia. Case report and review of literature. Acta Neuropathol (Berl) 49:231-235, 1980.
1006. Grisoli, F, Vincentelli, F, Foa, J, et al: Effect of bromocriptine on brain metastasis in breast cancer. Letter to the Editor. Lancet 2:745-746, 1981.
1007. Groeger, JS, Lucas, AB, and Coit, D: Venous access in the cancer patient. Principles and Practice of Oncology 5:1-14, 1991.
1008. Grondahl, TO and Langmoen, IA: Epileptogenic effect of antibiotic drugs. J Neurosurg 78:938-943, 1993.
1009. Grooms, GA, Eilber, FR, and Morton, DL: Failure of adjuvant immunotherapy to prevent central nervous system metastases in malignant melanoma patients. J Surg Oncol 9:147-153, 1977.
1010. Groothuis, D, Blasberg, RG, Molnar, P, et al: Regional blood flow in avian sarcoma virus (ASV)-induced brain tumors. Neurology 33:686-696, 1983.
1011. Groothuis, DR and Blasberg, RG: Rational brain tumor chemotherapy. The interaction of drug and tumor. Neurol Clin 3:801-816, 1985.
1012. Groothuis, DR, Lippitz, BE, Fekete, I, et al: The effect of an amino acid–lowering diet on the rate of melphalan entry into brain and xenotransplanted glioma. Cancer Res 52:5590-5596, 1992.
1013. Groothuis, DR and Mikhael, MA: Focal cerebral vasculitis associated with circulating immune complexes and brain irradiation. Ann Neurol 19:590-592, 1986.
1014. Groothuis, DR, Warnke, PC, Molnar, P, et al: Effect of hyperosmotic blood–brain barrier disruption on transcapillary transport in canine brain tumors. J Neurosurg 72:441-449, 1990.
1015. Grossman, DA, Finkelstein, DM, Ruckdeschel, JC, et al: Randomized prospective comparison of intraventricular methotrexate and thiotepa in patients with previously untreated neoplastic meningitis. Eastern Cooperative Oncology Group. J Clin Oncol 11:561-569, 1993.
1016. Grossman, SA and Lossignol, D: Diagnosis and treatment of epidural metastases. Oncology (Huntingt) 4:47-58, 1990.
1017. Grossman, SA and Moynihan, TJ: Neoplastic meningitis. Neurol Clin 9:843-856, 1991.
1018. Grossman, SA, Reinhard, CS, and Loats, HL: The intracerebral penetration of intraventricularly administered methotrexate: A quantitative autoradiographic study. J Neurooncol 7:319-328, 1989.
1019. Grossman, SA, Sheidler, VR, and Gilbert, MR: Decreased phenytoin levels in patients receiving chemotherapy. Am J Med 87:505-510, 1989.
1020. Grossman, SA, Trump, DL, Chen, DC, et al: Cerebrospinal fluid flow abnormalities in patients with neoplastic meningitis. An evaluation using ^{111}Indium-DTPA ventriculography. Am J Med 73:641-647, 1982.
1021. Grunberg, SM, Sonka, S, Stevenson, LL, et al: Progressive paresthesias after cessation of therapy with very high-dose cisplatin. Cancer Chemother Pharmacol 25:62-64, 1989.
1022. Grunberg, SM, Weiss, MH, Spitz, IM, et al: Treatment of unresectable meningiomas with the antiprogesterone agent mifepristone. J Neurosurg 74:861-866, 1991.
1023. Grunewald, RA, Chroni, E, Panayiotopoulos, CP, et al: Late onset radiation-induced motor neuron syndrome. Letter to the Editor. J Neurol Neurosurg Psychiatry 55:741-742, 1992.

1024. Grunwald, GB, Korngluth, SE, Towfighi, J, et al: Autoimmune basis for visual paraneoplastic syndrome in patients with small cell lung carcinoma. Retinal immune deposits and ablation of retinal ganglion cells. Cancer 60:780-786, 1987.
1025. Grucalp, R: Management of the febrile neutropenic patient with cancer. Oncology (Huntingt) 5:137-148, 1991.
1026. Gudesblatt, M, Cohen, JA, Gerber, O, et al: Truncal ataxia presumably due to malignant spinal cord compression. Letter to the Editor. Ann Neurol 21:511-512, 1987.
1027. Guess, HA, Resseguie, LJ, Melton, LJ, III, et al: Factors predictive of seizures among intensive care unit patients with gram-negative infections. Epilepsia 31:567-573, 1990.
1028. Guinee, VF, Guido, JJ, Pfalzgraf, KA, et al: The incidence of herpes zoster in patients with Hodgkin's disease. An analysis of prognostic factors. Cancer 56:642-648, 1985.
1029. Gullans, SR and Verbalis, JG: Control of brain volume during hyperosmolar and hypoosmolar conditions. Annu Rev Med 44:289-301, 1993.
1030. Gulya, AJ: Neurologic paraneoplastic syndromes with neurotologic manifestations. Laryngoscope 103:754-761, 1993.
1031. Guomundsson, KR: A survey of tumours of the central nervous system in Iceland during the 10-year period 1954-1963. Acta Neurol Scand 46:538-552, 1970.
1032. Gupta, SR, Zdonczyk, DE, and Rubino, FA: Cranial neuropathy in systemic malignancy in a VA population. Neurology 40:997-999, 1990.
1033. Gustafson, Y, Olsson, T, Asplund, K, et al: Acute confusional state (delirium) soon after stroke is associated with hypercortisolism. Cerebrovascular Diseases 3:33-38, 1993.
1034. Gustafsson, H, Rutberg, H, and Bengtsson, M: Spinal haematoma following epidural analgesia. Report of a patient with ankylosing spondylitis and a bleeding diathesis. Anaesthesia 43:220-222, 1988.
1035. Gutin, PH, Green, MR, Bleyer, WA, et al: Methotrexate pneumonitis induced by intrathecal methotrexate therapy: A case report with pharmacokinetic data. Cancer 38:1529-1534, 1976.
1036. Gutin, PH, Leibel, SA, and Sheline, GE (eds): Radiation Injury to the Nervous System. Raven Press, New York, 1991.
1037. Gutin, PH, Levi, JA, Wiernik, PH, et al: Treatment of malignant meningeal disease with intrathecal thioTEPA: A phase II study. Cancer Treat Rep 61:885-887, 1977.
1038. Gutin, PH, Levin, KJ, McDermott, MW, et al: Lipid peroxidation does not appear to be a factor in late radiation injury of the cervical spine cord of rats. Int J Radiat Oncol Biol Phys 25:67-72, 1993.
1039. Gutin, PH, Weiss, HD, Wiernik, PH, et al: Intrathecal N, N′, N″—triethylenethiophosphoramide [thio-TEPA (NSC 6396)] in the treatment of malignant meningeal disease: Phase I–II study. Cancer 38:1471-1475, 1976.
1040. Gutmann, DH, Cantor, CR, Piacente, GJ, et al: Cerebral vasculopathy and infarction in a woman with carcinomatous meningitis. Letter to the Editor. J Neurooncol 9:183-185, 1990.
1041. Guy, J, Mancuso, A, Beck, R, et al: Radiation-induced optic neuropathy: A magnetic resonance imaging study. J Neurosurg 74:426-432, 1991.
1042. Haaxma-Reiche, H, Daenen, S, and Witteveen, RJ: Experiences with the Ommaya reservoir for prophylaxis and treatment of the central nervous system in adult acute myelocytic leukemia. Blut 57:351-355, 1988.
1043. Haaxma-Reiche, H, Piers, A, and Beekhuis, H: Normal cerebrospinal fluid dynamics. A study with intraventricular injection of ^{111}In-DTPA in leukemia and lymphoma without meningeal involvement. Arch Neurol 46:997-999, 1989.
1044. Haberland, C, Cipriani, M, Kucuk, O, et al: Fulminant leukemic polyradiculoneuropathy in a case of B-cell prolymphocytic leukemia. Cancer 60:1454-1458, 1987.
1045. Habermalz, E, Habermalz, HJ, Stephani, U, et al: Cranial computed tomography of 64 children in continuous complete remission of leukemia I: Relations to therapy modalities. Neuropediatrics 14:144-148, 1983.
1046. Haddad, SF, Hitchon, PW, and Godersky, JC: Idiopathic and glucocorticoid-induced spinal epidural lipomatosis. J Neurosurg 74:38-42, 1991.
1047. Hadfield, MG, Vennart, GP, and Rosenblum, WI: Hypoglycemia: Invasion of the hypothalamus by lymphosarcoma. Metastasis to blood glucose regulating centers. Arch Pathol Lab Med 94:317-321, 1972.
1048. Haefeli, WE, Schoenenberger, RAZ, Weiss, P, et al: Acyclovir-induced neurotoxicity: Concentration–side effect relationship in acyclovir overdose. Am J Med 94:212-215, 1993.
1049. Hagen, N, Stulman, J, Krol, G, et al: The role of myelography and magnetic resonance imaging in cancer patients with symptomatic and asymptomatic epidural disease. Abstract. Neurology 39(Suppl I):309, 1989.
1050. Hagen, NA, Cirrincione, C, Thaler, HT, et al: The role of radiation therapy following resection of single brain metastasis from melanoma. Neurology 40:158-160, 1990.
1051. Hagen, NA, Stevens, CJ, and Michet, C: Trigeminal sensory neuropathy associated with connective tissue diseases. Neurology 40:891-896, 1990.
1052. Hagenau, C, Grosh, W, Currie, M, et al: Comparison of spinal magnetic resonance imaging and myelography in cancer patients. J Clin Oncol 5:1663-1669, 1987.
1053. Hagner, G, Iglesias-Rozas, JR, Kolmel, HW, et al: Hemorrhagic infarction of the basal ganglia. An unusual complication of acute leukemia. Oncology 40:387-391, 1983.
1054. Haie-Meder, C, Pellae-Cosset, B, Laplanche, A, et al: Results of a randomized clinical trial comparing two radiation schedules in the palliative treatment of brain metatases. Radiother Oncol 26:111-116, 1993.
1055. Haile-Mariam, T, Laws, E, and Tuazon, CU: Gram-negative meningitis associated with transsphenoidal surgery: Case reports and review. Clin Infect Dis 18:553-556, 1994.
1056. Haim, N, Barron, SA, and Robinson, E: Muscle cramps associated with vincristine therapy. Acta Oncol 30:707-711, 1991.

1057. Haimovic, IC, Arbit, E, and Posner, JB: Colonic ileus complicating laminectomy. Neurosurgery 3:369-372, 1978.

1058. Haimovitz-Friedman, A, et al: Activation of platelet heparitinase by tumor cell-derived factors. Blood 78:789-796, 1991.

1059. Haines, DE, Harkey, HL, and Al-Mefty, O: The "subdural" space: A new look at an outdated concept. Neurosurgery 32:111-120, 1993.

1060. Hainline, B, Tuzynski, MH, and Posner, JB: Ataxia in epidural spinal cord compression. Neurology 42:2193-2195, 1992.

1061. Hakansson, CH: Effect of irradiation of brain tumours on ventricular fluid pressure. Acta Radiologica: Therapy, Physics, Biology (Stockholm) 6:22-32, 1967.

1062. Halbach, M, Homberg, V, and Freund, HJ: Neuromuscular, autonomic and central cholinergic hyperactivity associated with thymoma and acethylcholine receptor-binding antibody. J Neurol 234:433-436, 1987.

1063. Hall, C, Dougherty, WG, Lebish, IJ, et al: Warning against use of intrathecal mitoxantrone. Letter to the Editor. Lancet 1:734, 1989.

1064. Hall, EJ: The Janeway Lecture 1992: Nine decades of radiobiology: Is radiation therapy any the better for it? Cancer 71:3753-3766, 1993.

1065. Hall, SM, Buzdar, AU, and Blumenschein, GR: Cranial nerve palsies in metastatic breast cancer due to osseous metastasis without intracranial involvement. Cancer 52:180-184, 1983.

1066. Halperin, EC: Concerning the inferior portion of the spinal radiotherapy field for malignancies that disseminate via the cerebrospinal fluid. Int J Radiat Oncol Biol Phys 26:357-362, 1992.

1067. Halperin, EC: Multiple-fraction-per-day external beam radiotherapy for adults with supratentorial malignant gliomas. J Neurooncol 14:255-262, 1992.

1068. Halperin, JR and Murphy, B: Extrapyramidal reaction to ondansetron. Cancer 69:1275, 1992.

1069. Hamers, FP, Brakkee, JH, Cavalletti, E, et al: Reduced glutathione protects against cisplatin-induced neurotoxicity in rats. Cancer Res 53:544-549, 1993.

1070. Hammack, J, Kotanides, H, Rosenblum, MK, et al: Paraneoplastic cerebellar degeneration: II. Clinical and immunologic findings in 21 patients with Hodgkin's disease. Neurology 42:1938-1943, 1992.

1071. Hammack, JE, Kimmel, DW, O'Neill, BP, et al: Paraneoplastic cerebellar degeneration: A clinical comparison of patients with and without Purkinje cell cytoplasmic antibodies. Mayo Clin Proc 65:1423-1431, 1990.

1072. Hamous, JE, Guffy, MM, and Aschenbrener, CA: Fatal acute respiratory failure following intrathecal methotrexate administration. Cancer Treat Rep 67:1025-1026, 1983.

1073. Hancock, SL, Cox, RS, and McDougall, IR: Thyroid diseases after treatment of Hodgkin's disease. N Engl J Med 325:599-605, 1991.

1074. Hande, KR and Garrow, GC: Acute tumor lysis syndrome in patients with high-grade non-Hodgkin's lymphoma. Am J Med 94:133-139, 1993.

1075. Handforth, A, Nag, S, Sharp, D, et al: Paraneoplastic subacute necrotic myelopathy. Can J Neurol Sci 10:204-207, 1983.

1076. Hankins, JR, Miller, JE, Salcman, M, et al: Surgical management of lung cancer with solitary cerebral metastasis. Ann Thorac Surg 46:24-28, 1988.

1077. Hanks, GW and Justins, DM: Cancer pain: Management. Lancet 339:1031-1035, 1992.

1078. Hansen, K, Gjerris, F, and Sorensen, PS: Absence of hydrocephalus in spite of impaired cerebrospinal fluid absorption and severe intracranial hypertension. Acta Neurochir (Wien) 86:93-97, 1987.

1079. Hansen, PB, Jensen, TH, Lykkegaard, S, et al: *Listeria monocytogenes* meningitis in adults. Sixteen consecutive cases. Scand J Infect Dis 19:55-60, 1987.

1080. Hansen, PB, Kjeldsen, L, Dalhoff, K, et al: Cerebrospinal fluid beta-2-microglobulin in adult patients with acute leukemia or lymphoma: A useful marker in early diagnosis and monitoring of CNS-involvement. Acta Neurol Scand 85:224-227, 1992.

1081. Hansen, RM and Borden, EC: Current status of interferons in the treatment of cancer. Oncology (Huntingt) 6:19-29, 1992.

1082. Hansen, SB, Galsgard, H, von Eyben, FE, et al: Tamoxifen for brain metastases from breast cancer. Letter to Editor. Ann Neurol 20:544, 1986.

1083. Hansen, SW, Helweg-Larsen, S, and Trojaborg, W: Long-term neurotoxicity in patients treated with cisplatin, vinblastine, and bleomycin for metastatic germ cell cancer. J Clin Oncol 7:1457-1461, 1989.

1084. Hantel, A, Dick, JD, and Karp, JE: Listeriosis in the setting of malignant disease. Changing issues in an unusual infection. Cancer 64:516-520, 1989.

1085. Harada, M, Shimizu, A, Nakamura, Y, et al: Role of the vertebral venous system in metastatic spread of cancer cells to the bone. In Karr, JP and Yamanaka, H (eds): Prostate Cancer and Bone Metastasis. Plenum Press, New York, 1992, pp 83-92.

1086. Harati, Y: Diabetic peripheral neuropathies. Ann Intern Med 107:546-559, 1987.

1087. Harbison, JW, Lessell, S, and Selhorst, JB: Neuro-ophthalmology of sphenoid sinus carcinoma. Brain 107:855-870, 1984.

1087a. Harbour, JW, DePotter, P, Shields, CL, et al: Uveal metastasis from carcinoid tumor: Clinical observations in nine cases. Opthalmology 101:1084-1090, 1994.

1088. Hardjasudarma, M, Husain, F, Fowler, M, et al: Central pontine myelinolysis as a manifestation of the paraneoplastic syndrome. South Med J 85:419-421, 1992.

1089. Hargreaves, KM and Pardridge, WM: Neutral amino acid transport at the blood–brain barrier. J Biol Chem 263:19392-19397, 1988.

1090. Harik, SI and Roessmann, U: The erythrocyte-type glucose transporter in blood vessels of primary and metastatic brain tumors. Ann Neurol 29:487-491, 1991.

1091. Harland, CC, Marsden, JR, Vernon, SA, et al: Dermatomyositis responding to treatment of associated toxoplasmosis. Br J Dermatol 125:76-78, 1991.

1092. Harper, CM, Jr, Thomas, JE, Cascino, TL, et al: Distinction between neoplastic and radiation-induced brachial plexopathy, with emphasis on the role of EMG. Neurology 39:502-506, 1989.
1093. Harrington, KD: Metastatic disease of the spine. In Harrington, KD (ed): Orthopaedic Management of Metastatic Bone Disease. CV Mosby, St Louis, 1988, pp 309-383.
1094. Harrington, KD (ed): Orthopaedic Management of Metastatic Bone Disease. CV Mosby, St Louis, 1988.
1095. Harrington, KD: Anterior decompression and stabilization of the spine as a treatment for vertebral collapse and spinal cord compression from metastatic malignancy. Clin Orthop 233:177-197, 1988.
1096. Harris, BE, Carpenter, JT, and Diasio, RB: Severe 5-fluorouracil toxicity secondary to dihydropyrimidine dehydrogenase deficiency. A potentially more common pharmacogenetic syndrome. Cancer 68:499-501, 1991.
1097. Harris, CP, Sigman, JD, and Jaeckle, KA: Intravascular malignant lymphomatosis: Amelioration of neurological symptoms with plasmapheresis. Ann Neurol 35:357-359, 1994.
1098. Harris, CP, Townshend, JJ, and Baringer, JR: Symptomatic hyponatraemia: Can myelinolysis be prevented by treatment? J Neurol Neurosurg Psychiatry 56:626-632, 1993.
1099. Harris, RL, Musher, DM, Bloom, K, et al: Manifestations of sepsis. Arch Intern Med 147:1895-1906, 1987.
1100. Harrison, KM, Muss, HB, Ball, MR, et al: Spinal cord compression in breast cancer. Cancer 55:2839-2844, 1985.
1101. Harrison, MJ, Wolfe, DE, Lau, T-S, et al: Radiation-induced meningiomas: Experience at the Mount Sinai Hospital and review of the literature. J Neurosurg 75:564-574, 1991.
1101a. Hart, IK, Vincent, A, Leys, K, et al: Serum autoantibodies bind to voltage-gated potassium channels in acquired neuromyotonia. Abstract. Ann Neurol 36:325, 1994.
1102. Hart, IR and Saini, A: Biology of tumour metastasis. Lancet 339:1453-1457, 1992.
1103. Hartmann, WH and Sherlock, P: Gastroduodenal metastases from carcinoma of the breast. Adrenal Steroid Metastases 14:426-431, 1960.
1104. Hartwell, RC and Sutton, LN: Mannitol, intracranial pressure, and vasogenic edema. Neurosurgery 32:444-450, 1993.
1105. Hashizume, Y and Hirano, A: Intramedullary spinal cord metastasis. Pathologic findings in five autopsy cases. Acta Neuropathol (Berl) 61:214-218, 1983.
1106. Hashizume, Y, Iljima, S, Kishimoto, H, et al: Pencil-shaped softening of the spinal cord. Pathologic study in 12 autopsy cases. Acta Neuropathol (Berl) 61:219-224, 1983.
1107. Hasle, H: Cerebellar toxicity during cytarabine therapy associated with renal insufficiency. Cancer Chemother Pharmacol 27:76-78, 1990.
1108. Hatam, A, Yu, Z, Bergstrom, M, et al: Effect of dexamethasone treatment on peritumoral brain edema: Evaluation by computed tomography. J Comput Assist Tomogr 6:586-592, 1982.
1109. Hattori, T, Hirayama, K, Imai, T, et al: Pontine lesion in opsoclonus-myoclonus syndrome shown by MRI. J Neurol Neurosurg Psychiatry 51:1572-1575, 1988.
1110. Hauben, M: Seizures after povidone-iodine mediastinal irrigation. Letter to the Editor. N Engl J Med 328:355-356, 1993.
1111. Hauch, TW, Shelbourne, JD, Cohen, HJ, et al: Meningeal mycosis fungoides: Clinical and cellular characteristics. Ann Intern Med 82:499-505, 1975.
1112. Hauge, MD, Cooper, KL, and Litin, SC: Insufficiency fractures of the pelvis that simulate metastatic disease. Mayo Clin Proc 63:807-812, 1988.
1112a. Haupt, R, Fears, TR, Robison, LL, et al: Educational attainment in long-term survivors of childhood acute lymphoblastic leukemia; JAMA 272:1427-1432, 1994.
1113. Hauzeur, JP, Pasteels, JL, Schoutens, A, et al: The diagnostic value of magnetic resonance imaging in non-traumatic osteonecrosis of the femoral head. J Bone Joint Surg [Am] 71-A:641-649, 1989.
1114. Haverkos, HW: Assessment of therapy for toxoplasma encephalitis. The TE Study Group. Am J Med 82:907-914, 1987.
1115. Hawke, SH, Davies, L, Pamphlett, R, et al: Vasculitis neuropathy. A clinical and pathological study. Brain 114:2175-2190, 1991.
1116. Hawkins, AR: Transport of essential nutrients across the blood–brain barrier of individual structures. Fed Proc 45:2055-2059, 1986.
1117. Hawkins, MM, Draper, GJ, and Kingston, JE: Incidence of second primary tumours among childhood cancer survivors. Br J Cancer 56:339-347, 1987.
1118. Hawley, RJ, Cohen, MH, Saini, N, et al: The carcinomatous neuromyopathy of oat cell lung cancer. Ann Neurol 7:65-72, 1980.
1119. Hayashi, M, Handa, Y, Kobayashi, H, et al: Plateau-wave phenomenon (I). Correlation between the appearance of plateau waves and CSF circulation in patients with intracranial hypertension. Brain 114:2681-2691, 1992.
1120. Hayashi, M, Kobayashi, H, Handa, Y, et al: Brain blood volume and blood flow in patients with plateau waves. J Neurosurg 63:556-561, 1985.
1121. Hayashi, M, Kobayashi, H, Handa, Y, et al: Plateau-wave phenomenon (II). Occurrence of brain herniation in patients with and without plateau waves. Brain 114:2693-2699, 1991.
1122. Hayes, FA, Thompson, EI, Hvizdala, E, et al: Chemotherapy as an alternative to laminectomy and radiation in the management of epidural tumor. J Pediatr 104:221-224, 1984.
1123. Haymaker, W and Lindgren, M: Nerve disturbances following exposure to ionizing radiation. In Vinken, PJ and Bruyn, GW (eds): Handbook of Clinical Neurology. Part I. Diseases of Nerves, vol 7. North-Holland Publishing Co, Amsterdam, 1970, pp 388-401.
1124. Hays, AP, Latov, N, Takatsu, M, et al: Experimental demyelination of nerve induced by serum of patients with neuropathy and an anti-MAG IgM protein. Neurology 37:242-256, 1987.
1125. Hazra, T, Mullins, GM, and Lott, S: Management

of cerebral metastases from bronchogenic carcinoma. Johns Hopkins Med J 130:377-383, 1972.

1126. Hazuka, MB, Burleson, WD, Stroud, DN, et al: Multiple brain metastases are associated with poor survival in patients treated with surgery and radiotherapy. J Clin Oncol 11:369-373, 1993.

1127. Hedley-Whyte, ET and Hsu, DW: Effect of dexamethasone on blood–brain barrier in the normal mouse. Ann Neurol 19:373-377, 1986.

1128. Heideman, RL, Cole, DE, Balis, F, et al: Phase I and pharmacokinetic evaluation of thiotepa in the cerebrospinal fluid and plasma of pediatric patients: Evidence for dose-dependent plasma clearance of thiotepa. Cancer Res 49:736-741, 1989.

1129. Heier, MS, Aass, N, Ous, S, et al: Asymmetrical autonomic dysfunction of the feet after retroperitoneal surgery in patients with testicular cancer: 2 case reports. J Urol 147:470-471, 1992.

1130. Heier, MS and Fossa, SD: Wernicke-Korsakoff-like syndrome in patients with colorectal carcinoma treated with high-dose doxifuridine (5′-dFUrd). Acta Neurol Scand 73:449-457, 1986.

1131. Heimdal, K, Hirschberg, H, Slettebo, H, et al: High incidence of serious side effects of high-dose dexamethasone treatment in patients with epidural spinal cord compression. J Neurooncol 12:141-144, 1992.

1132. Helfer, EL and Rose, LI: Corticosteroids and adrenal suppression. Characterising and avoiding the problem. Drugs 38(5):838-845, 1989.

1133. Heller, HM, Carnevale, NT, and Steigbigel, RT: Varicella zoster virus transverse myelitis without cutaneous rash. Case report. Am J Med 88:550-551, 1990.

1134. Helweg-Larsen, S, Rasmusson, B, and Sorensen, PS: Recovery of gait after radiotherapy in paralytic patients with metastatic epidural spinal cord compression. Neurology 40:1234-1236, 1990.

1134a. Helweg-Larsen, S and Sorensen, PS: Symptoms and signs in metastatic spinal cord compression: A study of progression from first symptoms until diagnosis in 153 patients. Eur J Cancer 30A:396-398, 1994.

1135. Helweg-Larsen, S, Wagner, A, Kjaer, L, et al: Comparison of myelography combined with post-myelographic spinal CT and MRI in suspected metastatic disease of the spinal canal. J Neurooncol 13:231-237, 1992.

1136. Hendrickson, FR: The optimum schedule for palliative radiotherapy for metastatic brain cancer. Int J Radiat Oncol Biol Phys 2:165-168, 1977.

1137. Hennerici, M, Rautenberg, W, Trockel, U, et al: Spontaneous progression and regression of small carotid atheroma. Lancet 1:1415-1419, 1985.

1138. Hennis, A, Corbin, D, and Fraser, H: Focal seizures and non-ketotic hyperglycaemia. J Neurol Neurosurg Psychiatry 55:195-197, 1992.

1139. Henson, JW, Cordon-Cardo, C, and Posner, JB: P-glycoprotein expression in brain tumors. J Neurooncol 14:37-43, 1992.

1140. Henson, JW, Jalaj, JK, Walker, RW, et al: *Pneumocystis carinii* pneumonia in patients with primary brain tumors. Arch Neurol 48:406-409, 1991.

1141. Henson, JW and Posner, JB: Neurological complications. In Holland, JF, Frei, El, Bast, RC, et al (eds): Cancer Medicine. Lea & Febiger, Philadelphia, 1993, pp 2268-2286.

1142. Henson, RA, Hoffman, HL, and Urich, H: Encephalomyelitis with carcinoma. Brain 88:449-464, 1965.

1143. Henson, RA, Russell, DS, and Wilkinson, M: Carcinomatous neuropathy and myopathy: A clinical and pathological study. Brain 77:82-121, 1954.

1144. Henson, RA and Urich, H (eds): Cancer and the Nervous System: The Neurological Manifestations of Systemic Malignant Disease. Blackwell Scientific, London, 1982.

1145. Heran, F, Defer, G, Brugieres, P, et al: Cortical blindness during chemotherapy: Clinical, CT, and MR correlations. J Comput Assist Tomogr 14:262-266, 1990.

1146. Hercbergs, A, Werner, A, and Brenner, HJ: Reduced thoracic vertebrae metastases following post mastectomy parasternal irradiation. Int J Radiat Oncol Biol Phys 11:773-776, 1985.

1147. Hermans, PE: The clinical manifestations of infective endocarditis. Mayo Clin Proc 57:15-21, 1982.

1148. Hersh, EM and Freireich, EJ: Host defense mechanisms and their modification by cancer chemotherapy. Methods in Cancer Research 4:355-435, 1968.

1149. Herzig, RH, Hines, JD, Herzig, GP, et al: Cerebellar toxicity with high-dose cytosine arabinoside. J Clin Oncol 5:927-932, 1987.

1150. Hetzel, DJ, Stanhope, CR, O'Neil, BP, et al: Gynecologic cancer in patients with subacute cerebellar degeneration predicted by anti-Purkinje cell antibodies and limited in metastatic volume. Mayo Clin Proc 65:1558-1563, 1990.

1151. Hewett, SJ and Atchison, WD: Specificity of Lambert-Eaton myasthenic syndrome immunoglobulin for nerve terminal calcium channels. Brain Res 599:324-332, 1992.

1152. Hickey, WF, Garnick, MB, Henderson, IC, et al: Primary cerebral venous thrombosis in patients with cancer—a rarely diagnosed paraneoplastic syndrome. Report of three cases and review of the literature. Am J Med 73:740-750, 1982.

1152a. Hida, C, Tsukamoto, T, Awano, H, et al: Ultrastructural localization of anti-Purkinje cell antibody-binding sites in paraneoplastic cerebellar degeneration. Arch Neurol 51:555-558, 1994.

1153. Hiesiger, EM, Picco-Del Bo, A, Lipschutz, LE, et al: Experimental meningeal carcinomatosis selectively depresses local cerebral glucose utilization in rat brain. Neurology 39:90-95, 1989.

1154. Hiesiger, EM, Voorhies, RM, Basler, GA, et al: Opening the blood–brain and blood–tumor barriers in experimental rat brain tumors: The effect of intracarotid hyperosmolar mannitol on capillary permeability and blood flow. Ann Neurol 19:50-59, 1986.

1155. Highley, M, Meller, ST, and Pinkerton, CR: Seizures and cortical dysfunction following high-dose cisplatin administration in children. Med Pediatr Oncol 20:143-148, 1992.

1156. Hildebrand, J: Lesions of the Nervous System in Cancer Patients. Monograph Series of the European Organization for Research on Treatment of Cancer, vol 5. Raven Press, New York, 1978.

1157. Hildebrand, J and Coers, C: The neuromuscular function in patients with malignant tumours. Electromyographic and histological study. Brain 90:67-82, 1967.
1158. Hildebrand, J, Leenaerts, L, Nubourgh, Y, et al: Epidural spinal cord compression in acute myelogenous leukemia. Arch Neurol 37:319, 1980.
1159. Hildebrand, J (ed): Neurological Adverse Reactions to Anticancer Drugs, European School of Oncology Monographs (Veronesi, U, series ed). Springer-Verlag, Berlin, 1990.
1160. Hilgard, P and Gordon-Smith, EC: Microangiopathic haemolytic anaemia and experimental tumour-cell emboli. Br J Haematol 26:651-659, 1974.
1161. Hilt, DC, Buchholz, D, Krumholz, A, et al: Herpes zoster ophthalmicus and delayed contralateral hemiparesis caused by cerebral angiitis: Diagnosis and management approaches. Ann Neurol 14:543-553, 1983.
1162. Hilton, E and Stroh, EM: Aseptic meningitis associated with administration of carbamazepine. J Infect Dis 159:363-364, 1989.
1163. Hindman, BJ (ed): Neurological and Psychological Complications of Surgery and Anesthesia. Little, Brown & Company, Boston, 1986.
1164. Hindo, WA, DeTrana, FA, III, Lee, M-S, et al: Large dose increment irradiation in treatment of cerebral metastases. Cancer 26:138-141, 1970.
1165. Hirano, A and Zimmerman, HM: Fenestrated blood vessels in a metastatic renal carcinoma in the brain. Lab Invest 26:465-468, 1972.
1166. Hirano, H, Suzuki, H, Sakakibara, T, et al: Foramen magnum and upper cervical cord tumors. Diagnostic problems. Clin Orthop 176:171-177, 1983.
1167. Hirano, M, Ott, BR, Raps, EC, et al: Acute quadriplegic myopathy: A complication of treatment with steroids, nondepolarizing blocking agents, or both. Neurology 42:2082-2087, 1992.
1167a. Hiromatsu, K, Kobayashi, T, Fujii, N, et al: Hypernatremic myopathy. J Neurol Sci 122:144-147, 1994.
1168. Hirose, G, Kosoegawa, H, Takado, M, et al: Spinal cord ischemia and left atrial myxoma. Arch Neurol 36:439, 1979.
1169. Hirsch, BE, Amodio, M, Einzig, AI, et al: Instillation of vancomycin into a cerebrospinal fluid reservoir to clear infection: Pharmacokinetic considerations. J Infect Dis 163:197-200, 1991.
1170. Hirschfeld, A: Stereotactic techniques in the management of cerebral neoplasms. Oncology (Huntingt) 3:25-40, 1989.
1171. Hitchins, RN, Bell, DR, Woods, RL, et al: A prospective randomized trial of single-agent versus combination chemotherapy in meningeal carcinomatosis. J Clin Oncol 5:1655-1662, 1987.
1171a. Hiyama, E, Yokoyama, T, Ichikawa, T, et al: Poor outcome in patients with advanced stage neuroblastoma and coincident opsomyoclonus syndrome. Cancer 74:1821-1826, 1994.
1172. Hoang-Xuan, K and Delattre, J-Y: Treatment of brain metastases. In Hildebrand, J (ed): Management in Neuro-oncology, European School of Oncology Monographs. Springer-Verlag, Berlin, 1992, pp 23-39.
1173. Hochberg, FH and Miller, DC: Primary central nervous system lymphoma. J Neurosurg 68:835-853, 1988.
1174. Hochberg, MC, Feldman, D, Stevens, MB, et al: Antibody to Jo-1 polymyositis/dermatomyositis: Association with interstitial pulmonary disease. J Rheumatol 11:663-665, 1984.
1175. Hockley, AD: Metastatic carcinoma in a spinal meningioma. J Neurol Neurosurg Psychiatry 38:695-697, 1975.
1176. Hoerni, B, Vallat, M, Durand, M, et al: Ocular toxoplasmosis and Hodgkin's disease: Report of two cases. Arch Ophthalmol 96:62-63, 1978.
1177. Hoerni-Simon, G, Suchaud, JP, Eghbali, H, et al: Secondary involvement of the central nervous system in malignant non-Hodgkin's lymphoma. A study of 30 cases in a series of 498 patients. Oncology 44:98-101, 1987.
1178. Hoffman, DL, Howard, JR, Jr, Sarma, R, et al: Encephalopathy, myelopathy, optic neuropathy, and anosmia associated with intravenous cytosine arabinoside. Clin Neuropharmacol 16:258-262, 1993.
1179. Hoffman, JC: Permanent paralysis of the accessory nerve after cannulation of the internal jugular vein. Letter to the Editor. Anesthesiology 58:583-584, 1983.
1180. Hoffman, JM, Waskin, HA, Schifter, T, et al: FDG-PET in differentiating lymphoma from nonmalignant central nervous system lesions in patients with AIDS. J Nucl Med 34:567-575, 1993.
1181. Hoffman, WF, Levin, VA, and Wilson, CB: Evaluation of malignant glioma patients during the post-irradiation period. J Neurosurg 50:624-628, 1979.
1182. Hofman, M, Rudy, W, Gunthert, U, et al: A link between ras and metastatic behavior of tumor cells: ras induces CD44 promoter activity and leads to low-level expression of metastasis-specific variants of CD44 in CREF cells. Cancer Res 53:1516-1521, 1993.
1183. Hofmann, T, Kasper, W, Meinertz, T, et al: Echocardiographic evaluation of patients with clinically suspected arterial emboli. Lancet 336:1421-1424, 1990.
1184. Holgersen, LO, Santulli, TV, Schulinger, IN, et al: Neuroblastoma with intraspinal (dumbbell) extension. J Pediatr Surg 18:406-411, 1983.
1185. Holland, JC, Morrow, GR, Schmale, A, et al: A randomized clinical trial of alprazolam versus progressive muscle relaxation in cancer patients with anxiety and depressive symptoms. J Clin Oncol 9:1004-1011, 1991.
1186. Holland, JC and Rowland, JH (eds): Handbook of Psychooncology: Psychological Care of the Patient with Cancer. Oxford University Press, New York, 1989.
1187. Holland, JF, Scharlau, C, Gailani, S, et al: Vincristine treatment of advanced cancer: A cooperative study of 392 cases. Cancer Res 33:1258-1264, 1973.
1188. Hollis, N, Marsh, RH, Marshall, RD, et al: Overwhelming pneumococcal sepsis in healthy adults years after splenectomy. Letter to the Editor. Lancet 1:110-111, 1987.
1189. Hollis, PH, Malis, LI, and Zappulla, RA: Neurological deterioration after lumbar puncture below

complete spinal subarachnoid block. J Neurosurg 64:253-256, 1986.
1190. Hollis, PH, Zappulla, RA, Spigelman, MK, et al: Physiological and electrophysiological consequences of etoposide-induced blood-brain barrier disruption. Neurosurgery 18:581-586, 1986.
1191. Holmes, VF, Adams, F, and Fernandez, F: Respiratory dyskinesia due to antiemetic therapy in a cancer patient. Cancer Treat Rep 71:415-416, 1987.
1192. Holoye, P, Libnoch, J, Cox, J, et al: Spinal cord metastasis in small cell lung carcinoma of the lung. Int J Radiat Oncol Biol Phys 10:349-356, 1984.
1193. Holte, H, Saeter, G, Dahl, IM, et al: Progressive loss of vision in patients with high-grade non-Hodgkin's lymphoma. Cancer 60:2521-2523, 1987.
1194. Holtz, A and Gerdin, B: Efficacy of the 21-aminosteroid U74006F in improving neurological recovery after spinal cord injury in rats. Neurol Res 14:49-52, 1992.
1195. Hong, F and Mayhew, E: Therapy of central nervous system leukemia in mice by liposome-entrapped 1-beta-D-arabinofuranosylcytosine. Cancer Res 49:5097-5102, 1989.
1196. Hoogenraad, TU, Sanders, E, and Tan, K: Paraneoplastic optic neuritis and encephalomyelitis, report of a case. Neuro-Ophthalmology 9:247-250, 1989.
1197. Hook, CC, Kimmel, DW, Kvols, LK, et al: Multifocal inflammatory leukoencephalopathy with 5-fluorouracil and levamisole. Ann Neurol 31:262-267, 1992.
1198. Hooper, DC, Pruitt, AA, and Rubin, RH: Central nervous system infection in the chronically immunosuppressed. Medicine (Baltimore) 61:166-188, 1982.
1199. Hopewell, JW and Wright, EA: The nature of latent cerebral irradiation damage and its modification by hypertension. Br J Radiol 43:161-167, 1970.
1200. Horber, FF, Scheidegger, JR, Grunig, BE, et al: Thigh muscle mass and function in patients treated with glucocorticoids. Eur J Clin Invest 15:302-307, 1985.
1201. Hormigo, A, Dalmau, J, Rosenblum, M, et al: Immunological and pathological study of a patient with anti-Ri-associated encephalopathy. Abstract. Ann Neurol 36:896-902, 1994.
1202. Hormigo, A, Lobo-Antunes, JL, Bravo-Marques, JM, et al: Syringomyelia secondary to compression of the cervical spinal cord by an extramedullary lymphoma. Neurosurgery 27:834-836, 1990.
1203. Hornbein, TF, Townes, BD, Schoene, RB, et al: The cost to the central nervous system of climbing to extremely high altitude. N Engl J Med 321:1714-1719, 1989.
1204. Horowitz, SH: Isolated facial numbness. Clinical significance and relation to trigeminal neuropathy. Ann Intern Med 80:49-53, 1974.
1205. Horowitz, SH: Peripheral nerve injury and causalgia secondary to routine venipuncture. Neurology 44:962-964, 1994.
1206. Horten, B, Price, RW, and Jimenez, D: Multifocal varicella-zoster virus leukoencephalitis temporally remote from herpes zoster. Ann Neurol 9:251-266, 1981.
1207. Horton, J, Baxter, DH, and Olson, KB: The management of metastases to the brain by irradiation and corticosteroids. Am J Roentgenol Radium Ther Nucl Med 3:334-336, 1971.
1208. Horton, J, Means, ED, Cunningham, TJ, et al: The numb chin in breast cancer. J Neurol Neurosurg Psychiatry 36:211-216, 1973.
1209. Horton, J, Olson, KB, Sullivan, J, et al: 5-Fluorouracil in cancer: An improved regimen. Ann Intern Med 73:897-900, 1970.
1209a. Horton, JC and Fishman, RA: Neurovisual findings in the syndrome of spontaneous intracranial hypotension from dural cerebrospinal fluid leak. Ophthalmology 101:244-251, 1994.
1210. Horwich, MS, Cho, L, Porro, RS, et al: Subacute sensory neuropathy: A remote effect of carcinoma. Ann Neurol 2:7-19, 1977.
1211. Horwitz, SJ, Boxerbaum, B, and O'Bell, J: Cerebral herniation in bacterial meningitis in childhood. Ann Neurol 7:524-528, 1980.
1212. Hoskin, PJ, Crow, J, and Ford, HT: The influence of extent and local management on the outcome of radiotherapy for brain metastases. Int J Radiat Oncol Biol Phys 19:111-115, 1990.
1213. Houck, JR and Murphy, K: Sudden bilateral profound hearing loss resulting from meningeal carcinomatosis. Otolaryngol Head Neck Surg 106:92-97, 1992.
1214. Houck, WA, Olson, KB, and Horton, J: Clinical features of tumor metastasis to the pituitary. Cancer 26:656-659, 1970.
1215. Houi, K, Mochio, S, and Kobayashi, T: Gangliosides attenuate vincristine neurotoxicity on dorsal root ganglion cells. Muscle Nerve 16:11-14, 1993.
1216. Hovestadt, A, van Woerkom, CM, and Vecht, CJ: Frequency of neurological disease in a cancer hospital. Letter to the Editor. Eur J Cancer 26:765-766, 1990.
1217. Hovi, L, Era, P, Rautonen, J, et al: Impaired muscle strength in female adolescents and young adults surviving leukemia in childhood. Cancer 72:276-281, 1993.
1218. Howard, GM, Jakobiec, FA, Trokel, SL, et al: Pulsating metastatic tumor of the orbit. Am J Ophthalmol 85:767-771, 1978.
1219. Howell, SB, Pfeifle, CE, and Wung, WE: Effect of allopurinol on the toxicity of high-dose 5-fluorouracil administered by intermittent bolus injection. Cancer 51:220-225, 1983.
1220. Hsu, CY, Hogan, EL, Wingfield, W, Jr, et al: Orthostatic hypotension with brainstem tumors. Neurology 34:1137-1143, 1984.
1221. Hu, D-S and Silberfarb, PM: Management of sleep problems in cancer patients. Oncology (Huntingt) 5:23-28, 1991.
1222. Huang, CY: Peripheral neuropathy in the elderly: A clinical and electrophysiologic study. J Am Geriatr Soc 29:49-54, 1981.
1223. Huang, PS and Koo, KE: Diffuse intravascular coagulation associated with brain tumor surgery in children. Pediatr Neurosurg 91:43-47, 1991.
1224. Huang, PS and Oz, M: Malignant carcinoid tumor metastatic to the dura mater simulating a meningioma. Neurosurgery 29:449-452, 1991.

1224a. Huang, T-Y, Arita, N, Ushio, Y, et al: Pharmacokinetics of intrathecal 1-(4-amino-2-methyl-5-pyrimidinyl)-methyl-3-(2-chloroethyl)-3-nitrosourea hydrochloride in rats. J Neurooncol 19:245-250, 1994.

1225. Hudson, CN, Curling, M, Potsides, P, et al: Paraneoplastic syndromes in patients with ovarian neoplasia. J R Soc Med 86:202-204, 1993.

1226. Hug, V, Keating, M, McCredie, K, et al: Clinical course and response to treatment of patients with acute myelogenous leukemia presenting with a high leukocyte count. Cancer 52:773-779, 1983.

1227. Hughes, BA, Kimmel, DW, and Aksamit, AJ: Herpes zoster-associated meningoencephalitis in patients with systemic cancer. Mayo Clin Proc 68:652-655, 1993.

1228. Hughes, M, Ahern, V, Kefford, R, et al: Paraneoplastic myelopathy at diagnosis in a patient with pathologic stage 1A Hodgkin disease. Cancer 70:1598-1600, 1992.

1229. Hughes, WT, Rivera, GK, Schell, MJ, et al: Successful intermittent chemoprophylaxis for *Pneumocystis carinii* pneumonitis. N Engl J Med 316:1627-1632, 1987.

1230. Hung, S, Hilsenback, S, and Feun, L: Seizure prophylaxis with phenytoin in patients with brain metastases. Abstract. Program/Proceedings American Society of Clinical Oncology 10:327, 1991.

1231. Hurwitz, BJ and Posner, JB: Cerebral infarction complicating subclavian vein catheterization. Ann Neurol 1:253-254, 1977.

1232. Hurwitz, RL, Mahoney, DH, Jr, Armstrong, DL, et al: Reversible encephalopathy and seizures as a result of conventional vincristine administration. Med Pediatr Oncol 16:216-219, 1988.

1233. Hutchings, M and Weller, RO: Anatomical relationships of the pia mater to cerebral blood vessels in man. J Neurosurg 65:316-325, 1986.

1234. Hwang, TL, Yung, WK, Lee, Y-Y, et al: High dose Ara-C related leukoencephalopathy. J Neurooncol 3:335-339, 1986.

1235. Hylton, PD, Reichman, OH, and Palutsis, R: Monitoring of transient central nervous system postirradiation effects by 133Xe inhalation regional cerebral blood flow measurements. Neurosurgery 21:843-848, 1987.

1236. Hyser, CL and Drake, ME, Jr: Myoclonus induced by metoclopramide therapy. Arch Intern Med 143:2201-2202, 1983.

1237. Icli, F, Karaoguz, H, Dincol, D, et al: Severe vascular toxicity associated with cisplatin-based chemotherapy. Cancer 72:587-593, 1993.

1238. Igarashi, M, Card, GG, Johnson, PE, et al: Bilateral sudden hearing loss and metastatic pancreatic adenocarcinoma. Arch Otolaryngol 105:196-199, 1979.

1239. Igarashi, M, Gilmartin, RC, Gerald, B, et al: Cerebral arteritis and bacterial meningitis. Arch Neurol 41:531-535, 1984.

1240. Illarramendi, JJ and Gallego, J: Cisplatin-based chemotherapy and acute cerebrovascular events. Letter to the Editor. Lancet 338:705, 1991.

1241. Ilyas, AA, Cook, SD, Dalakas, MC, et al: Anti-MAG IgM paraproteins from some patients with polyneuropathy associated with IgM paraproteinemia also react with sulfatide. J Neuroimmunol 37:85-92, 1992.

1241a. Inamura, T, Nomura, T, Bartus, RT, et al: Intracarotid infusion of RMP-7, a bradykinin analog: A method for selective drug delivery to brain tumors. J Neurosurg 81:752-758, 1994.

1242. Imaoka, S, Ueda, T, Shibata, H, et al: Fibrinolysis in patients with acute promyelocytic leukemia and disseminated intravascular coagulation during heparin therapy. Cancer 58:1736-1738, 1986.

1243. Inao, S, Kuchiwaki, H, Kanaiwa, H, et al: Magnetic resonance imaging assessment of brainstem distortion associated with a supratentorial mass. J Neurol Neurosurg Psychiatry 56:280-285, 1993.

1244. Ingber, D, Fujita, T, Kishimoto, S, et al: Synthetic analogues of fumagillin that inhibit angiogenesis and suppress tumour growth. Nature 348:555-557, 1990.

1245. Ingber, DE and Folkman, J: How does extracellular matrix control capillary morphogenesis? Cell 58:803-805, 1989.

1246. Ingram, LC, Fairclough, DL, Furman, WL, et al: Cranial nerve palsy in childhood acute lymphoblastic leukemia and non-Hodgkin's lymphoma. Cancer 67:2262-2268, 1991.

1247. Ingvar, DH and Lundberg, N: Paroxysmal systems in intracranial hypertension, studied with ventricular fluid pressure recording and electroencephalography. Brain 84:446-459, 1961.

1248. Inwards, DJ, Piepgras, DG, Lie, JT, et al: Granulomatous angiitis of the spinal cord associated with Hodgkin's disease. Cancer 68:1318-1322, 1991.

1249. Ischia, S, Ischia, A, Luzzani, A, et al: Results up to death in the treatment of persistent cervicothoracic (Pancoast) and thoracic malignant pain by unilateral percutaneous cervical cordotomy. Pain 21:339-355, 1985.

1250. Isensee, C, Reul, J, and Thron, A: Magnetic resonance imaging of thrombosed dural sinuses. Stroke 25:29-34, 1994.

1251. Iwasaki, Y, Sako, K, Ohara, Y, et al: Subacute panencephalitis associated with chronic graft-versus-host disease. Acta Neuropathol (Berl) 85:566-572, 1993.

1252. Jackson, CG, Netterville, JL, Glasscock, ME, III, et al: Defect reconstruction and cerebrospinal fluid management in neurotologic skull base tumors with intracranial extension. Laryngoscope 102:1205-1214, 1992.

1253. Jackson, DV, Jr, Castle, MC, Poplack, DG, et al: Pharmacokinetics of vincristine in the cerebrospinal fluid of subhuman primates. Cancer Res 40:722-724, 1980.

1254. Jackson, DV, Jr, McMahan, RA, Pope, EK, et al: Clinical trial of folinic acid to reduce vincristine neurotoxicity. Cancer Chemother Pharmacol 17:281-284, 1986.

1255. Jackson, DV, Jr, Pope, EK, McMahan, RA, et al: Clinical trial of pyridoxine to reduce vincristine neurotoxicity. J Neurooncol 4:37-41, 1986.

1256. Jackson, DV, Jr, Richards, F, II, Cooper, MR, et al: Prophylactic cranial irradiation in small cell carcinoma of the lung. A randomized study. JAMA 237:2730-2733, 1977.

1257. Jackson, M: Post radiation monomelic amyotrophy. Letter to the Editor. J Neurol Neurosurg Psychiatry 55:629, 1992.
1258. Jacobs, DH, Holmes, FF, and McFarlane, MJ: Meningiomas are not significantly associated with breast cancer. Arch Neurol 49:753-756, 1992.
1259. Jacobs, L, Kinkel, WR, and Vincent, RG: "Silent" brain metastasis from lung carcinoma determined by computerized tomography. Arch Neurol 34:690-693, 1977.
1260. Jacobs, M and Phuphanich, S: Seizures in brain metastasis and meningeal carcinomatosis. Abstract. Proc ASCO 9:96, 1990.
1261. Jacobs, RH, Awan, A, Bitran, JD, et al: Prophylactic cranial irradiation in adenocarcinoma of the lung. A possible role. Cancer 59:2016-2019, 1987.
1262. Jacobs, TP, Whitlock, RT, Edsall, J, et al: Addisonian crisis while taking high-dose glucocorticoids. An unusual presentation of primary adrenal failure in two patients with underlying inflammatory diseases. JAMA 260:2082-2084, 1988.
1263. Jacobson, DM, Thirkill, CE, and Tipping, SJ: A clinical triad to diagnose paraneoplastic retinopathy. Ann Neurol 28:162-167, 1990.
1264. Jacobson, DR and Fleming, BJ: Graves' disease with ophthalmopathy following radiotherapy for Hodgkin's disease. Case report. Am J Med Sci 288:217-220, 1984.
1265. Jacobson, SA, Leuchter, AF, and Walter, DO: Conventional and quantitative EEG in the diagnosis of delirium among the elderly. J Neurol Neurosurg Psychiatry 56:153-158, 1993.
1266. Jacquillat C, Khayat, D, Banzet, P, et al: Final report of the French multicenter phase II study of the nitrosourea fotemustine in 153 evaluable patients with disseminated malignant melanoma including patients with cerebral metastases. Cancer 66:1873-1878, 1990.
1267. Jaeckle, KA, Digre, KB, Jones, CR, et al: Central neurogenic hyperventilation: Pharmacologic intervention with morphine sulfate and correlative analysis of respiratory, sleep, and ocular motor dysfunction. Neurology 40:1715-1720, 1990.
1268. Jaeckle, KA, Krol, G, and Posner, JB: Evolution of computed tomographic abnormalities in leptomeningeal metastases. Ann Neurol 17:85-89, 1985.
1269. Jaeckle, KA, Stroop, WG, Price, M, et al: Autoimmune non-carcinomatous sensory-motor neuronopathy with posterior column degeneration. Abstract. Ann Neurol 20:140, 1986.
1270. Jaeckle, KA, Young, DF, and Foley, KM: The natural history of lumbosacral plexopathy in cancer. Neurology 35:8-15, 1985.
1271. Jain, S, Kotasek, D, Blumbergs, PC, et al: Aleukaemic leukostasis in a case of large cell non-Hodgkin's lymphoma: Report of a case with a distinctive central nervous system involvement. J Neurol Neurosurg Psychiatry 49:1079-1083, 1986.
1272. Jakobson, AM, Kreuger, A, Mortimer, O, et al: Cerebrospinal fluid exchange after intrathecal methotrexate overdose. A report of two cases. Acta Paediatr 81:359-361, 1992.
1273. Jamison, K, Wellisch, DK, Katz, RL, et al: Phantom breast syndrome. Arch Surg 114:93-95, 1979.
1274. Janecka, IP and Sekhar, LN: Surgical management of cranial base tumors: A report on 91 patients. Oncology (Huntingt) 3:69-80, 1989.
1275. Jankovic, J and Glass, JP: Metoclopramide-induced phantom dyskinesia. Neurology 35:432-435, 1985.
1275a. Jankovic, M, Brouwers, P, Valsecchi, MG, et al: Association of 1800 cGy cranial irradiation with intellectual function in children with acute lymphoblastic leukaemia. Lancet 344:224-227, 1994.
1276. Jankovic, M, Scotti, G, De Grandi, C, et al: Correlation between cranial computed tomographic scans at diagnosis in children with acute lymphoblastic leukaemia and central nervous system relapse. Lancet 2:1212-1214, 1988.
1277. Jann, S, Beretta, S, Moggio, M, et al: High-dose intravenous human immunoglobulin in polymyositis resistant to treatment. J Neurology Neurosurg Psychiatry 55:60-62, 1992.
1278. Jarden, JO, Dhawan, V, Moeller, JR, et al: The time course of steroid action on blood-to-brain and blood-to-tumor transport of 82Rb: A positron emission tomographic study. Ann Neurol 25:239-245, 1989.
1279. Jarosinski, PF, Moscow, JA, Alexander, MS, et al: Altered phenytoin clearance during intensive chemotherapy for acute lymphoblastic leukemia. J Pediatr 112:996-999, 1988.
1280. Jarrett, WH and Christy, JH: Retinal hole formation: From septic embolization in acute bacterial endocarditis. Am J Ophthalmol 64:472-474, 1967.
1281. Jellinger, K, Kothbauer, P, Sunder-Plassmann, E, et al: Intramedullary spinal cord metastases. J Neurol 220:31-41, 1979.
1282. Jellinger, K and Radiaszkiewicz, T: Involvement of the central nervous system in malignant lymphomas. Virchows Arch A Pathol Anat Histopathol 370:345-362, 1976.
1283. Jemsek, J, Greenberg, SB, Taber, L, et al: Herpes zoster-associated encephalitis: Clinicopathologic report of 12 cases and review of the literature. Medicine (Baltimore) 62:81-97, 1983.
1284. Jenkyn, LR, Kinlaw, WB, Bernat, JL, et al: Falsely localizing third-nerve palsy. Letter to the Editor. N Engl J Med 303:161-162, 1980.
1285. Jensen, TS, Krebs, B, Nielsen, J, et al: Immediate and long-term phantom limb pain in amputees: Incidence, clinical characteristics and relationship to pre-amputation limb pain. Pain 21:267-278, 1985.
1286. Jeppsson, B, Freund, HR, Gimmon, Z, et al: Blood–brain barrier derangement in sepsis: Cause of septic encephalopathy? Am J Surg 141:136-142, 1981.
1287. Jeremic, B, Djuric, L, and Mijatovic, L: Incidence of radiation myelitis of the cervical spinal cord at doses of 5500 cGy or greater. Cancer 68:2138-2141, 1991.
1288. Jeremic, B, Grujicic, D, Cirovic, V, et al: Radiotherapy of metastatic spinal cord compression. Acta Oncol 30:985-986, 1991.
1289. Jetmore, AB, Timmcke, AE, Gathright, JB, et al: Ogilvie's syndrome: Colonoscopic decompression and analysis of predisposing factors. Dis Colon Rectum 35:1135-1142, 1992.

1290. Jex, RK, van Heerden, JA, Carpenter, PC, et al: Ectopic ACTH syndrome. Diagnostic and therapeutic aspects. Am J Surg 149:276-282, 1985.
1291. Joffe, AM, Farley, JD, Linden, D, et al: Trimethoprim-sulfamethoxazole-associated aseptic meningitis: Case reports and review of the literature. Am J Med 87:332-338, 1989.
1292. Johanson, CE: Potential for pharmacologic manipulation of the blood-cerebrospinal fluid barrier. In Neuwelt, EA (ed): Implications of the Blood–Brain Barrier and Its Manipulation, vol 1, Basic Science Aspects. Plenum Medical Book Company, New York, 1989, pp 223-260.
1293. Johnson, BE, Becker, B, Goff, WB, II, et al: Neurologic, neuropsychologic, and computed cranial tomography scan abnormalities in 2- to 10-year survivors of small-cell lung cancer. J Clin Oncol 3:1659-1667, 1985.
1294. Johnson, BE, Patronas, N, Hayes, W, et al: Neurologic, computed cranial tomographic, and magnetic resonance imaging abnormalities in patients with small-cell lung cancer: Further follow-up of 6- to 13-year survivors. J Clin Oncol 8:48-56, 1990.
1295. Johnson, EM, Jr and Deckwerth, TL: Molecular mechanisms of developmental neuronal death. Annu Rev Neurosci 16:31-46, 1993.
1296. Johnson, PC, Rolak, LA, Hamilton, RH, et al: Paraneoplastic vasculitis of nerve: A remote effect of cancer. Ann Neurol 5:437-444, 1979.
1297. Johnston, EF, Hammond, AJ, and Cairncross, JG: Bilateral hypoglossal palsies: A late complication of curative radiotherapy. Can J Neurol Sci 16:198-199, 1989.
1298. Johnston, FG, Uttley, D, and Marsh, HT: Synchronous vertebral decompression and posterior stabilization in the treatment of spinal malignancy. Neurosurgery 25:872-876, 1989.
1299. Johnston, I, Gilday, DL, and Hendrick, EB: Experimental effects of steroids and steroid withdrawal on cerebrospinal fluid absorption. J Neurosurg 42:690-695, 1975.
1300. Jokelainen, M: The epidemiology of amyotrophic lateral sclerosis in Finland. J Neurol Sci 29:55-63, 1976.
1301. Jolicoeur, FB, Wayner, MJ, Rondeau, DB, et al: Effects of phenobarbital on taste aversion induced by X-radiation. Pharmacol Biochem Behav 11:709-712, 1979.
1302. Jolson, HM, Bosco, L, Bufton, MG, et al: Clustering of adverse drug events: Analysis of risk factors for cerebellar toxicity with high-dose cytarabine. J Natl Cancer Inst 84:500-505, 1992.
1303. Jones, A: Transient radiation myelopathy. Br J Radiol 37:727-744, 1964.
1304. Jones, GR, Mason, WH, Fishman, LS, et al: Primary central nervous system lymphoma without intracranial mass in a child. Diagnosis by documentation of monoclonality. Cancer 56:2804-2808, 1985.
1305. Jones, HR, Jr and Siekert, RG: Neurological manifestation of infective endocarditis. Review of clinical and therapeutic challenges. Brain 112:1295-1315, 1989.
1306. Jones, WB, Lewis, JL, Jr, and Lehr, M: Monitor of chemotherapy in gestational trophoblastic neoplasm by radioimmunoassay of the β-subunit of human chorionic gonadotropin. Am J Obstet Gynecol 121:669-673, 1975.
1307. Jonsson, B, Sjostrom, L, Jonsson, H, Jr, et al: Surgery for multiple myeloma of the spine. A retrospective analysis of 12 patients. Acta Orthop Scand 63:192-194, 1992.
1308. Jonsson, V, Schroder, HD, Trojaborg, W, et al: Autoimmune reactions in patients with M-component and peripheral neuropathy. J Intern Med 232:185-191, 1992.
1309. Jooma, R and Hayward, RD: Upward spinal coning: Impaction of occult spinal tumours following relief of hydrocephalus. J Neurol Neurosurg Psychiatry 47:386-390, 1984.
1310. Jortner, BS and Cho, E-S: Neurotoxicity of Adriamycin in rats: A low-dose effect. Cancer Treat Rep 64:257-261, 1980.
1311. Juacaba, SF, Jones, LD, and Tarin, D: Organ preferences in metastatic colony formation by spontaneous mammary carcinomas after intraarterial inoculation. Invasion Metastasis 3:208-220, 1983.
1312. Julien, J, Ferrer, X, Drouillard, J, et al: Cavernous sinus syndrome due to lymphoma. J Neurol Neurosurg Psychiatry 47:558-560, 1984.
1313. Julien, J, Vital, C, Aupy, G, et al: Guillain-Barré syndrome and Hodgkin's disease. Ultrastructural study of a peripheral nerve. J Neurol Sci 45:23-27, 1980.
1314. Junck, L and Marshall, WH: Neurotoxicity of radiological contrast agents. Ann Neurol 13:469-484, 1983.
1315. Juneau, P, Schoene, WC, and Black, P: Malignant tumors in the pituitary gland. Arch Neurol 49:555-558, 1992.
1316. Juvela, S, Heiskanen, O, Poranen, A, et al: The treatment of spontaneous intracerebral hemorrhage. A prospective randomized trial of surgical and conservative treatment. J Neurosurg 70:755-758, 1989.
1317. Kaczmarski, R, Pagliuca, A, Pullon, H, et al: Fulminant fungal sinusitis following intensive chemotherapy. Q J Med 75:365-370, 1990.
1318. Kaiko, RF, Foley, KM, Grabinski, PY, et al: Central nervous system excitatory effects of meperidine in cancer patients. Ann Neurol 13:180-185, 1983.
1319. Kakkar, VV, Corrigan, TP, Fossard, DP, et al: Prevention of fatal postoperative pulmonary embolism by low doses of heparin. Reappraisal of results of international multicentre trial. Lancet 1:567-569, 1977.
1320. Kakulas, BA, Harper, CG, Shibasaki, K, et al: Vertebral metastases and spinal cord compression. Clin Exp Neurol 15:98-113, 1978.
1321. Kalaria, RN, Gravina, SA, Schmidley, JW, et al: The glucose transporter of the human brain and blood–brain barrier. Ann Neurol 24:757-764, 1988.
1322. Kamada, K, Isu, T, Houkin, K, et al: Acute aggravation of subdural effusion associated with pachymeningitis carcinomatosa: Case report. Neurosurgery 29:464-466, 1991.
1323. Kamath, S, Booth, P, Lad, TE, et al: Taste thresholds of patients with cancer of the esophagus. Cancer 52:386-389, 1983.

1324. Kamby, C and Soerensen, PS: Characteristics of patients with short and long survivals after detection of intracranial metastases from breast cancer. J Neurooncol 6:37-45, 1988.
1325. Kamby, C, Vejborg, I, Daugaard, S, et al: Clinical and radiologic characteristics of bone metastases in breast cancer. Cancer 60:2524-2531, 1987.
1326. Kamen, BA, Holcenberg, JS, and Siegel, SE: Aziridinylbenzoquinone (AZQ) treatment of central nervous system leukemia. Letter to the Editor. Cancer Treat Rep 66:2105-2106, 1982.
1327. Kamen, BA, Moulder, JE, Kun, LE, et al: Effects of single-dose and fractionated cranial irradiation on rat brain accumulation of methotrexate. Cancer Res 44:5092-5094, 1984.
1328. Kamholtz, R and Sze, G: Current imaging in spinal metastatic disease. Semin Oncol 18:158-169, 1991.
1329. Kaminski, HJ, Diwan, VG, and Ruff, RL: Second occurrence of spinal epidural metastases. Neurology 41:744-746, 1991.
1330. Kanda, Y, Shigeno, K, Kinoshita, N, et al: Sudden hearing loss associated with interferon. Lancet 343:1134-1135, 1994.
1331. Kandel, RA, Bedard, YC, Pritzker, KP, et al: Lymphoma. Presenting as an intramuscular small cell malignant tumor. Cancer 53:1586-1589, 1984.
1332. Kaneda, A, Yamaura, I, Kamikozuru, M, et al: Paraplegia as a complication of corticosteroid therapy. J Bone Joint Surg [Am] 66:783-785, 1984.
1333. Kaniecki, R and Morris, JC: Reversible paraneoplastic limbic encephalitis. Neurology 43:2418-2419, 1993.
1334. Kanj, SS, Sharara, AI, Shpall, EJ, et al: Myocardial ischemia associated with high-dose carmustine infusion. Cancer 68:1910-1912, 1991.
1335. Kanner, RM, Martini, N, and Foley, KM: Incidence of pain and other clinical manifestations of superior pulmonary sulcus (Pancoast) tumors. In Bonica, JJ, Ventafridda, V, and Pagni, CA (eds): Advances in Pain Research and Therapy, vol 4. Raven Press, New York, 1982, pp 27-45.
1336. Kaplan, AM and Itabashi, HH: Encephalitis associated with carcinoma. Central hypoventilation syndrome and cytoplasmic inclusion bodies. J Neurol Neurosurg Psychiatry 37:1166-1176, 1974.
1337. Kaplan, ID, Adler, JR, Hicks, WL, Jr, et al: Radiosurgery for palliation of base of skull recurrences from head and neck cancers. Cancer 70:1980-1984, 1992.
1338. Kaplan, JG, DeSouza, TG, Farkash, A, et al: Leptomeningeal metastases: Comparison of clinical features and laboratory data of solid tumors, lymphomas and leukemias. J Neurooncol 9:225-229, 1990.
1339. Kaplan, JG, Portenoy, RK, Pack, DR, et al: Polyradiculopathy in leptomeningeal metastasis: The role of EMG and late response studies. J Neurooncol 9:219-224, 1990.
1340. Kaplan, MH, Rosen, PP, and Armstrong, D: Cryptococcosis in a cancer hospital. Clinical and pathological correlates in forty-six patients. Cancer 39:2265-2274, 1977.
1340a. Kappel, TJ, Manivel, KC, and Goswitz, JJ: Atypical lymphocytes in spinal fluid resembling posttransplant lymphoma in a cardia transplant recipient: A case report. Acta Cytol 38:470-474, 1994.
1341. Kardinal, CG, Loprinzi, CL, Schaid, DJ, et al: A controlled trial of cyprohepatidine in cancer patients with anorexia and/or cachexia. Cancer 65:2657-2662, 1990.
1342. Karp, G and Nahum, K: Hyperventilation as the initial manifestation of lymphomatous meningitis. J Neurooncol 13:173-175, 1992.
1343. Karpatkin, S and Pearlstein, E: Role of platelets in tumor cell metastases. Ann Intern Med 95:636-641, 1981.
1344. Kaspers, G-J, Kamphorst, W, van de Graaff, M, et al: Primary spinal epidural extraosseous Ewing's sarcoma. Cancer 68:648-654, 1991.
1345. Kato, A, Ushio, Y, Hayakawa, T, et al: Circulatory disturbance of the spinal cord with epidural neoplasm in rats. J Neurosurg 63:260-265, 1985.
1346. Kattah, JC, Suski, ET, Killen, JY, et al: Optic neuritis and systemic lymphoma. Am J Ophthalmol 89:431-436, 1980.
1347. Kawaguchi, T, Tobai, S, and Nakamura, K: Extravascular migration of tumor cells in the brain: An electron microscopic study. Invasion Metastasis 2:40-50, 1982.
1348. Kay, AC, Solberg, LA, Jr, Nichols, DA, et al: Prognostic significance of computed tomography of the brain in thrombotic thrombocytopenic purpura. Mayo Clin Proc 66:602-607, 1991.
1349. Kay, CL, Davies-Jones, GAB, Singal, R, et al: Paraneoplastic opsoclonus-myoclonus in Hodgkin's disease. Letter to the Editor. J Neurol Neurosurg Psychiatry 56:831-832, 1993.
1350. Kearsley, JH and Tattersall, MH: Cerebral embolism in cancer patients. Q J Med 51:279-291, 1982.
1351. Kelly, JJ, Jr: Peripheral neuropathies associated with monoclonal proteins: A clinical review. Muscle Nerve 8:138-150, 1985.
1352. Kelly, JJ, Jr, Kyle, RA, Miles, JM, et al: The spectrum of peripheral neuropathy in myeloma. Neurology 31:24-31, 1981.
1353. Kelly JJ, Jr, Kyle, RA, Miles, JM, et al: Osteosclerotic myeloma and peripheral neuropathy. Neurology 33:202-210, 1983.
1354. Kelly, PJ: Computer-assisted stereotaxis: New approaches for the management of intracranial intra-axial tumors. Neurology 36:535-541, 1986.
1355. Kelsey, SM, Williams, AC, and Corbin, D: Hyponatraemia as a cause of reversible ataxia. Short report. BMJ 293:1346, 1986.
1356. Keltner, JL, Thirkill, CE, Tyler, NK, et al: Management and monitoring of cancer-associated retinopathy. Arch Ophthalmol (Copenh) 110:48-53, 1992.
1357. Kende, G, Sirkin, SR, Thomas, PR, et al: Blurring of vision: A previously undescribed complication of cyclophosphamide therapy. Cancer 44:69-71, 1979.
1358. Kennedy, PGE: Neurological complications of varicella-zoster virus. In Kennedy, PGE and Johnson, RT (eds): Infections of the Nervous System. Butterworths, London, 1987, pp 177-208.
1359. Kepes, JJ: Large focal tumor-like demyelinating lesions of the brain: Intermediate entity between multiple sclerosis and acute disseminated encephalomyelitis? A study of 31 patients. Ann Neurol 33:18-27, 1993.
1360. Kerr, IG, Zimm, S, Collins, JM, et al: Effect of

intravenous dose and schedule on cerebrospinal fluid pharmacokinetics of 5-fluorouracil in the monkey. Cancer Res 44:4929-4932, 1984.
1361. Kestle, JRW, Hoffman, HJ, and Mock, AR: Moyamoya phenomenon after radiation for optic glioma. J Neurosurg 79:32-35, 1993.
1362. Khaleeli, AA, Edwards, RH, Gohil, K, et al: Corticosteroid myopathy: A clinical and pathological study. Clin Endocrinol (Oxf) 18:155-166, 1983.
1362a. Khandheria, BK, Seward, JB, and Tajik, AJ: Transesophageal echocardiography. Mayo Clin Proc 69:856-863, 1994.
1363. Khardori, N, Berkey, P, Hayat, S, et al: Spectrum and outcome of microbiologically documented *Listeria monocytogenes* infections in cancer patients. Cancer 64:1968-1970, 1989.
1364. Khoury, GF, Stein, C, and Ramming, KP: Neck and shoulder pain associated with hepatic arterial chemotherapy using an implantable infusion pump. Pain 32:275-277, 1988.
1365. Khurana, RK, Koski, CL, and Mayer, RF: Autonomic dysfunction in Lambert-Eaton myasthenic syndrome. J Neurol Sci 85:77-86, 1988.
1366. Kim, H-S, Suzuki, M, Lie, JT, et al: Clinically unsuspected disseminated intravascular coagulation (DIC). Am J Clin Pathol 66:31-39, 1976.
1367. Kim, H-S, Suzuki, M, Lie, JT, et al: Nonbacterial thrombotic endocarditis (NBTE) and disseminated intravascular coagulation (DIC): Autopsy study of 36 patients. Arch Pathol Lab Med 101:65-68, 1977.
1368. Kim, HK, Lee, SK, Hong, YS, et al: Cisplatin-induced peripheral neuropathy (PN) in patients with history of neurologic damage. Abstract. Program/Proceedings American Society of Clinical Oncology 10:A1224, 1991.
1369. Kim, S, Khatibi, S, Howell, SB, et al: Prolongation of drug exposure in cerebrospinal fluid by encapsulation into DepoFoam. Cancer Res 53:1596-1598, 1993.
1370. Kim, TH, Ramsay, NK, Steeves, RA, et al: Intermittent central nervous system irradiation and intrathecal chemotherapy for central nervous system leukemia in children. Int J Radiat Oncol Biol Phys 13:1451-1455, 1987.
1371. Kimmel, DW and Schutt, AJ: Multifocal leukoencephalopathy: Occurrence during 5-fluorouracil and levamisole therapy and resolution after discontinuation of chemotherapy. Mayo Clin Proc 68:363-365, 1993.
1372. Kimura, J (ed): Electrodiagnosis in Diseases of Nerve and Muscle: Principles and Practice, ed 2. FA Davis, Philadelphia, 1989, pp 519-534.
1373. King, DK, Loh, KK, Ayala, AG, et al: Eosinophilic meningitis and lymphomatous meningitis. Letter to the Editor. Ann Intern Med 82:228, 1975.
1374. King, KL and Boder, GB: Correlation of the clinical neurotoxicity of the vinca alkaloids vincristine, vinblastine, and vindesine with their effects on cultured rat midbrain cells. Cancer Chemother Pharmacol 2:239-242, 1979.
1375. King, RB and Stoops, WL: Cervical myelopathy with fasciculations in the lower extremities. J Neurosurg 20:948-952, 1963.
1376. King, WA, Black, KL, Ikezaki, K, et al: Tumor-associated neurological dysfunction prevented by lazaroids in rats. J Neurosurg 74:112-115, 1991.
1377. Kinn, A-C and Lantz, B: Vitamin B_{12} deficiency after irradiation for bladder carcinoma. J Urol 131:888-890, 1984.
1378. Kinsella, TJ, Sindelar, WF, DeLuca, AM, et al: Tolerance of peripheral nerve to intraoperative radiotherapy (IORT): Clinical and experimental studies. Int J Radiat Oncol Biol Phys 11:1579-1585, 1985.
1379. Kinsella, TJ, Weichselbaum, RR, and Sheline, GE: Radiation injury of cranial and peripheral nerves. In Gilbert, HA and Kagan, AR (eds): Radiation Damage to the Nervous System: A Delayed Therapeutic Hazard. Raven Press, New York, 1980, pp 145-153.
1380. Kinyoun, JL, Kalina, RE, Brower, SA, et al: Radiation retinopathy after orbital irradiation for Graves' ophthalmopathy. Arch Ophthalmol 102: 1473-1476, 1984.
1381. Kissel, JT, Halterman, RK, Rammohan, KW, et al: The relationship of complement-mediated microvasculopathy to the histologic features and clinical duration of disease in dermatomyositis. Arch Neurol 48:26-30, 1991.
1382. Kjellberg, RN, Shintani, A, Frantz, AG, et al: Proton-beam therapy in acromegaly. N Engl J Med 278:689-695, 1968.
1383. Klassen, AC, Loewenson, RB, and Resch, JA: Cerebral atherosclerosis in selected chronic disease states. Atherosclerosis 18:321-336, 1973.
1384. Klee, GG, Tallman, RD, Goellner, JR, et al: Elevation of carcinoembryonic antigen in cerebrospinal fluid among patients with meningeal carcinomatosis. Mayo Clin Proc 61:9-13, 1986.
1385. Klein, P, Haley, EC, Wooten, GF, et al: Focal cerebral infarctions associated with perivascular tumor infiltrates in carcinomatous leptomeningeal metastases. Arch Neurol 46:1149-1152, 1989.
1386. Klein, SL, Sanford, RA, and Muhlbauer, MS: Pediatric spinal epidural metastases. J Neurosurg 74:70-75, 1991.
1387. Kleinberg, L, Wallner, K, and Malkin, MG: Good performance status of long-term disease-free survivors of intracranial gliomas. Int J Radiat Oncol Biol Phys 26:129-133, 1993.
1388. Kleinschmidt-DeMasters, BK and Geier, JM: Pathology of high-dose intra-arterial BCNU. Surg Neurol 31:435-443, 1989.
1389. Kleinschmidt-DeMasters, BK and Yeh, M: "Locked-in syndrome" after intrathecal cytosine arabinoside therapy for malignant immunoblastic lymphoma. Cancer 70:2504-2507, 1992.
1390. Kleisbauer, JP, Vesco, D, Orehek, J, et al: Treatment of brain metastases of lung cancer with high doses of etoposide (VP16-213). Cooperative study from the Groupe Francais Pneumo-Cancerologie. Eur J Cancer Clin Oncol 24:131-135, 1988.
1391. Kline, DG, Kott, J, Barnes, G, et al: Exploration of selected brachial plexus lesions by the posterior subscapular approach. J Neurosurg 49:872-880, 1978.
1392. Kline, LB, Garcia, JH, and Harsh, GR, III: Lym-

phomatous optic neuropathy. Arch Ophthalmol 102:1655-1657, 1984.
1393. Klingele, TG, Gado, MH, Burde, RM, et al: Compression of the anterior visual system by the gyrus rectus. Case report. J Neurosurg 55:272-275, 1981.
1394. Klingon, GH: The Guillain-Barré syndrome associated with cancer. Cancer 18:157-163, 1965.
1395. Knerich, R, Robustelli Della Cuna, G, Butti, G, et al: Chemotherapy plus immunotherapy for patients with primary and metastatic brain tumors. J Neurosurg Sci 29:19-24, 1985.
1396. Knight, RS, Anslow, P, and Theaker, JM: Neoplastic angioendotheliosis: A case of subacute dementia with unusual cerebral CT appearances and a review of the literature. J Neurol Neurosurg Psychiatry 50:1022-1028, 1987.
1397. Kochi, M, Kuratsu, J, Mihara, Y, et al: Neurotoxicity and pharmacokinetics of intrathecal perfusion of ACNU in dogs. Cancer Res 50:3119-3123, 1990.
1397a. Kochi, M, Takaki, S, Kuratsu, J-I, et al: Neurotoxicity and pharmacokinetics of ventriculolumbar perfusion of methyl-6[3-(2-chloroethyl)-3-nitrosoureido]-6-deoxy-alpha-D-glucopyranoside (MCNU) in dogs. J Neurooncol 19:239-244, 1994.
1398. Koedel, U, Pfister, H-W, and Tomasz, A: Methylprednisolone attenuates inflammation, increase of brain water content and intracranial pressure, but does not influence cerebral blood flow changes in experimental pneumococcal meningitis. Brain Res 644:25-31, 1994.
1399. Koehler, PJ and Endtz, LJ: The Brown-Séquard syndrome. True or false? Arch Neurol 43:921-924, 1986.
1400. Koehler, PJ and Wijngaard, PR: Brown-Séquard syndrome due to spinal cord infarction after subclavian vein catheterisation. Letter to the Editor. Lancet 2:914-915, 1986.
1401. Kofman, S, Garvin, JS, Nagamani, D, et al: Treatment of cerebral metastases from breast carcinoma with prednisolone. JAMA 163:1473-1476, 1957.
1401a. Kohsyu, H, Aoyagi, M, Tojima, H, et al: Facial nerve enhancement in Gd-MRI in patients with Bell's palsy. Acta Otolaryngol 511:165-169, 1994.
1402. Kokkoris, CP: Leptomeningeal carcinomatosis. How does cancer reach the pia-arachnoid? Cancer 51:154-160, 1983.
1403. Komaki, R, Roh, J, Cox, JD, et al: Superior sulcus tumors: Results of irradiation of 36 patients. Cancer 48:1563-1568, 1981.
1404. Komarnicky, LT, Phillips, TL, Martz, K, et al: A randomized phase III protocol for the evaluation of misonidazole combined with radiation in the treatment of patients with brain metastases (RTOG-7916). Int J Radiat Oncol Biol Phys 20:53-58, 1991.
1405. Komori, S, Ludwig, J, Okazaki, H, et al: Reye's syndrome in Olmsted County, Minnesota: Did it exist before 1963? Mayo Clin Proc 67:871-875, 1992.
1406. Kondo, A, Inoue, T, Nagara, H, et al: Neurotoxicity of Adriamycin passed through the transiently disrupted blood-brain barrier by mannitol in the rat brain. Brain Res 412:73-83, 1987.
1407. Kondziolka, D, Bernstein, M, Resch, L, et al: Significance of hemorrhage into brain tumors: Clinicopathological study. J Neurosurg 67:852-857, 1987.
1408. Konefal, JB, Emami, B, and Pilipech, MV: Analysis of dose fractionation in the palliation of metastases from malignant melanoma. Cancer 61:243-246, 1988.
1409. Konotey-Ahulu, FI: Mental-nerve neuropathy: A complication of sickle-cell crisis. Letter to the Editor. Lancet 2:388, 1972.
1410. Kooistra, KL, Rodriguez, M, and Powis, G: Toxicity of intrathecally administered cytotoxic drugs and their antitumor activity against an intrathecal Walker 256 carciosarcoma model for meningeal carcinomatosis in the rat. Cancer Res 499:977-982, 1989.
1411. Kopelson, G, Parkinson, D, and Rudders, RA: Long-term survivors with leptomeningeal tumor involvement. Letter to the Editor. Int J Radiat Oncol Biol Phys 9:119-120, 1983.
1412. Kori, SH, Foley, KM, and Posner, JB: Brachial plexus lesions in patients with cancer: 100 cases. Neurology 31:45-50, 1981.
1413. Kornblau, SM, Cortes-Franco, J, and Estey, E: Neurotoxicity associated with fludarabine and cytosine arabinoside chemotherapy for acute leukemia and myelodysplasia. Leukemia 7:378-383, 1993.
1414. Koscielny, S, Tubiana, M, Le, MG, et al: Breast cancer: Relationship between the size of the primary tumour and the probability of metastatic dissemination. Br J Cancer 49:709-715, 1984.
1415. Kotagal, S, Shuter, E, and Horenstein, S: Chorea as a manifestation of bilateral subdural hematoma in an elderly man. Clinical note. Arch Neurol 38:195, 1981.
1416. Kraft, A, Zvibel, I, Doerr, R, et al: Matrix influences organ-site specificity of metastases by regulating production and response to autocrine growth factors. Contributions to Oncology 44:203-223, 1992.
1417. Kramer, ED, Rafto, S, Packer, RJ, et al: Comparison of myelography with CT follow-up versus gadolinium MRI for subarachnoid metastatic disease in children. Neurology 41:46-50, 1991.
1418. Kramer, JH, Norman, D, Brant-Zawadzki, B, et al: Absence of white matter changes on magnetic resonance imaging in children treated with CNS prophylaxis therapy for leukemia. Cancer 61:928-930, 1988.
1419. Kramer, RE, Luders, H, Lesser, RP, et al: Transient focal abnormalities of neuroimaging studies during focal status epilepticus. Epilepsia 28(5):528-532, 1987.
1420. Kranz, BR, Thierfelder, S, Gerl, A, et al: Cerebrospinal fluid immunocytology in primary central nervous system lymphoma. Letter to the Editor. Lancet 340:727, 1992.
1421. Krasna, MJ, Flancbaum, L, Cody, RP, et al: Vascular and neural invasion in colorectal carcinoma. Incidence and prognostic significance. Cancer 61:1018-1023, 1988.
1422. Krauth, D, Holden, A, Knapic, N, et al: Safety and efficacy of long-term oral anticoagulation in cancer patients. Cancer 59:983-985, 1987.

1423. Krendel, DA, Albright, RE, and Graham, DG: Infiltrative polyneuropathy due to acute monoblastic leukemia in hematologic remission. Neurology 37:474-477, 1987.
1424. Kretschmar, CS, Warren, MP, Lavally, BL, et al: Ototoxicity of preradiation cisplatin for children with central nervous system tumors. J Clin Oncol 8:1191-1198, 1990.
1425. Kristensen, CA, Kristjansen, PE, and Hansen, HH: Systemic chemotherapy of brain metastases from small-cell lung cancer: A review. J Clin Oncol 10:1498-1502, 1992.
1426. Kristensen, O, Melgard, B, and Schiodt, AV: Radiation myelopathy of the lumbo-sacral spinal cord. Acta Neurol Scand 56:217-222, 1977.
1427. Krol, G, Galicich, J, Arbit, E, et al: Preoperative localization of intracranial lesions on MR. AJNR 9:513-516, 1988.
1428. Krol, G, Heier, L, Becker, R, et al: MRI and myelography in the evaluation of epidural extension of primary and metastatic tumors. In Valk, J (ed): Neuroradiology 1985/1986. Proceedings of the XIIIth Congress of the European Society of Neuroradiology, Amsterdam, 11-15 September 1985. Elsevier, New York, 1986, pp 91-97.
1429. Krol, G, Sze, G, Malkin, M, et al: MR of cranial and spinal meningeal carcinomatosis: Comparison with CT and myelography. AJR 151:583-588, 1988.
1430. Krol, TC and O'Keefe, P: Brachial plexus neuritis and fatal hemorrhage following *Aspergillus* infection of a Hickman catheter. Cancer 50:1214-1217, 1982.
1431. Kroner, K, Krebs, B, Skov, J, et al: Immediate and long-term phantom breast syndrome after mastectomy: Incidence, clinical characteristics and relationship to pre-mastectomy breast pain. Pain 36:327-334, 1989.
1432. Kuberski, T: Eosinophils in the cerebrospinal fluid. Ann Intern Med 91:70-75, 1979.
1433. Kucharczyk, J, Fraser, CL, and Arieff, AI: Central nervous system manifestations of hyponatremia. In Arieff, AI and Griggs, RC (eds): Metabolic Brain Dysfunction in Systemic Disorders. Little, Brown & Company, Boston, 1992, pp 55-86.
1434. Kucuk, O, Kwaan, HC, Gunnar, W, et al: Thromboembolic complications associated with L-asparaginase therapy. Etiologic role of antithrombin III and plasminogen levels and therapeutic correction by fresh frozen plasma. Cancer 55:702-706, 1985.
1435. Kucuk, O, Noskin, G, Petersen, K, et al: Lower extremity vasospasm associated with ischemic neuropathy, dermal fibrosis, and digital gangrene in a patient with carcinoid syndrome. Cancer 62:1026-1029, 1988.
1436. Kumar, PP, Good, RR, Jones, EO, et al: Spine-sparing postmastectomy irradiation. Radiat Med 6:17-22, 1988.
1437. Kumar, PP, Good, RR, Leibrock, LG, et al: High activity iodine 125 endocurietherapy for recurrent skull base tumors. Cancer 61:1518-1527, 1988.
1438. Kunkler, RB and Cooksey, G: Carcinoma of the prostate presenting with a cerebral metastasis. Br J Urol 71:103-104, 1993.
1439. Kupersmith, MJ, Frohman, LP, Choi, IS, et al: Visual system toxicity following intra-arterial chemotherapy. Neurology 38:284-289, 1988.
1440. Kupfer, A, Aeschlimann, C, Wermuth, B, et al: Prophylaxis and reversal of ifosfamide encephalopathy with methylene-blue. Lancet 343:763-764, 1994.
1441. Kupfer, Y, Namba, T, Kaldawi, E, et al: Prolonged weakness after long-term infusion of vecuronium bromide. Ann Intern Med 117:484-486, 1992.
1442. Kuzel, T, Esparaz, B, Green, D, et al: Thrombogenicity of intravenous 5-fluorouracil alone or in combination with cisplatin. Cancer 65:885-889, 1990.
1443. Kuzuhara, S, Ohkoshi N, Kanemaru, K, et al: Subacute leucoencephalopathy induced by carmofur, a 5-fluorouracil derivative. J Neurol 234:365-370, 1987.
1444. Kyritsis, AP, Williams, EC, and Schutta, HS: Cerebral venous thrombosis due to heparin-induced thrombocytopenia. Stroke 21:1503-1505, 1990.
1445. La Mantia, L, Salmaggi, A, Tajoli, L, et al: Cryptococcal meningioencephalitis: Intrathecal immunological response. J Neurol 233:362-366, 1986.
1446. La Montagna, G, Manzo, C, Califano, E, et al: Absence of elevated creatine kinase in dermatomyositis does not exclude malignancy. Letter to the Editor. Scand J Rheumatol 17:73-74, 1988.
1447. La Rocca, RV, Meer, J, Gilliatt, RW, et al: Suramin-induced polyneuropathy. Neurology 40:954-960, 1990.
1448. Labadie, EL and Hamilton, RH: Survival improvement in coccidioidal meningitis by high-dose intrathecal amphotericin B. Arch Intern Med 146:2013-2018, 1986.
1449. Labadie, EL, Hamilton, RH, Lundell, DC, et al: Hypoliquorreic headache and pneumocephalus caused by thoraco-subarachnoid fistula. Neurology 27:993-995, 1977.
1450. Lachance, DH, O'Neill, BP, Harper, CM, Jr, et al: Paraneoplastic brachial plexopathy in a patient with Hodgkin's disease. Mayo Clin Proc 66:97-101, 1991.
1451. Lachance, DH, O'Neill, BP, Macdonald, DR, et al: Primary leptomeningeal lymphoma: Report of 9 cases, diagnosis with immunocytochemical analysis and review of the literature. Neurology 41:95-100, 1991.
1452. Lachmann, EA, Rook, JL, Tunkel, R, et al: Complications associated with intermittent pneumatic compression. Arch Phys Med Rehabil 73:482-485, 1992.
1453. Lackner, TE: Interaction of dexamethasone with phenytoin. Pharmacotherapy 11:344-347, 1991.
1454. Lacomis, D, Khosbin, S, and Schich, RM: MR imaging of paraneoplastic limbic encephalitis. J Comput Assist Tomogr 14:115-117, 1990.
1455. Lacomis, D, Smith, TW, and Chad, DA: Acute myopathy and neuropathy in status asthmaticus: Case report and literature review. Muscle Nerve 16:84-90, 1993.
1456. Lahr, MB: Hyponatremia during carbamazepine therapy. Clin Pharmacol Ther 37:693-696, 1985.
1457. Lakhanpal, S, Bunch, TW, Ilstrup, DM, et al: Polymyositis-dermatomyositis and malignant le-

sions: Does an association exist? Mayo Clin Proc 61:645-653, 1986.

1458. Lam, KS, Ho, JHC, Lee, AW, et al: Symptomatic hypothalamic-pituitary dysfunction in nasopharyngeal carcinoma patients following radiation therapy: A retrospective study. Int J Radiat Oncol Biol Phys 13:1343-1350, 1987.

1459. Lam, KS, Tse, VK, Wang, C, et al: Effects of cranial irradiation on hypothalamic-pituitary function—A 5-year longitudinal study in patients with nasopharyngeal carcinoma. Q J Med 286:165-176, 1991.

1460. Lambert, EH and Rooke, ED: Myasthenic state and lung cancer. In Brain, L and Norris, FH, Jr (eds): The Remote Effects of Cancer on the Nervous System. Grune & Stratton, New York, 1965, pp 67-80.

1461. Lampert, P, Tom, MI, and Rider, WD: Disseminated demyelination of the brain following Co^{60} (gamma) radiation. Arch Pathol 68:322-330, 1959.

1462. Lampert, PW and Davis, RL: Delayed effects of radiation on the human central nervous system: "Early" and "late" delayed reactions. Neurology 14:912-917, 1964.

1463. Lampl, Y, Paniri, Y, Eshel, Y, et al: Alkaline phosphatase level in CSF in various brain tumors and pulmonary carcinomatous meningitis. J Neurooncol 9:35-40, 1990.

1464. Lamy, C, Mas, JL, Varet, B, et al: Postradiation lower motor neuron syndrome presenting as monomelic amyotrophy. J Neurol Neurosurg Psychiatry 64:648-649, 1991.

1465. Lance, JW and Anthony, M: Neck-tongue syndrome in sudden turning of the head. J Neurol Neurosurg Psychiatry 43:97-101, 1980.

1466. Lane, RJ and Mastaglia, FL: Drug-induced myopathies in man. Lancet 2:562-566, 1978.

1467. Lang, B, Newsom-Davis, J, and Wray, D: Autoimmune aetiology for myasthenic (Eaton-Lambert) syndrome. Lancet 1:224-226, 1981.

1468. Lange, OF, Scheef, W, and Haase, KD: Palliative radio-chemotherapy with ifosfamide and BCNU for breast cancer patients with cerebral metastases. A 5-year experience. Cancer Chemother Pharmacol 26(Suppl):S78-S80, 1990.

1469. Langston, JW, Dorfman, LJ, and Forno, LS: "Encephalomyeloneuritis" in the absence of cancer. Neurology 25:633-637, 1975.

1470. Lanser, JB, van Seters, AP, Moolenaar, AJ, et al: Neuropsychologic and neurologic side effects of mitotane and reversibility of symptoms. Letter to the Editor. J Clin Oncol 10:1504, 1992.

1471. Lantos, G: Cortical blindness due to osmotic disruption of the blood–brain barrier by angiographic contrast material: CT and MRI studies. Neurology 39:567-571, 1989.

1472. Larson, SJ, Sances, A, Jr, Baker, JB, et al: Herniated cerebellar tonsils and cough syncope. J Neurosurg 40:524-528, 1974.

1473. Larson, SM, Schall, GL, and Di Chiro, G: The influence of previous lumbar puncture and pneumoencephalography on the incidence of unsuccessful radioisotope cisternography. J Nucl Med 12:555-557, 1971.

1474. Lashford, LS, Davies, AG, Richardson, RB, et al: A pilot study of 131I monoclonal antibodies in the therapy of leptomeningeal tumors. Cancer 61:857-868, 1988.

1475. Latchaw, RE, Gabrielsen, TO, and Seeger, JF: Cerebral angiography in meningeal sarcomatosis and carcinomatosis. Neuroradiology 8:131-139, 1974.

1476. Latini, P, Maranzano, E, Ricci, S, et al: Role of radiotherapy in metastatic spinal cord compression: Preliminary results from a prospective trial. Radiother Oncol 15:227-233, 1989.

1477. Latov, N: Neuropathy and anti-GM1 antibodies. Ann Neurol 27(Suppl):S41-S43, 1990.

1478. Lauer, SJ, Kirchner, PA, and Camitta, BM: Identification of leukemic cells in the cerebrospinal fluid from children with acute lymphoblastic leukemia: Advances and dilemmas. Am J Pediatr Hematol Oncol 11(1):64-73, 1989.

1479. Laukkanen, E, Klonoff, H, Allan, B, et al: The role of prophylactic brain irradiation in limited stage small cell lung cancer: Clinical, neuropsychologic, and CT sequelae. Int J Radiat Oncol Biol Phys 14:1109-1117, 1988.

1480. Launay, M, Fredy, D, Merland, JJ, et al: Narrowing and occlusion of arteries by intracranial tumors. Review of the literature and report of 25 cases. Neuroradiology 14:117-126, 1977.

1481. Lavenstein, BL and Cantor, FK: Acute dystonia. An unusual reaction to diphenhydramine. JAMA 236:291, 1976.

1482. LaVenuta, F and Moore, JA: Involvement of the inner ear in acute stem cell leukemia. Report of two cases. Ann Otol Rhinol Laryngol 81:132-137, 1972.

1483. Lavey, RS, Johnstone, AK, Taylor, JM, et al: The effect of hyperfractionation on spinal cord response to radiation. Int J Radiat Oncol Biol Phys 24:681-686, 1992.

1484. Lawson, LA, Blouin, RA, Smith, RB, et al: Phenytoin-dexamethasone interaction: A previously unreported observation. Surg Neurol 16:23-24, 1981.

1485. Le Chevalier, T, Smith, FP, Caille, P, et al: Sites of primary malignancies in patients presenting with cerebral metastases: A review of 120 cases. Cancer 56:880-882, 1985.

1486. Le Quesne, PM, Fowler, CJ, and Harding, AE: A study of the effects of isaxonine on vincristine-induced peripheral neuropathy in man and regeneration following peripheral nerve crush in the rat. J Neurol Neurosurg Psychiatry 48:933-935, 1985.

1487. Leach, W: Irradiation of the ear. J Laryngol Otol 79:870-880, 1965.

1488. Lebeau, B, Chastang, C, Muir, JF, et al: No effect of an antiaggregant treatment with aspirin in small cell lung cancer treated with CCAVP16 chemotherapy. Results from a randomized clinical trial of 303 patients. Cancer 71:1741-1745, 1993.

1489. Lebeau, B, Chastang, CI, Brechot, JM, et al: Subcutaneous heparin treatment increases complete response rate and overall survival in small cell lung cancer. Abstract. Lung Cancer 7(Suppl):129, 1991.

1490. LeBerthon, B, Khawli, LA, Alauddin, M, et al: Enhanced tumor uptake of macromolecules induced by a novel vasoactive interleukin 2 immunoconjugate. Cancer Res 51:2694-2698, 1991.

1491. Leblanc, RA: Metastasis of bronchogenic carcinoma to acoustic neurinoma. J Neurosurg 41:614-617, 1974.

1492. Lecky, BR, Murray, NM, and Berry, RJ: Transient radiation myelopathy: Spinal somatosensory evoked responses following incidental cord exposure during radiotherapy. J Neurol Neurosurg Psychiatry 43:747-750, 1980.

1493. Lederman, RJ, Bukowski, RM, and Nickerson, P: Carcinoid myopathy. Cleve Clin J Med 54:299-303, 1987.

1494. Lederman, RJ and Wilbourn, AJ: Brachial plexopathy: Recurrent cancer or radiation? Neurology 34:1331-1335, 1984.

1495. Lee, AW, Ng, SH, Ho, JH, et al: Clinical diagnosis of late temporal lobe necrosis following radiation therapy for nasopharyngeal carcinoma. Cancer 61:1535-1542, 1988.

1496. Lee, BI, Lee, BC, Hwang, YM, et al: Prolonged ictal amnesia with transient focal abnormalities on magnetic resonance imaging. Epilepsia 33:1042-1046, 1992.

1497. Lee, J-P, and Lee, S-T: Hepatocellular carcinoma presenting as intracranial metastasis. Surg Neurol 30:316-320, 1988.

1498. Lee, JS, Murphy, WK, Glisson, BS, et al: Primary chemotherapy of brain metastasis in small-cell lung cancer. J Clin Oncol 7:916-922, 1989.

1499. Lee, JS, Umsawasdi, T, Barkley, HT, Jr, et al: Timing of elective brain irradiation: A critical factor for brain metastasis-free survival in small cell lung cancer. Int J Radiat Oncol Biol Phys 13:697-704, 1987.

1500. Lee, JS, Umsawasdi, T, Dhingra, HM, et al: Effects of brain irradiation and chemotherapy on myelosuppression in small-cell lung cancer. J Clin Oncol 4:1615-1619, 1986.

1501. Lee, JS, Unsawasdi, T, Lee, Y-Y, et al: Neurotoxicity in long-term survivors of small cell lung cancer. Int J Radiat Oncol Biol Phys 12:313-321, 1986.

1502. Lee, PW, Hung, BK, Woo, EK, et al: Effects of radiation therapy on neuropsychological functioning in patients with nasopharyngeal carcinoma. J Neurol Neurosurg Psychiatry 52:488-492, 1989.

1503. Lee, RJ, Bartzokis, T, Yeoh, T-K, et al: Enhanced detection of intracardiac sources of cerebral emboli by transesophageal echocardiography. Stroke 22:734-739, 1991.

1504. Lee, SH: Cancer cell estrogen receptor of human mammary carcinoma. Cancer 44:1-12, 1979.

1505. Lee, Y-T: Breast carcinoma: Pattern of metastasis at autopsy. J Surg Oncol 23:175-180, 1983.

1506. Lee, Y-Y, Glass, JP, Geoffray, A, et al: Cranial computed tomographic abnormalities in leptomeningeal metastasis. AJR 143:1035-1039, 1984.

1507. Lee, YY, Glass, JP, and Wallace, S: Myelography in cancer patients: Modified technique. AJR 145: 791-795, 1985.

1508. Leenders, KL, Beaney, RP, Brooks, DJ, et al: Dexamethasone treatment of brain tumor patients: Effects on regional cerebral blood flow, blood volume and oxygen utilization. Neurology 35:1610-1616, 1985.

1509. Leff, RS, Thompson, JM, Daly, MB, et al: Acute neurologic dysfunction after high-dose etoposide therapy for malignant glioma. Cancer 62:32-35, 1988.

1510. Legha, SS, Brodey, GP, Keating, MJ, et al: Early clinical evaluation of acridinylaminomethanesulfon-*m*-anisidide (AMSA) in patients with advanced breast cancer and acute leukemia. Abstract No. C-518. Proceedings American Association for Cancer Research 20:416, 1979.

1511. Lehmann, J: Tryptophan deficiency stupor—A new psychiatric syndrome. Acta Psychiatr Scand 300(Suppl):1-57, 1982.

1512. Lehne, G and Lote, K: Pulmonary toxicity of cytotoxic and immunosuppressive agents. A review. Acta Oncol 29:113-124, 1990.

1513. Lehrer, RI, Ganz, T, Selsted, ME, et al: Neutrophils and host defense [clinical conference]. Ann Intern Med 109:127-142, 1988.

1514. Lehrer, S, Levine, E, and Bloomer, WD: Abnormally diminished sense of smell in women with oestrogen receptor positive breast cancer. Letter to the Editor. Lancet 2:333, 1985.

1515. Leibel, SA and Fuks, Z: Is local failure a cause of or a marker for metastatic dissemination in carcinoma of the uterine cervix? Int J Radiat Oncol Biol Phys 24:377-380, 1992.

1516. Leibel, SA, Gutin, PH, Sneed, PK, et al: Interstitial irradiation for the treatment of primary and metastatic brain tumors. In DeVita, VT, Jr, Hellman, S, and Rosenberg, SA (eds): Cancer. Principles & Practice of Oncology, vol 3. JB Lippincott, Philadelphia, 1989, pp 1-11.

1517. Leibel, SA, Ling, CC, Kutcher, GJ et al: The biological basis for conformal three-dimensional radiation therapy. Int J Radiat Oncol Biol Phys 21:805-811, 1991.

1518. Leibel, SA, Scott, CB, and Loeffler, JS: Contemporary approaches to the treatment of malignant gliomas with radiation therapy. Semin Oncol 21:198-219, 1994.

1519. Leigh, RJ and Zee, DS: The Neurology of Eye Movements, ed 2. FA Davis, Philadelphia, 1991.

1520. Leikensohn, J, Milko, D, and Cotton, R: Carotid artery rupture. Management and prevention of delayed neurologic sequelae with low-dose heparin. Arch Otolaryngol 104:307-310, 1978.

1521. Leinung, MC, Young, WF, Jr, Whitaker, MD, et al: Diagnosis of corticotropin-producing bronchial carcinoid tumors causing Cushing's syndrome. Mayo Clin Proc 65:1314-1321, 1990.

1521a. Lekos, A, Katirji, BM, Cohen, ML, et al: Mononeuritis multiplex. A harbinger of acute leukemia in relapse. Arch Neurol 51:618-622, 1994.

1522. Lemann, W, Wiley, RG, and Posner, JB: Leukoencephalopathy complicating intraventricular catheters: Clinical, radiographic and pathologic study of 10 cases. J Neurooncol 6:67-74, 1988.

1522a. Lennon, VA: Paraneoplastic autoantibodies: The case for a descriptive generic nomenclature. Neurology 44:2236-2240, 1994.

1523. Lennon, VA, Sas, DF, Busk, MF, et al: Enteric neuronal autoantibodies in pseudoobstruction with small-cell lung carcinoma. Gastroenterology 100:137-142, 1991.

1524. Lentnek, A, Sande, MA, Whitley, RJ, et al: Evaluation of new anti-infective drugs for the treatment of cryptococcal meningitis. Infectious Diseases Society of America and the Food and Drug Administration. Clin Infect Dis 15(Suppl 1):S189-S194, 1992.

1525. Lenz, M and Freid, JR: Metastases to the skeleton, brain, spinal cord from cancer of the breast and the effect of radiotherapy. Ann Surg 93:278-293, 1931.
1526. Leonard, JV and Kay, JD: Acute encephalopathy and hyperammonaemia complicating treatment of acute lymphoblastic leukemia with asparaginase. Lancet 1:162-163, 1986.
1527. LeQuang, C: Postirradiation lesions of the brachial plexus. Results of surgical treatment. Hand Clin 5(1):23-32, 1989.
1528. Lerner, PI: Neurologic complications of infective endocarditis. Med Clin North Am 69:385-398, 1985.
1529. LeRoux, PD, Berger, MS, Elliott, JP, et al: Cerebral metastases from ovarian carcinoma. Cancer 67:2194-2199, 1991.
1530. Lessell, S, Lessell, IM, and Rizzo, JF, III: Ocular neuromyotonia after radiation therapy. Am J Ophthalmol 102:766-770, 1986.
1531. Lester, EP, Feld, E, Kinzie, JJ, et al: Necrotizing myelopathy complicating Hodgkin's disease. Arch Neurol 36:583-585, 1979.
1532. Levi, J and Wiernik, P: A comparative clinical trial of 5-azacytidine and guanazole in previously treated adults with acute nonlymphocytic leukemia. Cancer 38:36-41, 1976.
1533. Levi, M, ten Cate, H, van der Poll, T, et al: Pathogenesis of disseminated intravascular coagulation in sepsis. JAMA 270:975-979, 1993.
1534. Levin, B and Posner, JB: Swallow syncope: Report of a case and review of the literature. Neurology 22:1086-1093, 1972.
1535. Levin, JM, Schiff, D, Loeffler, JS, et al: Complications of therapy for venous thromboembolic disease in patients with brain tumors. Neurology 43:1111-1114, 1993.
1536. Levin, S, Nelson, KE, Spies, HW, et al: Pneumococcal meningitis: The problem of the unseen cerebrospinal fluid leak. Am J Med Sci 264:319-327, 1972.
1537. Levin, VA, Chamberlain, M, Silver, P, et al: Phase I/II study of intraventricular and intrathecal ACNU for leptomeningeal neoplasia. Cancer Chemother Pharmacol 23:301-307, 1989.
1538. Levin, VA, Edwards, MS, and Byrd, A: Quantitative observations of the acute effects of x-irradiation on brain capillary permeability: Part I. Int J Radiat Oncol Biol Phys 5:1627-1631, 1979.
1539. Levin, VA, Gutin, PH, and Leibel, S: Neoplasms of the central nervous system. In DeVita, VT, Jr, Hellman, S, and Rosenberg, SA (eds): Cancer, Principles & Practice of Oncology, ed 4. JB Lippincott, Philadelphia, 1993, pp 1679-1737.
1540. Levin, VA and Prados, MD: Treatment of recurrent gliomas and metastatic brain tumors with a polydrug protocol designed to combat nitrosourea resistance. J Clin Oncol 10:766-771, 1992.
1541. Levin, VA, Stearns, J, Byrd, A, et al: The effect of phenobarbital pretreatment on the antitumor activity of 1,3-Bis(2-chloroethyl)-l-nitrosourea (BCNU), 1-(2-chloroethyl)-3-(2,6-cyclohexyl-l-nitrosourea (CCNU) and 1-(2-chloroethyl)-3-dioxo-3-piperidyl-l-nitrosourea (PCNU), and on the plasma pharmacokinetics and biotransformation of BCNU. J Pharmacol Exp Ther 208:1-6, 1979.
1542. Levine, M, Jones, MW, and Sheppard, I: Differential effect of cimetidine on serum concentrations of carbamazepine and phenytoin. Neurology 35:562-565, 1985.
1543. Levine, MN, Gent, M, Hirsh, J, et al: The thrombogeneic effect of anticancer drug therapy in women with stage II breast cancer. N Engl J Med 318:404-407, 1988.
1544. Levitt, LP and Prager, D: Mononeuropathy due to vincristine toxicity. Neurology 25:894-895, 1975.
1545. Levitz, RE and Quintiliani, R: Trimethoprim-sulfamethoxazole for bacterial meningitis. Ann Intern Med 100:881-890, 1984.
1546. Levkoff, S, Cleary, P, Liptzin, B, et al: Epidemiology of delirium: An overview of research issues and findings. Int Psychogeriatr 3:149-167, 1991.
1547. Levkoff, S, Liptzin, B, Cleary, P, et al: Review of research instruments and techniques used to detect delirium. Int Psychogeriatr 3:253-271, 1991.
1548. Levkoff, SE, Evans, DA, Liptzin, B, et al: Delirium. The occurrence and persistence of symptoms among elderly hospitalized patients. Arch Intern Med 152:334-340, 1992.
1549. Levy, DE: Transient CNS deficits: A common, benign syndrome in young adults. Neurology 38:831-836, 1988.
1550. Levy, MH and Catalano, RB: Control of common physical symptoms other than pain in patients with terminal disease. Semin Oncol 12:411-430, 1985.
1551. Lewis, AJ:Sarcoma metastatic to the brain. Cancer 61:593-601, 1988.
1552. Lewis, DA: Unrecognized chronic lithium neurotoxic reactions. JAMA 250:2029-2030, 1983.
1553. Lewis, DA and Smith, RE: Steroid-induced psychiatric syndrome: A report of 14 cases and review of the literature. J Affective Disord 5:319-332, 1983.
1554. LeWitt, PA, Barton, NW, and Posner, JB: Hiccup with dexamethasone therapy. Letter to the Editor. Ann Neurol 12:405-406, 1982.
1555. Leys, K, Lang, B, Johnston, I, et al: Calcium channel autoantibodies in the Lambert-Eaton myasthenic syndrome. Ann Neurol 29:307-314, 1991.
1556. Li, CY, Witzig, TE, Phyliky, RL, et al: Diagnosis of B-cell non-Hodgkin's lymphoma of the central nervous system by immunocytochemical analysis of cerebrospinal fluid lymphocytes. Cancer 57:737-744, 1986.
1557. Li, KC and Poon, PY: Sensitivity and specificity of MRI in detecting malignant spinal cord compression and in distinguishing malignant from benign compression fractures of vertebrae. Magn Reson Imaging 6:547-556, 1988.
1558. Li, MH and Holtas, S: MR imaging of spinal intramedullary tumors. Acta Radiol [Diagn] (Stockh) 32:505-513, 1991.
1559. Li, MH, Holtas, S, and Larsson, E-M: MR imaging of intradural extramedullary tumors. Acta Radiol [Diagn] (Stockh) 33:207-212, 1992.
1560. Li, MH, Holtas, S, and Larsson, E-M: MR imag-

ing of spinal lymphoma. Acta Radiol [Diagn] (Stockh) 33:338-342, 1992.

1561. Liang, D-C, Lin, JC-T, Shih, S-L, et al: Cranial computed tomography in children with acute lymphoblastic leukemia after prophylactic treatment with cranial radiation therapy and intrathecal methotrexate. Cancer 71:2105-2108, 1993.

1562. Libshitz, HI, Jing, B-S, Wallace, S, et al: Sterilized metastases: A diagnostic and therapeutic dilemma. AJR 140:15-19, 1983.

1563. Lichtenstein, PK, Heubi, JE, Daugherty, CC, et al: Grade I Reye's syndrome. A frequent cause of vomiting and liver dysfunction after varicella and upper-respiratory-tract infection. N Engl J Med 309:133-139, 1983.

1564. Lieberman, A, LeBrun, Y, Glass, P, et al: Use of high-dose corticosteroids in patients with inoperable brain tumors. J Neurol Neurosurg Psychiatry 40:678-682, 1977.

1565. Lieberman, A, Ruoff, M, Estey, E, et al: Irreversible pulmonary toxicity after single course of BCNU. Am J Med Sci 279:53-56, 1980.

1565a. Liedtke, W, Quabeck, K, Beelen, DW, et al: Recurrent acute inflammatory demyelinating polyradiculitis after allogeneic bone marrow transplantation. J Neurol Sci 125:110-111, 1994.

1566. Lien, EA, Wester, K, Lonning, PE, et al: Distribution of tamoxifen and metabolites into brain tissue and brain metastases in breast cancer patients. Br J Cancer 63:641-645, 1991.

1567. Lien, HH, Blomlie, V, Saeter, G, et al: Osteogenic sarcoma: MR signal abnormalities of the brain in asymptomatic patients treated with high-dose methotrexate. Radiology 179:547-550, 1991.

1568. Lim, V, Sobel, DF, and Zyroff, J: Spinal cord pial metastases: MR imaging with gadopentetate dimeglumine. AJNR 11:975-982, 1990.

1569. Limper, AH, Prakash, UB, Kokmen, E, et al: Cardiopulmonary metastatic lesions of osteosarcoma and associated cerebral infarction. Mayo Clin Proc 63:592-595, 1988.

1570. Lindquist, L, Linne, T, Hansson, L-O, et al: Value of cerebrospinal fluid analysis in the differential diagnosis of meningitis: A study of 710 patients with suspected central nervous system infection. Eur J Clin Microbiol Infect Dis 7:374-380, 1988.

1571. Lindsley, H, Teller, D, Noonan, B, et al: Hyperviscosity syndrome in multiple myeloma. Am J Med 54:682-688, 1973.

1572. Linnemann, CC, Jr and Alvira, MM: Pathogenesis of varicella-zoster angiitis in the CNS. Arch Neurol 37:239-240, 1980.

1573. Liotta, LA: Tumor invasion and metastases. Advances in Oncology 4:3-11, 1988.

1574. Liotta, LA, Kleinerman, J, and Saidel, GM: Quantitative relationships of intravascular tumor cells, tumor vessels and pulmonary metastases following tumor implantation. Cancer Res 34:997-1004, 1974.

1575. Liotta, LA and Kohn, E: Cancer invasion and metastases [clinical conference]. JAMA 263:1123-1126, 1990.

1576. Liposwki, ZJ: Delirum: Acute Confusional States. Oxford University Press, New York, 1990.

1577. Lippman, SM, Buzaid, AC, Iacono, RP, et al: Cranial metastases from prostate cancer simulating meningioma: Report of two cases and review of the literature. Neurosurgery 19:820-823, 1986.

1578. Lipton, RB, Apfel, SC, Dutcher, JP, et al: Taxol produces a predominantly sensory neuropathy. Neurology 39:368-373, 1989.

1579. Lipton, RB, Galer, BS, Dutcher, JP, et al: Quantitative sensory testing demonstrates that subclinical sensory neuropathy is prevalent in patients with cancer. Arch Neurol 44:944-946, 1987.

1580. Lipton, RB, Galer, BS, Dutcher, JP, et al: Large and small fibre type sensory dysfunction in patients with cancer. J Neurol Neurosurg Psychiatry 54:706-709, 1991.

1581. Liptzin, B and Levkoff, SE: An empirical study of delirium subtypes. Br J Psychiatry 161:843-845, 1992.

1582. Liptzin, B, Levkoff, SE, Cleary, PD, et al: An empirical study of diagnostic criteria for delirium. Am J Psychiatry 148:454-457, 1991.

1583. Lisak, RP, Mitchell, M, Zweiman, B, et al: Guillain-Barré syndrome and Hodgkin's disease: Three cases with immunological studies. Ann Neurol 1:72-78, 1977.

1584. Lishner, M, Scheinbaum, R, and Messner, HA: Intrathecal vancomycin in the treatment of Ommaya reservoir infection by *Staphylococcus epidermidis*. Scand J Infect Dis 23:101-104, 1991.

1585. Liskow, A, Chang, CH, DeSanctis, P, et al: Epidural cord compression in association with genitourinary neoplasms. Cancer 58:949-954, 1986.

1586. Liss, RH and Chadwick, M: Correlation of 5-fluorouracil (NSC-19893) distribution in rodents with toxicity and chemotherapy in man. Cancer Chemother Biol Response Modif 58:777-786, 1974.

1587. List, AF and Kummet, TD: Spinal cord toxicity complicating treatment with cisplatin and etoposide. Am J Clin Oncol 13:256-258, 1990.

1588. Little, JR, Dale, AJ, and Okazaki, H: Meningeal carcinomatosis. Clinical manifestations. Arch Neurol 30:138-143, 1974.

1589. Littley, MD, Shalet, SM, and Beardwell, CG: Radiation and the hypothalamic-pituitary axis. In Gutin, PH, Leibel, SA, and Sheline, GE (eds): Radiation Injury to the Nervous System. Raven Press, New York, 1991, pp 303-324.

1590. Littman, P, Coccia, P, Bleyer, WA, et al: Central nervous system (CNS) prophylaxis in children with low risk acute lymphoblastic leukemia (ALL). Int J Radiat Oncol Biol Phys 13:1443-1449, 1987.

1591. Littman, P, Rosenstock, J, Gale, G, et al: The somnolence syndrome in leukemic children following reduced daily dose fractions of cranial radiation. Int J Radiat Oncol Biol Phys 10:1851-1853, 1984.

1591a. Liu, GT, Schatz, NJ, Curtin, VT, et al: Bilateral extraocular muscle metastases in Zollinger-Ellison syndrome. Arch Opththalmol 112:451-452, 1994.

1592. Livrea, P, Trojano, M, Simone, IL, et al: Acute changes in blood-CSF barrier permselectivity to serum proteins after intrathecal methotrexate and CNS irradiation. J Neurol 231:336-339, 1985.

1593. Lodrini, S and Savoiardo, M: Metastases of carcinoma to intracranial meningioma: Report of two cases and review of the literature. Cancer 48:2668-2673, 1981.

1594. Loeffler, JS and Alexander, E, III: The role of stereotactic radiosurgery in the management of intracranial tumors. Oncology (Huntingt) 4:21-41, 1990.

1595. Loeffler, JS, Kooy, HM, Wen, PY, et al: The treatment of recurrent brain metastases with stereotactic radiosurgery. J Clin Oncol 8:576-582, 1990.

1596. Loftus, CM, Biller, J, Hart, MN, et al: Management of radiation-induced accelerated carotid atherosclerosis. Arch Neurol 44:711-714, 1987.

1597. Loh, FL, Herskovitz, S, Berger, AR, et al: Brachial plexopathy associated with interleukin-2 therapy. Neurology 42:462-463, 1992.

1598. Lokich, JJ: The frequency and clinical biology of the ectopic hormone syndromes of small cell carcinoma. Cancer 50:2111-2114, 1982.

1599. Long, DM: Capillary ultrastructure in human metastatic brain tumors. J Neurosurg 51:53-58, 1979.

1600. Longeval, E, Hildebrand, J, and Vollont, GH: Early diagnosis of metastasis in the epidural space. Acta Neurochir (Wien) 31:177-184, 1975.

1601. Loprinzi, CL, Duffy, J, and Ingle, JN: Postchemotherapy rheumatism. J Clin Oncol 11:768-770, 1993.

1602. Lord, CF and Herndon, JH: Spinal cord compression secondary to kyphosis associated with radiation therapy for metastatic disease. Clin Orthop 210:120-127, 1986.

1603. Lossos, A and Siegal, T: Numb chin syndrome in cancer patients: Etiology, response to treatment, and prognostic significance. Neurology 42:1181-1184, 1992.

1604. Lossos, A and Siegal, T: Spinal subarachnoid hemorrhage associated with leptomeningeal metastases. J Neurooncol 12:167-171, 1992.

1604a. Lossos, A and Siegal, T: Thiamine (B_1) deficiency in cancer out-patients: Possible causes and neurological manifestations. J Neurooncol 21:73, 1994.

1605. Louis, DN, Hamilton, AJ, Sobel, RA, et al: Pseudopsammomatous meningioma with elevated serum carcinoembryonic antigen: A true secretory meningioma. J Neurosurg 74:129-132, 1991.

1606. Love, JG and Rivers, MH: Spinal cord tumors simulating protruded intervertebral disks. JAMA 179:878-881, 1962.

1607. Love, RR: Tamoxifen therapy in primary breast cancer: Biology, efficacy, and side effects. J Clin Oncol 7:803-815, 1989.

1608. Lowe, J and Russell, NH: Cerebral vasculitis associated with hairy cell leukemia. Cancer 60:3025-3028, 1987.

1609. Lowe, JT, Jr and Hudson, WR: Rhinocerebral phycomycosis and internal carotid artery thrombosis. Arch Otolaryngol 101:100-103, 1975.

1610. Lowe, SW, Schmitt, EM, Smith, SW, et al: p53 is required for radiation-induced apoptosis in mouse thymocytes. Nature 362:847-849, 1993.

1611. Lowry, SF and Moldawer, LL: Tumor necrosis factor and other cytokines in the pathogenesis of cancer cachexia. Principles and Practice of Oncology 4(8):1-12, 1990.

1612. Ludwig, H, Fruhwald, F, Tscholakoff, D, et al: Magnetic resonance imaging of the spine in multiple myeloma. Lancet 2:364-366, 1987.

1613. Ludwig, R, Calvo, W, Kober, B, et al: Effects of local irradiation and i.v. methotrexate on brain morphology in rabbits: Early changes. J Cancer Res Clin Oncol 113:235-240, 1987.

1614. Lukert, BP and Raisz, LG: Glucocorticoid-induced osteoporosis: Pathogenesis and management. Ann Intern Med 22:352-364, 1990.

1615. Lukes, SA, Posner, JB, Nielsen, S, et al: Bacterial infections of the CNS in neutropenic patients. Neurology 34:269-275, 1984.

1616. Lundberg, N: Continuous recording and control of ventricular fluid pressure in neurosurgical practice. Acta Psychiatr Neurol Scand 36(Suppl 149):1-193, 1960.

1617. Lundberg, N and West, KA: Leakage as a source of error in measurement of the cerebrospinal fluid pressure by lumbar puncture. Acta Neurol Scand Suppl 41:115-121, 1965.

1618. Lundberg, WB, Cadman, EC, and Skeel, RT: Leptomeningeal mycosis fungoides. Cancer 38:2149-2153, 1976.

1619. Luo, QL, Orcutt, JC, and Seifter, LS: Orbital mucormycosis with retinal and ciliary artery occlusions. Br J Ophthalmol 73:680-683, 1989.

1620. Luque, FA, Furneaux, HM, Ferziger, R, et al: Anti-Ri: An antibody associated with paraneoplastic opsoclonus and breast cancer. Ann Neurol 29:241-251, 1991.

1621. Luque, FA, Selhorst, JB, and Petruska, P: Parkinsonism induced by high-dose cytosine arabinoside. Mov Disord 2:219-222, 1987.

1622. Lustman, F, Flament-Durant, J, Colle, H, et al: Paraplegia due to epidural infiltration in a case of chronic lymphocytic leukemia. J Neurooncol 5:259-260, 1988.

1622a. Lutz, J and Coleman, MP: Trends in primary cerebral lymphoma. Br J Cancer 70:716-718, 1994.

1623. Luxton, G, Petrovich, Z, Jozsef, G, et al: Stereotactic radiosurgery: Principles and comparison of treatment methods. Neurosurgery 32(2):241-259, 1993.

1624. Luzzatto, G and Schafer, AI: The prethrombotic state in cancer. Semin Oncol 17:147-159, 1990.

1625. Lyding, JM, Tseng, A, Newman, A, et al: Intramedullary spinal cord metastasis in Hodgkin's disease. Rapid diagnosis and treatment resulting in neurologic recovery. Cancer 60:1741-1744, 1987.

1626. Lynch, HT, Droszcz, CP, Albano, WA, et al: "Organic brain syndrome" secondary to 5-fluorouracil toxicity. Dis Colon Rectum 24:130-131, 1981.

1627. Lyons, MK, O'Neill, BP, Marsh, WR, et al: Primary spinal epidural non-Hodgkin's lymphoma: Report of eight patients and review of the literature. Neurosurgery 30:675-680, 1992.

1628. Ma, SK, Chan, JC, and Wong, KF: Diagnosis of spinal extramedullary hemopoiesis by magnetic resonance imaging. Am J Med 95:111-112, 1993.

1629. Maat-Schieman, ML, Bots, GT, Thomeer, RT, et al: Malignant astrocytoma following radiotherapy for craniopharyngioma. Br J Radiol 58:480-482, 1985.

1630. Macchi, PJ, Grossman, RI, Gomori, JM, et al: High field MR imaging of cerebral venous thrombosis. J Comput Assist Tomogr 10:10-15, 1986.

1631. Macchiarini, P, Buonaguidi, R, Hardin, M, et al: Results and prognostic factors of surgery in the management of non-small cell lung cancer with solitary brain metastasis. Cancer 68:300-304, 1991.
1632. Macchiarini, P, Fontanini, G, Hardin, MJ, et al: Relation of neovascularisation to metastasis of non-small-cell lung cancer. Lancet 340:145-146, 1992.
1633. MacDonald, DR: Neurologic complications of chemotherapy. Neurol Clin 9:955-967, 1991.
1634. MacDonald, DR, Rottenberg, DA, Schutz, JS, et al: Radiation-induced optic neuropathy. In Rottenberg, DA (ed): Neurological Complications of Cancer Treatment. Butterworth-Heinemann, Boston, 1991, pp 37-61.
1635. MacDonald, DR, Strong, E, Nielsen, S, et al: Syncope from head and neck cancer. J Neurooncol 1:257-268, 1983.
1636. MacDonald, JS and Schnall, SF: The role of 5-FU plus levamisole in the therapy of colon cancer. Principles and Practice of Oncology 5(1):1-9, 1991.
1637. MacDonell, LA, Potter, PE, and Leslie, RA: Localized changes in blood–brain barrier permeability following the administration of antineoplastic drugs. Cancer Res 38:2930-2934, 1978.
1638. Machado, M, Sacman, M, Kaplan, RS, et al: Expanded role of the cerebrospinal fluid reservoir in neurooncology: Indications, causes of revision, and complications. Neurosurgery 17:600-603, 1985.
1639. Mack, EE and Gomez, EC: Neurotropic melanoma. A case report and review of the literature. J Neurooncol 13:165-171, 1992.
1640. Mack, EE and Wilson, CB: Meningiomas induced by high-dose cranial irradiation. J Neurosurg 79:28-31, 1993.
1641. Mackay-Sim, A: Changes in smell and taste function in thyroid, parathyroid, and adrenal diseases. In Getchell, TV, Bartoshuk, LM, Doty, RL, et al (eds): Smell and Taste in Health and Disease. Raven Press, New York, 1991, pp 817-827.
1642. MacKenzie, JR, LaBan, MM, and Sackeyfio, AH: The prevalence of peripheral neuropathy in patients with anorexia nervosa. Arch Phys Med Rehabil 70:827-830, 1989.
1643. Madajewicz, S, Chowhan, N, Iliya, A, et al: Intracarotid chemotherapy with etoposide and cisplatin for malignant brain tumors. Cancer 67:2844-2849, 1991.
1644. Madajewicz, S, West, CR, Park, HC, et al: Phase II study—Intra-arterial BCNU therapy for metastatic brain tumors. Cancer 47:653-657, 1981.
1645. Madow, L and Alpers, BJ: Encephalitic form of metastatic carcinoma. Archives of Neurology and Psychiatry 65:161-173, 1951.
1646. Magnaes, B: Body position and cerebrospinal fluid pressure. Part I: Clinical studies on the effect of rapid postural changes. J Neurosurg 44:687-697, 1976.
1647. Mahajan, SL, Ikeda, Y, Myers, TJ, et al: Acute acoustic nerve palsy associated with vincristine therapy. Cancer 47:2404-2406, 1981.
1648. Mahaley, MS, Jr, Mettlin, C, Natarajan, N, et al: National survey of patterns of care for brain-tumor patients. J Neurosurg 71:826-836, 1989.
1649. Mahaley, MS, Jr, Whaley, RA, Blue, M, et al: Central neurotoxicity following intracarotid BCNU chemotherapy for malignant gliomas. J Neurooncol 3:297-314, 1986.
1650. Mahmoud, HH, Rivera, GK, Hancock, ML, et al: Low leukocyte counts with blast cells in cerebrospinal fluid of children with newly diagnosed acute lymphoblastic leukemia. N Engl J Med 329:312-319, 1993.
1651. Mahoney, DH, Jr, Fernbach, DJ, Glaze, DG, et al: Elevated myelin basic protein levels in the cerebrospinal fluid of children with acute lymphoblastic leukemia. J Clin Oncol 2:58-61, 1984.
1652. Maiche, AG, Kajanti, MJ, and Pyrhonen, S: Simultaneous disseminated herpes zoster and bacterial infection in cancer patients. Letter to the Editor. Acta Oncol 31:681-683, 1992.
1653. Maiese, K, Walker, RW, Gargan, R, et al: Intra-arterial cisplatin–associated optic and otic toxicity. Arch Neurol 49:83-86, 1992.
1654. Maitland, CG, Scherokman, BJ, Schiffman, J, et al: Paraneoplastic tonic pupils. J Clin Neuro-ophthalmol 5:99-104, 1985.
1655. Majolino, I, Caponetto, A, Scime, R, et al: Wernicke-like encephalopathy after autologous bone marrow transplantation. Haematologica 75:282-284, 1990.
1656. Major, LF, Brown, GL, and Wilson, WP: Carcinoid and psychiatric symptoms. South Med J 66:787-790, 1973.
1657. Major, PP, Agarwal, RP, and Kufe, DW: Deoxycoformycin: Neurological toxicity. Cancer Chemother Pharmacol 5:193-196, 1981.
1658. Malamud, N: Psychiatric disorder with intracranial tumors of limbic system. Arch Neurol 17:113-123, 1967.
1659. Malamut, RI, Marques, W, England, JD, et al: Postsurgical idiopathic brachial neuritis. Muscle Nerve 17:320-324, 1994.
1660. Malapert, D, Brugieres, P, and Degos, JD: Motor neuron syndrome in the arms after radiation treatment. J Neurol Neurosurg Psychiatry 54:1123-1124, 1991.
1661. Malapert, D and Degos, JD: Painful legs and moving toes. Neuropathy caused by cytarabine. Rev Neurol (Paris) 145:869-871, 1989.
1662. Maldonado, JE, Kyle, RA, Ludwig, J, et al: Meningeal myeloma. Arch Intern Med 126:660-663, 1970.
1663. Malherbe, C, Burrill, K, Levin, SR, et al: Effect of diphenylhydantoin on insulin secretion in man. N Engl J Med 286:339-342, 1972.
1664. Malkin, MG and Posner, JB: Cerebrospinal fluid tumor markers for the diagnosis and management of leptomeningeal metastases. A Review. Eur J Cancer Clin Oncol 23(1):1-4, 1987.
1665. Mallat, Z, Vassal, T, Naouri, JF, et al: Aseptic meningoencephalitis after iopamidol myelography. Letter to the Editor. Lancet 338:252, 1991.
1666. Malow, BA and Dawson, DM: Neuralgic amyotrophy in association with radiation therapy for Hodgkin's disease. Neurology 41:440-441, 1991.
1667. Man, A and Brock, PG: Intrathecal mitozantrone. Letter to the Editor. Lancet 1:327, 1987.

1668. Mancall, EL and Rosales, RK: Necrotizing myelopathy associated with visceral carcinoma. Brain 87:639-656, 1964.
1669. Mancebo, J, Domingo, P, Blanch, L, et al: Postneurosurgical and spontaneous gram-negative bacillary meningitis in adults. Scand J Infect Dis 18:533-538, 1986.
1670. Manchul, LA, Jin, A, Pritchard, KI, et al: The frequency of malignant neoplasms in patients with polymyositis-dermatomyositis. A controlled study. Arch Intern Med 145:1835-1839, 1985.
1671. Mandell, LR, Walker, RW, Steinherz, P, et al: Reduced incidence of the somnolence syndrome in leukemic children with steroid coverage during prophylactic cranial radiation therapy. Results of a pilot study. Cancer 63:1975-1978, 1989.
1672. Mandler, RN, Kerrigan, DP, Smart, J, et al: Castleman's disease in POEMS syndrome with elevated interleukin-6. Cancer 69:2697-2703, 1992.
1673. Mandybur, TI: Intracranial hemorrhage caused by metastatic tumors. Neurology 27:650-655, 1977.
1674. Manishen, WJ, Sivananthan, K, and Orr, FW: Resorbing bone stimulates tumor cell growth. A role for the host microenvironment in bone metastasis. Am J Pathol 123:39-45, 1986.
1675. Mant, MJ, Fisk, RL, and Amy, RW: Case report: Chronic disseminated intravascular coagulation due to occult carcinoma. Am J Med Sci 274:69-74, 1977.
1676. Manz, HJ, Phillips, TM, and McCullough, DC: Herpes simplex type 2 encephalitis concurrent with known cerebral metastases. Acta Neuropathol (Berl) 47:237-240, 1979.
1677. Maor, MH, Frias, AE, and Oswald, MJ: Palliative radiotherapy for brain metastases in renal carcinoma. Cancer 62:1912-1917, 1988.
1678. Mapstone, TB, Rekate, HL, and Shurin, SB: Quadriplegia secondary to hematoma after lateral C-1, C-2 puncture in a leukemic child. Neurosurgery 12:230-231, 1983.
1679. Maranzano, E, Latini, P, Checcaglini, F, et al: Radiation therapy in metastatic spinal cord compression. A prospective analysis of 105 consecutive patients. Cancer 67:1311-1317, 1991.
1679a. Marcantonio, ER, Juarez, G, Goldman, L et al: The relationship of postoperative delirium with psychoactive medications. JAMA 272:1518-1522, 1994.
1680. Mareel, MM, Van Roy, FM, and De Baetselier, P: The invasive phenotypes. Cancer Metastasis Rev 9:45-62, 1990.
1681. Margileth, DA, Poplack, DG, Pizzo, PA, et al: Blindness during remission in two patients with acute lymphoblastic leukemia: A possible complication of multimodality therapy. Cancer 39:58-61, 1977.
1682. Marina, NM, Pratt, CB, Shema, SJ, et al: Brain metastases in osteosarcoma. Report of a long-term survivor and review of the St. Jude Children's Research Hospital experience. Cancer 71:3656-3660, 1993.
1683. Mark, RJ, Poen, J, Tran, LM, et al: Postirradiation sarcomas. A single-institution study and review of the literature. Cancer 73:2653-2662, 1994.
1684. Markesbery, WR, Brooks, WH, Gupta, GD, et al: Treatment for patients with cerebral metastases. Arch Neurol 35:754-756, 1978.
1685. Markham, M and Abeloff, MD: Small-cell lung cancer and limbic encephalitis. Letter to the Editor. Ann Intern Med 96:785, 1982.
1686. Markman, M, Sheidler, V, Ettinger, DS, et al: Antiemetic efficacy of dexamethasone. Randomized double-blind, crossover study with prochlorperazine in patients receiving cancer chemotherapy. N Engl J Med 311:549-552, 1984.
1687. Marks, JE and Wong, J: The risk of cerebral radionecrosis in relation to dose, time and fractionation: A follow-up study. Prog Exp Tumor Res 29:210-218, 1985.
1687a. Marmarou, A, Hochwald, G, Nakamura, T, et al: Brain edema resolution by CSF pathways and brain vasculature in cats. Am J Physiol Heart Circ Physiol 267:H514-H520, 1994.
1688. Marr, WG and Chambers, RG: Pseudotumor cerebri syndrome. Following unilateral radical neck dissection. Am J Ophthalmol 51:605-611, 1961.
1689. Marsano, L and McClain, C: How to manage both acute and chronic hepatic encephalopathy. Journal of Critical Illness 8:579-600, 1993.
1690. Marsh, WL, Jr, Bylund, DJ, Heath, VC, et al: Osteoarticular and pulmonary manifestations of acute leukemia. Case report and review of the literature. Cancer 57:385-390, 1986.
1691. Marshall, LF, King, J, and Langfitt, TW: The complications of high-dose corticosteroid therapy in neurosurgical patients: A prospective study. Ann Neurol 1:201-203, 1977.
1692. Marshall, PC, Brett, EM, and Wilson, J: Myoclonic encephalopathy of childhood (the dancing eye syndrome): A long-term follow-up study. Abstract. Neurology 28:348, 1978.
1693. Martin, DS, Benecke, J, and Maas, C: Metastatic tumor presenting as chronic otitis and facial paralysis. Ann Otol Rhinol Laryngol 101:280-281, 1992.
1694. Martin, R, Schwulera, U, Menke, G, et al: Interleukin-2 and blood brain barrier in cats: pharmacokinetics and tolerance following intrathecal and intravenous administration. Eur Cytokine Netw 3:399-406, 1992.
1695. Martin, RA, Handel, SF, and Aldama, AE: Inability to sneeze as a manifestation of medullary neoplasm. Neurology 41:1675-1676, 1991.
1696. Martin, WG, Brown, GC, Parrish, RK, et al: Ocular toxoplasmosis and visual field defects. Am J Ophthalmol 90:25-29, 1980.
1697. Martino, RL, Benson, AB, III, Merritt, JA, et al: Transient neurologic dysfunction following moderate-dose methotrexate for undifferentiated lymphoma. Cancer 54:2003-2005, 1984.
1698. Masdeu, JC, Breuer, AC, and Schoene, WC: Spinal subarachnoid hematomas: Clue to a source of bleeding in traumatic lumbar puncture. Neurology 29:872-876, 1979.
1699. Masi, AT and Hochberg, MC: Temporal association of polymyositis-dermatomyositis with malignancy: Methodologic and clinical considerations. Mt Sinai J Med 55:471-478, 1988.
1700. Masse, SR, Wolk, RW, and Conklin, RH: Peripituitary gland involvement in acute leukemia in adults. Arch Pathol 96:141-142, 1973.

1701. Massey, EW, Moore, J, and Schold, SC, Jr.: Mental neuropathy from systemic cancer. Neurology 31:1277-1281, 1981.
1702. Masur, H, Hood, E, III, and Armstrong, D: A trichomonas species in a mixed microbial meningitis. JAMA 236:1978-1979, 1976.
1703. Matsuda, M, Yoneda, S, Handa, H, et al: Cerebral hemodynamic changes during plateau waves in brain-tumor patients. J Neurosurg 50:483-488, 1979.
1704. Mattes, RD, Curran, WJ, Jr, Alavi, J, et al: Clinical implications of learned food aversions in patients with cancer treated with chemotherapy or radiation therapy. Cancer 70:192-200, 1992.
1705. Mattioli Belmonte, M, Gugliotta, L, Delvos, U, et al: A regimen for antithrombin III substitution in patients with acute lymphoblastic leukemia under treatment with L-asparaginase. Haematologica 76:209-214, 1991.
1706. Mattle, H, Sieb, JP, Rohner, M, et al: Nontraumatic spinal epidural and subdural hematomas. Neurology 37:1351-1356, 1987.
1707. Mattson, RH, Cramer, JA, Collins, JF, et al: Comparison of carbamazepine, phenobarbital, phenytoin, and primidone in partial and secondarily generalized tonic-clonic seizures. N Engl J Med 313:145-151, 1985.
1708. Maurice-Williams, RS: Mechanism of production of gait unsteadiness by tumours in the posterior fossa. J Neurol Neurosurg Psychiatry 38:143-148, 1975.
1709. Mauskop, A and Foley, KM: Control of Pain. In Harrington, KD (ed): Orthopaedic Management of Metastatic Bone Disease. CV Mosby, St Louis, 1988, pp 121-137.
1710. Mavligit, GM, Stuckey, SE, Cabanillas, FF, et al: Diagnosis of leukemia or lymphoma in the central nervous system by beta-2-microglobulin determination. N Engl J Med 303:718-722, 1980.
1711. Max, MB, Deck, MDF, and Rottenberg, DA: Pituitary metastasis: Incidence in cancer patients and clinical differentiation from pituitary adenoma. Neurology 31:998-1002, 1981.
1712. Maxon, HR: Radiation-induced thyroid disease. Med Clin North Am 69:1049-1061, 1985.
1713. Mayer, RJ, Berkowitz, RS, and Griffiths, CT: Central nervous system involvement by ovarian carcinoma: A complication of prolonged survival with metastatic disease. Cancer 41:776-783, 1978.
1714. Mayo, DR and Booss, J: Varicella zoster-associated neurologic disease without skin lesions. Arch Neurol 46:313-315, 1989.
1715. Mayr, NA, Yuh, WT, Muhonen, MG, et al: Pituitary metastases: MR findings. J Comput Assist Tomogr 17:432-437, 1993.
1716. Mazur, EM and Bertino, JR: Myeloblastoma and acute myelogenous leukemia: Presentation with a cervical neuropathy and complete response to chemotherapy. Cancer 49:637-639, 1982.
1717. McAlhany, HJ and Netsky, MG: Compression of the spinal cord by extramedullary neoplasms. A clinical and pathologic study. J Neuropathol Exp Neurol 14:276-287, 1955.
1718. McCartney, JR and Boland, R: Understanding and managing behavioral disturbances in the ICU. Journal of Critical Illness 8:87-97, 1993.
1719. McCracken, GH, Sande, MA, Lentnek, A, et al: Evaluation of new anti-infective drugs for the treatment of acute bacterial meningitis. Infectious Diseases Society of America and the Food and Drug Administration. Clin Infect Dis 15(Suppl 1):S182-S188, 1992.
1720. McCue, JD and Zandt, JR: Acute psychoses associated with the use of ciprofloxacin and trimethoprim-sulfamethoxazole. Am J Med 90:528-529, 1991.
1720a. McCutcheon, IE, Baranco, RA, Katz, DA, et al: Adoptive immunotherapy of intracerebral metastases in mice. J Neurosurg 72:102-109, 1994.
1721. McDonald, LW, Donovon, MP, Plantz, RG, et al: Radiosensitivity of the vestibular apparatus of the rabbit. Radiat Res 27:510-511, 1966.
1722. McEvoy, KM, Windebank, AJ, Daube, JR, et al: 3,4-Diaminopyridine in the treatment of the Lambert-Eaton myasthenic syndrome. N Engl J Med 321:1567-1571, 1989.
1723. McGehee, WG, Klotz, TA, Epstein, DJ, et al: Coumadin necrosis associated with hereditary protein C deficiency. Ann Intern Med 100:59-60, 1984.
1724. McGuire, SA, Gospe, SM, Jr, and Dahl, G: Acute vincristine neurotoxicity in the presence of hereditary motor and sensory neuropathy type I. Med Pediatr Oncol 17:520-523, 1989.
1725. McGuirt, WF, Feehs, RS, Strickland, JL, et al: Irradiation-induced atherosclerosis: A factor in therapeutic planning. Ann Otol Rhinol Laryngol 101:222-228, 1992.
1726. McIntosh, TK, Thomas, M, Smith, D, et al: The novel 21-aminosteroid U74006F attenuates cerebral edema and improves survival after brain injury in the rat. J Neurotrauma 9:33-46, 1992.
1727. McKee, LC, Jr and Collins, RD: Intravascular leukocyte thrombi and aggregates as a cause of morbidity and mortality in leukemia. Medicine (Baltimore) 53:463-478, 1974.
1728. McKenney, SA and Fehir, KM: Myelofibrosis following treatment with a nitrosourea for malignant glioma. Cancer 58:1426-1427, 1987.
1729. McKenzie, MR, Souhami, L, Podgorsak, EB, et al: Photon radiosurgery: A clinical review. Can J Neurol Sci 19:212-221, 1992.
1730. McKeown, CA, Swartz, M, Blom, J, et al: Tamoxifen retinopathy. Br J Ophthalmol 65:177-179, 1981.
1731. McLean, DR, Clink, HM, Enst, P, et al: Myelopathy after intrathecal chemotherapy. A case report with unique magnetic resonance imaging changes. Cancer 73:3037-3040, 1994.
1732. McLeod, JG: Peripheral neuropathy associated with lymphomas, leukemias, and polycythemia vera. In Dyck, PJ and Thomas, PK (eds): Peripheral Neuropathy, vol 2, ed 3. WB Saunders, Philadelphia, 1993, pp 1591-1598.
1733. McLeod, JG: Paraneoplastic neuropathies. In Dyck, PJ and Thomas, PK (eds): Peripheral Neuropathy, vol 2, ed 3. WB Saunders, Philadelphia, 1993, pp 1583-1590.
1734. McLeod, JG and Penny, R: Vincristine neuropathy: An electrophysiological and histological study. J Neurol Neurosurg Psychiatry 32:297-304, 1969.
1735. McLeod, JG and Pollard, JD: Peripheral neurop-

athy associated with paraproteinemia. In Vinken, PJ, Bruyn, GW, Klawans, HL, et al (eds): Neuropathies. Revised Series 7/Handbook of Clinical Neurology, vol 51. Elsevier Science Publishers, Amsterdam, 1987, pp 429-444.
1736. McMahon, MM, Farnell, MB, and Murray, MJ: Nutritional support of critically ill patients. Mayo Clin Proc 68:911-920, 1993.
1737. Mead, GM, Arnold, AM, Green, JA, et al: Epileptic seizures associated with cisplatin administration. Cancer Treat Rep 66:1719-1722, 1982.
1737a. Melki, PS, Halimi, P, Wibault, P, et al: MRI in chronic progressive radiation myelopathy. J Comput Assist Tomogr 18:1-6, 1994.
1738. Meessen, S, Riedel, RR, and Bruhl, P: Status epilepticus in MVEC chemotherapy of urothelial cancer. Urologe [A] 29:348-349, 1990.
1739. Mehta, BM, Glass, JP, and Shapiro, WR: Serum and cerebrospinal fluid distribution of 5-methyltetrahydrofolate after intravenous calcium leucovorin and intra-Ommaya methotrexate administration in patients with meningeal carcinomatosis. Cancer Res 43:435-438, 1983.
1740. Melgaard, B, Kohler, O, Sand Hansen, H, et al: Misonidazole neuropathy. A prospective study. J Neurooncol 6:227-230, 1988.
1741. Melick, EP and Hjorth, RJ: Improvement in paraplegia with vertebral Paget's disease treated with calcitonin. BMJ 1:627-628, 1976.
1742. Melki, PS, Halimi, P, Wibault, P, et al: MRI in chronic progressive radiation myelopathy. J Comput Assist Tomogr 18:1-6, 1994.
1743. Meltzer, RS, Singer, C, Armstrong, D, et al: Case report: Antemortem diagnosis of central nervous system strongyloidiasis. Am J Med Sci 277:91-98, 1979.
1744. Melzack, R: Phantom limbs and the concept of a neuromatrix. Trends Neurosci 13:88-92, 1990.
1744a. Mencel, PJ, DeAngelis, LM, and Motzer, RJ: Hormonal ablation as effective therapy for carcinomatous meningitis from prostatic carcinoma. Cancer 73:1892-1894, 1994.
1745. Mendez, IM and Del Maestro, RF: Cerebral metastases from malignant melanoma. Can J Neurol Sci 15:119-123, 1988.
1746. Mendez, MF: Pavor nocturnus from a brainstem glioma. Letter to the Editor. J Neurol Neurosurg Psychiatry 55:860, 1992.
1747. Merchut, MP: Brain metastases from undiagnosed systemic neoplasms. Arch Intern Med 149:1076-1080, 1989.
1748. Merimsky, O, Inbar, M, Reider-Groswasser, I, et al: Brain metastases of malignant melanoma in interferon complete responders: Clinical and radiological observations. J Neurooncol 12:137-140, 1992.
1749. Merimsky, O, Reider-Groswasser, IR, Inbar, M, et al: Interferon-related mental deterioration and behavioral changes in patients with renal cell carcinoma. Eur J Cancer 26:596-600, 1990.
1750. Merrill, CF, Kaufman, DI, and Dimitrov, NV: Breast cancer metastatic to the eye is a common entity. Cancer 68:623-627, 1991.
1751. Merrill, JE: Interleukin-2 effects in the central nervous system. Ann N Y Acad Sci 594:188-199, 1990.
1752. Messer, J, Reitman, D, Sacks, HS, et al: Association of adrenocorticosteroid therapy and peptic-ulcer disease. N Engl J Med 309:21-24, 1983.
1753. Mesulam, M-M and Geschwind, N: Disordered mental states in the postoperative period. Urol Clin North Am 3:199-215, 1976.
1754. Metz, O, Stoll, W, and Plenert, W: Meningiosis prophylaxis with intrathecal ^{198}Au-colloid and methotrexate in childhood acute lymphocytic leukemia. Cancer 49:224-228, 1982.
1755. Mewis, L and Young, SE: Breast carcinoma metastatic to the choroid. Analysis of 67 patients. Ophthalmology 89:147-151, 1982.
1756. Meyer, MA, Kelly, PJ, and Yanagihara, T: Stereotactic biopsy of possible brain tumors: Nonmalignant diagnoses. Abstract No. 49P. Neurology 40(Suppl 1):129, 1990.
1757. Meyer, RD, Rosen, P, and Armstrong, D: Phycomycosis complicating leukemia and lymphoma. Ann Intern Med 77:871-879, 1972.
1758. Meyer, SL, Font, RL, and Shaver, RP: Intraocular nocardiosis: Report of three cases. Arch Ophthalmol 83:536-541, 1970.
1759. Meyer, WH, Ayers, D, McHaney, VA, et al: Ifosfamide and exacerbation of cisplatin-induced hearing loss. Letter to the Editor. Lancet 341:754-755, 1993.
1760. Meyers, CA and Abbruzzese, JL: Cognitive functioning in cancer patients: Effect of previous treatment. Neurology 42:434-436, 1992.
1761. Meyers, CA, Scheibel, RS, and Forman, AD: Persistent neurotoxicity of systemically administered interferon-alpha. Neurology 41:672-676, 1991.
1762. Meyers, CA, Weitzner, M, Byrne, K, et al: Evaluation of the neurobehavioral functioning of patients before, during, and after bone marrow transplantation. J Clin Oncol 12:820-826, 1994.
1763. Michel, O and Brusis, T: Hearing loss as a sequel of lumbar puncture. Ann Otol Rhinol Laryngol 101:390-394, 1992.
1764. Michikawa, M, Wada, Y, Sano, M, et al: Radiation myelopathy: Significance of gadolinium-DPTA enhancement in the diagnosis. Neuroradiology 33:286-289, 1991.
1765. Milam, AH, Saari, CJ, Jacobson, SG, et al: Autoantibodies against retinal bipolar cells in cutaneous melanoma-associated retinopathy. Invest Ophthalmol Vis Sci 34:91-100, 1993.
1766. Mildenberger, M, Beach, TG, McGeer, EG, et al: An animal model of prophylactic cranial irradiation: Histologic effects at acute, early and delayed stages. Int J Radiat Oncol Biol Phys 18:1051-1060, 1990.
1767. Millay, RH, Klein, ML, Shults, WT, et al: Maculopathy associated with combination chemotherapy and osmotic opening of the blood–brain barrier. Am J Ophthalmol 102:626-632, 1986.
1768. Millburn, L, Hibbs, GG, and Hendrickson, FR: Treatment of spinal cord compression from metastatic carcinoma. Review of literature and presentation of a new method of treatment. Cancer 21:447-452, 1968.
1769. Miller, DR and Bergstrom, L: Vascular complications of head and neck surgery. Arch Otolaryngol 100:136-140, 1974.
1770. Miller, JW, Klass, DW, Mokri, B, et al: Triphasic

waves in cerebral carcinomatosis. Another nonmetabolic cause. Arch Neurol 43:1191-1193, 1986.
1771. Miller, L, Link, MP, Bologna, S, et al: Cerebellar atrophy caused by high-dose cytosine arabinoside: CT and MR findings. AJR 152:343-344, 1989.
1772. Miller, LJ and Eaton, VE: Ifosfamide-induced neurotoxicity: A case report and review of the literature. Ann Pharmacother 26:183-187, 1992.
1772a. Millot, R, Rubie, H, Mazingue, F, et al: Cerebrospinal fluid drug levels of leukemic children receiving intravenous 5 g/m^2 methotrexate. Leuk Lymphoma 14:141-144, 1994.
1773. Mills, RP, Insalaco, SJ, and Joseph, A: Bilateral cavernous sinus metastasis and ophthalmoplegia. Case report. J Neurosurg 55:463-466, 1981.
1774. Milman, N, Vig, L, Pedersen, NS, et al: Cerebrospinal fluid ferritin in patients with leukaemia and malignant lymphoma. Scand J Haematol 35:132-136, 1985.
1775. Minamisawa, T, Tsuchiya, T, and Eto, H: Changes in the averaged evoked potential of the rabbit during and after fractionated x-irradiation. Electroencephalogr Clin Neurophysiol 33:591-601, 1972.
1776. Minette, SE and Kimmel, DW: Subdural hematoma in patients with systemic cancer. Mayo Clin Proc 64:637-642, 1989.
1777. Minniti, CP, Maggi, M, and Helman, LJ: Suramin inhibits the growth of human rhabdomyosarcoma by interrupting the insulin-like growth factor II autocrine growth loop. Cancer Res 52:1830-1835, 1992.
1778. Miralles, GD, O'Fallon, JR, and Talley, NJ: Plasma-cell dyscrasia with polyneuropathy. N Engl J Med 327:1919-1923, 1992.
1779. Mirimanoff, RO and Choi, NC: The risk of intradural spinal metastases in patients with brain metastases from bronchogenic carcinomas. Int J Radiat Oncol Biol Phys 12:2131-2136, 1986.
1780. Mirimanoff, RO and Choi, NC: Intradural spinal metastases in patients with posterior fossa brain metastases from various primary cancers. Oncology 44:232-236, 1987.
1781. Mitchell, D, Fisher, J, Irving, D, et al: Lateral sinus thrombosis and intracranial hypertension in essential thrombocythaemia. Letter to the Editor. J Neurol Neurosurg Psychiatry 49:218-219, 1986.
1782. Mitchell, DM and Olczak, SA: Remission of a syndrome indistinguishable from motor neurone disease after resection of bronchial carcinoma. BMJ 2:176-177, 1979.
1783. Mitchell, MS: Relapse in the central nervous system in melanoma patients successfully treated with biomodulators. J Clin Oncol 7:1701-1709, 1989.
1784. Mitchell, RB, Wagner, JE, Karp, JE, et al: Syndrome of idiopathic hyperammonemia after high-dose chemotherapy. Review of nine cases. Am J Med 85:662-667, 1988.
1785. Mittal, MM, Gupta, NC, and Sharma, ML: Spinal epidural meningioma associated with increased intracranial pressure. Neurology 20:818-820, 1970.
1786. Miyatake, S-I, Kikuchi, H, Oda, Y, et al: A case of treatment-related leukoencephalopathy: Sequential MRI, CT and PET findings. J Neurooncol 14:143-149, 1992.
1787. Mizock, BA, Sabelli, HC, Dubin, A, et al: Septic encephalopathy. Evidence for altered phenylalanine metabolism and comparison with hepatic encephalopathy. Arch Intern Med 150:443-449, 1990.
1788. Mizusawa, H, Takagi, A, Sugita, H, et al: Mounding phenomenon: An experimental study in vitro. Neurology 33:90-93, 1983.
1789. Moberg, A and Reis, GV: Carcinosis meningum. Acta Med Scand 170:747-755, 1961.
1790. Modhi, G, Bauman, W, and Nicolis, G: Adrenal failure associated with hypothalamic and adrenal metastases: A case report and review of the literature. Cancer 47:2098-2101, 1981.
1791. Modhi, G and Nicolis, G: Hypoglycemia associated with carcinoid tumors. A case report and review of the literature. Cancer 53:1804-1806, 1984.
1792. Moertel, CG, Fleming, TR, MacDonald, JS, et al: Levamisole and fluorouracil for adjuvant therapy of resected colon carcinoma. N Engl J Med 322:352-358, 1990.
1793. Moertel, CG, Kvols, LK, and Rubin, J: A study of cyproheptadine in the treatment of metastatic carcinoid tumor and the malignant carcinoid syndrome. Cancer 67:33-36, 1991.
1794. Molgaard, CP, Yucel, EK, Geller, SC, et al: Access-site thrombosis after placement of inferior vena cava filters with 12-14-F delivery sheaths. Radiology 185:257-261, 1992.
1795. Molinatti, PA, Scheithauer, BW, Randall, RV, et al: Metastasis to pituitary adenoma. Arch Pathol Lab Med 109:287-289, 1985.
1796. Moll, JW, Henzen-Logmans, SC, Van der Meche, FG, et al: Early diagnosis and intravenous immune globulin therapy in paraneoplastic cerebellar degeneration. Letter to the Editor. J Neurol Neurosurg Psychiatry 56:112, 1993.
1796a. Moll, JWB, Markusse, HM, Pijnenburg, JJJM, et al: Antineuronal antibodies in patients with neurologic complications of primary Sjögren's syndrome. Neurology 43:2574-2581, 1993.
1797. Mollman, JE, Hogan, WM, Glover, DJ, et al: Unusual presentation of *cis*-platinum neuropathy. Neurology 38:488-490, 1988.
1798. Molnar, P, Blasberg, RG, Groothuis, D, et al: Regional blood-to-tissue transport in avian sarcoma virus (ASV)-induced brain tumors. Neurology 33:702-711, 1983.
1799. Monreal, M, Lafoz, E, Casals, A, et al: Occult cancer in patients with deep venous thrombosis. A systematic approach. Cancer 67:541-545, 1991.
1800. Monro, P and Mair, WG: Radiation effects on the human central nervous system 14 weeks after x-radiation. Acta Neuropathol (Berl) 11:267-274, 1968.
1801. Montpetit, VJA, Stewart, D, Dancea, S, et al: Pathology of dorsal root ganglia (DRG) in *cis*-platinum therapy. Abstract No. 34. J Neuropathol Exp Neurol 47:312, 1988.
1802. Moore, AP and Humphrey, PR: Man-in-the-barrel syndrome caused by cerebral metastases. Neurology 39:1134-1135, 1989.

1803. Moore, EW, Thomas, LB, Shaw, RK, et al: The central nervous system in acute leukemia. A postmortem study of 117 consecutive cases, with particular reference to hemorrhages, leukemic infiltrations, and the syndrome of meningeal leukemia. Arch Intern Med 105:141-158, 1960.
1804. Moots, PL, Walker, RW, Sze, G, et al: Diagnosis of dural venous sinus thrombosis by magnetic resonance imaging. Ann Neurol 22:431-432, 1987.
1805. Moretti, JA: Sensorineural hearing loss following radiotherapy to the nasopharynx. Laryngoscope 86:598-602, 1976.
1806. Morgan, WE, III, Malmgren, RA, and Albert, DM: Metastatic carcinoma of the ciliary body simulating uveitis. Diagnosis by cytologic examination of aqueous humor. Arch Ophthalmol 83:54-58, 1970.
1807. Mori, E and Yamadori, A: Acute confusional state and acute agitated delirium. Occurrence after infarction in the right middle cerebral artery territory. Arch Neurol 44:1139-1143, 1987.
1808. Mori, K, Takeuchi, J, Ishikawa, M, et al: Occlusive arteriopathy and brain tumor. J Neurosurg 49:22-35, 1978.
1809. Mori, M, Aoki, N, Shimada, H, et al: Detection of JC virus in the brains of aged patients without progressive multifocal leukoencephalopathy by the polymerase chain reaction and Southern hybridization analysis. Neurosci Lett 141:151-155, 1992.
1810. Mori, M, Yamaguchi, K, Honda, S, et al: Cancer cachexia syndrome developed in nude mice bearing melanoma cells producing leukemia-inhibitory factor. Cancer Res 51:6656-6659, 1991.
1811. Moroso, MJ and Blair, RL: A review of *cis*-platinum ototoxicity. J Otolaryngol 12:365-369, 1983.
1812. Morris, AD and Hopewell, JW: Combined effects of radiation and methotrexate on the cells of the rat subependymal plate. J R Soc Med 76:848-852, 1983.
1813. Morris, JG, Grattan-Smith, P, Panegyres, PK, et al: Delayed cerebral radiation necrosis. Q J Med 87:119-129, 1994.
1814. Morris, JG and Joffe, R: Perineural spread of cutaneous basal and squamous cell carcinomas. The clinical appearance of spread into the trigeminal and facial nerves. Arch Neurol 40:424-429, 1983.
1815. Morrison, RE, Brown, J, and Gooding, RS: Spinal cord abscess caused by *Listeria monocytogenes*. Arch Neurol 37:243-244, 1980.
1816. Morrison, VA, Haake, RJ, and Weisdorf, DJ: The spectrum of non-*Candida* fungal infections following bone marrow transplantation. Medicine (Baltimore) 72:78-88, 1993.
1817. Morrow, CS and Cowan, KH: Mechanisms and clinical significance of multidrug resistance. Oncology (Huntingt) 2:55-68, 1988.
1818. Morse, HG Moore, GE, Ortiz, LM, et al: Malignant melanoma: From subcutaneous nodule to brain metastasis. Cancer Genet Cytogenet 72:16-23, 1994.
1819. Morse, RM and Litin, EM: The anatomy of a delirium. Am J Psychiatry 128:111-116, 1971.
1820. Mortensen, ME, Cecalupo, AJ, Lo, WD, et al: Inadvertent intrathecal injection of daunorubicin with fatal outcome. Med Pediatr Oncol 20:249-253, 1992.
1821. Moseley, RP, Davies, AG, Richardson, RB, et al: Intrathecal administration of ^{131}I radiolabelled monoclonal antibody as a treatment for neoplastic meningitis. Br J Cancer 62:637-642, 1990.
1822. Moseley, RP, Oge, K, Shafqat, S, et al: HMFGA1 antigen: A new marker for carcinomatous meningitis. Int J Cancer 44:440-444, 1989.
1823. Moser, RP and Johnson, ML: Surgical management of brain metastases: How aggressive should we be? Oncology 3:123-127, 1989.
1824. Moskovskaya, NU: Effects of ionizing radiation on the functioning of the vestibular analyser. Vestn Otorinolaringol 21:59-62, 1960.
1825. Mossman, KL: Quantitative radiation dose-response relationships for normal tissues in man. Radiat Res 95:392-398, 1993.
1826. Mossman, KL, Chencharick, JD, Scheer, AC, et al: Radiation-induced changes in gustatory function: comparison of effects of neutron and photon irradiation. Int J Radiat Oncol Biol Phys 5:521-528, 1979.
1827. Mossman, KL and Henkin, RI: Radiation-induced changes in taste acuity in cancer patients. Int J Radiat Oncol Biol Phys 4:663-670, 1978.
1828. Moster, ML, Savino, PJ, Sergott, RC, et al: Isolated sixth-nerve palsies in young adults. Arch Ophthalmol 102:1328-1330, 1984.
1828a. Motomura, M, Johnston, I, Lang, B, et al: Anti-calcium channel antibodies detected using *Conus Magnus* toxin in Lambert-Eaton myasthenic syndrome sera. Abstract. Ann Neurology 36:324, 1994.
1829. Mott, MG, Stevenson, P, and Wood, CB: Methotrexate meningitis. Letter to the Editor. Lancet 2:656, 1972.
1830. Mueller, BU, Skelton, J, Callender, DP, et al: A prospective randomized trial comparing the infectious and noninfectious complications of an externalized catheter versus a subcutaneously implanted device in cancer patients. J Clin Oncol 10:1943-1948, 1992.
1831. Mueller, J, Hotson, JR, and Lanston, JW: Hyperviscosity-induced dementia. Neurology 33:101-103, 1983.
1832. Muggia, FM, Camacho, FJ, Kaplan, BH, et al: Weekly 5-fluorouracil combined with PALA: Toxic and therapeutic effects in colorectal cancer. Cancer Treat Rep 71:253-256, 1987.
1833. Mulhern, RK, Ochs, J, Fairclough, D, et al: Intellectual and academic achievement status after CNS relapse: A retrospective analysis of 40 children treated for acute lymphoblastic leukemia. J Clin Oncol 5:933-940, 1987.
1834. Mulligan, MJ, Vasu, R, Grossi, CE, et al: Case report: Neoplastic meningitis with eosinophilic pleocytosis in Hodgkin's disease: A case with cerebellar dysfunction and a review of the literature. Am J Med Sci 296(5):322-326, 1988.
1835. Mullin, JM and Snock, KV: Effect of tumor necrosis factor on epithelial tight junctions and transepithelial permeability. Cancer Res 50:2172-2176, 1990.

1836. Munier, F, Perentes, E, Herbort, CP, et al: Selective loss of optic nerve β-tubulin in vincristine-induced blindness. Letter to the Editor. Am J Med 93:232-234, 1992.

1837. Murata, J-I, Sawamura, Y, Takahashi, A, et al: Intracerebral hemorrhage caused by a neoplastic aneurysm from small-cell lung carcinoma: Case report. Neurosurgery 32:124-126, 1993.

1838. Murgo, AJ: Thrombotic microangiopathy in the cancer patient including those induced by chemotherapeutic agents. Semin Hematol 24:161-177, 1987.

1839. Murphy, KC, Feld, R, Evans, WK, et al: Intramedullary spinal cord metastases from small cell carcinoma of the lung. J Clin Oncol 1:99-106, 1983.

1840. Murray, JJ, Greco, FA, Wolff, SN, et al: Neoplastic meningitis. Marked variations of cerebrospinal fluid composition in the absence of extradural block. Am J Med 75:289-294, 1983.

1841. Murros, KE and Toole, JF: The effect of radiation on carotid arteries. A review article. Arch Neurol 46:449-455, 1989.

1842. Musto, P, Modini, S, Ladogana, S, et al: Increased risk of neurological relapse in acute lymphoblastic leukemias with high levels of cerebrospinal fluid thymidine kinase at diagnosis. Leuk Lymphoma 9:121-124, 1993.

1843. Mutoh, S, Aikou, I, and Ueda, S: Spinal coning after lumbar puncture in prostate cancer with asymptomatic vertebral metastasis: A case report. J Urol 145:834-835, 1991.

1844. Myers, C, Cooper, M, Stein, C, et al: Suramin: A novel growth factor antagonist with activity in hormone-refractory metastatic prostate cancer. J Clin Oncol 10:881-889, 1992.

1845. Myers, EN and Conley, J: Gustatory sweating after radical neck dissection. Arch Otolaryngol 91:534-542, 1970.

1846. Myklebust, AT, Godal, A, and Fodstad, O: Targeted therapy with immunotoxins in a nude rat model for leptomeningeal growth of human small cell lung cancer. Cancer Res 54:2146-2150, 1994.

1847. Nadelson, T: The psychiatrist in the surgical intensive care unit: I. Postoperative delirium. Arch Surg 111:113-117, 1976.

1848. Nader, S, Schultz, PN, Fuller, LM, et al: Calcium status following neck radiation therapy in Hodgkin's disease. Arch Intern Med 144:1577-1578, 1984.

1849. Nagahiro, S, Yamamoto, YL, Diksic, M, et al: Neurotoxicity after intracarotid 1,3-bis(2-chloroethyl)-1-nitrosourea administration in the rat: Hemodynamic changes studied by double-tracer autoradiography. Neurosurgery 29:19-25, 1991.

1850. Nagourney, RA, Hedaya, R, Linnoila, M, et al: Carcinoid carcinomatous meningitis. Ann Intern Med 102:779-782, 1985.

1851. Nakagawa, H, Groothuis, DR, Owens, ES, et al: Dexamethasone effects on [1251] albumin distribution in experimental RG-2 gliomas and adjacent brain. J Cereb Blood Flow Metab 7:687-701, 1987.

1852. Nakagawa, H, Kubo, S, Murasawa, A, et al: Measurements of CSF biochemical tumor markers in patients with meningeal carcinomatosis and brain tumors. J Neurooncol 12:111-120, 1992.

1852a. Nakagawa, H, Miyawaki, Y, Fujita, T, et al: Surgical treatment of brain metastases of lung cancer: Retrospective analysis of 89 cases. J Neurol Neurosurg Psychiatry 57:950-956, 1994.

1853. Nakagawa, H, Murasawa, A, Kubo, S, et al: Diagnosis and treatment of patients with meningeal carcinomatosis. J Neurooncol 13:81-89, 1992.

1853a. Nagakawa, H, Yamada, M, Kanayama, T, et al: Myelin basic protein in the cerebrospinal fluid of patients with brain tumors. Neurosurgery 34:825-833, 1994.

1854. Nakagawa, Y, Tashiro, K, Isu, T, et al: Occlusion of cerebral artery due to metastasis of chorioepithelioma. Case report. J Neurosurg 51:247-250, 1979.

1855. Nakanishi, T, Sobue, I, Toyokura, Y, et al: The Crow-Fukase syndrome: A study of 102 cases in Japan. Neurology 34:712-720, 1984.

1856. Nand, S, Fisher, SG, Salgia, R, et al: Hemostatic abnormalities in untreated cancer: Incidence and correlation with thrombotic and hemorrhagic complications. J Clin Oncol 5:1998-2003, 1987.

1857. Nand, S and Messmore, H: Hemostasis in malignancy. Am J Hematol 35:45-55, 1990.

1858. Narakas, AO: Operative treatment for radiation-induced and metastatic brachial plexopathy in 45 cases, 15 having an omentoplasty. Bull Hosp Jt Dis Orthop Inst 44(2):354-375, 1984.

1859. Naschitz, JE, Abrahamson, J, and Yeshurun, D: Clinical significance of paraneoplastic syndrome. Oncology 46:40-44, 1989.

1860. Naschitz, JE, Yeshurun, D, Abrahamson, J, et al: Ischemic heart disease precipitated by occult cancer. Cancer 69:2712-2720, 1992.

1861. Naschitz, JE, Yeshurun, D, and Lev, LM: Thromboembolism in cancer. Changing trends. Cancer 71:1384-1390, 1993.

1862. Naul, LG, Peet, GJ, and Maupin, WB: Avascular necrosis of the vertebral body: MR imaging. Radiology 172:219-222, 1989.

1863. Nausieda, PA, Tanner, CM, and Weiner, WJ: Opsoclonic cerebellopathy: A paraneoplastic syndrome responsive to thiamine. Arch Neurol 38:780-781, 1981.

1864. Navia, BA, Petito, CK, Gold, JW, et al: Cerebral toxoplasmosis complicating the acquired immune deficiency syndrome: Clinical and neuropathological findings in 27 patients. Ann Neurol 19:224-238, 1986.

1865. Needham, PR, Daley, AG, and Lennard, RF: Steroids in advanced cancer: Survey of current practice. BMJ 305:999, 1992.

1866. Neef, C and de Voodg-van der Straaten, I: An interaction between cytostatic and anticonvulsant drugs. Clin Pharmacol Ther 43:372-375, 1988.

1867. Nelson, DA: Dangers from methylprednisolone acetate therapy by intraspinal injection. Arch Neurol 45:804-806, 1988.

1868. Nelson, E, Blinzinger, K, and Hager, H: An electron-microscopic study of bacterial meningitis. Arch Neurol 6:390-403, 1962.

1869. Nelson, KR and McQuillen, MP: Neurologic complications of graft-versus-host disease. Neurol Clin 6:389-403, 1988.

1870. Nesbit, ME, Sather, H, Robison, LL, et al: Sanctuary therapy: A randomized trial of 724 children with previously untreated acute lymphoblastic leukemia. A report from Children's Cancer Study Group. Cancer Res 42:674-680, 1982.
1871. Nestor, JJ: Unilateral facial pain in lung cancer. Letter to the Editor. Lancet 338:1149, 1991.
1872. Neta, R and Oppenheim, JJ: IL-1: Can we exploit Jekyll and subjugate Hyde? Biological Therapy of Cancer Updates 2:1-11, 1992.
1873. Neuwelt, EA, Barnett, PA, Hellstrom, I, et al: Delivery of melanoma-associated immunoglobulin monoclonal antibody and Fab fragments to normal brain utilizing osmotic blood–brain barrier disruption. Cancer Res 48:4725-4729, 1988.
1874. Neuwelt, EA and Dahlborg, SA: Chemotherapy administered in conjunction with osmotic blood–brain barrier modification in patients with brain metastases. J Neurooncol 4:195-207, 1987.
1875. Neuwelt, EA, Pagel, M, Barnett, P, et al: Pharmacology and toxicity of intracarotid Adriamycin administration following osmotic blood–brain barrier modification. Cancer Res 41:4466-4470, 1981.
1876. Neuwelt, EA, Specht, HD, Barnett, PA, et al: Increased delivery of tumor-specific monoclonal antibodies to brain after osmotic blood–brain barrier modification in patients with melanoma metastatic to the central nervous system. Neurosurgery 20:885-895, 1987.
1877. Neuwelt, EA (ed): Implications of the Blood-Brain Barrier and Its Manipulation, vol 1, Basic Science Aspects. Plenum Medical Book Company, New York, 1989.
1878. Nevill, TJ, Benstead, TJ, McCormick, CW, et al: Horner's syndrome and demyelinating peripheral neuropathy caused by high-dose cytosine arabinoside. Am J Hematol 32:314-315, 1989.
1879. Neville, AJ, Robins, HI, Martin, P, et al: Effect of whole body hyperthermia and BCNU on the development of radiation myelitis in the rat. Int J Radiat Biol Rel Std Phys Chem Med 46:417-420, 1984.
1880. New, P, Barohn, R, Gales, T, et al: Taxol neuropathy after long-term administration. Abstract. Proceedings American Association for Cancer Research 32:A1226, 1991.
1881. Newsome, DA, Eong VG, and Cameron TP: "Steroid-induced" mydriasis and ptosis. Invest Ophthalmol Vis Sci 10:424-429, 1971.
1882. Newton, HB, Fleisher, M, Schwartz, MK, et al: Glucose-phosphate isomerase as a CSF marker for leptomeningeal metastasis. Neurology 41:395-398, 1991.
1883. Newton, HB, Page, MA, Junck, L, et al: Intra-arterial cisplatin for the treatment of malignant gliomas. J Neurooncol 7:39-45, 1989.
1884. Newton, JC, Barsa-Newton, MC, and Wardly, J: The effects of X radiation on the retina of the albino rabbit as viewed with the scanning electron microscope. Radiat Res 81:311-318, 1980.
1885. Newton, LK: Neurologic complications of polycythemia and their impact on therapy. Oncology (Huntingt) 4:59-66, 1990.
1886. Ng,THK, Chan, YW, Yu, YL, et al: Encephalopathy and neuropathy following ingestion of a Chinese herbal broth containing podophyllin. J Neurol Sci 101:107-113, 1991.
1887. Nicholas, DS and Weller, RO: The fine anatomy of the human spinal meninges. A light and scanning electron microscopy study. J Neurosurg 69:276-282, 1988.
1888. Nichols, CR, Roth, BJ, Williams, SD, et al: No evidence of acute cardiovascular complications of chemotherapy for testicular cancer: An analysis of the Testicular Cancer Intergroup Study. J Clin Oncol 10:760-765, 1992.
1889. Nichols, M, Bergevin, PR, Vyas, AC, et al: Neurotoxicity from 5-fluorouracil (NSC-19893) administration reproduced by mitomycin C (NSC-26980). Cancer Treat Rep 60:293-294, 1976.
1890. Nicola, GC and Nizzoli, V: Increased intracranial pressure and papilloedema associated with spinal tumors. Neurochirurgia 12:138-144, 1969.
1891. Nicolson, GL: Organ specificity of tumor metastasis: Role of preferential adhesion, invasion and growth of malignant cells at specific secondary sites. Cancer Metastasis Rev 7:143-188, 1988.
1892. Nicolson, GL: Cancer metastasis: Tumor cell and host organ properties important in metastasis to specific secondary sites. Biochim Biophys Acta 948:175-224, 1988.
1893. Nicolson, GL: Gene expression, cellular diversification and tumor progression to the metastatic phenotype. Bioessays 13:337-342, 1991.
1894. Nicolson, GL, Kawaguchi, T, Kaweguchi, M, et al: Brain surface invasion and metastasis of murine malignant melanoma variants. J Neurooncol 4:209-218, 1987.
1895. Nielsen, OS, Munro, AJ, and Tannock, JF: Bone metastases: Pathophysiology and management policy. J Clin Oncol 9:509-524, 1991.
1896. Nielson, SL and Posner, JB: Brain metastasis localized to an area of infarction. J Neurooncol 1:191-195, 1983.
1897. Nightingale, S, Schofield, IS, and Dawes, PJ: Visual, cortical somatosensory and brainstem auditory evoked potentials following incidental irradiation of the rhombencephalon. J Neurol Neurosurg Psychiatry 47:91-93, 1984.
1898. Ninane, J, Taylor, D, and Day, S: The eye as a sanctuary in acute lymphoblastic leukaemia. Lancet 2:452-453, 1980.
1899. Nishi, Y, Yufu, Y, Shinomiya, S, et al: Polyneuropathy in acute megakaryoblastic leukemia. Cancer 68:2033-2036, 1991.
1900. Nishikai, M and Sato, A: Low incidence of antinuclear antibodies in dermatomyositis with malignancy. Letter to the Editor. Ann Rheum Dis 49:422, 1990.
1901. Nitsch, C and Klatzo, J: Regional patterns of blood–brain barrier breakdown during epileptiform seizures induced by various convulsive agents. J Neurol Sci 59:305-322, 1983.
1902. Nitzan, DW, Azaz, B, and Constantini, S: Severe limitation in mouth opening following transtemporal neurosurgical procedures: Diagnosis, treatment, and prevention. J Neurosurg 76:623-625, 1992.
1903. Noetzel, MJ, Cawley, LP, James, VL, et al: Anti-

neurofilament protein antibodies in opsoclonus-myoclonus. J Neuroimmunol 15:137-145, 1987.

1903a. Noordjik, EM, Vecht, CJ, Haaxma-Reiche, H, et al: The choice of treatment of single brain metastasis should be based on extracranial tumor activity and age. Int J Radiat Oncol Biol Phys 29:711-717, 1994.

1904. Nordstrom, B and Strang, P: Microangiopathic hemolytic anemias (MAHA) in cancer. A case report and review. Anticancer Res 13:1845-1850, 1993.

1905. Novak, LJ: Radiotherapy of the central nervous system in acute leukemia. Am J Pediatr Hematol Oncol 11(1):87-92, 1989.

1906. Nugent, JL, Bunn, PA, Matthews, MJ, et al: CNS metastases in small cell bronchogenic carcinoma: Increasing frequency and changing pattern with lengthening survival. Cancer 44:1885-1893, 1979.

1907. Null, JA, LiVolsi, VA, and Glenn, WW: Hodgkin's disease of the thymus (granulomatous thymoma) and myasthenia gravis: A unique association. Am J Clin Pathol 67:521-525, 1977.

1908. O'Brien, MER, Tonge, K, Blake, P, et al: Blindness associated with high-dose carboplatin. Letter to the Editor. Lancet 339:558, 1992.

1909. O'Brien, TJ and Mack, GR: Multifocal osteonecrosis after short-term high-dose corticosteroid therapy. A case report. Clin Orthop 279:176-179, 1992.

1910. O'Callaghan, MJ and Ekert, H: Vincristine toxicity unrelated to dose. Arch Dis Child 51:289-292, 1976.

1911. O'Dwyer, PJ, Alonso, MT, Leyland-Jones, B, et al: Teniposide: A review of 12 years experience. Cancer Treat Rep 68:1455-1466, 1984.

1912. O'Keeffe, ST, Tormey, WP, Glasgow, R, et al: Thiamine deficiency in hospitalized elderly patients. Gerontology 40:18-24, 1994.

1913. O'Laoire, SA, Crockard, HA, Thomas, DG, et al: Brain-stem hematoma: A report of six surgically treated cases. J Neurosurg 56:222-227, 1982.

1914. O'Neill, BP, DiNapoli, RP, and Okazaki, H: Cerebral infarction as a result of tumor emboli. Cancer 60:90-95, 1987.

1915. O'Neill, JH, Murray, NM, and Newsom-Davis, J: The Lambert-Eaton myasthenic syndrome. A review of 50 cases. Brain 111:577-596, 1988.

1916. O'Rourke, T, George, CB, Redmond, J, III, et al: Spinal computed tomography and computed tomographic metrizamide myelography in the early diagnosis of metastatic disease. J Clin Oncol 4:576-583, 1986.

1917. Obbens, EA, Leavens, ME, Beal, JW, et al: Ommaya reservoirs in 387 cancer patients: A 15-year experience. Neurology 35:1274-1278, 1985.

1918. Obbens, EAMT and Posner, JB: Systemic cancer involving the spinal cord. In Davidoff, RA (ed): Handbook of the Spinal Cord, vol 4. Marcel Dekker, New York, 1987, pp 451-489.

1919. Obrist, R, Paravicini, U, Hartmann, D, et al: Vindesine. A clinical trial with special reference to neurological side effects. Cancer Chemother Pharmacol 2:233-237, 1979.

1920. Ochs, J, Mulhern, R, Fairclough, D, et al: Comparison of neuropsychologic functioning and clinical indicators of neurotoxicity in long-term survivors of childhood leukemia given cranial radiation or parenteral methotrexate: A prospective study. J Clin Oncol 9:145-151, 1991.

1921. Odio, CM, Faingezicht, I, Paris, M, et al: The beneficial effects of early dexamethazone administration in infants and children with bacterial meningitis. N Engl J Med 324:1525-1531, 1991.

1922. Ogasawara, H, Kiya, K, Kurisu, K, et al: Effect of intracarotid infusion of etoposide with angiotensin II–induced hypertension on the blood–brain barrier and the brain tissue. J Neurooncol 13:111-117, 1992.

1923. Ogihara, Y, Sekiguchi, K, and Tsuruta, T: Osteogenic sarcoma of the fourth thoracic vertebra. Long-term survival by chemotherapy only. Cancer 53:2615-2618, 1984.

1924. Oh, SJ, Slaughter, R, and Harrell, L: Paraneoplastic vasculitic neuropathy: A treatable neuropathy. Muscle Nerve 14:152-156, 1991.

1925. Ohkubo, C, Bigos, D, and Jain, RK: Interleukin 2 induced leukocyte adhesion to the normal and tumor microvascular endothelium in vivo and its inhibition by dextran sulfate: Implications for vascular leak syndrome. Cancer Res 51:1561-1563, 1991.

1926. Ohnishi, T, Posner, JB, and Shapiro, WR: Vasogenic brain edema induced by arachidonic acid: Role of extracellular arachidonic acid in blood–brain barrier dysfunction. Neurosurgery 30:545-551, 1992.

1927. Ohnishi, T, Sher, PB, Posner, JB, et al: Increased capillary permeability in rat brain induced by factors secreted by cultured C6 glioma cells: Role in peritumoral brain edema. J Neurooncol 10:13-25, 1991.

1928. Oikarinen, AI, Uitto, J, and Oikarinen, J: Glucocorticoid action on connective tissue: From molecular mechanisms to clinical practice. Med Biol 64:221-230, 1986.

1929. Ojeda, VJ: Necrotizing myelopathy associated with malignancy. A clinicopathologic study of two cases and literature review. Cancer 53:1115-1123, 1984.

1930. Ojeda, VJ and Walters, MNI: Spinal cord disorders in patients with cancer. Pathol Annu 19:63-88, 1984.

1931. Oka, K and Shimodaira, H: Telepharmacodynamics to predict therapeutic effects of glucocorticoids. Letter to the Editor. Lancet 338:385, 1991.

1931a. Okamoto, H, Shinkai, T, Matsuno, Y, et al: Intradural parenchymal involvement in the spinal subarachnoid space associated with primary lung cancer. Cancer 72:2583-2588, 1993.

1932. Okeda, R, Karakama, T, Kimura, S, et al: Neuropathologic study on chronic neurotoxicity of 5-fluorouracil and its masked compounds in dogs. Acta Neuropathol (Berl) 63:334-343, 1984.

1933. Okeda, R, Shibutani, M, Matsuo, T, et al: Subacute neurotoxicity of 5-fluorouracil and its derivative, carmofur, in cats. Acta Pathologica Japonica (Tokyo) 38:1255-1266, 1988.

1933a. O'Keeffe, ST, Tormey, WP, Glasgow, R, et al: Thiamine deficiency in hospitalized elderly patients. Gerontology 40:18-24, 1994.

1934. Oldendorf, WH, Cornford, ME, and Brown, WJ: The large apparent work capability of the blood–

brain barrier: A study of the mitochondrial content of capillary endothelial cells in brain and other tissues of the rat. Ann Neurol 1:409-417, 1977.

1935. Oliff, A, Bleyer, WA, and Poplack, DG: Acute encephalopathy after initiation of cranial irradiation for meningeal leukaemia. Lancet 2:13-15, 1978.

1936. Olin, JW, Young, R, Graor, RA, et al: Treatment of deep vein thrombosis and pulmonary emboli in patients with primary and metastatic brain tumors. Anticoagulants or inferior vena cava filter? Arch Intern Med 147:2177-2179, 1987.

1937. Olinger, CP and Ohlhaber, RL: Eighteen-gauge microscopic-telescopic needle endoscope with electrode channel: Potential clinical and research application. Surg Neurol 2:151-160, 1974.

1938. Olivi, A, Duncan, KL, Corden, BJ, et al: Comparison of the CNS toxicity of cisplatin, iproplatin and carboplatin given by intrathecal administration in a rat model. Abstract. Proceedings American Association for Cancer Research 30:A1852, 1989.

1939. Olsen, KS: Epidural blood patch in the treatment of post-lumbar puncture headache. Pain 30:293-301, 1987.

1940. Olsen, NK, Pfeiffer, P, Johannsen, L, et al: Radiation-induced brachial plexopathy: Neurological follow-up in 161 recurrence-free breast cancer patients. Int J Radiat Oncol Biol Phys 26:43-49, 1993.

1941. Olsen, NK, Pfeiffer, P, Mondrup, K, et al: Radiation-induced brachial plexus neuropathy in breast cancer patients. Acta Oncol 29:885-890, 1990.

1942. Olson, ME, Chernik, NL, and Posner, JB: Infiltration of the leptomeninges by systemic cancer. A clinical and pathologic study. Arch Neurol 30:122-137, 1974.

1943. Olsson, Y: Vascular permeability in the peripheral nervous system. In Dyck, PJ, Thomas, PK, Lambert, EH, and Bunge, R (eds): Peripheral Neuropathy, vol 1, ed 2. WB Saunders, Philadelphia, 1984, pp 579-597.

1944. Omland, H and Fossa, SD: Spontaneous regression cerebral and pulmonary metastases in renal cell carcinoma. Scand J Urol Nephrol 23:159-160, 1989.

1945. Ongerboer de Visser, BW, Somers, R, Nooyen, WH, et al: Intraventricular methotrexate therapy of leptomeningeal metastasis from breast carcinoma. Neurology 33:1565-1572, 1983.

1946. Ongerboer de Visser, BW and Tiessens, G: Polyneuropathy induced by cisplatin. Prog Exp Tumor Res 29:190-196, 1985.

1947. Onorato, IM, Wormser, GP, and Nicholas, P: "Normal" CSF in bacterial meningitis. JAMA 244:1469-1471, 1980.

1948. Onrot, J, Wiley, RG, Fogo, A, et al: Neck tumour with syncope due to paroxysmal sympathetic withdrawal. J Neurol Neurosurg Psychiatry 50:1063-1066, 1987.

1949. Ophir, D, Guterman, A, and Gross-Isseroff, R: Changes in smell acuity induced by radiation exposure of the olfactory mucosa. Arch Otolaryngol Head Neck Surg 114:853-855, 1988.

1950. Oppenheim, H: Uber Hirnsymptome bei Carcinomatose ohne nachweisbare. Veranderungen im Gehirn. Charité-Annalen (Berlin) 13:335-344, 1888.

1951. Ortega, P, Malamud, N, and Shimkin, MB: Metastasis to pineal body. Arch Pathol 52:518-528, 1951.

1952. Oshiro, H and Perlman, HB: Subarachnoid spread of tumor to the labyrinth. Arch Otolaryngol 81:328-334, 1965.

1953. Osswald, S and Trouton, TG: Neurocardiogenic (vasodepressor) syncope. N Engl J Med 329:30, 1993.

1954. Oster, JR, Perez, GO, Larios, O, et al: Cerebral salt wasting in a man with carcinomatous meningitis. Arch Intern Med 143:2187-2188, 1983.

1955. Ostrow, S, Hahn, D, Wiernik, PH, et al: Ophthalmologic toxicity after *cis*-dichlorodiammineplatinum(II) therapy. Cancer Treat Rep 62:1591-1594, 1978.

1955a. Ottinger, H, Cyrus, C, Belka, C, et al: Meningeal involvement in acute leukaemia and high-grade non-Hodgkin's lymphoma is associated with elevated activities of galactosyltransferases in the cerebrospinal fluid. Onkologie 17:180-183, 1994.

1956. Overby, MC and Rothman, AS: Anterolateral decompression for metastatic epidural spinal cord tumors. Results of a modified costotransversectomy approach. J Neurosurg 62:344-348, 1985.

1957. Ovesen, L, Sorensen, M, Hannibal, J, et al: Electrical taste detection thresholds and chemical smell detection thresholds in patients with cancer. Cancer 68:2260-2265, 1991.

1958. Ovesen, P, Kroner, K, Ornsholt, J, et al: Phantom-related phenomena after rectal amputation: Prevalence and clinical characteristics. Pain 44:289-291, 1991.

1959. Oviatt, DL, Kirshner, HS, and Stein, RS: Successful chemotherapeutic treatment of epidural compression in non-Hodgkin's lymphoma. Cancer 49:2446-2448, 1982.

1960. Owellen, RJ, Hartke, CA, Dickerson, RM, et al: Inhibition of tubulin-microtubule polymerization by drugs of the Vinca alkaloid class. Cancer Res 36:1499-1502, 1976.

1961. Paakko, E, Vainiopaa, L, Lanning, M, et al: White matter changes in children treated for acute lymphoblastic leukemia. Cancer 70:2728-2733, 1992.

1962. Packer, RJ, Sutton, LN, Atkins, TE, et al: A prospective study of cognitive function in children receiving whole-brain radiotherapy and chemotherapy: 2-year results. J Neurosurg 70:707-713, 1989.

1963. Packer, RJ, Zimmerman, RA, Rosenstock, J, et al: Focal encephalopathy following methotrexate therapy. Administration via a misplaced intraventricular catheter. Arch Neurol 38:450-452, 1981.

1964. Pagani, JJ, Hayman, LA, Bigelow, RH, et al: Diazepam prophylaxis of contrast media–induced seizures during computed tomography of patients with brain metastases. AJNR 140:787-792, 1983.

1965. Page, KA, Vogel, H, and Horoupian, DS: Intracerebral (parenchymal) infusion of methotrexate: Report of a case. J Neurooncol 12:181-186, 1992.

1966. Pages, M, Pages, AM, and Bories-Azeau, L: Severe sensorimotor neuropathy after cis-platin therapy.

Letter to the Editor. J Neurol Neurosurg Psychiatry 49:333-334, 1986.

1967. Paget, S: The distribution of secondary growths in cancer of the breast. Lancet 1:571-573, 1889.

1968. Pai, LH, Bookman, MA, Ozols, RF, et al: Clinical evaluation of intraperitoneal *Pseudomonas* exotoxin immunoconjugate OVB3-PE in patients with ovarian cancer. J Clin Oncol 9:2095-2103, 1991.

1969. Paillas, JE and Pellet, W: Brain metastases. In Vinken, PJ and Bruyn, GW (eds): Handbook of Clinical Neurology, vol 18. Elsevier, New York, 1975, pp 201-232.

1969a. Palackharry, CS: The epidemiology of non-Hodgkin's lymphoma: Why the increased incidence? Oncology (Huntingt) 8:67-78, 1994.

1970. Paladine, W, Belle, N, and Weaver, JW: Reduction of vincristine (VCR) paresthesias of the hand. Abstract. Program/Proceedings American Society of Clinical Oncology 8:A1290, 1989.

1971. Paling, MR, Black, WC, Levine, PA, et al: Tumor invasion of the anterior skull base: A comparison of MR and CT studies. J Comput Assist Tomogr 11:824-830, 1987.

1972. Pamphlett, R: Carcinoma metastasis to meningioma. J Neurol Neurosurg Psychiatry 47:561-563, 1984.

1973. Pannullo, S and Posner, JB: Seizures after bone marrow transplant. Abstract. Ann Neurol 32:287, 1992.

1974. Panullo, SC, Reich, JB, Krol, G, et al: MRI changes in intracranial hypotension. Neurology 43:919-926, 1993.

1975. Paone, JF and Jeyasingham, K: Remission of cerebellar dysfunction after pneumonectomy for bronchogenic carcinoma. N Engl J Med 302:156, 1980.

1976. Paparella, MM, Berlinger, NT, Oda, M, et al: Otological manifestations of leukemia. Laryngoscope 83:1510-1526, 1973.

1977. Pardridge, WM, Boado, RJ, and Farrell, CR: Brain-type glucose transporter (GLUT-1) is selectively localized to the blood–brain barrier. Studies with quantitative western blotting and in situ hybridization. J Biol Chem 265:18035-18040, 1990.

1978. Pardridge, WM, Oldendorf, WH, Cancilla, P, et al: Blood–brain barrier: Interface between internal medicine and the brain. Ann Intern Med 105:82-95, 1986.

1979. Paredes, JP, Puente, JL, and Potel, J: Variations in sensitivity after sectioning the intercostobrachial nerve. Am J Surg 160:525-528, 1990.

1979a. Parent, JM and Lowenstein, DH: Treatment of refractory generalized status epilepticus with continuous infusion of midazolam. Neurology 44:1837-1840, 1994.

1980. Park, Y, Oster, MW, and Olarte, MR: Prostatic cancer with an unusual presentation: Polymyositis and mediastinal adenopathy. Cancer 48:1262-1264, 1981.

1981. Parkinson, DR, Cano, PO, Jerry, LM, et al: Complications of cancer immunotherapy with Levamisole. Lancet 1:1129-1132, 1977.

1982. Parks, BJ: Postoperative peripheral neuropathies. Surgery 74:348-357, 1973.

1983. Parlow, JL and Einarson, DW: An unusual cause of delayed postmyelogram headache. Anesthesiology 75:145-146, 1991.

1984. Parry, BR: Radiation recall induced by tamoxifen. Letter to the Editor. Lancet 340:49, 1992.

1985. Parsons, JT: The effect of radiation on normal tissues of the head and neck. In Million, RR and Cassisi, NJ (eds): Management of Head and Neck Cancer: A Multidisciplinary Approach, ed 2. JB Lippincott, Philadelphia, 1994, pp 245-290.

1986. Parsons, JT, Fitzgerald, CR, Hood, CI, et al: The effects of irradiation on the eye and optic nerve. Int J Radiat Oncol Biol Phys 9:609-622, 1983.

1987. Parsons, M: The spinal form of carcinomatous meningitis. Q J Med 41:509-519, 1972.

1988. Partanen, VSJ, Soininen, H, Saksa, M, et al: Electromyographic and nerve conduction findings in a patient with neuromyotonia, normocalcemic tetany and small-cell lung cancer. Acta Neurol Scand 61:216-226, 1980.

1989. Pasqualini, T, McCalla, J, Berg, S, et al: Subtle primary hypothyroidism in patients treated for acute lymphoblastic leukemia. Acta Endocrinol (Copenh) 124:375-380, 1991.

1989a. Patchell, RA: Neurological complications of organ transplantation. Ann Neurol 36:688-703, 1994.

1990. Patchell, R and Perry, MC: Eosinophilic meningitis in Hodgkin's disease. Neurology 31:887-888, 1981.

1991. Patchell, RA: Brain metastases. In Patchell, RA (ed): Neurologic Complications of Systemic Cancer. Neurologic Clinics. WB Saunders, Philadelphia, 1991, pp 817-824.

1992. Patchell, RA, Cirrincoine, C, Thaler, HT, et al: Single brain metastases: Surgery plus radiation or radiation alone. Neurology 36:447-453, 1986.

1993. Patchell, RA, Tibbs, PA, Walsh, JW, et al: A randomized trial of surgery in the treatment of single metastases to the brain. N Engl J Med 322:494-500, 1990.

1994. Patel, SR, Forman, AD, and Benjamin, RS: High-dose ifosfamide-induced exacerbation of peripheral neuropathy. J Natl Cancer Inst 86:305-306, 1994.

1995. Paterson, AH, Agarwal, M, Lees, A, et al: Brain metastases in breast cancer patients receiving adjuvant chemotherapy. Cancer 49:651-654, 1982.

1996. Paterson, AHG and McPherson, TA: A possible neurologic complication of DTIC. Letter to the Editor. Cancer Treat Rep 61:105-106, 1978.

1997. Patterson, WP and Ringenberg, QS: The pathophysiology of thrombosis in cancer. Semin Oncol 17:140-146, 1990.

1998. Pavlidis, NA, Petris, C, Briassoulis, E, et al: Clear evidence that long-term, low-dose tamoxifen treatment can induce ocular toxicity. A prospective study of 63 patients. Cancer 69:2961-2964, 1992.

1999. Pavlovsky, S, Fismann, N, Arizaga, R, et al: Neuropsychological study in patients with ALL: Two different CNS prevention therapies—Cranial irradiation plus IT methotrexate vs. IT methotrexate alone. Am J Pediatr Hematol Oncol 5:79-86, 1983.

2000. Payne, DG: Radiation therapy of tumours involving the skull base. Can J Neurol Sci 12:363-365, 1985.
2001. Payne, R and Foley, KM (eds): Cancer pain. Med Clin North Am 71:153-352, 1987.
2001a. Pearce, SHS, Rees, CJ: Coma in Wernicke's encephalopathy. Postgrad Med 70:597, 1994.
2001b. Peckham, M: Clinical aspects of metastases. In: Bock, G and Whelan, J (eds): Metastasis. John Wiley & Sons, Chichester, 1988, pp 223-243.
2002. Pellettieri, L, Sjolander, U, and Jakobsson, K-E: Prognostic evaluation before operative extirpation and radiotherapy of solitary brain metastasis. Acta Neurochir (Wien) 86:6-11, 1987.
2003. Penar, PL and Wilson, JT: Cost and survival analysis of metastatic cerebral tumors treated by resection and radiation. Neurosurgery 34:888-894, 1994.
2004. Pepin, EP: Cerebral metastasis presenting as migraine with aura. Letter to the Editor. Lancet 336:127-128, 1990.
2005. Percy, AK, Elveback, LR, Okazaki, H, et al: Neoplasms of the central nervous system. Epidemiologic considerations. Neurology 22:40-48, 1972.
2006. Peress, NS, Su, PC, and Turner, I: Combined myelopathy and radiculoneuropathy with malignant lymphoproliferative disease. Arch Neurol 36:311-313, 1979.
2007. Perfect, JR and Wright, KA: Amphotericin B lipid complex in the treatment of experimental cryptococcal meningitis and disseminated candidosis. J Antimicrob Chemother 33:73-81, 1994.
2008. Perling, LH, Laurent, JP, and Cheek, WR: Epidural hibernoma as a complication of corticosteroid treatment. Case report. J Neurosurg 69:613-616, 1988.
2009. Perrault, DJ, Turley, J, Quirt, I, et al: A prospective study of vincristine neuropathy. Abstract. Program/Proceedings American Society of Clinical Oncology 7:A1115, 1988.
2010. Perrin, RG, Livingston, KE, and Aarabi, B: Intradural extramedullary spinal metastasis. A report of 10 cases. J Neurosurg 56:835-837, 1982.
2011. Perrin, RG and McBroom, RJ: Anterior versus posterior decompression for symptomatic spinal metastasis. Can J Neurol Sci 14:75-80, 1987.
2012. Perrin, RG and McBroom, RJ: Spinal fixation after anterior decompression for symptomatic spinal metastasis. Neurosurgery 22:324-327, 1988.
2013. Perry, JR, Bilbao, JM, and Gray, T: Fatal basilar vasculopathy complicating bacterial meningitis. Stroke 23:1175-1178, 1992.
2014. Perry, JR, Deodhare, SS, Bilbao, JM, et al: The significance of spinal cord compression as the initial manifestation of lymphoma. Neurosurgery 32:157-162, 1993.
2015. Perry, MC (ed): Toxicity of chemotherapy. Semin Oncol 19:453-457, 1992.
2016. Peters, WP, Holland, JF, Senn, H, et al: Corticosteroid administration and localized leukocyte mobilization in man. N Engl J Med 282:342-345, 1972.
2017. Petersdorf, RG, Swarner, DR, and Garcia, M: Studies on the pathogenesis of meningitis during pneumococcal bacteremia. J Clin Invest 41:320-327, 1962.
2018. Peterslund, NA, Black, FT, Geil, JP, et al: Beta-2-microglobulin in the cerebrospinal fluid of patients with infections of the central nervous system. Acta Neurol Scand 80:579-583, 1989.
2019. Peterson, K, Forsyth, PA, and Posner, JB: Paraneoplastic sensorimotor neuropathy associated with breast cancer. J Neurooncol 21:159-170, 1994.
2020. Peterson, K, Rosenblum, MK, Powers, JM, et al: Effect of brain irradiation on demyelinating lesions. Neurology 43:2105-2112, 1993.
2021. Peterson, K, Rosenblum, MK, Kotanides, H, et al: Paraneoplastic cerebellar degeneration. I. A clinical analysis of 55 anti-Yo antibody positive patients. Neurology 42:1931-1937, 1992.
2021a. Petren-Mallmin, M: Clinical and experimental imaging of breast cancer metastases in the spine. Acta Radiol 391:1-23, 1994.
2022. Pettersson, CA, Sharma, HS, and Olsson, Y: Vascular permeability of spinal nerve roots. A study in the rat with Evans blue and lanthanum as tracers. Acta Neuropathol (Berl) 81:148-154, 1990.
2023. Peylan-Ramu, N, Poplack, DG, Pizzo, PA, et al: Abnormal CT scans of the brain in asymptomatic children with acute lymphocytic leukemia after prophylactic treatment of the central nervous system with radiation and intrathecal chemotherapy. N Engl J Med 298:815-818, 1978.
2024. Pezner, RD and Archambeau, JO: Brain tolerance unit: A method to estimate risk of radiation brain injury for various dose schedules. Int J Radiat Oncol Biol Phys 7:397-402, 1981.
2025. Pezzimenti, JF, Bruckner, HW, and DeConti, RC: Paralytic brachial neuritis in Hodgkin's disease. Cancer 31:626-632, 1973.
2026. Pfeffer, MR, Wygoda, M, and Siegal, T: Leptomeningeal metastases—treatment results in 98 consecutive patients. Isr J Med Sci 24:611-618, 1988.
2027. Pfister, HW, Borasio, GD, Dirnagl, U, et al: Cerebrovascular complications of bacterial meningitis in adults. Neurology 42:1497-1504, 1992.
2028. Pfister, HW, Koedel, U, Haberl, RL, et al: Microvascular changes during the early phase of experimental bacterial meningitis. J Cereb Blood Flow Metab 10:914-922, 1990.
2029. Pfister, HW, Koedel, U, Lorenzl, S, et al: Antioxidants attenuate microvascular changes in the early phase of experimental pneumococcal meningitis in rats. Stroke 23:1798-1804, 1992.
2030. Phanthumchinda, K, Intragumtornchai, T, and Kasantikul, V: Stroke-like syndrome, mineralizing microangiopathy, and neuroaxional dystrophy following intrathecal methotrexate therapy. Neurology 41:1847-1848, 1991.
2031. Phillips, MH, Stelzer, KJ, Griffin, TW, et al: Stereotactic radiosurgery: A review and comparison of methods. J Clin Oncol 12:1085-1099, 1994.
2032. Phillips, PC, Delattre, J-Y, Berger, CA, et al: Early and progressive increases in regional brain capillary permeability following single- and fractionated-dose cranial radiation in the rat. Abstract. Neurology 37(Suppl 1):301, 1987.
2033. Phillips, PC, Dhawan, V, Strother, SC, et al: Reduced cerebral glucose metabolism and increased brain capillary permeability following high-dose

methotrexate chemotherapy: A positron emission tomographic study. Ann Neurol 21:59-63, 1987.
2034. Phillips, PC, Thaler, HT, Berger, CA, et al: Acute high-dose methotrexate neurotoxicity in the rat. Ann Neurol 20:583-589, 1986.
2035. Phillips, PC, Than, TT, Cork, LC, et al: Intrathecal 4-hydroperoxycyclophosphamide: Neurotoxicity, cerebrospinal fluid pharmacokinetics, and antitumor activity in a rabbit model of VX2 leptomeningeal carcinomatosis. Cancer Res 52:6168-6174, 1992.
2036. Pichini, S, Altieri, I, Bacosi, A, et al: High-performance liquid chromatographic-mass spectrometic assay of busulfan in serum and cerebrospinal fluid. J Chromatogr 581:143-146, 1992.
2037. Pickren, JW, Lopez, G, Tsukada, Y, et al: Brain metastases: An autopsy study. Cancer Treatment Symposia 2:295-313, 1983.
2038. Pies, R: Persistent bipolar illness after steroid administration. Arch Intern Med 141:1087, 1981.
2039. Pihko, H, Tyni, T, Virkola, K, et al: Transient ischemic cerebral lesions during induction chemotherapy for acute lymphoblastic leukemia. J Pediatr 123:718-724, 1993.
2040. Pillay, N, Gilbert, JJ, Ebers, GC, et al: Internuclear ophthalmoplegia and "optic neuritis": paraneoplastic effects of bronchial carcinoma. Neurology 34:788-791, 1984.
2041. Pinedo, HM and Peters, GF: Fluorouracil: Biochemistry and pharmacology. J Clin Oncol 6: 1653-1664, 1988.
2042. Plant, GT, Donald, JJ, Jackowski, A, et al: Partial, non-thrombotic, superior sagittal sinus occlusion due to occipital skull tumours. J Neurol Neurosurg Psychiatry 54:520-523, 1991.
2043. Pleet, DL, Mandel, S, and Neilan, B: Paroxysmal unilateral hyperhidrosis and malignant mesothelioma. Case report. Arch Neurol 40:256, 1983.
2044. Ploner, F, Saltuari, L, Marosi, MJ, et al: Cerebral air emboli with use of central venous catheter in mobile patient. Letter to the Editor. Lancet 338:1331, 1991.
2045. Plotz, PH, Dalakas, M, Leff, RL, et al: Current concepts in the idiopathic inflammatory myopathies: Polymyositis, dermatomyositis, and related disorders. Ann Intern Med 111:143-157, 1989.
2046. Plouffe, JF and Fass, RJ: Histoplasma meningitis: Diagnostic value of cerebrospinal fluid serology. Ann Intern Med 92:189-191, 1980.
2047. Plum, F and Posner, JB: The pathologic physiology of signs and symptoms of coma. In Plum, F and Posner, JB (eds): The Diagnosis of Stupor and Coma. FA Davis, Philadelphia, 1980, pp 1-86.
2048. Pluss, JL and DiBella, NJ: Reversible central nervous system dysfunction due to tamoxifen in a patient with breast cancer. Ann Intern Med 101:652, 1984.
2049. Pochedly, C: Neurological manifestations in acute leukemia. II. Involvement of cranial nerves and hypothalamus. N Y State J Med 75:715-721, 1975.
2050. Pocock, NA, Eisman, JA, Dunstan, CR, et al: Recovery from steroid-induced osteoporosis. Ann Intern Med 107:319-323, 1987.
2051. Poduslo, JF: Albumin and the blood–nerve barrier. In Dyck, PJ and Thomas, PK (eds): Peripheral Neuropathy, vol 1, ed 3, WB Saunders, Philadelphia, 1993, pp 446-452.
2052. Poisson, M, Hauw, JJ, Pouillart, P, et al: Malignant gliomas treated after surgery by combination chemotherapy and delayed radiation therapy. Part II. Tolerance to irradiation after chemotherapy. Acta Neurochir (Wien) 51:27-42, 1979.
2053. Polans, AS, Burton, MD, Haley, TL, et al: Recoverin, but not visinin, in an autoantigen in the human retina identified with a cancer-associated retinopathy. Invest Ophthalmol Vis Sci 34:81-90, 1993.
2054. Pollard, RB, Egbert, PR, Gallagher, JG, et al: Cytomegalovirus retinitis in immunosuppressed hosts. I. Natural history and effects of treatment with adenine arabinoside. Ann Intern Med 93:655-664, 1980.
2055. Pollay, M, Fullenwider, C, Roberts, PA, et al: Effect of mannitol and furosemide on blood–brain osmotic gradient and intracranial pressure. J Neurosurg 59:945-950, 1983.
2056. Polo, JM, Fabrega, E, Casafont, F, et al: Treatment of cerebral aspergillosis after liver transplantation. Neurology 42:1817-1819, 1992.
2057. Polsky, B and Armstrong, D: Infectious complications of neoplastic disease. Am J Infect Control 13:199-209, 1985.
2058. Polsky, B, Depman, MR, and Gold, JW: Intraventricular therapy of cryptococcal meningitis via a subcutaneous reservoir. Am J Med 81:25-28, 1986.
2058a. Ponta, H, Sleeman, J, Herrlich, P: Tumor metastasis formation: Cell-surface proteins confer metastasis-promoting or -suppressing properties. Biochim Biophys Acta 1198:1-10, 1994.
2059. Popiela, T, Lucchi, R, and Giongo, F: Methylprednisolone as palliative therapy for female terminal cancer patients. The Methyprednisolone Female Preterminal Cancer Study Group. Eur J Cancer Clin Oncol 25:1823-1829, 1989.
2060. Pors, H, von Eyben, FE, Sorensen, OS, et al: Long-term remission of multiple brain metastases with tamoxifen. J Neurooncol 10:173-177, 1991.
2061. Portenoy, RK: Cancer pain: Pathophysiology and syndromes. Lancet 339:1026-1031, 1992.
2062. Portenoy, RK, Galer, BS, Salamon, O, et al: Identification of epidural neoplasm: Radiography and bone scintigraphy in the symptomatic and asymptomatic spine. Cancer 64:2207-2213, 1989.
2063. Portenoy, RK, Lipton, RB, and Foley, KM: Back pain in the cancer patient: An algorithm for evaluation and management. Neurology 37:134-138, 1987.
2064. Posner, JB: The role of the neurologist in the management of cancer. Am J Med 65:4-6, 1978.
2065. Posner, JB: Neurologic complications of systemic cancer. Disease-a-Month 25:1-60, 1978.
2066. Posner, JB: Clinical manifestations of brain metastasis. In Weiss, L, Gilbert, HA, and Posner, JB (eds): Brain Metastasis. G.K. Hall & Co., Boston, 1980, pp 189-207.
2067. Posner, JB: Back pain and epidural spinal cord compression. Med Clin North Am 71:185-205, 1987.
2068. Posner, JB: Surgery for metastases to the brain. Editorial. N Engl J Med 322:544-545, 1990.

2069. Posner, JB: Paraneoplastic cerebellar degeneration. Prin Pract Oncol Updates 5:(11):1-13, 1991.
2070. Posner, JB: Paraneoplastic syndromes. Neurol Clin 9:919-936, 1991.
2071. Posner, JB: Supportive care of the neuro-oncology patient. In Hildebrand, J (ed): Management in Neuro-Oncology, European School of Oncology Monographs. Springer-Verlag, Berlin, 1992, pp 89-103.
2072. Posner, JB: Pathogenesis of central nervous system paraneoplastic syndromes. Rev Neurol (Paris) 148:505-512, 1992.
2073. Posner, JB and Chernik, NL: Intracranial metastases from systemic cancer. Adv Neurol 19:575-587, 1978.
2074. Posner, JB and Furneaux, HM: Paraneoplastic syndromes. In Waksman, BH (ed): Immunologic Mechanisms in Neurologic and Psychiatric Disease. Raven Press Ltd, New York, 1990, pp 187-219.
2075. Posner, JB, Howieson, J, and Cvitkovic, E: "Disappearing" spinal cord compression: Oncolytic effect of glucocorticosteroids (and other chemotherapeutic agents) on epidural metastases. Ann Neurol 2:409-413, 1977.
2076. Post, MJD, Mendez, DR, Kline, LB, et al: Metastatic disease to the cavernous sinus: Clinical syndrome and CT diagnosis. J Comput Assist Tomogr 9:115-120, 1985.
2077. Post, MJD, Quencer, RM, Green, BA, et al: Intramedullary spinal cord metastases, mainly of nonneurogenic origin. AJR 148:1015-1022, 1987.
2078. Potter, KM, Juacaba, SF, Price, JE, et al: Observations on organ distribution of fluorescein-labelled tumour cells released intravascularly. Invasion Metastasis 3:221-233, 1983.
2079. Potts, DG and Zimmerman, RD: Nuclear magnetic resonance imaging of skull base lesions. Can J Neurol Sci 12:327-331, 1985.
2080. Poungvarin, N, Bhoopat, W, Viriyavejakul, A, et al: Effects of dexamethasone in primary supratentorial intracerebral hemorrhage. N Engl J Med 316:1229-1233, 1987.
2081. Powell, BL, Capizzi, RL, Lyerly, ES, et al: Peripheral neuropathy after high-dose cytosine arabinoside, daunorubicin, and asparaginase consolidation for acute nonlymphocytic leukemia. J Clin Oncol 4:95-97, 1986.
2082. Powell, HC, Gibbs, CJ, Jr, Lorenzo, AM, et al: Toxoplasmosis of the central nervous system in the adult. Electron microscopic observations. Acta Neuropath (Berl) 41:211-216, 1978.
2083. Powell, N: Metastatic carcinoma in association with Paget's disease of bone. Br J Radiol 56:582-585, 1983.
2084. Powers, BE, Beck, ER, Gillette, EL, et al: Pathology of radiation injury to the canine spinal cord. Int J Radiat Oncol Biol Phys 23:539-549, 1992.
2085. Powers, SK and Edwards, MS: Prophylaxis of thromboembolism in the neurosurgical patient: A review. Neurosurgery 10:509-513, 1982.
2086. Prados, M, Leibel, S, Barnett, CM, et al: Interstitial brachytherapy for metastatic brain tumors. Cancer 63:657-660, 1989.
2087. Prandoni, P, Lensing, AW, Buller, HR, et al: Deep-vein thrombosis and the incidence of subsequent symptomatic cancer. N Engl J Med 327:1128-1133, 1992.
2088. Pratt, CB, Goren, MP, Meyer, WH, et al: Ifosfamide neurotoxicity is related to previous cisplatin treatment for pediatric solid tumors. J Clin Oncol 8:1399-1401, 1990.
2089. Pratt, CB, Green, AA, Horowitz, ME, et al: Central nervous system toxicity following the treatment of pediatric patients with ifosfamide/mesna. J Clin Oncol 4:1253-1261, 1986.
2090. Preston, FE, Sokol, RJ, Lilleyman, JS, et al: Cellular hyperviscosity as a cause of neurological symptoms in laeukemia. BMJ 1:476-768, 1978.
2091. Price, JE: The biology of metastatic breast cancer. Cancer 66(Suppl 6):1313-1320, 1990.
2092. Price, R, Chernik, NL, Horta-Barbosa, L, et al: Herpes simplex encephalitis in an anergic patient. Am J Med 54:222-228, 1973.
2093. Price, RA and Birdwell, DA: The central nervous system in childhood leukemia. III. Mineralizing microangiopathy and dystrophic calcification. Cancer 42:717-728, 1978.
2094. Price, RA and Jamieson, PA: The central nervous system in childhood leukemia. II. Subacute leukoencephalopathy. Cancer 35:306-318, 1975.
2095. Price, RA and Johnson, WW: The central nervous system in childhood leukemia. I. The arachnoid. Cancer 31:520-533, 1973.
2096. Priest, JR, Ramsay, NK, Steinherz, PG, et al: A syndrome of thrombosis and hemorrhage complicating L-asparaginase therapy for childhood acute lymphoblastic leukemia. J Pediatr 100:984-989, 1982.
2097. Pringle, CE, Hudson, AJ, Munoz, DG, et al: Primary lateral sclerosis. Clinical features, neuropathology and diagnostic criteria. Brain 115:495-520, 1992.
2098. Prinz, RA, Barbato, AL, Braithwaite, SS, et al: Prior irradiation and the development of coexistent differentiated thyroid cancer and hyperparathyroidism. Cancer 49:874-877, 1982.
2099. Prioleau, PG and Katzenstein, AL: Major peripheral arterial occlusion due to malignant tumor embolism: Histologic recognition and surgical management. Cancer 42:2009-2014, 1978.
2100. Pruitt, AA: Opportunistic central nervous system infections. In Rottenberg, DA (ed): Neurological Complications of Cancer Treatment. Butterworth-Heinemann, Boston, 1991, pp 195-218.
2101. Pruitt, AA: Central nervous system infections in cancer patients. Neurol Clin 9:867-888, 1991.
2102. Pruitt, AA, Rubin, RH, Karchmer, AW, et al: Neurologic complications of bacterial endocarditis. Medicine (Baltimore) 57:329-343, 1978.
2103. Pruzanski, W and Watt, JG: Serum viscosity and hyperviscosity syndrome in IgG multiple myeloma. Ann Intern Med 77:853-860, 1972.
2104. Pullar, M, Blumbergs, PC, Phillips, GE, et al: Neoplastic cerebral aneurysm from metastatic gestational choriocarcinoma. J Neurosurg 63:644-647, 1985.
2105. Pullen, J, Boyett, J, Shuster, J, et al: Extended triple intrathecal chemotherapy trial for prevention of

CNS relapse in good-risk and poor-risk patients with B-progenitor acute lymphoblastic leukemia: A Pediatric Oncology Group study. J Clin Oncol 11:839-849, 1993.

2106. Punt, J, Pritchard, J, Pincott, JR, et al: Neuroblastoma: A review of 21 cases presenting with spinal cord compression. Cancer 45:3095-3101, 1980.

2107. Purohit, DP, Dick, DJ, Perry, RH, et al: Solitary extranodal lymphoma of sciatic nerve. J Neurol Sci 74:23-34, 1986.

2108. Quagliarello, VJ, Ma, A, Stukenbrok, H, et al: Ultrastructural localization of albumin transport across the cerebral microvasculature during experimental meningitis in the rat. J Exp Med 174:657-672, 1991.

2109. Quagliarello, V and Scheld, WM: Bacterial meningitis: Pathogenesis, pathophysiology, and progress. N Engl J Med 327:864-872, 1992.

2110. Quagliarello, VJ, Wispelwey, B, Long, WJ, Jr, et al: Recombinant human interleukin-1 induces meningitis and blood–brain barrier injury in the rat. Characterization and comparison with tumor necrosis factor. J Clin Invest 87:1360-1366, 1991.

2111. Quigley, MR, Reigel, DH, and Kortyna, R: Cerebrospinal fluid shunt infections. Report of 41 cases and a critical review of the literature. Pediatr Neurosurg 15:111-120, 1989.

2112. Quinn, JP, Weinstein, RA, and Caplan, LR: Eosinophilic meningitis and ibuprofen therapy. Neurology 34:108-109, 1984.

2113. Ra'anani, P, Shpilberg, O, Berezin, M, et al: Acute leukemia relapse presenting as central diabetes insipidus. Cancer 73:2312-2316, 1994.

2114. Raasveld, MHM, Surachno, S, Hack, CE, et al: Thromboembolic complications and dose of monoclonal OKT3 antibody. Letter to the Editor. Lancet 339:1363-1364, 1992.

2115. Radinsky, R and Fidler, IJ: Regulation of tumor cell growth at organ-specific metastases. In Vivo 6:325-331, 1992.

2116. Ragab, AH, Frech, RS, and Vietti, TJ: Osteoporotic fractures secondary to methotrexate therapy of acute leukemia in remission. Cancer 25:580-585, 1970.

2117. Raichle, ME, Eichling, JO, and Grubb, RL, Jr: Brain permeability of water. Arch Neurol 30:319-321, 1974.

2118. Ram, Z, Walbridge, S, Oshiro, EM, et al: Intrathecal gene therapy for malignant leptomeningeal neoplasia. Cancer Res 54:2141-2145, 1994.

2119. Rampling, R and Catterall, M: Facial nerve damage in the treatment of tumours of the parotid gland. Clin Oncol 10:345-351, 1984.

2120. Rando, TA and Fishman, RA: Spontaneous intracranial hypotension. Report of two cases and review of the literature. Neurology 42:481-487, 1992.

2121. Raney, B, Tefft, M, Heyn, R, et al: Ascending myelitis after intensive chemotherapy and radiation therapy in children with cranial parameningeal sarcoma. Cancer 69:1498-1506, 1992.

2122. Ransom, DT, DiNapoli, RP, and Richardson, RL: Cranial nerve lesions due to base of the skull metastases in prostate carcinoma. Cancer 65:586-589, 1990.

2123. Raoult, D, Brouqui, P, Marchou, B, et al: Acute and chronic Q fever in patients with cancer. Clin Infect Dis 14:127-130, 1992.

2124. Rapoport, SI: Quantitative aspects of osmotic opening of the blood–brain barrier. In Weiss, L, Gilbert, HA, and Posner, JB (eds): Brain Metastases. GK Hall & Co, Boston, 1980, pp 100-114.

2125. Rapoport, SI and Robinson, PJ: Blood–tumor barrier disruption controversies. Letter to the Editor. J Cereb Blood Flow Metab 11:165-168, 1991.

2126. Raroque, HG, Jr, Mandler, RN, Griffey, MS, et al: Neoplastic angioendotheliomatosis. Arch Neurol 47:929-930, 1990.

2127. Rashiq, S, Briewa, L, Mooney, M, et al: Distinguishing acyclovir neurotoxicity from encephalomyelitis. J Intern Med 234:507-511, 1993.

2128. Raskin, NH and Prusiner, S: Carotidynia. Neurology 27:43-46, 1977.

2129. Ratanatharathorn, V and Powers, WE: Epidural spinal cord compression from metastatic tumor: Diagnosis and guidelines for management. Cancer Treat Rev 18:55-71, 1991.

2130. Rate, WR, Solin, LJ, and Turrisi, AT: Palliative radiotherapy for metastatic malignant melanoma: Brain metastases, bone metastases, and spinal cord compression. Int J Radiat Oncol Biol Phys 15:859-864, 1988.

2131. Ravits, J: Myasthenia gravis: A well-understood neuromuscular disorder. Postgrad Med 83:219-223, 1988.

2132. Ravussin, P, Abou-Madi, M, Archer, D, et al: Changes in CSF pressure after mannitol in patients with and without elevated CSF pressure. J Neurosurg 69:869-876, 1988.

2133. Rawanduzy, A, Sarkis, A, and Rovit, RL: Severe phenytoin-induced bone marrow depression and agranulocytosis treated with human recombinant granulocyte-macrophage colony-stimulating factor. Case report. J Neurosurg 79:121-124, 1993.

2134. Raymond, PL and Balaa, MA: Diplopia and diarrhea: Ileal carcinoid metastatic to the central nervous system. Am J Gastroenterol 87:240-243, 1992.

2135. Recht, L, Straus, DJ, Cirrincione, C, et al: Central nervous system metastases from non-Hodgkin's lymphoma: Treatment and prophylaxis. Am J Med 84:425-435, 1988.

2136. Rechthand, E and Rapoport, SI: Regulation of the microenvironment of peripheral nerve: Role of the blood–nerve barrier. Prog Neurobiol 28:303-343, 1987.

2137. Rechthand, E, Smith, QR, Latker, CH, et al: Altered blood–nerve barrier permeability to small moleculares in experimental diabetes mellitus. J Neuropathol Exp Neurol 46:302-314, 1987.

2138. Reddel, RR, Kefford, RF, Grant, JM, et al: Ototoxicity in patients receiving cisplatin: Importance of dose and method of drug administration. Cancer Treat Rep 66:19-23, 1982.

2139. Reddy, RV and Vakili, ST: Midbrain encephalitis as a remote effect of a malignant neoplasm. Arch Neurol 38:781-782, 1981.

2140. Redman, BG, Tapazoglou, E, and Al-Sarraf, M: Meningeal carcinomatosis in head and neck can-

cer. Report of six cases and review of the literature. Cancer 58:2656-2661, 1986.
2141. Redmon, B, Pyzdrowski, KL, Elson, MK, et al: Hypoglycemia due to an insulin-binding monoclonal antibody in multiple myeloma. N Engl J Med 326:994-998, 1992.
2142. Redmond, J, III, Friedl, KE, Cornett, P, et al: Clinical usefulness of an algorithm for the early diagnosis of spinal metastatic disease. J Clin Oncol 6:154-157, 1988.
2143. Reece, DE, Frei-Lahr, DA, Shepherd, JD, et al: Neurologic complications in allogeneic bone marrow transplant patients receiving cyclosporin. Bone Marrow Transplant 8:393-401, 1991.
2144. Reeder, GS, Khandheria, BK, Seward, JB, et al: Transesophageal echocardiography and cardiac masses. Mayo Clin Proc 66:1101-1109, 1991.
2145. Reese, TS and Karnovsky, MJ: Fine structural localization of a blood–brain barrier to exogenous peroxidase. J Cell Biol 34:207-217, 1967.
2146. Reich, JB, Sierra, J, Camp, W, et al: Magnetic resonance imaging measurements and clinical changes accompanying transtentorial and foramen magnum brain herniation. Ann Neurol 33:159-170, 1993.
2147. Reichman, HR, Farrell, CL, and Del Maestro, RF: Effects of steroids and nonsteroid antiinflammatory agents on vascular permeability in a rat glioma model. J Neurosurg 65:233-237, 1986.
2148. Reid, IR, King, AR, Alexander, CJ, et al: Prevention of steroid-induced osteoporosis with (3-amino-1-hydroxypropylidene)-1, 1-biphosphonate (APD). Lancet 1:143-146, 1988.
2149. Reid, IR, Teitelbaum, SL, Dusso, A, et al: Hypercalcemic hyperparathyroidism complicating oncogenic osteomalacia. Effect of successful tumor resection on mineral homeostasis. Am J Med 83:350-354, 1987.
2150. Reid, JM, Pendergrass, TW, Krailo, MD, et al: Plasma pharmacokinetics and cerebrospinal fluid concentrations of idarubicin and idarubicinol in pediatric leukemia patients: A Children's Cancer Study Group report. Cancer Res 50:6525-6528, 1990.
2151. Reinhold, HS, Kaalen, JG, and Unger-Gils, K: Radiation myelopathy of the thoracic spinal cord. Int J Radiat Oncol Biol Phys 1:651-657, 1976.
2152. Reisner, SA, Rinkevich, D, Markiewicz, W, et al: Cardiac involvement in patients with myeloproliferative disorders. Am J Med 93:498-504, 1992.
2153. ReMine, SG and McIlrath, DC: Bowel perforation in steroid-treated patients. Ann Surg 192:581-586, 1980.
2154. Remler, MP, Marcussen, WH, and Tiller-Borsich, J: The late effects of radiation on the blood–brain barrier. Int J Radiat Oncol Biol Phys 12:1965-1969, 1986.
2155. Renaudin, J, Fewer, D, Wilson, CB, et al: Dose dependency of decadron in patients with partially excised brain tumors. J Neurosurg 39:302-305, 1973.
2156. Rennick, G, Shann, F, and de Campo, J: Cerebral herniation during bacterial meningitis in children. BMJ 306:953-955, 1993.
2157. Requena, I, Arias, M, Lopez-Ibor, L, et al: Cavernomas of the central nervous system: Clinical and neuroimaging manifestations in 47 patients. J Neurol Neurosurg Psychiatry 54:590-594, 1991.
2158. Resar, LM, Phillips, PC, Kastan, MB, et al: Acute neurotoxicity after intrathecal cytosine arabinoside in two adolescents with acute lymphoblastic leukemia of B-cell type. Cancer 71:117-123, 1993.
2159. Reske, SN, Karstens, JH, Gloeckner, W, et al: Radioimmunoimaging for diagnosis of bone marrow involvement in breast cancer and malignant lymphoma. Lancet 1:299-301, 1989.
2160. Retsas, S and Gershuny, AR: Central nervous system involvement in malignant melanoma. Cancer 61:1926-1934, 1988.
2161. Rex, JH, Larsen, RA, Dismukes, WE, et al: Catastrophic visual loss due to *Cryptococcus neoformans* meningitis. Medicine (Baltimore) 72:207-224, 1993.
2162. Ribeiro, RC and Pui, C-H: The clinical and biological correlates of coagulopathy in children with acute leukemia. J Clin Oncol 4:1212-1218, 1986.
2163. Ribeiro, RC, Pui, CH, and Schell, MJ: Vertebral compression fracture as a presenting feature of acute lymphoblastic leukemia in children. Cancer 61:589-592, 1988.
2164. Riccardi, R, Chabner, B, Glaubiger, DL, et al: Influence of tetrahydrouridine on the pharmacokinetics of intrathecally administered 1-β-D-arabinofuranosylcytosine. Cancer Res 42:1736-1739, 1982.
2165. Riccardi, R, Holcenberg, JS, Glaubiger, DL, et al: L-asparaginase pharmacokinetics and asparagine levels in cerebrospinal fluid of rhesus monkeys and humans. Cancer Res 41:4554-4558, 1981.
2166. Riccardi, R, Riccardi, A, Di Rocco, C, et al: Cerebrospinal fluid pharmacokinetics of carboplatin in children with brain tumors. Cancer Chemother Pharmacol 30:21-24, 1992.
2167. Richardson, JB and Callen, JP: Dermatomyositis and malignancy. Med Clin North Am 73:1211-1220, 1989.
2168. Rickles, FR and Edwards, RL: Activation of blood coagulation in cancer: Trousseau's syndrome revisited. Blood 62:14-31, 1983.
2169. Rider, WD: Radiation damage to the brain—A new syndrome. J Can Assoc Radiol 14:67-69, 1963.
2170. Ridgway, EW, Jaffe, N, and Walton, DS: Leukemic ophthalmopathy in children. Cancer 38:1744-1749, 1976.
2171. Ridley, A, Kennard, C, Scholtz, CL, et al: Omnipause neurons in two cases of opsoclonus associated with oat cell carcinoma of the lung. Brain 110:1699-1709, 1987.
2172. Riehl, J-L and Brown, WJ: Acute cerebellar syndrome secondary to 5-fluorouracil therapy. Neurology 14:961-967, 1965.
2173. Riggs, JE: Distinguishing between extrinsic and intrinsic tongue muscle weakness in unilateral hypoglossal palsy. Neurology 34:1367-1368, 1984.
2174. Riggs, JE, Ashraf, M, Snyder, RD, et al: Prospective nerve conduction studies in cisplatin therapy. Ann Neurol 23:92-94, 1988.
2175. Ripps, H, Carr, RE, Siegel, IM, et al: Functional abnormalities in vincristine-induced night blindness. Invest Ophthalmol Vis Sci 25:787-794, 1984.
2176. Ritch, PS: Cis-dichlorodiammineplatinum II-

induced syndrome of inappropriate secretion of antidiuretic hormone. Cancer 61:448-450, 1988.
2177. Ritch, PS, Hansen, RM, and Heuer, DK: Ocular toxicity from high-dose cytosine arabinoside. Cancer 51:430-432, 1983.
2177a. River, Y, Averbuch-Heller, L, Weinberger, M, et al: Antibiotic induced meningitis. J Neurol Neurosurg Psychiatry 57:705-708, 1994.
2178. Rizzo, JF, III and Gittinger, JW, Jr: Selective immunohistochemical staining in the paraneoplastic retinopathy syndrome. Ophthalmology 99:1286-1295, 1992.
2179. Rizzoli, HV and Pagnanelli, DM: Treatment of delayed radiation necrosis of the brain. A clinical observation. J Neurosurg 60:589-594, 1984.
2180. Rizzuto, N and Gambetti, PL: Status spongiosus of rat central nervous system induced by actinomycin D. Acta Neuropathol (Berl) 36:21-30, 1976.
2181. Robb, RM, Ervin, LD, and Sallan, SE: An autopsy study of eye involvement in acute leukemia of childhood. Med Pediatr Oncol 6:171-177, 1979.
2182. Robertson, GL, Bhoopalam, N, and Zelkowitz, LJ: Vincristine neurotoxicity and abnormal secretion of antidiuretic hormone. Arch Intern Med 132:717-720, 1973.
2183. Robinson, HJ, Jr, Hartleben, PD, Lund, G, et al: Evaluation of magnetic resonance imaging in the diagnosis of osteonecrosis of the femoral head. J Bone Joint Surg Am 71:650-663, 1989.
2184. Robinson, WR and Muderspach, LI: Spinal cord compression in metastatic cervical cancer. Gynecol Oncol 48:269-271, 1993.
2185. Rodesch, G, Van Bogaert, P, Mavroudakis, N, et al: Neuroradiologic findings in leptomeningeal carcinomatosis: The value of interest gadolinium-enhanced MRI. Neuroradiology 32:26-32, 1990.
2186. Rodgers, H, Veale, D, Smith, P, et al: Spinal cord compression in polyarteritis nodosa. J R Soc Med 85:707-708, 1992.
2187. Rodichok, LD, Ruckdeschel, JC, and Harper, GR: Early detection and treatment of spinal epidural metastases: The role of myelography. Ann Neurol 20:696-702, 1986.
2188. Rodriguez, GC, Soper, JT, Berchuck, A, et al: Improved palliation of cerebral metastases in epithelial ovarian cancer using a combined modality approach including radiation therapy, chemotherapy, and surgery. J Clin Oncol 10:1553-1560, 1992.
2189. Rodriguez, M, Truh, LI, O'Neill, BP, et al: Autoimmune paraneoplastic cerebellar degeneration: Ultrastructural localization of antibody-binding sites in Purkinje cells. Neurology 38:1380-1386, 1988.
2190. Roessmann, U, Kaufman, B, and Friede, RL: Metastatic lesions in the sella turcica and pituitary gland. Cancer 25:478-480, 1970.
2191. Rogers, LR: Cerebrovascular Complications in Cancer Patients. Oncology 8:23-30, 1994.
2192. Rogers, LR and Barnett, G: Percutaneous aspiration of brain tumor cysts via the Ommaya reservoir system. Neurology 41:279-282, 1991.
2193. Rogers, LR, Borkowski, GP, Albers, JW, et al: Obturator mononeuropathy caused by pelvic cancer: Six cases. Neurology 43:1489-1492, 1993.
2194. Rogers, LR, Cho, E-S, Kempin, S, et al: Cerebral infarction from non-bacterial thrombotic endocarditis. Clinical and pathological study including the effects of anticoagulation. Am J Med 83:746-756, 1987.
2195. Rogers, LR, Duchesneau, PM, Nunez, C, et al: Comparison of cisternal and lumbar CSF examination in leptomeningeal metastasis. Neurology 42:1239-1241, 1992.
2195a. Romero, A, Rabinovich, MG, Vallejo, CT, et al: Vinorelbine as first-line chemotherapy for metastatic breast carcinoma. J Clin Oncol 12:336-341, 1994.
2196. Ron, E, Modan, B, Boice, JD, Jr, et al: Tumors of the brain and nervous system after radiotherapy in childhood. N Engl J Med 319:1033-1039, 1988.
2197. Ron, IG, Inbar, MJ, Barak, Y, et al: Organic delusional syndrome associated with tamoxifen treatment. Cancer 69:1415-1417, 1992.
2198. Roobol, TH, Kazzaz, BA, and Vecht, CJ: Segmental rigidity and spinal myoclonus as a paraneoplastic syndrome. J Neurol Neurosurg Psychiatry 50:628-631, 1987.
2199. Ropper, A: Neurological and Neurosurgical Intensive Care, ed 3. Raven Press, New York, 1993.
2200. Ropper, AH: Lateral displacement of the brain and level of consciousness in patients with an acute hemispheral mass. N Engl J Med 314:953-958, 1986.
2201. Ropper, AH: Treatment of intracranial hypertension. In Ropper, AH (ed): Neurological and Neurosurgical Intensive Care, ed 3. Raven Press, New York, 1993, pp 29-52.
2202. Ropper, AH: Seronegative, non-neoplastic acute cerebellar degeneration. Neurology 43:1602-1605, 1993.
2203. Rosen, P and Armstrong, D: Infective endocarditis in patients treated for malignant neoplastic diseases: A postmortem study. Am J Clin Pathol 60:241-250, 1973.
2204. Rosen, P and Armstrong, D: Nonbacterial thrombotic endocarditis in patients with malignant neoplastic diseases. Am J Med 54:23-29, 1973.
2205. Rosen, ST, Aisner, J, Makuch, RW, et al: Carcinomatous leptomeningitis in small cell lung cancer: A clinicopathologic review of the National Cancer Institute experience. Medicine 61:45-53, 1982.
2206. Rosenberg, SA: Adoptive cellular therapy in patients with advanced cancer. An update. Biological Therapy of Cancer Updates 1:1-15, 1991.
2207. Rosenblum, MK: Paraneoplasia and autoimmunologic injury of the nervous system: The anti-Hu syndrome. Brain Pathol 3:199-212, 1993.
2208. Rosenblum, MK, Delattre, J-Y, Walker, RW, et al: Fatal necrotizing encephalopathy complicating treatment of malignant gliomas with intra-arterial BCNU and irradiation: A pathological study. J Neurooncol 7:269-281, 1989.
2209. Rosenblum, WI: Biology of disease. Aspects of endothelial malfunction and function in cerebral microvessels. Lab Invest 55:252-268, 1986.
2210. Rosenfeld, CS and Broder, LE: Cisplatin-induced autonomic neuropathy. Cancer Treat Rep 68:659-660, 1984.
2211. Rosenfeld, MR and Posner, JB: Paraneoplastic motor neuron disease. In Rowland, LP (ed): Advances in Neurology, vol 56: Amyotrophic Lateral

Sclerosis and Other Motor Neuron Diseases. Raven Press, New York, 1991, pp 445-459.

2212. Rosenfeld, MR, Wong, E, Dalmau, J, et al: Cloning and characterization of a Lambert-Eaton myasthenic syndrome antigen. Ann Neurol 33:113-120, 1993.

2213. Rosenstein, M, Armstrong, J, Kris, M, et al: A reappraisal of the role of prophylactic cranial irradiation in limited small cell lung cancer. Int J Radiat Oncol Biol Phys 24:43-48, 1992.

2214. Rosner, D, Nemoto, T, and Lane, WW: Chemotherapy induces regression of brain metastases in breast carcinoma. Cancer 58:832-839, 1986.

2215. Ross, AT and Zeman, W: Opsoclonus, occult carcinoma, and chemical pathology in dentate nuclei. Arch Neurol 17:546-551, 1967.

2216. Ross, HS, Rosenberg, S, and Friedman, AH: Delayed radiation necrosis of the optic nerve. Am J Ophthalmol 76:683-686, 1973.

2217. Ross, JS, Masaryk, TJ, Modic, MT, et al: Vertebral hemangiomas: MR imaging. Radiology 165:165-169, 1987.

2218. Ross, MH, Abend, WK, Schwartz, RB, et al: A case of C2 herpes zoster with delayed bilateral pontine infarction. Neurology 41:1685-1686, 1991.

2219. Roth, G, Magistris, MR, Le-Fort, D, et al: Post-radiation brachial plexopathy. Persistent conduction block. Myokymic discharges and cramps. Rev Neurol (Paris) 144(3):173-180, 1988.

2220. Rothman, AL, Cheeseman, SH, Lehrman, SN, et al: Herpes simplex encephalitis in a patient with lymphoma: Relapse following acyclovir therapy. JAMA 259:1056-1057, 1988.

2221. Rotstein, J and Good, RA: Steroid pseudorheumatism. Arch Intern Med 99:545-555, 1957.

2222. Rottenberg, DA (ed): Neurological Complications of Cancer Treatment. Butterworth-Heinemann, Boston, 1991.

2223. Rottenberg, DA, Chernik, NL, Deck, MD, et al: Cerebral necrosis following radiotherapy of extracranial neoplasms. Ann Neurol 1:339-357, 1977.

2224. Rottenberg, DA, Hurwitz, BJ, and Posner, JB: The effect of oral glycerol on intraventricular pressure in man. Neurology 27:600-608, 1977.

2225. Rottenberg, DA and Posner, JB: Intracranial pressure control. In Cottrell, JE and Turndorf, H (eds): Anesthesia and Neurosurgery. CV Mosby, St Louis, 1980, pp 89-118.

2226. Rowed, DW, Kassel, EE, and Lewis, AJ: Transorbital intracavernous needle biopsy in painful ophthalmoplegia. Case report. J Neurosurg 62:776-780, 1985.

2227. Rowinsky, EK, Eisenhauer, EA, Chaudhry, V, et al: Clinical toxicities encountered with paclitaxel (TAXOL). Semin Oncol 20(No 4, Suppl 3):1-15, 1993.

2228. Rowland, LP and Schneck, SA: Neuromuscular disorders associated with malignant neoplastic disease. J Chronic Dis 16:777-795, 1963.

2229. Rowland, LP, Sherman, WH, Latov, N, et al: Amyotrophic lateral sclerosis and lymphoma: Bone marrow examination and other diagnostic tests. Neurology 42:1101-1102, 1992.

2230. Roy, PH and Beahrs, OH: Spinal accessory nerve in radical neck dissections. Am J Surg 118:800-804, 1969.

2231. Rozental, JM, Levine, RL, Nickles, RJ, et al: Cerebral diaschisis in patients with malignant glioma. J Neurooncol 8:153-161, 1990.

2232. Rubenstein, CL, Varni, JW, and Katz, ER: Cognitive functioning in long-term survivors of childhood leukemia: A prospective analysis. J Dev Behav Pediatr 11:301-305, 1990.

2233. Rubin, AM and Kang, H: Cerebral blindness and encephalopathy with cyclosporin A toxicity. Neurology 37:1072-1076, 1987.

2234. Rubin, EH, Andersen, JW, Berg, DT, et al: Risk factors for high-dose cytarabine neurotoxicity: An analysis of a Cancer and Leukemia Group B trial in patients with acute myeloid leukemia. J Clin Oncol 10:948-953, 1992.

2235. Rubin, J and Yu, VL: Malignant external otitis: Insights into pathogenesis, clinical manifestations, diagnosis, and therapy. Am J Med 85:391-398, 1988.

2236. Rubin, P: Extradural spinal cord compression by tumor. I. Experimental production and treatment trials. Radiology 93:1243-1248, 1969.

2237. Rubin, P, Whitaker, JN, Ceckler, TL, et al: Myelin basic protein and magnetic resonance imaging for diagnosing radiation myelopathy. Int J Radiat Oncol Biol Phys 15:1371-1381, 1988.

2238. Rubin, RH and Young, LS (eds): Clinical Approach to Infection in the Compromised Host. Plenum Press, New York, 1987.

2239. Rubinstein, AB, Schein, M, and Reichenthal, E: The association of carcinoma of the breast with meningioma. Surg Gynecol Obstet 169:334-336, 1989.

2240. Rubinstein, LJ, Herman, MM, Long, TG, et al: Disseminated necrotizing leukoencephalopathy: A complication of treated central nervous system leukemia and lymphoma. Cancer 35:291-305, 1975.

2241. Rubinstein, MK: Cranial mononeuropathy as the first sign of intracranial metastases. Ann Intern Med 70:49-54, 1969.

2242. Rudd, A, McKenzie, JG, and Millard, PH: Carcinoma of the bronchus presenting with hemichorea. Letter to the Editor. J Neurol Neurosurg Psychiatry 49:1210-1211, 1986.

2243. Ruff, RL and Lanska, DJ: Epidural metastases in prospectively evaluated veterans with cancer and back pain. Cancer 63:2234-2241, 1989.

2244. Ruff, RL and Posner, JB: The incidence of systemic venous thrombosis and the risk of anticoagulation in patients with malignant gliomas. Trans Am Neurol Assoc 106:223-226, 1981.

2245. Ruff, RL, Wiener, SN, and Leigh, RJ: Magnetic resonance imaging in patients with diplopia. A review. Invest Radiol 21:311-319, 1986.

2246. Ruifrok, AC, Stephens, LC, and van der Kogel, AJ: Radiation response of the rat cervical spinal cord after irradiation at different ages: Tolerance, latency and pathology. Int J Radiat Oncol Biol Phys 29:73-79, 1994.

2247. Ruifrok, ACC, Kleiboer, BJ, and van der Kogel, AJ: Radiation tolerance and fractionation sensitivity of the developing rat cervical spinal cord. Int J Radiat Oncol Biol Phys 24:505-510, 1992.

2248. Ruiz, L, Gilden, J, Jaffe, N, et al: Auditory function in pediatric osteosarcoma patients treated with multiple dose of cis-diamminedichloroplatinum (II). Cancer Res 49:742-744, 1989.

2249. Ruiz, MA, Marugan, I, Estelles, A, et al: The influence of chemotherapy on plasma coagulation and fibrinolytic systems in lung cancer patients. Cancer 63:643-648, 1989.

2250. Rush, JA and Younge, BR: Paralysis of cranial nerves III, IV, and VI. Cause and prognosis in 1,000 cases. Arch Ophthalmol 99:76-79, 1981.

2251. Rushton, JG and Rooke, ED: Brain tumor headache. Headache 2:147-152, 1962.

2252. Russell, DM, Prendergast, PJ, Darby, PL, et al: A comparison between muscle function and body composition in anorexia nervosa: The effect of refeeding. Am J Clin Nutr 38:229-237, 1983.

2252a. Russell, JW, Windebank, AJ, and Podratz, JL: Role of nerve growth factor in suramin neurotoxicity studies in vitro. Ann Neurol 36:221-228, 1994.

2253. Russell, NA, Belanger, G, Benoit, BG, et al: Spinal epidural lipomatosis: A complication of glucocorticoid therapy. Can J Neurol Sci 11:383-386, 1984.

2254. Russell, RWR and Wade, JPH: Haematological causes of cerebrovascular disease. In Toole, JF (ed): Handbook of Clinical Neurology, vol 55, Vascular Diseases, Part III. Elsevier, New York, 1989, pp 463-481.

2255. Rustin, GJS, Newlands, ES, Begent, RHJ, et al: Weekly alternating etoposide, methotrexate, and actinomycin/vincristine and cyclophosphamide chemotherapy for the treatment of CNS metastases of choriocarcinoma. J Clin Oncol 7:900-903, 1989.

2256. Ryback, RS, Eckardt, MH, and Paulter, CP: Clinical relationships between serum phosphorus and other blood chemistry values in alcoholics. Arch Intern Med 140:673-677, 1980.

2257. Sabbagh, R, Shields, CL, Shields, JA, et al: Spontaneous hyphema. Initial manifestation of lung carcinoma. JAMA 266:3194, 1991.

2258. Sack, GH, Jr, Levin, J, and Bell, WR: Trousseau's syndrome and other manifestations of chronic disseminated coagulopathy in patients with neoplasms: Clinical, pathophysiologic, and therapeutic features. Medicine 56:1-37, 1977.

2259. Sackellares, JC, Lee, SI, and Dreifuss, FE: Stupor following administration of valproic acid to patients receiving other antiepileptic drugs. Epilepsia 20:697-703, 1979.

2260. Sacks, JG and O'Grady, RB: Painful ophthalmoplegia and endophthalmos due to metastatic carcinoma: Simulation of essential facial hemiatrophy. Transactions–American Academy of Ophthalmology and Otolaryngology 75:351-354, 1971.

2261. Sadiq, SA, Thomas, FP, Kilidireas, K, et al: The spectrum of neurologic disease associated with anti-GM1 antibodies. Neurology 40:1067-1072, 1990.

2262. Sadowsky, CH, Sachs, E, Jr, and Ochoa, J: Postradiation motor neuron syndrome. Arch Neurol 33:786-787, 1976.

2263. Saengnipanthkul, S, Jiraraltanaphochai, K, Rojviroj, S, et al: Metastatic adenocarcinoma of the spine. Spine 17:427-430, 1992.

2264. Sagar, HJ and Read, DJ: Subacute sensory neuropathy with remission: An association with lymphoma. J Neurol Neurosurg Psychiatry 45:83-85, 1982.

2265. Sagar, SM, Thomas, RJ, Loverock, LT, et al: Olfactory sensations produced by high-energy photon irradiation of the olfactory receptor mucosa in humans. Int J Radiat Oncol Biol Phys 20:771-776, 1991.

2266. Sage, MR: Blood–brain barrier: Phenomenon of increasing importance to the imaging clinician. AJR 138:887-898, 1982.

2267. Sahenk, Z, Brady, ST, and Mendell, JR: Studies on the pathogenesis of vincristine-induced neuropathy. Muscle Nerve 10:80-84, 1987.

2268. Said, G, Lacroix, C, Chemouilli, P, et al: Cytomegalovirus neuropathy in acquired immunodeficiency syndrome: A clinical and pathological study. Ann Neurol 29:139-146, 1991.

2269. Sakai, K, Mitchell, DJ, Tsukamoto, T, et al: Isolation of a complementary DNA clone encoding an autoantigen recognized by an anti-neuronal cell antibody from a patient with paraneoplastic cerebellar degeneration. Ann Neurol 28:692-698, 1990.

2270. Sakai, Y, Kobayashi, K, and Iwata, N: Effects of an anabolic steroid and vitamin B complex upon myopathy induced by corticosteroids. Eur J Pharmacol 52:353-359, 1978.

2271. Salahuddin, TS, Johansson, BB, Kalimo, H, et al: Structural changes in the rat brain after carotid infusions of hyperosmolar solutions. An electron microscopic study. Acta Neuropathol (Berl) 77:5-13, 1988.

2272. Salaki, JS, Louria, DB, and Chmel, H: Fungal and yeast infections of the central nervous system. A clinical review. Medicine (Baltimore) 63:108-132, 1984.

2273. Salata, RA, King RE, Gose, F, et al: *Listeria monocytogenes* cerebritis, bacteremia, and cutaneous lesions complicating hairy cell leukemia. Am J Med 81:1068-1072, 1986.

2274. Salbeck, R, Grau, HC, and Artmann, H: Cerebral tumor staging in patients with bronchial carcinoma by computed tomography. Cancer 66:2007-2011, 1990.

2275. Salcman, M and Broadwell, RD: The blood-brain barrier. In Salcman, M (ed): Neurobiology of Brain Tumors, vol 4, Concepts in Neurosurgery. Williams & Wilkins, Baltimore, 1991, pp 229-249.

2276. Saleh, MN, Christian, ES, and Diamond, BR: Intrathecal cytosine arabinoside-induced acute, rapidly reversible paralysis. Am J Med 86:729-730, 1989.

2277. Salick, AI and Pearson, CM: Electrical silence of myoedema. Neurology 17:899-901, 1967.

2278. Salner, AL, Botnick, LE, Herzog, AG, et al: Reversible brachial plexopathy following primary radiation therapy for breast cancer. Cancer Treat Rep 65:797-802, 1981.

2279. Samaan, NA, Pham, FK, Sellin, RV, et al: Successful treatment of hypoglycemia using glucagon in a patient with an extrapancreatic tumor. Ann Intern Med 113:404-406, 1990.

2280. Samlowski, WE, Park, KJ, Galinsky, RE, et al: Intrathecal administration of interleukin-2 for meningeal carcinomatosis due to malignant melanoma: Sequential evaluation of intracranial pressure, cerebrospinal fluid cytology, and cytokine induction. J Immunother 13:49-54, 1993.

2281. Samuels, BL, Vogelzang, NJ, and Kennedy, BJ: Vascular toxicity following vinblastine, bleomycin, and cisplatin therapy for germ cell tumours. Int J Androl 10:363-369, 1987.

2282. Samuels, ML, Leary, WV, Alexanian, R, et al: Clinical trials with N-isopropyl-alpha-(2-methylhydrazino)-p-tolnamide hydrochloride in malignant lymphoma and other disseminated neoplasia. Cancer 20:1187-1194, 1967.

2283. Sanchez-Reyes, A, Farrus, B, and Biete, A: A new theoretical formula for fractionated radiotherapy based on a saturable cellular repair mechanism. Acta Oncol 32:57-62, 1993.

2284. Sanda, MG, Yang, JC, Topalian, SL, et al: Intravenous administration of recombinant human macrophage colony-stimulating factor to patients with metastatic cancer: A phase I study. J Clin Oncol 10:1643-1649, 1992.

2285. Sande, MA, Whitley, RJ, McCracken, GH, et al: Evaluation of new anti-infective drugs for the treatment of toxoplasma encephalitis. Infectious Diseases Society of America and the Food and Drug Administration. Clin Infect Dis 15(Suppl 1):S200-S205, 1992.

2286. Sanderson, IR, Pritchard, J, and Marsh, HT: Chemotherapy as the initial treatment of spinal cord compression due to disseminated neuroblastoma. J Neurosurg 70:688-690, 1989.

2287. Sanderson, PA, Kuwabara, T, and Cogan, DG: Optic neuropathy presumably caused by vincristine therapy. Am J Ophthalmol 81:146-150, 1976.

2288. Saphner, T, Gallion, HH, van Nagell, JR, et al: Neurologic complications of cervical cancer. A review of 2261 cases. Cancer 64:1147-1151, 1989.

2289. Saphner, T, Tormey, DC, and Gray, R: Venous and arterial thrombosis in patients who received adjuvant therapy for breast cancer. J Clin Oncol 9:286-294, 1991.

2290. Sapozink, MD and Kaplan, HS: Intracranial Hodgkin's disease. A report of 12 cases and review of the literature. Cancer 52:1301-1307, 1983.

2291. Saris, SC, Patronas, NJ, Rosenberg, SA, et al: The effect of intravenous interleukin-2 on brain water content. J Neurosurg 71:169-174, 1989.

2292. Sarma, DP and Godeau, L: Brain metastasis from prostatic cancer. J Surg Oncol 23:173-174, 1983.

2293. Sarpel, S, Sarpel, G, Yu, E, et al: Early diagnosis of spinal-epidural metastasis by magnetic resonance imaging. Cancer 59:1112-1116, 1987.

2293a. Sasso, E, Delsoldato, S, Negrotti, A, et al: Reversible valproate-induced extrapyramidal disorders. Epilepsia 35:391-393, 1994.

2294. Sato, S, Inuzuka, T, Nakano, R, et al: Antibody to a zinc finger protein in a patient with paraneoplastic cerebellar degeneration. Biochem Biophys Res Commun 178:198-206, 1991.

2295. Sauer, EG, Dearing, WH, and Wollaeger, EE: Serious untoward gastrointestinal manifestations possibly related to administration of cortisone and corticotropin. Proc Staff Meet Mayo Clin 28:641-649, 1953.

2296. Sause, WT, Crowley, J, Eyre, HJ, et al: Whole brain irradiation and intrathecal methotrexate in the treatment of solid tumor leptomeningeal metastases—a Southwest Oncology Group study. J Neurooncol 6:107-112, 1988.

2297. Sauter, NP, Atkins, MB, Mier, JW, et al: Transient thyrotoxicosis and persistent hypothyroidism due to acute autoimmune thyroiditis after interleukin-2 and interferon-alpha therapy for metastatic carcinoma: A case report. Am J Med 92:441-444, 1992.

2298. Savaraj, N, Feun, LG, Lu, K, et al: Pharmacology of intrathecal VP-16-213 in dogs. J Neurooncol 13:211-215, 1992.

2299. Savino, PJ, Hilliker, JK, Casell, GH, et al: Chronic sixth nerve palsies. Are they really harbingers of serious intracranial disease? Arch Ophthalmol 100:1442-1444, 1982.

2300. Savitz, MH and Anderson, PJ: Primary melanoma of the leptomeninges: A review. Mt Sinai J Med 41:774-791, 1974.

2301. Sawaya, R and Donlon, JA: Chronic disseminated intravascular coagulation and metastatic brain tumor: A case report and review of the literature. Neurosurgery 12:580-584, 1983.

2302. Sawaya, R and Glas-Greenwalt, P: Postoperative venous thromboembolism and brain tumors: Part II. Hemostatic profile. J Neurooncol 14:127-134, 1992.

2302a. Sawaya, R, Rayford, A, Kona, S, et al: Plasminogen activator inhibitor-1 in the pathogenesis of delayed radiation damage in rat spinal cord *in vivo*. J Neurosurg 81:381-387, 1994.

2303. Sawaya, R, Zuccarello, M, Elkalliny, M, et al: Postoperative venous thromboembolism and brain tumors: Part I. Clinical profile. J Neurooncol 14:119-125, 1992.

2304. Schabet, M, Ohneseit, P, Buchholz, R, et al: Intrathecal ACNU treatment of B16 melanoma leptomeningeal metastasis in a new athymic rat model. J Neurooncol 14:169-175, 1992.

2305. Schachter, S and Freeman, R: Transient ischemic attack and Adriamycin cardiomyopathy. Neurology 32:1380-1381, 1982.

2306. Schackert, G, Price, JE, Bucana, CD, et al: Unique patterns of brain metastasis produced by different human carcinomas in athymic nude mice. Int J Cancer 44:892-897, 1989.

2307. Scheithauer, W, Ludwig, H, and Maida, E: Acute encephalopathy associated with continuous vincristine sulfate combination therapy: Case report. Invest New Drugs 3:315-318, 1985.

2308. Scheld, WM, Whitley, RJ, and Durack, DT: Infections of the Central Nervous System. Raven Press, New York, 1991.

2309. Schell, MJ, McHaney, VA, Green, AA, et al: Hearing loss in children and young adults receiving cisplatin with or without prior cranial irradiation. J Clin Oncol 7:754-760, 1989.

2310. Scher, HI and Yagoda, A: Bone metastases: Pathogenesis, treatment and rationale for use of resorption inhibitors. Am J Med 82(2A):6-28, 1987.

2311. Scherokman, B, Filling-Katz, MR, and Tell, D: Brachial plexus neuropathy following high-dose cytarabine in acute monoblastic leukemia. Cancer Treat Rep 69:1005-1006, 1985.

2312. Schiff, D and DeAngelis, LM: Therapy of venous thromboembolism in patients with brain metastasis. Cancer 73:493-498, 1994.

2312a. Schiff, D, Shaw, EG, and Cascino, TL: Outcome after spinal re-irradiation for malignant epidural spinal cord compression. Ann Neurol. In press, 1995.

2313. Schiller, JH and Witt, PL: Levamisole: Clinical and biological effects. Biological Therapy of Cancer Updates 2(9):1-14, 1992.

2314. Schimandle, JH and Levine, AM: An isolated nonosseous metastasis to the epidural space from an osteogenic sarcoma. Cancer 69:103-107, 1992.

2315. Schimpff, S, Serpick, A, Stoler, B, et al: Varicella-zoster infection in patients with cancer. Ann Intern Med 765:241-254, 1972.

2315a. Schinkel, AH, Smit, JJM, van Tellingen, O, et al: Disruption of the mouse mdrla-P-Glycoprotein gene leads to a deficiency in the blood–brain barrier and to increased sensitivity to drugs. Cell 77:491-502, 1994.

2316. Schiodt, AV and Kristensen, O: Neurologic complications after irradiation of malignant tumors of the testis. Acta Radiol Oncol Radiat Phys Biol 17:369-378, 1978.

2317. Schipper, HI, Bardosi, A, Jacobi, C, et al: Meningeal carcinomatosis: Origin of local IgG production in the CSF. Neurology 38:413-416, 1988.

2318. Schirner, M, Lichtner, RB, and Schneider, MR: The stable prostacyclin analogue Cicaprost inhibits its metastasis to lungs and lymph nodes in the 13762NF MTLn3 rat mammary carcinoma. Clin Exp Metastasis 12:24-30, 1994.

2319. Schlesinger, JJ, Salit, IE, and McCormack, G: Streptococcal meningitis after myelography. Arch Neurol 39:576-577, 1982.

2320. Schlesinger, LS, Ross, SC, and Schaberg, DR: *Staphylococcus aureus* meningitis: A broad-based epidemiologic study. Medicine (Baltimore) 66:148-156, 1987.

2321. Schlitt, M, Morawetz, RB, Bonnin, J, et al: Progressive multifocal leukoencephalopathy: Three patients diagnosed by brain biopsy, with prolonged survival in two. Neurosurgery 18:407-414, 1986.

2322. Schmidbauer, M, Budka, H, Pilz, P, et al: Presence, distribution and spread of productive varicella zoster virus infection in nervous tissues. Brain 115:383-398, 1992.

2323. Schmidbauer, M, Budka, H, and Shah, KV: Progressive multifocal leukoencephalopathy (PML) in AIDS and in the pre-AIDS era. A neuropathological comparison using immunocytochemistry and in situ DNA hybridization for virus detection. Acta Neuropathol (Berl) 80:375-380, 1990.

2324. Schmidley, JW and Galloway, P: Polymyositis following autologous bone marrow transplantation in Hodgkin's disease. Neurology 40:1003-1004, 1990.

2325. Schmidt, D, Einicke, I, and Haenel, F: The influence of seizure type on the efficacy of plasma concentrations of phenytoin, phenobarbital, and carbamazepine. Arch Neurol 43:263-265, 1986.

2326. Schmidt, T and Tauber, MG: Pharmacodynamics of antibiotics in the therapy of meningitis: Infection model observations. J Antimicrob Chemother 31(Suppl D):61-70, 1993.

2327. Schold, SC, Cho, ES, Somasundaram, M, et al: Subacute motor neuronopathy: A remote effect of lymphoma. Ann Neurol 5:271-287, 1979.

2328. Schold, SC, Wasserstrom, WR, Fleisher, M, et al: Cerebrospinal fluid biochemical markers of central nervous system metastases. Ann Neurol 8:597-604, 1980.

2329. Schor, JD, Levkoff, SE, Lipsitz, LA, et al: Risk factors for delirium in hospitalized elderly. JAMA 267:827-831, 1992.

2330. Schramm, J and Umbach, W: Simultaneous occurrence of spinal tumor and lumbar disk herniation. Neurochirurgica 20:22-28, 1977.

2331. Schriner, RW, Ryu, JH, and Edwards, WD: Microscopic pulmonary tumor embolism causing subacute cor pulmonale: A difficult antemortem diagnosis. Mayo Clin Proc 66:143-148, 1991.

2332. Schubiger, O and Haller, D: Metastases to the pituitary-hypothalamic axis. An MR study of 7 symptomatic patients. Neuroradiology 34:131-134, 1992.

2333. Schuchter, LM, Luginbuhl, WE, and Meropol, NJ: The current status of toxicity protectants in cancer therapy. Semin Oncol 19:742-751, 1992.

2334. Schukneckt, B, Huber, P, Buller, B, et al: Spinal leptomeningeal neoplastic disease. Evaluation by MR, myelography and CT myelography. Eur Neurol 32:11-16, 1992.

2335. Schulman, P, Kerr, LD, and Spiera, H: A reexamination of the relationship between myositis and malignancy. J Rheumatol 18:1689-1692, 1991.

2336. Schultheiss, TE: Spinal cord radiation "tolerance": Doctrine versus data. Int J Radiat Oncol Biol Phys 19:219-221, 1991.

2337. Schultheiss, TE, Higgins, EM, and El-Mahdi, AM: The latent period in clinical radiation myelopathy. Int J Radiat Oncol Biol Phys 10:1109-1115, 1984.

2338. Schultheiss, TE, Stephens, LC, and Maor, MH: Analysis of the histopathology of radiation myelopathy. Int J Radiat Oncol Biol Phys 14:27-32, 1988.

2339. Schultheiss, TE, Stephens, LC, and Peters, LJ: Survival in radiation myelopathy. Int J Radiat Oncol Biol Phys 12:1765-1769, 1986.

2340. Schumann, GB and Crisman, LG: Cerebrospinal fluid cytopathology. Clin Lab Med 5:275-302, 1985.

2341. Schwartz, CL, Miller, NR, Wharam, MD, et al: The optic nerve as the site of initial relapse in childhood acute lymphoblastic leukemia. Cancer 63:1616-1620, 1989.

2342. Schwartzmann, RJ and Hill, JB: Neurologic complications of disseminated intravascular coagulation. Neurology 32:791-797, 1982.

2343. Schweinle, JE and Alperin, JB: Central nervous system recurrence ten years after remission of acute lymphoblastic leukemia. Cancer 45:16-18, 1980.

2344. Schwid, S, Ketonen, L, Betts, R, et al: Cerebrovascular complications after primary varicella-zoster infection. Letter to the Editor. Lancet 340:669, 1992.

2345. Scott, M: Lower extremity pain simulating sciatica. Tumors of the high thoracic and cervical cord as causes. JAMA 160:528-534, 1956.

2346. Scott, TF: A new cause of cerebrospinal fluid eosinophilia: Neurosarcoidosis. Letter to the Editor. Am J Med 84:973-974, 1988.

2347. Scott, WW, Jr, Siegelman, SS, Harrington, DP, et al: Diagnosis and pathophysiology of paradoxical embolism. Radiology 121:59-62, 1976.

2348. Scott-Moncrieff, JCR, Chan, TCK, Samuels, ML, et al: Plasma and cerebrospinal fluid pharmacokinetics of cytosine arabinoside in dogs. Cancer Chemother Pharmacol 29:13-18, 1991.

2349. Sculier, J-P, Feld, R, Evans, WK, et al: Neurologic disorders in patients with small cell lung cancer. Cancer 60:2275-2283, 1987.

2350. Scully, RE, Mark, EJ, McNeely, WF, et al: Case records of the Massachusetts General Hospital. Case 14—1988. N Engl J Med 318:903-915, 1988.

2351. Scully, RE, Mark, EJ, McNeely, WF, et al: Case records of the Massachusetts General Hospital. Case 9—1988. N Engl J Med 318:563-570, 1988.

2352. Segal, GM and Duckert, LG: Reversible mechlorethamine-associated hearing loss in a patient with Hodgkin's disease. Cancer 57:1089-1091, 1986.

2353. Segredo, V, Caldwell, JE, Matthay, MA, et al: Persistent paralysis in critically ill patients after long-term administration of vecuronium. N Engl J Med 327:524-528, 1992.

2353a. Seidman, AD and Barrett, S: Photopsia during 3-hour paclitaxel administration at doses >250 mg/m^2. J Clin Oncol 12:1741-1742, 1994.

2354. Seifter, EJ, Parker, RI, Gralnick, HR, et al: Abnormal coagulation results in patients with Hodgkin's disease. Am J Med 78:942-950, 1985.

2355. Seiter, S, Arch, R, Reber, S, et al: Prevention of tumor metastasis formation by anti-variant CD44. J Exp Med 177:443-455, 1993.

2356. Sekas, G and Paul, HS: Hyperammonemia and carnitine deficiency in a patient receiving sulfadiazine and pyrimethamine. Am J Med 95:112-113, 1993.

2357. Sengupta, RP, So, SC, and Perry, RH: Nodular fasciitis: An unusual cause of extradural spinal cord compression. Br J Surg 62:573-575, 1975.

2358. Sepkowitz, KA, Brown, AE, and Telzak, EE: *Pneumocystis carinii* pneumonia among patients without AIDS at a cancer hospital. JAMA 267:832-837, 1992.

2359. Seyfert, S, Kabbeck-Kupijai, D, Marx, P, et al: Cerebrospinal fluid cell preparation methods. An evaluation. Acta Cytol 36:927-931, 1992.

2360. Seymour, JF and Rodriguez, MA: Mental neuropathy (numb chin syndrome): A harbinger of tumor progression or relapse. Letter to the Editor. Cancer 71:874-875, 1993.

2361. Shaikh, BS, Appelbaum, PC, and Aber, RC: Vertebral disk space infection and osteomyelitis due to *Candida albicans* in a patient with acute myelomonocytic leukemia. Cancer 45:1025-1028, 1980.

2362. Shalev, O and Silverberg, R: Dexamethasone for acute radiation encephalopathy. Letter to the Editor. Lancet 2:574-575, 1978.

2363. Shapiro, ET, Bell, GI, Polonsky, KS, et al: Tumor hypoglycemia: Relationship to high molecular weight insulin-like growth factor-II. J Clin Invest 85:1672-1679, 1990.

2364. Shapiro, R and Janzen, AH: Osteoblastic metastases to floor of skull simulating meningioma en plaque. AJR 81:964-966, 1959.

2365. Shapiro, WR, Chernik, NL, and Posner, JB: Necrotizing encephalopathy following intraventricular instillation of methotrexate. Arch Neurol 28:96-102, 1973.

2366. Shapiro, WR, Hiesiger, EM, Cooney, GA, et al: Temporal effects of dexamethasone on blood-to-brain and blood-to-tumor transport of 14C-alpha-aminoisobutyric acid in rat C6 glioma. J Neurooncol 8:197-204, 1990.

2367. Shapiro, WR, Posner, JB, Ushio, Y, et al: Treatment of meningeal neoplasms. Cancer Treat Rep 61:733-743, 1977.

2368. Shapiro, WR, Voorhies, RM, Hiesiger, EM, et al: Pharmacokinetics of tumor cell exposure to [14C]methotrexate after intracarotid administration without and with hyperosmotic opening of the blood–brain and blood–tumor barriers in rat brain tumors: A quantitative autoradiographic study. Cancer Res 48:694-701, 1988.

2369. Shapiro, WR, Young, DF, and Mehta, BM: Methotrexate: Distribution in cerebrospinal fluid after intravenous, ventricular and lumbar injections. N Engl J Med 293:161-166, 1975.

2370. Sharfstein, SS, Sack, DS, and Fauci, AS: Relationship between alternate-day corticosteroid therapy and behavioral abnormalities. JAMA 248:2987-2989, 1982.

2371. Sharpe, JA: Visual dysfunction with basal skull tumours. Can J Neurol Sci 12:332-335, 1985.

2372. Shaw, B, Mansfield, FL, and Borges, L: One-stage posterolateral decompression and stabilization for primary and metastatic vertebral tumors in the thoracic and lumbar spine. J Neurosurg 70:405-410, 1989.

2372a. Shaw, EG, Su, JQ, Eagan, RT, et al: Prophylactic cranial irradiation in complete responders with small-cell lung cancer: Analysis of the Mayo Clinic and North Central Cancer Treatment Group databases. J Clin Oncol 12:2327-2332, 1994.

2373. Shaw, PJ and Bates, D: Conservative treatment of delayed cerebral radiation necrosis. J Neurol Neurosurg Psychiatry 47:1338-1341, 1984.

2374. Shaw, PJ, Procopis, PG, Menser, MA, et al: Bulbar and pseudobulbar palsy complicating therapy with high-dose cytosine arabinoside in children with leukemia. Med Pediatr Oncol 19:122-125, 1991.

2375. Shay, M, Braester, A, and Cohen, I: Dermatomyositis as presenting symptom of Hodgkin's disease. Ann Hematol 63:116-118, 1991.

2376. Sheeler, LR, Myers, JH, Eversman, JJ, et al: Adrenal insufficiency secondary to carcinoma metastatic to the adrenal gland. Cancer 52:1312-1316, 1983.

2377. Sheldon, R and Slaughter, D: A syndrome of microangiopathic hemolytic anemia, renal impair-

ment, and pulmonary edema in chemotherapy-treated patients with adenocarcinoma. Cancer 58:1428-1436, 1986.
2378. Sheline, GE and Brady, LW: Radiation therapy for brain metastases. J Neurooncol 4:219-225, 1987.
2379. Sheline, GE, Wara, WM, and Smith, V: Therapeutic irradiation and brain injury. Int J Radiat Oncol Biol Phys 6:1215-1228, 1980.
2380. Shepherd, FA, Laskey, J, Evans, WK, et al: Cushing's syndrome associated with ectopic corticotropin production and small-cell lung cancer. J Clin Oncol 10:21-27, 1992.
2381. Sheppeard, H, Cleak, DK, Ward, DJ, et al: A review of early mortality and morbidity in elderly patients following Charnley total hip replacement. Arch Orthop Trauma Surg 97:243-248, 1980.
2382. Sherlock, P and Hartmann, WH: Adrenal steroids and the pattern of metastases of breast cancer. JAMA 181:313-317, 1962.
2383. Shevell, MI and Rosenblatt, DS: The neurology of cobalamin. Can J Neurol Sci 19:472-486, 1992.
2384. Shewmon, DA and Masdeu, JC: Delayed radiation necrosis of the brain contralateral to original tumor. Arch Neurol 37:592-594, 1980.
2385. Shibata, S: Ultrastructure of capillary walls in human brain tumors. Acta Neuropathol (Berl) 78:561-571, 1989.
2386. Shibutani, M and Okeda, R: Experimental study on subacute neurotoxicity of methotrexate in cats. Acta Neuropathol (Berl) 78:291-300, 1989.
2387. Shibutani, M, Okeda, R, Hori, A, et al: Methotrexate-related multifocal axonopathy. Report of an autopsy case. Acta Neuropathol (Berl) 79:333-335, 1989.
2388. Shimamura, K, Oka, K, Nakazawa, M, et al: Distribution patterns of microthrombi in disseminated intravascular coagulation. Arch Pathol Lab Med 107:543-547, 1983.
2389. Shimamura, Y, Chikama, M, Tanimoto, T, et al: Optic nerve degeneration caused by supraophthalmic carotid artery infusion with cisplatin and ACNU. Case report. J Neurosurg 72:285-288, 1990.
2390. Shimizu, K, Okamoto, Y, Miyao, Y, et al: Adoptive immunotherapy of human meningeal gliomatosis and carcinomatosis with LAK cells and recombinant interleukin-2. J Neurosurg 66:519-521, 1987.
2391. Shimizu, K, Ushio, Y, Hayakawa, T, et al: Combination chemotherapy with 1-(4-amino-2-methyl-5-pyrimidinyl)methyl-3-(2-choroethyl)-3-nitrosourea hydrochloride and bleomycin in meningeal carcinomatosis in rats. Cancer Res 40:1341-1343, 1980.
2392. Shingleton, BJ, Bienfang, DC, Albert, DM, et al: Ocular toxicity associated with high-dose carmustine. Arch Ophthalmol 100:1766-1772, 1982.
2393. Shinonaga, M, Chang, CC, Suzuki, N, et al: Immunohistological evaluation of macrophage infiltrates in brain tumors. Correlation with peritumoral edema. J Neurosurg 68:259-265, 1988.
2394. Shivers, RR, Kavaliers, M, Teskey, GC, et al: Magnetic resonance imaging temporarily alters blood–brain barrier permeability in the rat. Neurosci Lett 76:25-31, 1987.
2395. Shoenfeld, Y, Aderka, D, Sandbank, U, et al: Fatal peripheral neurolymphomatosis after remission of histiocytic lymphoma. Neurology 33:243-245, 1983.
2396. Shome, DK, Gupta, NK, Prajapati, NC, et al: Orbital granulocytic sarcomas (myeloid sarcomas) in acute nonlymphocytic leukemia. Cancer 70:2298-2301, 1992.
2397. Shortliffe, EH and Crapo, LM: Thyroid carcinoma with spinal cord compression. Letter to the Editor. JAMA 247:1565-1566, 1982.
2398. Shuangshoti, S, Tangchai, P, and Netsky, MG: Primary adenocarcinoma of choroid plexus. Arch Pathol 91:101-106, 1971.
2399. Shuffler, MD, Baird, HW, Fleming, CR, et al: Intestinal pseudo-obstruction as the presenting manifestation of small-cell carcinoma of the lung. A paraneoplastic neuropathy of the gastrointestinal tract. Ann Intern Med 98:129-134, 1983.
2400. Shukovsky, LJ and Fletcher, GH: Retinal and optic nerve complications in a high dose irradiation technique of ethmoid sinus and nasal cavity. Radiology 104:629-634, 1972.
2401. Siatkowski, RM, Lam, BL, Schatz, NJ, et al: Optic neuropathy in Hodgkin's disease. Am J Ophthalmol 114:625-629, 1992.
2402. Sidi, Y, Douer, D, and Pinkhas, J: Sicca syndrome in a patient with toxic reaction to busulfan. Case report. JAMA 238:1951, 1977.
2403. Sieben, GM, De Reuck, JL, De Bruyne, JC, et al: Subacute necrotic myelopathy. Its appearance eight years after cure of a breast carcinoma. Arch Neurol 38:775-777, 1981.
2404. Siefert, E: Uber die multiple Karzinomatose des Zentralnervensystems. Münchener Medizinische Wochenschrift 49:826-828, 1902.
2404a. Siegal, T, Lossos, A, and Pfeffer, MR: Leptomeningeal metastases: Analysis of 31 patients with sustained off-therapy response following combined-modality therapy. Neurology 44:1463-1469, 1994.
2405. Siegal, T and Siegal, T: Current considerations in the management of neoplastic spinal cord compression. Spine 14:223-228, 1989.
2406. Siegal, T and Siegal, T: Participation of serotonergic mechanisms in the pathophysiology of experimental neoplastic spinal cord compression. Neurology 41:574-580, 1991.
2407. Siegal, T and Siegal, T: Serotonergic manipulations in experimental neoplastic spinal cord compression. J Neurosurg 78:929-937, 1993.
2408. Siegal, T and Haim, N: Cisplatin-induced peripheral neuropathy. Frequent off-therapy deterioration, demyelinating syndromes, and muscle cramps. Cancer 66:1117-1123, 1990.
2409. Siegal, T, Siegal, T, and Lossos, F: Experimental neoplastic spinal cord compression: Effect of anti-inflammatory agents and glutamate receptor antagonists on vascular permeability. Neurosurgery 26:967-970, 1990.
2410. Siegal, T, Mildworf, B, Stein, D, et al: Leptomeningeal metastases: Reduction of regional cerebral blood flow and cognitive impairment. Ann Neurol 17:100-102, 1985.
2411. Siegal, T, Siegal, T, Robin, G, et al: Anterior decompression of the spine for metastatic epidural cord compression: A promising avenue of therapy? Ann Neurol 11:28-34, 1982.

2412. Siegal, T, Shohami, E, Shapira, Y, et al: Indomethacin and dexamethasone treatment in experimental neoplastic spinal cord compression. Part 2: Effect on edema and prostaglandin synthesis. Neurosurgery 22:334-339, 1988.
2413. Siegal, T, Shorr, J, Lubetzki-Korn, I, et al: Myeloma protein synthesis within the CNS by plasma cell tumors. Ann Neurol 10:271-273, 1981.
2414. Siegal, T, Siegel, T, Shapira, Y, et al: Indomethacin and dexamethasone treatment in experimental neoplastic spinal cord compression: Part 1. Effect on water content and specific gravity. Neurosurgery 22:328-333, 1988.
2415. Siegal, T and Tiqva, P: Vertebral body resection for epidural compression by malignant tumors. J Bone Joint Surg Am 67:375-382, 1985.
2416. Siegel, JP and Puri, RK: Interleukin-2 toxicity. J Clin Oncol 9:694-704, 1991.
2417. Siemsen, JK and Meister, L: Bronchogenic carcinoma with severe orthostatic hypotension. Ann Intern Med 58:669-676, 1963.
2418. Sigsbee, B, Deck, MD, and Posner, JB: Nonmetastatic superior sagittal sinus thrombosis complicating systemic cancer. Neurology 29:139-146, 1979.
2419. Silber, JH, Radcliffe, J, Peckham, V, et al: Whole-brain irradiation and decline in intelligence: The influence of dose and age on IQ score. J Clin Oncol 10:1390-1396, 1992.
2420. Silberfarb, PM: Chemotherapy and cognitive defects in cancer patients. Annu Rev Med 34:35-46, 1983.
2421. Silbergeld, DL and Ali-Osman, F: Isolation and characterization of microvessels from normal brain and brain tumors. J Neurooncol 11:49-55, 1991.
2422. Silbert, PL, Knezevic, WV, and Bridge, DT: Cerebral infarction complicating intravenous immunoglobulin therapy for polyneuritis cranialis. Neurology 42:257-259, 1992.
2423. Silbert, SW, Smith, KR, Jr, and Horenstein, S: Primary leptomeningeal melanoma. An ultrastructural study. Cancer 41:519-527, 1978.
2423a. Sillevis-Smitt, P and Posner, JB: Paraneoplastic peripheral neuropathy. Bailliere's Clinical Neurology. In press: 1995.
2424. Silvis, SE and Paragas, PD, Jr: Paresthesias, weakness, seizures, and hypophosphatemia in patients receiving hyperalimentation. Gastroenterology 62:513-520, 1972.
2425. Simberkoff, MS, Cross, AP, Al-Ibrahim, M, et al: Efficacy of pneumococcal vaccine in high-risk patients. Results of a Veterans Administration Cooperative Study. N Engl J Med 315:1318-1327, 1986.
2426. Simmons, ED and Somberg, KA: Acute tumor lysis syndrome after intrathecal methotrexate administration. Cancer 67:2062-2065, 1991.
2427. Simon, RP and Abele, JS: Spinal-fluid pleocytosis estimated by the Tyndall effect. Ann Intern Med 89:75-76, 1978.
2428. Simonescu, ME: Metastatic tumors of the brain. A follow-up study of 195 patients with neurosurgical considerations. J Neurosurg 17:361-373, 1960.
2429. Simpson, CJ and Kellett, JM: The relationship between pre-operative anxiety and post-operative delirium. J Psychosom Res 31:491-497, 1987.
2430. Simpson, RK, Jr, Sirbasku, DM, and Baskin, DS: Solitary brainstem metastasis: Comparisons of x-ray computed tomography and magnetic resonance imaging to pathology. J Neurooncol 5:57-63, 1987.
2431. Sinha, AA, Lopez, MT, and McDevitt, HO: Autoimmune diseases: The failure of self tolerance. Science 248:1380-1388, 1990.
2432. Siniscalco, M, Obele, I, Melis, P, et al: Physical and genetic mapping of the CDR gene with particular reference to its position with respect to the FRAXA site. Am J Med Genet 38:357-362, 1991.
2433. Sinniah, D, Looi, LM, Ortega, JA, et al: Cerebellar coning and uncal herniation in childhood acute leukaemia. Lancet 2:702-704, 1982.
2434. Sinoff, CL and Blumsohn, A: Spinal cord compression in myelomatosis: Response to chemotherapy alone. Eur J Cancer Clin Oncol 25:197-200, 1989.
2435. Slack, J: Coning and lumbar puncture. Letter to the Editor. Lancet 2:474-475, 1980.
2436. Slansky, HH, Kolbert, G, and Gartner, S: Exophthalmos induced by steroids. Arch Ophthalmol 77:578-581, 1967.
2437. Slatkin, NE and Posner, JB: Management of spinal epidural metastases. Clin Neurosurg 30:698-716, 1983.
2438. Slevin, ML: The clinical pharmacology of etoposide. Cancer 67:319-329, 1991.
2439. Slevin, ML, Piall, EM, Aherne, GW, et al: Effect of dose and schedule on pharmacokinetics of high-dose cytosine arabinoside in plasma and cerebrospinal fluid. J Clin Oncol 1:546-551, 1983.
2440. Slivka, A, Wen, PY, Shea, WM, et al: *Pneumocystis carinii* pneumonia during steroid taper in patients with primary brain tumors. Am J Med 94(2):216-219, 1993.
2441. Sloan, MA, Mueller, JD, Adelman, LS, et al: Fatal brainstem stroke following internal jugular vein catherization. Neurology 41:1092-1095, 1991.
2442. Smalley, SR, Laws, ER, Jr, O'Fallon, JR, et al: Resection for solitary brain metastasis. Role of adjuvant radiation and prognostic variables in 229 patients. J Neurosurg 77:531-540, 1992.
2443. Smalley, SR, Schray, MF, Laws, ER, Jr, et al: Adjuvant radiation therapy after surgical resection of solitary brain metastasis: Association with pattern of failure and survival. Int J Radiat Oncol Biol Phys 13:1611-1616, 1987.
2444. Smets, EMA, Garssen, B, Schuster-Uitterhoeve, ALJ, et al: Fatigue in cancer patients. Br J Cancer 68(2):220-224, 1993.
2445. Smith, DB, Howell, A, Harris, M, et al: Carcinomatous meningitis associated with infiltrating lobular carcinoma of the breast. Eur J Surg Oncol 11:33-36, 1985.
2446. Smith, FP, Slavik, M, and Macdonald, JS: Association of breast cancer with meningioma. Report of two cases and review of the literature. Cancer 42:1992-1994, 1978.
2447. Smith, MA, Adamson, PC, Balis, FM, et al: Phase I and pharmacokinetic evaluation of all-*trans*-retinoic acid in pediatric patients with cancer. J Clin Oncol 10:1666-1673, 1992.

2448. Smith, MT, Armbrustmacher, VM, and Violett, TW: Diffuse meningeal rhabdomyosarcoma. Cancer 47:2081-2086, 1981.
2449. Smith, R: An evaluation of surgical treatment for spinal cord compression due to metastatic carcinoma. J Neurol Neurosurg Psychiatry 28:152-158, 1965.
2450. Smith, WD, Sinar, J, and Carey, M: Sagittal sinus thrombosis and occult malignancy. Letter to the Editor. J Neurol Neurosurg Psychiatry 46:187-188, 1983.
2451. Smoker, WR, Godersky, JC, Knutzon, RK, et al: The role of MR imaging in evaluating metastatic spinal disease. AJR 149:1241-1248, 1987.
2452. Snider, S, Bashir, R, and Bierman, P: Neurologic complications after high-dose chemotherapy and autologous bone marrow transplantation for Hodgkin's disease. Neurology 44:681-684, 1994.
2453. Snooks, SJ and Swash, M: Motor conduction velocity in the human spinal cord: Slowed conduction in multiple sclerosis and radiation myopathy. J Neurol Neurosurg Psychiatry 48:1135-1139, 1985.
2454. Snyder, NA, Fiegal, DW, and Arieff, AI: Hypernatremia in elderly patients. A heterogeneous, morbid, and iatrogenic entity. Ann Intern Med 107:309-319, 1987.
2455. Snyder, RD, Stovring, J, Cushing, AH, et al: Cerebral infarction in childhood bacterial meningitis. J Neurol Neurosurg Psychiatry 44:581-585, 1981.
2455a. Solenski, NJ and Bleck, TP: Managing secondary neurologic dysfunction in the ICU. Prompt detection and reversal may avoid permanent sequelae. Journal of Critical Illness 9:843-853, 1994.
2456. Solomon, A: Neurological manifestations of macroglobulinemia. In Brain, L and Norris, FH, Jr (eds): The Remote Effects of Cancer on the Nervous System. Grune & Stratton, New York, 1965, pp 112-124.
2457. Solomon, GE and Chutorian, AM: Opsoclonus and occult neuroblastoma. N Engl J Med 279:475-477, 1968.
2458. Solymosi, L and Wappenschmidt, J: A new neuroradiologic method for therapy of spinal epidural hematomas. Neuroradiology 27:67-69, 1985.
2459. Somer, T: Hyperviscosity syndrome in plasma cell dyscrasias. Advances in Microcirculation 6:1-55, 1975.
2460. Son, YH: Effectiveness of irradiation therapy in peripheral neuropathy caused by malignant disease. Cancer 20:1447-1451, 1967.
2461. Sonksen, PH, Ayres, AB, Braimbridge, M, et al: Acromegaly caused by pulmonary carcinoid tumours. Clin Endocrinol (Oxf) 5:503-513, 1976.
2462. Sorensen, JB, Hansen, HH, Hansen, M, et al: Brain metastases in adenocarcinoma of the lung: Frequency, risk groups, and prognosis. J Clin Oncol 6:1474-1480, 1988.
2463. Sorensen, JM, Chun, HG, Vena, D, et al: Pentostatin (DCF) therapy for hairy cell leukemia (HCL): Update of a group C protocol of 208 patients (PTS) who have failed interferon alpha (IFNA). Abstract. Program/Proceedings American Society of Clinical Oncology 10:A787, 1991.
2464. Sorensen, PS, Helweg-Larsen, S, Mouridsen, H, et al: Effect of high-dose dexamethasone in carcinomatous metastatic spinal cord compression treated with radiotherapy: A randomised trial. Eur J Cancer 30A:22-27, 1994.
2465. Sorensen, S, Borgesen, SE, Rohde, K, et al: Metastatic epidural spinal cord compression. Results of treatment and survival. Cancer 65:1502-1508, 1990.
2466. Sotaniemi, KA: Slimmer's paralysis—Peroneal neuropathy during weight reduction. J Neurol Neurosurg Psychiatry 47:564-566, 1984.
2467. Sparano, JA, Gucalp, R, Llena, JF, et al: Cerebral infection complicating systemic aspergillosis in acute leukemia: Clinical and radiographic presentation. J Neurooncol 13:91-100, 1992.
2468. Spears, WT, Morphis, JG, II, Lester, SG, et al: Brain metastases and testicular tumors: Long-term survival. Int J Radiat Oncol Biol Phys 22:17-22, 1992.
2469. Spector, R: Micronutrient homeostasis in mammalian brain and cerebrospinal fluid. J Neurochem 53:1667-1674, 1989.
2470. Spiegel, D, Bloom, JR, Kraemer, HC, et al: Effect of psychosocial treatment on survival of patients with metastatic breast cancer. Lancet 2:888-891, 1989.
2471. Spigelman, MK, Zappulla, RA, Johnson, J, et al: Etoposide-induced blood–brain barrier disruption. Effect of drug compared with that of solvents. J Neurosurg 61:674-678, 1984.
2472. Spigelman, MK, Zappulla, RA, Strauchen, JA, et al: Etoposide induced blood–brain barrier disruption in rats: Duration of opening and histological sequelae. Cancer Res 46:1453-1457, 1986.
2473. Spivack, SD: Drugs five years later: Procarbazine. Ann Intern Med 81:795-800, 1974.
2474. Spriggs, DR, Stopa, E, Mayer, RJ, et al: Fludarabine phosphate (NSC 312878) infusions for the treatment of acute leukemia: Phase I and neuropathological study. Cancer Res 46:5953-5958, 1986.
2475. Stackpole, CW, Valle, EF, and Alterman, AL: B12 melanoma metastasis to an "Artificial Organ" implant. Cancer Res 51:2444-2450, 1991.
2476. Stark, RJ and Henson, RA: Cerebral compression by myeloma. J Neurol Neurosurg Psychiatry 44:833-836, 1981.
2477. Stark, RJ, Henson, RA, and Evans, SJ: Spinal metastases. A retrospective survey from a general hospital. Brain 105:189-213, 1982.
2478. Steck, AJ and Schluep, M: Neuromuscular manifestations of plasma cell dyscrasias. Curr Neurol 9:219-244, 1989.
2479. Steeg, PS, Bevilacqua, G, Kopper, L, et al: Evidence for a novel gene associated with low tumor metastatic potential. J Natl Cancer Inst 80:200-204, 1988.
2480. Steel, GG: Radiobiology of human tumour cells. In Steel, GG, Adams, GE, and Horwich, A (eds): The Biological Basis of Radiotherapy, ed 2. Elsevier Science Publishers BV, Amsterdam, The Netherlands, 1989, pp 163-179.
2481. Stefansson, K, Antel, JP, Wollman, RL, et al: Antineuronal antibodies in serum of a patient with Hodgkin's disease and cerebellar ataxia. Abstract. Neurology 31(4, part 2):126, 1981.
2482. Stein, DA and Chamberlain, MC: Evaluation and management of seizures in the patient with cancer. Oncology (Huntingt) 5:33-47, 1991.
2483. Stein, M, Steiner, M, Klein, B, et al: Involvement of

the central nervous system by ovarian carcinoma. Cancer 58:2066-2069, 1986.

2484. Steiner, I and Siegal, T: Muscle cramps in cancer patients. Cancer 63:574-577, 1989.

2485. Steinherz, P, Jereb, B, and Galicich, J: Therapy of CNS leukemia with intraventricular chemotherapy and low-dose neuraxis radiotherapy. J Clin Oncol 3:1217-1226, 1985.

2486. Stephani, U, Harten, G, Langermann, H-J, et al: Cranial computed tomography of 64 children in continuous complete remission of leukemia II: Relations to patient data and neurological complications. Neuropediatrics 14:149-154, 1983.

2487. Sternberger, NH and Sternberger, LA: Blood–brain barrier protein recognized by monoclonal antibody. Proc Natl Acad Sci U S A 84:8169-8173, 1987.

2488. Sternby, NH: Atherosclerosis and malignant tumours. Bull WHO 53:555-561, 1976.

2489. Sternby, NH and Berge, T: Atherosclerosis and malignant tumours. Acta Pathologica et Microbiologica Scandinavia Section A Pathology (Copenhagen) 236:34-44, 1973.

2490. Sterns, RH: Severe symptomatic hyponatremia: Treatment and outcome. A study of 64 cases. Ann Intern Med 107:656-664, 1987.

2491. Stetler-Stevenson, WG, Aznavoorian, S, and Liotta, LA: Tumor cell interactions with the extracellular matrix during invasion and metastasis. Annu Rev Cell Biol 9:541-573, 1993.

2492. Stevenson, GC and Hoyt, WF: Metastasis to midbrain from mammary carcinoma. JAMA 186:514-516, 1963.

2493. Stewart, DJ, Belanger, G, Grahovac, Z, et al: Phase I study of intracarotid administration of carboplatin. Neurosurgery 30:512-517, 1992.

2494. Stewart, DJ, Leavens, M, Friedman, J, et al: Penetration of N-(phosphonacetyl)-L-aspartate into human central nervous system and intracerebral tumor. Cancer Res 40:3163-3166, 1980.

2495. Stewart, DJ, Maroun, JA, Hugenholtz, H, et al: Combined intra-Ommaya methotrexate, cytosine arabinoside, hydrocortisone and thio-TEPA for meningeal involvement by malignancies. J Neurooncol 5:315-322, 1987.

2496. Stewart, PA, Hayakawa, K, Farrell, CL, et al: Quantitative study of microvessel ultrastructure in human peritumoral brain tissue. Evidence for a blood–brain barrier defect. J Neurosurg 67:697-705, 1987.

2497. Stewart, PA and Wiley, MJ: Developing nervous tissue induces formation of blood–brain barrier characteristics in invading endothelial cells: A study using quail-chick transplantation chimeras. Dev Biol 84:183-192, 1981.

2498. Stiefel, FC, Breitbart, WS, and Holland, JC: Corticosteroids in cancer: Neuropsychiatric complications. Cancer Invest 7(5):479-491, 1989.

2499. Stiller, C: Survival of patients in clinical trials and at specialist centres. In Williams, CJ (ed): Introducing New Treatments for Cancer. Practical, Ethical and Legal Problems. John Wiley & Sons, New York, 1992, pp 119-136.

2499a. Stiller, CA: Centralised treatment, entry to trials and survival. Br J Cancer 70:352-362, 1994.

2500. Stillman, MJ, Christensen, W, Payne, R, et al: Leukemic relapse presenting as sciatic nerve involvement by chloroma (granulocytic sarcoma). Cancer 62:2047-2050, 1988.

2501. Stillwagon, GB, Lee, DJ, Moses, H, et al: Response of cranial nerve abnormalities in nasopharyngeal carcinoma to radiation therapy. Cancer 57:2272-2274, 1986.

2502. Stilman, N and Masdeu, JC: Incidence of seizures with phenytoin toxicity. Neurology 35:1769-1772, 1985.

2503. Stoll, DB, Lublin, F, Brodovsky, H, et al: Association of subacute motor neuronopathy with thymoma. Cancer 54:770-772, 1984.

2504. Storey, P and Trumble, M: Rectal doxepin and carbamazepine therapy in patients with cancer. Letter to the Editor. N Engl J Med 327:1318-1319, 1992.

2505. Storm, AJ, van der Kogel, AJ, and Nooter, K: Effect of X-irradiation on the pharmacokinetics of methotrexate in rats: Alteration of the blood–brain barrier. Eur J Cancer Clin Oncol 21:759-764, 1985.

2506. Stotka, VL, Barcay, SJ, Bell, HS, et al: Intractable hiccough as the primary manifestation of brain stem tumor. Am J Med 32:313-315, 1962.

2507. Stracke, ML and Liotta, LA: Multi-step cascade of tumor cell metastasis. In Vivo 6:309-316, 1992.

2508. Straus, SE, Ostrove, JM, Inchauspe, G, et al: NIH Conference. Varicella-zoster virus infections. Biology, natural history, treatment, and prevention. Ann Intern Med 108:221-237, 1988.

2509. Strausbaugh, LJ: Intracarotid infusions of protamine sulfate disrupt the blood–brain barrier of rabbits. Brain Res 409:221-226, 1987.

2510. Stridsklev, IC, Hagen, S, and Klepp, O: Radiation therapy for brain metastases from malignant melanoma. Acta Radiologica: Oncology, Radiation, Physics, Biology (Stockholm) 23:231-235, 1984.

2511. Strong, JM, Collins, JM, Lester, C, et al: Pharmacokinetics of intraventricular and intravenous N,N′,N″-triethylenethiophosphoramide (thiotepa) in rhesus monkeys and humans. Cancer Res 46:6101-6104, 1986.

2512. Strother, DR, Glynn-Barnhart, A, Kovnar, E, et al: Variability in the disposition of intraventricular methotrexate: A proposal for rational dosing. J Clin Oncol 7:1741-1747, 1989.

2512a. Strugar, J, Rothbart, D, Harrington, W, et al: Vascular permeability factor in brain metastases: Correlation with vasogenic brain edema and tumor angiogenesis. J Neurosurg 81:560-566, 1994.

2513. Sudarsky, L and Ronthal, M: Gait disorders among elderly patients. A survey of 50 patients. Arch Neurol 40:740-743, 1983.

2514. Sugarbaker, EV: Patterns of metastasis in human malignancies. Cancer Biology Reviews 2:235-278, 1981.

2515. Sugarbaker, EV and Chretien, PB: A tumor shunt syndrome. Transient cerebral ischemia induced by a large thyroid adenoma. Arch Surg 104:213-215, 1972.

2516. Sugiura, M, Hiraoka, K, Ohkawa, S, et al: A clinicopathological study on cardiac lesions in 64 cases of disseminated intravascular coagulation. Jpn Heart J 18:57-69, 1977.

2517. Sullivan, MP, Moon, TE, Trueworthy, R, et al:

Combination intrathecal therapy for meningeal leukemia: Two versus three drugs. Blood 50:471-479, 1977.
2518. Sumi, SM, Farrell, DF, and Knauss, TA: Lymphoma and leukemia manifested by steroid-responsive polyneuropathy. Arch Neurol 40:577-582, 1983.
2519. Sundaresan, N, Choi, IS, Hughes, JE, et al: Treatment of spinal metastases from kidney cancer by presurgical embolization and resection. J Neurosurg 73:548-554, 1990.
2520. Sundaresan, N, DiGiacinto, GV, Hughes, JE, et al: Treatment of neoplastic spinal cord compression: Results of a prospective study. Neurosurgery 29:645-650, 1991.
2521. Sundaresan, N, Rosen, G, Fortner, JG, et al: Preoperative chemotherapy and surgical resection in the management of posterior paraspinal tumors. Report of three cases. J Neurosurg 58:446-450, 1983.
2522. Sundaresan, N, Sachdev, VP, DiGiacinto, GV, et al: Reoperation for brain metastases. J Clin Oncol 6:1625-1629, 1988.
2523. Sundaresan, N and Suite, ND: Optimal use of the Ommaya reservoir in clinical oncology. Oncology (Huntingt) 3:15-23, 1989.
2523a. Sung, C, Blaney, SM, Cole, DE, et al: A pharmacokinetic model of topotecan clearance from plasma and cerebrospinal fluid. Cancer Res 54:5118-5122, 1994.
2524. Sung, JP, Campbell, GD, and Grendahl, JG: Miconazole therapy for fungal meningitis. Arch Neurol 35:443-447, 1978.
2525. Supler, ML and Friedman, WA: Acute bilateral ophthalmoplegia secondary to cavernous sinus metastasis: A case report. Neurosurgery 31:783-786, 1992.
2526. Sutherland, GE, Palitang, EG, Marr, JJ, et al: Sterilization of Ommaya reservoir by instillation of vancomycin. Am J Med 71:1068-1070, 1981.
2527. Sutherland, JE, Persky, VW, and Brody, JA: Proportionate mortality trends: 1950 through 1986. JAMA 264:3178-3184, 1990.
2528. Suzuki, N, Sako, K, and Yonemasu, Y: Effects of induced hypertension on blood flow and capillary permeability in rats with experimental brain tumors. J Neurooncol 10:213-218, 1991.
2529. Suzuki, T, Koizumi, J, Uchida, K, et al: Carmofur-induced organic mental disorders. Jpn J Psychiatry Neurol 44:723-727, 1990.
2530. Suzumiya, J, Marutsuka, K, Ueda, S, et al: An autopsy case of necrotizing ventriculo-encephalitis caused by cytomegalovirus in Hodgkin's disease. Acta Pathol Jpn 41:291-298, 1991.
2531. Svien, HJ, Baker, HL, and Rivers, MH: Jugular foramen syndrome and allied syndromes. Neurology 13:797-809, 1963.
2532. Swann, KW, Black, PM, and Baker, MF: Management of symptomatic deep venous thrombosis and pulmonary embolism on a neurosurgical service. J Neurosurg 64:563-567, 1986.
2533. Swash, M, Fox, KP, and Davidson, AR: Carcinoid myopathy: Serotonin-induced muscle weakness in man? Arch Neurol 32:572-574, 1975.
2534. Sweeney, JD, Ziegler, P, Pruet, C, et al: Hyperzincuria and hypozincemia in patients treated with cisplatin. Cancer 63:2093-2095, 1989.
2535. Swift, PS, Phillips, T, Martz, K, et al: CT characteristics of patients with brain metastases treated in RTOG study 79-16. Int J Radiat Oncol Biol Phys 25:209-214, 1993.
2536. Swift, TR: Involvement of peripheral nerves in radical neck dissection. Am J Surg 119:694-698, 1970.
2537. Sykes, NP: Oral naloxone in opioid-associated constipation. Letter to the Editor. Lancet 337: 1475, 1991.
2538. Sylvestre, DL, Sandson, TA, and Nachmanoff, DB: Transient brachial plexopathy as a complication of internal jugular vein cannulation. Letter to the Editor. Neurology 41:760, 1991.
2539. Szabo, A, Dalmau, J, Manley, G, et al: HuD, a paraneoplastic encephalomyelitis antigen, contains RNA-binding domains and is homologous to Elav and Sex-lethal. Cell 67:325-333, 1991.
2540. Sze, G: Magnetic resonance imaging in the evaluation of spinal tumors. Cancer 67(Suppl 4):1229-1241, 1991.
2541. Sze, G, Abramson, A, Krol, G, et al: Gadolinium-DTPA in the evaluation of intradural extramedullary spinal disease. AJR 150:911-921, 1988.
2542. Taira, M, Kojima, K, and Takeuchi, H: A comparative study of the action of actinomycin D and actinomycinic ACID on the central nervous system when injected into the cerebrospinal fluid of higher animals. Epilepsia 13:649-662, 1972.
2543. Tajima, A, Yen, M-H, Nakata, H, et al: Effects of dexamethasone on blood flow and volume of perfused microvessels in traumatic brain edema. Adv Neurol 52:343-350, 1990.
2544. Takakura, K, Sano, K, Hojo, S, et al: Metastatic Tumors of the Central Nervous System. Igaku-Shoin Ltd, Tokyo, 1982.
2545. Tallman, RD, Kimbrough, SM, O'Brien, JF, et al: Assay for β-glucuronidase in cerebrospinal fluid: Usefulness for the detection of neoplastic meningitis. Mayo Clin Proc 60:293-298, 1985.
2546. Tally, PW, Laws, ER, Jr, and Scheithauer, BW: Metastases of central nervous system neoplasms. Case report. J Neurosurg 68:811-816, 1988.
2547. Tamargo, RJ, Sills, AK, Jr, Reinhard, CS, et al: Interstitial delivery of dexamethasone in the brain for the reduction of peritumoral edema. J Neurosurg 74:956-961, 1991.
2548. Tanabe, CT and Hill, CL: Dysphagia secondary to anterior cervical osteophytes. J Neurosurg 35:338-341, 1971.
2549. Tanabe, KK, Ellis, LM, and Saya, H: Expression of CD44R1 adhesion molecule in colon carcinomas and metastases. Lancet 341:725-726, 1993.
2550. Tang, RA, Kellaway, J, and Young, SE: Ophthalmic manifestations of systemic cancer. Oncology (Huntingt) 5:59-71, 1991.
2551. Tannock, I, Gospodarowicz, M, Meakin, W, et al: Treatment of metastatic prostatic cancer with low-dose prednisone: Evaluation of pain and quality of life as pragmatic indices of response. J Clin Oncol 7:590-597, 1989.
2552. Targoff, IN, Trieu, EP, Plotz, PH, et al: Antibodies to glycl-transfer RNA synthetase in patients with myositis and interstitial lung disease. Arthritis Rheum 35:821-830, 1992.
2553. Tarind, D: Biological and clinical studies relevant

to metastases of breast cancer. Cancer Metastasis Rev 5:95-108, 1986.

2554. Tarlov, IM and Klinger, H: Spinal cord compression studies. II: Time limits for recovery after acute compression in dogs. Archives of Neurology and Psychiatry 71:271-290, 1954.

2555. Tashima, CK: Immediate cerebral symptoms during rapid intravenous administration of cyclophosphamide (NSC-26271). Cancer Chemotherapy Reports 59:441-442, 1975.

2556. Tauber, MG, Kennedy, SI, Tureen, JH, et al: Experimental pneumococcal meningitis causes central nervous system pathology without inducing the 72-kd heat shock protein. Am J Pathol 141:53-60, 1992.

2557. Tauber, MG, Sachdeva, M, Kennedy, SL, et al: Toxicity in neuronal cells caused by cerebrospinal fluid from pneumococcal gram-negative meningitis. J Infect Dis 166:1045-1050, 1992.

2558. Taylor, CW, Lui, R, Fanta, P, et al: Effects of suramin on in vitro growth of fresh human tumors. J Natl Cancer Inst 84:489-494, 1992.

2559. Taylor, D and Lewis, S: Delirium. J Neurol Neurosurg Psychiatry 56:742-751, 1993.

2560. Taylor, LP and Posner, JB: Steroid myopathy in cancer patients treated with dexamethasone. Abstract. Neurology 39(Suppl 1):129, 1989.

2561. Taylor, LP and Posner, JB: Phenobarbital rheumatism in patients with brain tumor. Ann Neurol 25:92-94, 1989.

2562. Taylor, SA, Crowley, J, Pollock, TW, et al: Objective antitumor activity of Acivicin in patients with recurrent CNS malignancies: A Southwest Oncology Group trial. J Clin Oncol 9:1476-1479, 1991.

2563. Tchekmedyian, NS, Cella, DF, and Mooradian, AD (eds): Proceedings of the Second International Quality of Life Symposium, February 23 and 24, 1991: Care of the older patient: Clinical and quality of life issues. Oncology 6(2 Suppl):1-160, 1992.

2564. Tchekmedyian, NS, Hichman, M, Siau, J, et al: Megestrol acetate in cancer anorexia and weight loss. Cancer 69:1268-1274, 1992.

2565. Teears, RJ and Silverman, EM: Clinicopathologic review of 88 cases of carcinoma metastatic to the pituitary gland. Cancer 36:216-220, 1975.

2566. Teele, DW, Dashefsky, B, Rakusan, T, et al: Meningitis after lumbar puncture in children with bacteremia. N Engl J Med 305:1079-1081, 1981.

2567. Tefft, M, Mitus, A, and Schulz, MD: Initial high dose irradiation for metastases causing spinal cord compression in children. AJR 106:385-393, 1969.

2568. Teichmann, KD and Dabbagh, N: Severe visual loss after a single dose of vincristine in a patient with spinal cord astrocytoma. J Ocul Pharmacol 4:117-121, 1988.

2569. Ten Hoeve, RF and Twijnstra, A: A lethal neurotoxic reaction after intraventricular methotrexate administration. Cancer 62:2111-2113, 1988.

2570. Teravainen, H and Larsen, A: Some features of the neuromuscular complications of pulmonary carcinoma. Ann Neurol 2:495-502, 1977.

2571. Tessitore, L, Costelli, P, and Baccino, FM: Humoral mediation for cachexia in tumour-bearing rats. Br J Cancer 67:15-23, 1993.

2572. Tham, LC, Millward, MJ, Lind, MJ, et al: Metastatic breast cancer presenting with diabetes insipidus. Letter to the Editor. Acta Oncol 31(6):679-683, 1992.

2573. Thant, M, Hawley, RJ, Smith, MT, et al: Possible enhancement of vincristine neuropathy by VP-16. Cancer 49:859-864, 1982.

2574. Theodore, WH and Gendelman, S: Meningeal carcinomatosis. Arch Neurol 38:696-699, 1981.

2575. Theologides, A: Anorexins, asthenins, and cachectins in cancer. Am J Med 81:696-698, 1986.

2576. Theriault, RL: Hypercalcemia of malignancy: Pathophysiology and implications for treatment. Oncology (Huntingt) 7:47-55, 1993.

2577. Thibadoux, GM, Pereira, WV, Hodges, JM, et al: Effects of cranial radiation on hearing in children with acute lymphocytic leukemia. J Pediatr 96:403-406, 1980.

2578. Thirkill, CE, Fitzgerald, P, Sergott, RC, et al: Cancer-associated retinopathy (CAR syndrome) with antibodies reacting with retinal, optic nerve, and cancer cells. N Engl J Med 321:1589-1594, 1989.

2579. Thomas, JE, Cascino, TL, and Earle, JD: Differential diagnosis between radiation and tumor plexopathy of the pelvis. Neurology 35:1-7, 1985.

2580. Thomas, JE and Colby, MY: Radiation-induced or metastatic brachial plexopathy? JAMA 222:1392-1395, 1972.

2581. Thomas, JE and Howard, FM, Jr: Segmental zoster paresis—A disease profile. Neurology 22:459-466, 1972.

2582. Thomas, JE and Waltz, AG: Neurological manifestations of nasopharyngeal malignant tumors. JAMA 192:103-106, 1965.

2583. Thomas, JE and Yoss, RE: The parasellar syndrome: Problems in determining etiology. Mayo Clin Proc 45:617-623, 1970.

2584. Thompson, GM, Migdal, CS, and Whittle, RJ: Radiation retinopathy following treatment of posterior nasal space carcinoma. Br J Ophthalmol 67:609-614, 1983.

2585. Thompson, PD: Stiff muscles. Editorial. J Neurol Neurosurg Psychiatry 56:121-124, 1993.

2586. Thompson, PD, Wise, RJS, and Kendall, BE: Enophthalmos and metastatic carcinoma of the breast. Letter to the Editor. J Neurol Neurosurg Psychiatry 48:1305-1306, 1985.

2587. Thompson, SW, Davis, LE, Kornfeld, M, et al: Cisplatin neuropathy. Clinical, electrophysiologic, morphologic, and toxicologic studies. Cancer 54:1269-1275, 1984.

2588. Thompson, T and Evans, W: Paradoxical embolism. Q J Med 23:135-150, 1930.

2589. Thordarson, H and Talstad, I: Acute meningitis and cerebellar dysfunction complicating high-dose cytosine arabinoside therapy. Acta Medica Scandinavica 220:493-495, 1986.

2589a. Thoron, L and Arbit, E: Hemostatic changes in patients with brain tumors and systemic malignancy. J Neurooncol. In press, 1995.

2590. Tien, R, Arieff, AI, Kucharczyk, W, et al: Hyponatremic encephalopathy: Is central pontine myelinolysis a component? Am J Med 92:513-522, 1992.

2591. Tien, RD, Tuori, SL, Pulkingham, N, et al: Ganglioglioma with leptomeningeal and subarachnoid spread: Results of CT, MR, and PET imaging. AJR 159:391-393, 1992.

2592. Tjia, TL, Yeow, YK, and Tan, CB: Cryptococcal meningitis. J Neurol Neurosurg Psychiatry 48:853-858, 1985.

2592a. Tjuvajev, J, Uehara, H, Desai, R, et al: Corticotropin releasing factor as an alternative treatment of peritumoral brain edema. In Ito, S (ed): Intracranial Pressure IX. Tokyo, Springer-Verlag, 1994, pp 120-124.

2593. Tobias, JS: Clinical practice of radiotherapy. Lancet 339:159-163, 1992.

2594. Tomlinson, BE, Perry, RH, and Stewart-Wynne, EG: Influence of site of origin of lung carcinomas on clinical presentation and central nervous system metastases. J Neurol Neurosurg Psychiatry 42:82-88, 1979.

2595. Toner, GC, Pike, J, and Schwarz, MA: The blood–brain barrier and response of CNS metastases to chemotherapy. J Neurooncol 7:21-24, 1989.

2596. Tontsch, U and Bauer, H-C: Glial cells and neurons induce blood–brain barrier related enzymes in cultured cerebral endothelial cells. Brain Res 539:247-253, 1991.

2597. Toole, JF: Cerebrovascular Disorders, ed 3. Raven Press, New York, 1984, pp 187-198.

2598. Tornatore, C, Berger, JR, Houff, SA, et al: Detection of JC virus DNA in peripheral lymphocytes from patients with and without progressive multifocal leukoencephalopathy. Ann Neurol 31:454-462, 1992.

2599. Torvik, A and Berntzen, AE: Necrotizing vasculitis without visceral involvement. Postmortem examination of three cases with affection of skeletal muscles and peripheral nerves. Acta Med Scand 184:69-77, 1968.

2600. Toyokuni, S, Ebina, Y, Okada, S, et al: Report of a patient with POEMS Takatsuki/Crow-Fukase syndrome associated with focal spinal pachymeningeal amyloidosis. Cancer 70:882-886, 1992.

2601. Traynelis, VC, Powell, RG, Koss, W, et al: Cerebrospinal fluid eosinophilia and sterile shunt malfunction. Neurosurgery 23:645-649, 1988.

2602. Triozzi, PL, Kinney, P, and Rinehart, JJ: Central nervous system toxicity of biological response modifiers. Ann N Y Acad Sci 594:347-354, 1990.

2603. Trivedi, NS, Eddi, D, and Shevde, K: Headache prevention following accidental dural puncture in obstetric patients. J Clin Anesth 5:42-45, 1993.

2604. Trivedi, S: Psychiatric symptoms in carcinoid syndrome. J Indian Med Assoc 82:292-294, 1984.

2605. Trosch, RM and Ransom, BR: Levodopa-responsive parkinsonism following central herniation due to bilateral subdural hematomas. Neurology 40:376-377, 1990.

2606. Trotter, JL, Hendin, BA, and Osterland, K: Cerebellar degeneration with Hodgkin's disease. An immunological study. Arch Neurol 33:660-661, 1976.

2607. Trousseau, A: Phlegmasia alba dolens. Clinique Medicale de L'Hotel Dieu de Paris 3:94 , 1865.

2608. Trump, DL, Grossman, SA, Thompson, G, et al: CSF infections complicating the management of neoplastic meningitis. Clinical features and results of therapy. Arch Intern Med 142:583-586, 1982.

2609. Trump, DL, Grossman, SA, Thompson, G, et al: Treatment of neoplastic meningitis with intraventricular thiotepa and methotrexate. Cancer Treat Rep 66:1549-1551, 1983.

2610. Trump, DL, Tutsch, KD, Koeller, JM, et al: Phase I clinical study with pharmacokinetic analysis of 2-beta-D-ribofuranosylthiazole-4-carboxamide (NSC 186193) administered as a 5-day infusion. Cancer Res 45:2853-2858, 1985.

2611. Tryba, M: Side effects of stress bleeding prophylaxis. Am J Med 86:85-93, 1989.

2612. Tsukada, Y, Fouad, A, Pickren, JW, et al: Central nervous system metastasis from breast carcinoma. Autopsy study. Cancer 52:2349-2354, 1983.

2613. Tsukamoto, T, Mochizuki, R, Mochizuki, H, et al: Paraneoplastic cerebellar degeneration and limbic encephalitis in a patient with adenocarcinoma of the colon. J Neurol Neurosurg Psychiatry 56:713-716, 1993.

2614. Tuchman, M, Stoeckeler, JS, Kiang, DT, et al: Familial pyrimidinemia and pyrimidinuria associated with severe fluorouracil toxicity. N Engl J Med 313:245-249, 1985.

2615. Tuchman, RF, Alvarez, LA, Kantrowitz, AB, et al: Opsoclonus-myoclonus syndrome: Correlation of radiographic and pathological observations. Neuroradiology 31:250-252, 1989.

2616. Tucker, RM, Denning, DW, Dupont, B, et al: Itraconazole therapy for chronic coccidioidal meningitis. Ann Intern Med 112:108-112, 1990.

2617. Tuma, R and DeAngelis, LM: Acute encephalopathy in patients with systemic cancer. Abstract. Ann Neurol 32:288, 1992.

2618. Tung, H, Raffel, C, and McComb, JG: Ventricular cerebrospinal fluid eosinophilia in children with ventriculoperitoneal shunts. J Neurosurg 75:541-544, 1991.

2619. Tunkel, AR, Wispelwey, B, and Scheld, WM: Bacterial meningitis: Recent advances in pathophysiology and treatment. Ann Intern Med 112:610-623, 1990.

2620. Tureen, JH, Dworkin, RJ, Kennedy, SL, et al: Loss of cerebrovascular autoregulation in experimental meningitis rabbits. J Clin Invest 85:577-581, 1990.

2621. Turgman, J, Braham, J, Modan, B, et al: Neurological complications in patients with malignant tumors of the nasopharynx. Eur Neurol 17:149-154, 1978.

2622. Turnbull, DM, Rawlins, MD, Weightman, D, et al: "Therapeutic" serum concentration of phenytoin: The influence of seizure type. J Neurol Neurosurg Psychiatry 47:231-234, 1984.

2623. Turner, DM and Graf, CJ: Nontraumatic subdural hematoma secondary to dural metastasis: Case report and review of the literature. Neurosurgery 11:678-680, 1982.

2624. Turner, S, Marosszeky, B, Timms, I, et al: Malignant spinal cord compression: A prospective evaluation. Int J Radiat Oncol Biol Phys 26:141-146, 1993.

2625. Turpie, AG, Hirsh, J, Gent, M, et al: Prevention of deep vein thrombosis in potential neurosurgical patients. A randomized trial comparing graduated compression stockings alone or graduated compression stockings plus intermittent pneu-

matic compression with control. Arch Intern Med 149:679-681, 1989.
2626. Twijnstra, A, Keyser, A, and Ongerboer de Visser, BW (eds): Neurooncology. Primary Tumors and Neurological Complications of Cancer. Elsevier, Amsterdam, The Netherlands, 1993.
2627. Twijnstra, A, Ongerboer de Visser, BW, van Zanten, AP, et al: Serial lumbar and ventricular cerebrospinal fluid biochemical marker measurements in patients with leptomeningeal metastases from solid and hematological tumors. J Neurooncol 7:57-63, 1989.
2628. Tyler, KL and Martin, JB: Infectious Diseases of the Central Nervous System, Contemporary Neurology Series, No. 41. FA Davis, Philadelphia, 1993.
2629. Uchiyama, R, Matsumoto, M, and Kobayashi, N: Studies on the pathogenesis of coagulopathy in patients with arterial thromboembolism and malignancy. Thromb Res 59:955-965, 1990.
2630. Uematsu, Y, Yukawa, S, Yokote, H, et al: Meningeal melanocytoma: Magnetic resonance imaging characteristics and pathological features. Case report. J Neurosurg 76:705-709, 1992.
2631. Ueunten, D, Tobias, J, Sochat, M, et al: An unusual cause of bacterial meningitis in the elderly. *Propionibacterium acnes.* Arch Neurol 40:388-389, 1983.
2632. Ueyama, H, Kumamoto, T, and Araki, S: Circulating autoantibody to muscle protein in a patient with paraneoplastic myositis and colon cancer. Eur Neurol 32:281-284, 1992.
2633. Uldry, PA, Teta, D, and Regli, L: Focal cerebral necrosis caused by intraventricular chemotherapy with methotrexate. Neurochirurgie 37:72-74, 1991.
2634. Unsold, R, Safran, AB, Safran, E, et al: Metastatic infiltration of nerves in the cavernous sinus. Arch Neurol 37:59-61, 1980.
2635. Unterberg, A, Schmidt, W, Wahl, M, et al: Evidence against leukotrienes as mediators of brain edema. J Neurosurg 74:773-780, 1991.
2636. Urba, WJ, Steis, RG, Longo, DL, et al: Immunomodulatory properties and toxicity of interleukin 2 in patients with cancer. Cancer Res 50:185-192, 1990.
2637. Urban, C, Nirenberg, A, Caparros, B, et al: Chemical pleuritis as the cause of acute chest pain following high-dose methotrexate treatment. Cancer 51:34-37, 1983.
2638. Urbano-Marquez, A, Casademont, J, and Grau, JM: Polymyositis/dermatomyositis: The current position. Ann Rheum Dis 50:191-195, 1991.
2639. Urch, CE, George, AJT, Stevenson, GT, et al: Intrathecal treatment of leptomeningeal lymphoma with immunotoxin. Int J Cancer 47:909-915, 1991.
2640. Ushio, Y, Arita, N, Hayakawa, T, et al: Chemotherapy of brain metastases from lung carcinoma: A controlled randomized study. Neurosurgery 28:201-205, 1991.
2641. Ushio, Y, Chernik, NL, Posner, JB, et al: Meningeal carcinomatosis: Development of an experimental model. J Neuropathol Exp Neurol 36:228-244, 1977.
2642. Ushio, Y, Chernik, NL, Shapiro, WR, et al: Metastatic tumor of the brain: Development of an experimental model. Ann Neurol 2:20-29, 1977.
2643. Ushio, Y, Posner, JB, and Shapiro, WR: Chemotherapy of experimental meningeal carcinomatosis. Cancer Res 37:1232-1237, 1977.
2644. Ushio, Y, Posner, R, Kim, J-H, et al: Treatment of experimental spinal cord compression by extradural neoplasms. J Neurosurg 47:380-390, 1977.
2645. Ushio, Y, Posner, R, Posner, JB, et al: Experimental spinal cord compression by epidural neoplasm. Neurology 27:422-429, 1977.
2646. Ushio, Y, Shimizu, K, Aragaki, Y, et al: Alteration of blood–CSF barrier by tumor invasion into the meninges. J Neurosurg 55:445-449, 1981.
2647. Valdez, IH, Wolff, A, Atkinson, JC, et al: Use of pilocarpine during head and neck radiation therapy to reduce xerostomia and salivary dysfunction. Cancer 71:1848-1851, 1993.
2648. Valk, PE, Budinger, TF, Levin, VA, et al: PET of malignant cerebral tumors after interstitial brachytherapy. Demonstration of metabolic activity and correlation with clinical outcome. J Neurosurg 69:830-838, 1988.
2649. Valk, PE and Dillon, WP: Radiation injury of the brain. AJNR 12:45-62, 1991.
2650. Vallat, JM, Leboutet, MJ, Hugon, J, et al: Acute pure sensory paraneoplastic neuropathy with perivascular endoneurial inflammation: Ultrastructural study of capillary walls. Neurology 36:1395-1399, 1986.
2651. Van Amelsvoort, T, Bakshi, R, Devaux, CB, et al: Hyponatremia associated with carbamazepine and oxcarbazepine therapy: A review. Epilepsia 35:181-188, 1994.
2652. Van Coster, RN, De Vivo, DC, Blake, D, et al: Adult Reye's syndrome: A review with new evidence for a generalized defect in intramitochondrial enzyme processing. Neurology 41:1815-1821, 1991.
2653. Van Crevel, H: RIHSA cisternography in cerebral tumours. Neuroradiology 18:133-138, 1979.
2654. Van Crevel, H: Papilloedema, CSF pressure, and CSF flow in cerebral tumours. J Neurol Neurosurg Psychiatry 42:493-500, 1979.
2655. Van Crevel, H: Pathogenesis of raised cerebrospinal fluid pressure. Doc Ophthalmol 52:251-257, 1982.
2655a. Van den Aardweg, GJMJ, Hopewell, JW, Whitehouse, EM, et al: A new model of radiation-induced myelopathy: A comparison of the response of mature and immature pigs. Int J Radiat Oncol Biol Phys 29:763-770, 1994.
2656. Van den Bogaet, W, Horiot, J-C, and van der Schueren, E: Radiotherapy with multiple fractions per day. In Steel, GG, Adams, GE, and Horwich, A (eds): The Biological Basis of Radiotherapy, ed 2. Elsevier Science Publishers, Amsterdam, 1989, pp 209-222.
2656a. Vanden Driessche, T, Geldhof, A, Bakkus, M, et al: Metastasis of mouse T lymphoma cells is controlled by the level of major histocompatibility complex class IH-2D^k antigens. Int J Cancer 58:217-225, 1994.
2657. Van der Hoop, RG, van der Burg, MEL, ten Bokkel Huinink, WW, et al: Incidence of neuropathy in 395 patients with ovarian cancer treated with or without cisplatin. Cancer 66:1697-1702, 1990.

2658. Van der Hoop, RG, Vecht, CJ, van der Burg, ME, et al: Prevention of cisplatin neurotoxicity with an ACTH (4-9) analogue in patients with ovarian cancer. N Engl J Med 322:89-94, 1990.
2659. Van der Kogel, AJ (ed): Late Effects of Radiation on the Spinal Cord. Dose-Effect Relationships and Pathogenesis. The Radiobiological Institute of the Organization for Health Research, Tno Rijswijk, The Netherlands, 1979, pp 1-160.
2660. Van der Mast, RC, Fekkes, D, Moleman, P, et al: Is postoperative delirium related to reduced plasma tryptophan? Lancet 338:851-852, 1991.
2661. Van der Sande, JJ, Kroger, R, and Boogerd, W: Multiple spinal epidural metastases: An unexpectedly frequent finding. J Neurol Neurosurg Psychiatry 53:1001-1003, 1990.
2662. Van der Sande, JJ, Veltkamp, JJ, and Bouwhuis-Hoogerwerf, ML: Hemostasis and intracranial surgery. J Neurosurg 58:693-698, 1983.
2663. Van der Steen-Banasik, E, Hermans, J, Tjho-Heslinga, R, et al: The objective response of brain metastases on radiotherapy. A prospective study using computer tomography. Acta Oncol 31:777-780, 1992.
2664. Van Echo, DA, Chiuten, DF, Gormley, PE, et al: Phase 1 clinical and pharmacological study of 4'-(9-acridinylamino)-methanesulfon-m-anisidide using an intermittent biweekly schedule. Cancer Res 39:3881-3884, 1979.
2665. Van Eck, JHM, Go, KG, and Ebels, EJ: Metastatic tumours of the brain. Psychiatria, Neurologica, Neurochirurgia (Amsterdam) 68:443-462, 1965.
2666. Van Hazel, GA, Scott, M, and Eagan, RT: The effect of CNS metastases on the survival of patients with small cell cancer of the lung. Cancer 51:933-937, 1983.
2667. Van Kooten, B, van Diemen, HA, Groenhout, KM, et al: A pilot study on the influence of a corticotropin (4-9) analogue on *Vinca* alkaloid-induced neuropathy. Arch Neurol 49:1027-1031, 1992.
2668. Van Laethem, JL, Gay, F, Franck, N, et al: Hyperammoniemic coma in a patient with ureterosigmoidostomy and normal liver function. Dig Dis Sci 37:1754-1756, 1992.
2669. Van Lieshout, JJ, Wieling, W, Van Montfrans, GA, et al: Acute dysautonomia associated with Hodgkin's disease. J Neurol Neurosurg Psychiatry 49:830-832, 1986.
2670. Van Rossum, J, Zwaan, FE, and Bots, GT: Facial palsy as the initial symptom of lymphoreticular malignancy. Case report. Eur Neurol 18:212-216, 1979.
2671. Van Uitert, RL and Eisenstadt, ML: Venous pulsations not always indicative of normal intracranial pressure. Letter to the Editor. Arch Neurol 35:550, 1978.
2672. Van Zanten, AP: Central Nervous System Metastases from Extracranial Malignancies. Diagnostic Value of Clinical Chemical Parameters. Rodopi, Amsterdam, 1986, pp 1-99.
2673. Van Zanten, AP, Twijnstra, A, Ongerboer de Visser, BW, et al: Cerebrospinal fluid tumour markers in patients treated for meningeal malignancy. J Neurol Neurosurg Psychiatry 54:119-123, 1991.
2674. Vandenberg, SA, Kulig, K, Spoerke, DG, et al: Chlorambucil overdose: Accidental ingestion of an antineoplastic drug. J Emerg Med 6:495-498, 1988.
2675. Vanneste, J, Augustijn, P, Dirven, P, et al: Shunting normal-pressure hydrocephalus: Do the benefits outweigh the risks? A multicenter study and literature review. Neurology 42:54-59, 1992.
2676. Varney, NR, Alexander, B, and MacIndoe, JH: Reversible steroid dementia in patients without steroid psychosis. Am J Psychiatry 141:369-372, 1984.
2677. Vassal, G, Deroussent, A, Hartmann, O, et al: Dose-dependent neurotoxicity of high-dose busulfan in children: A clinical and pharmacological study. Cancer Res 50:6203-6207, 1990.
2678. Vecht, CHJ and Van Doorn, JL: Het gevaar van spinale inklemming bij myelumcompressie; lumbale of cervicale myelografie. Ned Tijdschr Geneeskd 129:171-174, 1985.
2679. Vecht, CJ: Evaluation and management of metastatic spinal cord compression. In Hildebrand, J (ed): Management in Neuro-Oncology, European School of Oncology Monographs (Veronesi, U [series ed]). Springer-Verlag, Berlin, 1992, pp 63-75.
2680. Vecht, CJ, Haaxma-Reiche, H, Noordijk, EM, et al: Treatment of single brain metastasis: Radiotherapy alone or combined with neurosurgery? Ann Neurol 33:583-590, 1993.
2681. Vecht, CJ, Haaxma-Reiche, H, van Putten, WLJ, et al: Initial bolus of conventional versus high-dose dexamethasone in metastatic spinal cord compression. Neurology 39:1255-1257, 1989.
2682. Vecht, CJ, Hoff, AM, Kansen, PJ, et al: Types and causes of pain in cancer of the head and neck. Cancer 70:178-184, 1992.
2683. Vecht, CJ, Hovestadt, A, Verbiest, HBC, et al: Dose-effect relationship of dexamethasone on Karnofsky performance in metastatic brain tumors: A randomized study of doses of 4, 8, and 16 mg per day. Neurology 44:675-680, 1994.
2684. Vecht, CJ, Van de Brand, HJ, and Wajer, OJ: Post-axillary dissection pain in breast cancer due to a lesion of the intercostobrachial nerve. Pain 38:171-176, 1989.
2685. Veilleux, M, Bernier, JP, and Lamarche, JB: Paraneoplastic encephalomyelitis and subacute dysautonomia due to an occult atypical carcinoid tumour of the lung. Can J Neurol Sci 17:324-328, 1990.
2686. Venger, BH and Aldama, EA: Mycotic vasculitis with repeated intracranial aneurysmal hemorrhage. Case report. J Neurosurg 69:775-779, 1988.
2687. Ventafridda, V, Caraceni, A, Martini, C, et al: On the significance of Lhermitte's sign in oncology. J Neurooncol 10:133-137, 1991.
2688. Ventura, GJ, Keating, MJ, Castellanos, AM, et al: Reversible bilateral lateral rectus muscle palsy associated with high-dose cytosine arabinoside and mitoxantrone therapy. Cancer 58:1633-1635, 1986.
2689. Verghese, A, Widrich, WC, and Arbeit, RD: Central venous septic thrombophlebitis—the role of medical therapy. Medicine (Baltimore) 64:394-400, 1985.

2690. Verma, P and Oger, J: Treatment of acquired autoimmune myasthenia gravis: A topic review. Can J Neurol Sci 19:360-375, 1992.
2691. Verweij, J, Schornagel, J, de Mulder, P, et al: Toxic dermatitis induced by 10-ethyl-10-deazaaminopterin (10-EdAM), a novel antifolate. Cancer 66:1910-1913, 1990.
2692. Viadana, E, Bross, ID, and Pickren, JW: An autopsy study of some routes of dissemination of cancer of the breast. Br J Cancer 27:336-340, 1973.
2693. Viadana, E, Cotter, R, Pickren, JW, et al: An autopsy study of metastatic sites of breast cancer. Cancer Res 33:179-181, 1973.
2694. Vick, NA: Letter to the Editor. J Neurooncol 6:199, 1988.
2695. Victor, M: The effects of nutritional deficiency on the nervous system. A comparison with the effects of carcinoma. In Brain, L and Norris, FH, Jr (eds): Contemporary Neurology Symposia, vol 1, The Remote Effects of Cancer on the Nervous System. Grune & Stratton, New York, 1965, pp 134-161.
2696. Vikram, B and Chu, FC: Radiation therapy for metastases to the base of the skull. Radiology 130:465-468, 1979.
2697. Vincent, D, Dubas, F, Hauw, JJ, et al: Nerve and muscle microvasculitis in peripheral neuropathy: A remote effect of cancer? J Neurol Neurosurg Psychiatry 49:1007-1010, 1986.
2698. Viollier, A-F, Peterson, DE, DeJongh, CA, et al: *Aspergillus* sinusitis in cancer patients. Cancer 58:366-371, 1986.
2699. Viswanathan, R and Glickman, L: Clonazepam in the treatment of steroid-induced mania in a patient after renal transplantation. N Engl J Med 320:319-320, 1989.
2700. Vital, A, Vital, C, Julien, J, et al: Polyneuropathy associated with IgM monoclonal gammopathy. Immunological and pathological study in 31 patients. Acta Neuropathol (Berl) 79:160-167, 1989.
2701. Vital, C, Vital, A, Julien, J, et al: Peripheral neuropathies and lymphoma without monoclonal gammopathy: A new classification. J Neurol 237:177-185, 1990.
2702. Vitale, V, Scolaro, T, and Orsatti, M: Prophylactic brain irradiation: Still an open question (Review). Anticancer Res 14:295-300, 1994.
2703. Vizel, M and Oster, MW: Ocular side effects of cancer chemotherapy. Cancer 49:1999-2002, 1982.
2704. Vock, P, Mattle, H, Studer, M, et al: Lumbosacral plexus lesions: Correlation of clinical signs and computed tomography. J Neurol Neurosurg Psychiatry 51:72-79, 1988.
2705. Vogel, H and Horoupian, DS: Filamentous degeneration of neurons. A possible feature of cytosine arabinoside neurotoxicity. Cancer 71:1303-1308, 1993.
2706. Vogelzang, NJ: Vascular and other complications of chemotherapy for testicular cancer. World J Urol 2:32-37, 1984.
2707. Vogelzang, NJ, Bosl, GJ, Johnson, K, et al: Raynaud's phenomenon: A common toxicity after combination chemotherapy for testicular cancer. Ann Intern Med 95:288-292, 1981.
2707a. Volm, M, van Kaick, G, and Mattern, J: Analysis of c-*fos*, c-*jun*, c-*erb1*, c-*erb2* and c-*myc* in primary lung carcinomas and their lymph node metastases. Clin Exp Metastasis 12:329-334, 1994.
2708. Vonofakos, D, Zieger, A, and Marcu, H: Subdural hematoma associated with dural metastatic tumor. Neuroradiology 20:213-218, 1980.
2709. Voorhies, RM, Engel, I, Gamache, FW, Jr, et al: Intraoperative localization subcortical brain tumors: Further experience with B-mode realtime sector scanning. Neurosurgery 12(2):189-194, 1983.
2710. Voorhies, RM, Sundaresan, N, and Thaler, HT: The single supratentorial lesion. An evaluation of preoperative diagnostic tests. J Neurosurg 53:364-368, 1980.
2711. Vorbrodt, AW, Lossinsky, AS, Wisniewski, HM, et al: Ultrastructural observations on the transvascular route of protein removal in vasogenic brain edema. Acta Neuropathol (Berl) 66:265-273, 1985.
2712. Vortmeyer, AO, Hagel, C, and Lass, R: Haemorrhagic thiamine deficient encephalopathy following prolonged parenteral nutrition. J Neurol Neurosurg Psychiatry 55:826-829, 1992.
2713. Vosskamper, M, Korf, B, Frank, F, et al: Paraneoplastic necrotizing myopathy: A rare disorder to be differentiated from polymyositis. Letter to the Editor. J Neurol 236:489-492, 1989.
2714. Vu, T, Amin, J, Ramos, M, et al: New assay for the rapid determination of plasma holotranscobalamin II levels: Preliminary evaluation in cancer patients. Am J Hematol 42:202-211, 1993.
2715. Vugrin, D, Cvitkovic, E, Posner, J, et al: Neurological complications of malignant germ cell tumors of testis: Biology of brain metastases (I). Cancer 44:2349-2353, 1979.
2716. Waber, DP, Gioia, G, Paccia, J, et al: Sex differences in cognitive processing in children treated with CNS prophylaxis for acute lymphoblastic leukemia. J Pediatr Psychol 15:105-122, 1990.
2717. Waber, DP, Tarbell, NJ, Kahn, CM, et al: The relationship of sex and treatment modality to neuropsychologic outcome in childhood acute lymphoblastic leukemia. J Clin Oncol 10:810-817, 1992.
2718. Waerness, E: Neuromyotonia and bronchial carcinoma. Electromyogr Clin Neurophysiol 14:527-535, 1974.
2719. Wahl, M, Unterberg, A, Baethmann, A, et al: Mediators of blood–brain barrier dysfunction and formation of vasogenic brain edema. J Cereb Blood Flow Metab 8:621-634, 1988.
2720. Wakai, S, Andoh, Y, Ochiai, C, et al: Postoperative contrast enhancement in brain tumors and intracerebral hematomas: CT study. J Comput Assist Tomogr 14(2):267-271, 1990.
2720a. Walbridge, S and Rybak, SM: Immunotoxin therapy of leptomeningeal neoplasia. J Neurooncol 20:59-65, 1994.
2721. Wald, SL and McLaurin, RL: Oral glycerol for the treatment of traumatic intracranial hypertension. J Neurosurg 56:323-331, 1982.
2722. Walker, AE and Adamkiewitcz, JJ: Pseudotumor cerebri associated with prolonged corticosteroid

therapy: Reports of four cases. JAMA 188:779-784, 1964.

2723. Walker, AE, Robins, M, and Weinfeld, FD: Epidemiology of brain tumors: The national survey of intracranial neoplasms. Neurology 35:219-226, 1985.

2724. Walker, MC, Masters, JR, and Margison, GP: 06-alkylguanine-DNA-alkyltransferase activity and nitrosourea sensitivity in human cancer cell lines. Br J Cancer 66:840-843, 1992.

2725. Walker, RW, Allen, JC, Rosen, G, et al: Transient cerebral dysfunction secondary to high-dose methotrexate. J Clin Oncol 4:1845-1850, 1986.

2726. Walker, RW and Brochstein, JA: Neurologic complications of immunosuppressive agents. Neurol Clin 6:261-278, 1988.

2727. Walker, RW, Cairncross, JG, and Posner, JB: Cerebral herniation in patients receiving cisplatin. J Neurooncol 6:61-65, 1988.

2728. Walker, RW and Rosenblum, MK: Amphotericin B–associated leukoencephalopathy. Neurology 42:2005-2010, 1992.

2729. Walker, RW, Rosenblum, MK, Kempin, SJ, et al: Carboplatin-associated thrombotic microangiopathic hemolytic anemia. Cancer 64:1017-1020, 1989.

2730. Wall, JG, Weiss, RB, Norton, L, et al: Arterial thrombosis associated with adjuvant chemotherapy for breast carcinoma: A Cancer and Leukemia Group B study. Am J Med 87:501-504, 1989.

2731. Walls, TJ: Metabolic and toxic peripheral neuropathies including diabetes. Curr Opin Neurol Neurosurg 5:375-378, 1992.

2732. Walsh, DB, Downing, S, Nauta, R, et al: Metastatic cancer. A relative contraindication to vena cava filter placement. Cancer 59:161-163, 1987.

2733. Walsh, JC: Neuromyotonia: An unusual presentation of intrathoracic malignancy. J Neurol Neurosurg Psychiatry 39:1086-1091, 1976.

2734. Walsh, JC, Low, PA, and Allsop, JL: Localized sympathetic overactivity: An uncommon complication of lung cancer. J Neurol Neurosurg Psychiatry 39:93-95, 1976.

2735. Walsh, TJ, Clark, AW, Parhad, IM, et al: Neurotoxic effects of cisplatin therapy. Arch Neurol 39:719-720, 1982.

2736. Walsh, TJ, Hier, DB, and Caplan, LR: Fungal infections of the central nervous system: Comparative analysis of risk factors and clinical signs in 57 patients. Neurology 35:1654-1657, 1985.

2737. Walther, PJ, Rossitch, E, Jr, and Bullard, DE: The development of Lhermitte's sign during cisplatin chemotherapy. Possible drug-induced toxicity causing spinal cord demyelination. Cancer 60:2170-2172, 1987.

2738. Walton, JN, Tomlinson, BE, and Pearce, GW: Subacute "poliomyelitis" and Hodgkin's disease. J Neurol Sci 6:435-445, 1968.

2739. Walzer, PD, Armstrong, D, Weisman, P, et al: Serum immunoglobulin levels in childhood Hodgkin's disease. Effect of splenectomy and long-term follow-up. Cancer 45:2084-2089, 1980.

2740. Wara, WM, Phillips, TL, Sheline, GE, et al: Radiation tolerance of the spinal cord. Cancer 35:1558-1562, 1975.

2741. Ward, PH, Hanson, DG, and Abemayor, E: Transcutaneous Teflon injection of the paralyzed vocal cord: A new technique. Laryngoscope 95:644-649, 1985.

2742. Warner, E: Type B lactic acidosis and metastatic breast cancer. Breast Cancer Res Treat 24:75-79, 1992.

2743. Warpeha, RL: Head and neck surgery. Surg Clin North Am 57:1357-1363, 1977.

2744. Warrell, RP, Jr: Etiology and current management of cancer-related hypercalcemia. Oncology (Huntingt) 6:37-43, 1992.

2745. Warrell, RP, Jr and Berman, E: Phase I and II study of fludarabine phosphate in leukemia: Therapeutic efficacy with delayed central nervous system toxicity. J Clin Oncol 4:74-79, 1986.

2746. Warrell, RP, Jr, De Thé, H, Wang, Z-Y, et al: Acute promyelocytic leukemia. N Engl J Med 329:177-189, 1993.

2747. Warren, BA and Vales, O: The adhesion of thromboplastic tumor emboli to vessel walls in vivo. Br J Exp Pathol 53:301-313, 1972.

2748. Warren, RD and Bender, RA: Drug interactions with antineoplastic agents. Cancer Treat Rep 61:1231-1241, 1977.

2749. Waskin, H, Stehr-Green, JK, Helmick, CG, et al: Risk factors for hypoglycemia associated with pentamidine therapy for *Pneumocystis* pneumonia. JAMA 260:345-347, 1988.

2750. Wasserstrom, W, Glass, JP, and Posner, JB: Diagnosis and treatment of leptomeningeal metastases from solid tumors: Experience with 90 patients. Cancer 49:759-772, 1982.

2751. Wasserstrom, WR, Schwartz, MK, Fleisher, M, et al: Cerebrospinal fluid biochemical markers in central nervous system tumors: A review. Ann Clin Lab Sci 11:239-251, 1981.

2752. Watanabe, M, Sugimoto, T, and Tsuruo, T: Expression of a Mr 41,000 glycoprotein associated with throbin-independent platelet aggregation in high metastatic variants of murine B16 melanoma. Cancer Res 50:6657-6662, 1990.

2753. Waterston, JA and Gilligan, BS: Paraneoplastic optic neuritis and external ophthalmoplegia. Aust N Z J Med 16:703-704, 1986.

2754. Watkin, SW, Husband, DJ, Green, JA, et al: Ifosfamide encephalopathy: A reappraisal. Eur J Cancer Clin Oncol 25:1303-1310, 1989.

2755. Watkins, SM and Griffin, JP: High incidence of vincristine-induced neuropathy in lymphomas. BMJ 1:610-612, 1978.

2756. Watne, K, Hager, B, Heier, M, et al: Reversible oedema and necrosis after irradiation of the brain. Diagnosis procedures and clinical manifestations. Acta Oncol 29:891-895, 1990.

2757. Watson, CP, Evans, RJ, and Watt, VR: The postmastectomy pain syndrome and the effect of topical capsaicin. Pain 38:177-186, 1989.

2758. Watson, GW, Fuller, TJ, Elms, J, et al: *Listeria* cerebritis: Relapse of infection in renal transplant patients. Arch Intern Med 138:83-87, 1978.

2759. Watson, JD, Gibson, J, Joshua, DE, et al: Aseptic meningitis associated with high dose intravenous immunoglobulin therapy. J Neurol Neurosurg Psychiatry 54:275-276, 1991.

2760. Watts, RG: Combination chemotherapy with ifosfamide and etoposide is effective in the treatment of central nervous system metastasis of childhood neuroblastoma. Cancer 69:3012-3014, 1992.

2761. Waxman, SG, Sabin, TD, and Embree, LJ: Subacute brain-stem encephalitis. J Neurol Neurosurg Psychiatry 37:811-816, 1974.

2762. Weaver, DD, Winn, HR, and Jane, JA: Differential intracranial pressure in patients with unilateral mass lesions. J Neurosurg 56:660-665, 1982.

2763. Weaver, DF, Heffernan, LP, Purdy, RA, et al: Eosinophil-induced neurotoxicity: Axonal neuropathy, cerebral infarction, and dementia. Neurology 38:144-146, 1988.

2764. Weber, DM, Dimopoulos, MA, and Alexanian, R: Increased neurotoxicity with VAD-cyclosporin in multiple myeloma. Letter to the Editor. Lancet 341:558-559, 1993.

2765. Weber, JD and Rutala, WA: Epidemiology of hospital-acquired fungal infections. In Holmberg, K and Meyer, RD (eds): Diagnosis and Therapy of Systemic Fungal Infections. Raven Press, New York, 1989, pp 1-24.

2766. Weber, P, Shepard, KV, and Vijayakumar, S: Metastases to pineal gland. Cancer 63:164-165, 1989.

2767. Weber, T, Turner, RW, Frye, S, et al: Progressive multifocal leukoencephalopathy diagnosed by amplification of JC virus-specific DNA from cerebrospinal fluid. AIDS 8:49-57, 1994.

2768. Weber, W, Tackmann, W, Freund, HJ, et al: The evaluation of neurotoxicity in cancer patients treated with vinca alkaloids with special reference to vindesine. Anticancer Res 1:31-34, 1981.

2769. Weed, JC, Jr and Creasman, WT: Meningeal carcinomatosis secondary to advanced squamous cell carcinoma of the cervix: A case report. Meningeal metastasis of advanced cervical cancer. Gynecol Oncol 3:201-204, 1975.

2770. Weiden, PL: Intracarotid cisplatin as therapy for melanoma metastatic to brain: Ipsilateral response and contralateral progression. Am J Med 85:439-440, 1988.

2770a. Weidmann, B, Mulleneisen, N, Bojko, P, et al: Hypersensitivity reactions to carboplatin. Cancer 73:2218-2222, 1994.

2771. Weijl, NI, Van Der Harst, D, Brand, A, et al: Hypothyroidism during immunotherapy with interleukin-2 is associated with antithyroid antibodies and response to treatment. J Clin Oncol 11(7):1376-1383, 1993.

2772. Weiner, HL, Rezai, AR, and Cooper, PR: Sigmoid diverticular perforation in neurosurgical patients receiving high-dose corticosteroids. Neurosurgery 33:40-43, 1993.

2773. Weingarten, JS, O'Sheal, SF, and Margolis, WS: Eosinophilic meningitis and the hypereosinophilic syndrome. Case report and review of the literature. Am J Med 78:674-676, 1985.

2773a. Weinrich, S and Sarna, L: Delirium in the older person with cancer. Cancer 74:2079-2091, 1994.

2773b. Weinstat-Saslow, D and Steeg, PS: Angiogenesis and colonization in the tumor metastatic process: Basic and applied advances. FASEB J 8:401-407, 1994.

2774. Weisberg, LA and Nice, CN: Intracranial tumors simulating the presentation of cerebrovascular syndromes. Early detection with cerebral computed tomography (CCT). Am J Med 63:517-524, 1977.

2775. Weisenthal, R, Frayer, WC, Nichols, CW, et al: Bilateral ocular disease as the initial presentation of malignant lymphoma. Br J Ophthalmol 72:248-252, 1988.

2776. Weiss, L: Analysis of the incidence of intraocular metastasis. Br J Ophthalmol 77:149-151, 1993.

2777. Weiss, L, Gilbert, HA, and Posner, JB (eds): Brain Metastasis. GK Hall & Co, Boston, 1980.

2778. Weiss, L and Gilbert, HA (eds): Bone Metastasis. GK Hall & Co, Boston, 1981.

2779. Weiss, L, Harlos, JP, Torhorst, J, et al: Metastatic patterns of renal carcinoma: An analysis of 687 necropsies. J Cancer Res Clin Oncol 114:605-612, 1988.

2780. Weiss, L, Mayhew, E, Rapp, DG, et al: Metastatic inefficiency in mice bearing B16 melanoma. Br J Cancer 45:44-53, 1982.

2781. Weiss, L, Nannmark, U, Johansson, BR, et al: Lethal deformation of cancer cells in the microcirculation: A potential rate regulator of hematogenous metastasis. Int J Cancer 50:103-107, 1992.

2782. Weiss, L, Orr, FW, and Honn, KV: Interactions of cancer cells with the microvasculature during metastasis. FASEB J 2:12-21, 1988.

2783. Weiss, LW and Ward, PM: Effects of metastatic cascades on metastatic patterns: Studies on colon-26 carcinomas in mice. Int J Cancer 41:450-455, 1988.

2784. Weissman, DE: Glucocorticoid treatment for brain metastases and epidural spinal cord compression: A review. J Clin Oncol 6:543-551, 1988.

2785. Weissman, DE, Dufer, D, Vogel, V, et al: Corticosteroid toxicity in neuro-oncology patients. J Neurooncol 5:125-128, 1987.

2786. Weissman, DE, Janjan, NA, Erickson, B, et al: Twice-daily tapering dexamethasone treatment during cranial radiation for newly diagnosed brain metastases. J Neurooncol 11:235-239, 1991.

2787. Weissman, DE, Negendank, WG, Al-Katib, AM, et al: Bone marrow necrosis in lymphoma studied by magnetic resonance imaging. Am J Hematol 40:42-46, 1992.

2788. Weissman, DE and Stewart, C: Experimental drug therapy of peritumoral brain edema. J Neurooncol 6:339-342, 1988.

2789. Weller, M, Sommer, N, Stevens, A, et al: Increased intrathecal synthesis of fibronectin in bacterial and carcinomatous meningitis. Acta Neurol Scand 82:138-142, 1990.

2790. Weller, M, Stevens, A, Sommer, N, et al: Tumor cell dissemination triggers an intrathecal immune response in neoplastic meningitis. Cancer 69:1475-1480, 1992.

2791. Weller, M, Stevens, A, Sommer, N, et al: Tumour necrosis factor-alpha in malignant melanomatous meningitis. Letter to the Editor. J Neurol Neurosurg Psychiatry 55:74, 1992.

2792. Weller, PF: The immunobiology of eosinophils. N Engl J Med 324:1110-1118, 1991.

2793. Wen, PY, Blanchard, KL, Block, CC, et al: Development of Lhermitte's sign after bone marrow transplantation. Cancer 69:2262-2266, 1992.

2794. Wendling, LR, Cromwell, LD, and Latchaw, RE: Computed tomography of intracerebral leukemic masses. AJR 132:217-220, 1979.
2795. Werner, MH, Burger, PC, Heinz, ER, et al: Intracranial atherosclerosis following radiotherapy. Neurology 38:1158-1160, 1988.
2796. Wernick, R and Smith, DL: Central nervous system toxicity associated with weekly low-dose methotrexate treatment. Arthritis Rheum 32:770-775, 1989.
2797. Wessel, K, Diener, HC, Dichgans, J, et al: Cerebellar dysfunction in patients with bronchogenic carcinoma: Clinical and posturographic findings. J Neurol 235:290-296, 1988.
2798. Westbrook, KC, Ballantyne, AJ, Eckles, NE, et al: Breast cancer and vocal paralysis. South Med J 67:805-807, 1974.
2798a. Wheeler, A and Rubenstein, EB: Current management of disseminated intravascular coagulation. Oncology (Huntingt) 8:69-79, 1994.
2799. Whitaker, JN, Lisak, RP, Rifaat, MB, et al: Immunoreactive myelin basic protein in the cerebrospinal fluid in neurological disorders. Ann Neurol 7:58-64, 1978.
2800. White, FA, III, Ishaq, M, Stoner, GL, et al: JC virus DNA is present in many human brain samples from patients without progressive multifocal leukoencephalopathy. J Virol 66:5726-5734, 1992.
2801. White, M, Cirrincione, C, Blevins, A, et al: Cryptococcal meningitis: Outcome in patients with AIDS and patients with neoplastic disease. J Infect Dis 165:960-963, 1992.
2802. Whitley, RJ: Viral encephalitis. N Engl J Med 323:242-250, 1990.
2803. Whitley, RJ, Lentnek, A, McCracken, GH, et al: Evaluation of new anti-infective drugs for the treatment of viral encephalitis. Infectious Diseases Society of America and the Food and Drug Administration. Clin Infect Dis 15(Suppl 1):S195-S199, 1992.
2804. Whittaker, JA, Parry, DH, Bunch, C, et al: Coma associated with vincristine therapy. BMJ 4:335-337, 1973.
2805. Whittet, HB and Boscoe, MJ: Isolated palsy of the hypoglossal nerve after central venous catheterisation. Case report. BMJ 288:1042-1043, 1984.
2806. Wiederkehr, F, Bueler, MR, and Vonderschmitt, DJ: Analysis of circulating immune complexes isolated from plasma, cerebrospinal fluid and urine. Electrophoresis 12:478-486, 1991.
2806a. Wijdicks, EFM, Litchy, WJ, Harrison, BA, et al: The clinical spectrum of critical illness polyneuropathy. Mayo Clin Proc 69:955-959, 1994.
2807. Wijdicks, EF and Sharbrough, FW: New-onset seizures in critically ill patients. Neurology 43: 1042-1044, 1993.
2808. Wijdicks, EF and Stevens, M: The role of hypotension in septic encephalopathy following surgical procedures. Arch Neurol 49:653-656, 1992.
2809. Wilbourn, AJ: Electrodiagnosis of plexopathies. Neurol Clin 3:511-529, 1985.
2810. Wilding, G, Caruso, R, Lawrence, TS, et al: Retinal toxicity after high-dose cisplatin therapy. J Clin Oncol 3:1683-1689, 1985.
2811. Wiley, RG, Gralla, RJ, Casper, ES, et al: Neurotoxicity of the pyrimidine synthesis inhibitor N-phosphonocetyl-L-aspartate. Ann Neurol 12: 175-183, 1982.
2812. Wilkins, DE and Samhouri, AM: Isolated bilateral oculomotor paresis due to lymphoma. Neurology 29:1425-1428, 1979.
2813. Wilkinson, PC and Zeromski, J: Immunofluorescent detection of antibodies against neurons in sensory carcinomatous neuropathy. Brain 88:529-538, 1965.
2814. Williams, CL, Hay, JE, Huiatt, TW, et al: Paraneoplastic IgG striational autoantibodies produced by clonal thymic B cells and in serum of patients with myasthenia gravis and thymoma react with titin. Lab Invest 66:331-336, 1992.
2815. Williams, ME, Walker, AN, Bracikowski, JP, et al: Ascending myeloencephalopathy due to intrathecal vincristine sulfate. A fatal chemotherapeutic error. Cancer 51:2041-2047, 1983.
2816. Williams, MG, Earhart, RH, Bailey, H, et al: Prevention of central nervous system toxicity of the antitumor antibiotic acivicin by concomitant infusion of an amino acid mixture. Cancer Res 50:5475-5480, 1990.
2817. Williams, SD, Birch, R, Einhorn, LH, et al: Treatment of disseminated germ-cell tumors with cisplatin, bleomycin and either vinblastine or etoposide. N Engl J Med 315:1435-1440, 1987.
2818. Williams, TJ and Yarwood, H: Effect of glucocorticosteroids on microvascular permeability. Am Rev Respir Dis 141:S39-S43, 1990.
2819. Willner, C and Low, PA: Pharmacologic approaches to neuropathic pain. In Dyck, PJ and Thomas, PK (eds): Peripheral Neuropathy, vol 2, ed 3. WB Saunders, Philadelphia, 1993, pp 1709-1720.
2820. Wilson, CB, Larson, DA, and Gutin, PH: Radiosurgery: A new application? Editorial. J Clin Oncol 10:1373-1374, 1992.
2821. Wilson, DA, Nitschke, R, Bowman, ME, et al: Transient white matter changes on MR images in children undergoing chemotherapy for acute lymphocytic leukemia: Correlation with neuropsychologic deficiencies. Radiology 180:205-209, 1991.
2822. Wilson, JR, Conwit, RA, Eidelman, BH, et al: Sensorimotor neuropathy resembling CIDP in patients receiving FK506. Muscle Nerve 17:528-532, 1994.
2823. Wilson, JWL, Morales, A, and Sharp, D: Necrotizing myelopathy associated with renal cell carcinoma. Urology 21:390-392, 1983.
2824. Wilson, LM: Intensive care delirium. The effect of outside deprivation in a windowless unit. Arch Intern Med 130:225-226, 1972.
2825. Wilson, PJ, Turner, HR, Kirchner, KA, et al: Nocardial infections in renal transplant recipients. Medicine (Baltimore) 68:38-57, 1989.
2826. Wilson, WB, Perez, GM, and Kleinschmidt-DeMasters, BK: Sudden onset of blindness in patients treated with oral CCNU and low-dose cranial irradiation. Cancer 59:901-907, 1987.
2827. Wilson, WH, Jain, V, Bryant, G, et al: Phase I and II study of high-dose ifosfamide, carboplatin, and etoposide with autologous bone marrow rescue in

lymphomas and solid tumors. J Clin Oncol 10:1712-1722, 1992.
2828. Windebank, AJ, Smith, AG, and Russell, JW: The effect of nerve growth factor, ciliary neurotrophic factor, and ACTH analogs on cisplatin neurotoxicity in vitro. Neurology 44:488-494, 1994.
2829. Wingard, JR: Management of infectious complications of bone marrow transplantation. Oncology (Huntingt) 4:69-82, 1990.
2830. Winick, N, Buchanan, GR, Murphy, SB, et al: Deoxycoformycin causes profound T cell dysfunction in patients with hairy cell leukemia. Abstract. Program/Proceedings American Society of Clinical Oncology 6:152, 1987.
2831. Winick, NJ, Bowman, WP, Kamen, BA, et al: Unexpected acute neurological toxicity in the treatment of children with acute lymphoblastic leukemia. J Natl Cancer Inst 84:252-256, 1992.
2832. Winkelman, MD, Adelstein, DJ, and Karlins, NL: Intramedullary spinal cord metastasis. Diagnostic and therapeutic considerations. Arch Neurol 44:526-531, 1987.
2833. Winkelman, MD and Hines, JD: Cerebellar degeneration caused by high-dose cytosine arabinoside: A clinicopathological study. Ann Neurol 14:520-527, 1983.
2834. Wispelwey, B, Dacey, RG, Jr, and Scheld, WM: Brain abscess. In Scheld, WM, Whitley, RJ, and Durack, DT (eds): Infections of the Central Nervous System. Raven Press, New York, 1991, pp 457-486.
2835. Withers, HR: Biological basis of radiation therapy for cancer. Lancet 339:156-159, 1992.
2836. Wokke, JHJ, Jennekens, FG, van den Oord, CJ, et al: Histological investigations of muscle atrophy and end plates in two critically ill patients with generalized weakness. J Neurol Sci 88:95-106, 1988.
2837. Wolf, AL, Adcock, LL, Hachiya, JT, et al: Choriocarcinoma with brain metastases. Successful management of increased intracranial pressure with barbiturates. Cancer 57:1432-1436, 1986.
2838. Wolf, DG and Spector, SA: Diagnosis of human cytomegalovirus central nervous system disease in AIDS patients by DNA amplification from cerebrospinal fluid. J Infect Dis 166:1412-1415, 1992.
2839. Wolf, PA, Rosman, NP, and New, PFJ: Multiple small cryptic venous angiomas of brain mimicking cerebral metastases. Neurology 17:491-501, 1967.
2840. Wolff, L, Zighelboim, J, and Gale, RP: Paraplegia following intrathecal cytosine arabinoside. Cancer 43:83-85, 1979.
2841. Wolinsky, JS, Swoveland, P, Johnson, KP, et al: Subacute measles encephalitis complicating Hodgkin's disease in an adult. Ann Neurol 1:452-457, 1977.
2842. Wolkowitz, OM, Reus, VI, Weingartner, H, et al: Cognitive effects of corticosteroids. Am J Psychiatry 147:1297-1303, 1990.
2843. Womack, LW and Liesegang, TJ: Complications of herpes zoster ophthalmicus. Arch Ophthalmol 101:42-45, 1983.
2844. Wong, DA, Fornasier, VL, and MacNab, I: Spinal metastases: The obvious, the occult, and the imposters. Spine 15:1-4, 1990.
2845. Wong, MC, Krol, G, and Rosenblum, MK: Occult epidural chloroma complicated by acute paraplegia following lumbar puncture. Ann Neurol 31:110-112, 1992.
2846. Woo, E, Lam, K, Yu, YL, et al: Temporal lobe and hypothalamic-pituitary dysfunctions after radiotherapy for nasopharyngeal carcinoma: A distinct clinical syndrome. J Neurol Neurosurg Psychiatry 51:1302-1307, 1988.
2847. Woo, E, Yu, YL, Ng, M, et al: Spinal cord compression in multiple myeloma: Who gets it? Aust N Z J Med 16:671-675, 1986.
2848. Woolsey, RM and Young, RR (eds): Disorders of the Spinal Cord. Neurol Clin 9:503-816, 1991.
2849. Word, JA, Kalokhe, UP, Aron, BS, et al: Transient radiation myelopathy (Lhermitte's sign) in patients with Hodgkin's disease treated by mantle irradiation. Int J Radiat Oncol Biol Phys 6:1731-1733, 1980.
2850. Wright, CG and Schaefer, SD: Inner ear histopathology in patients treated with *cis*-platinum. Laryngoscope 92:1408-1413, 1982.
2851. Wright, DC: Surgical treatment of brain metastases. In Rosenberg, SA (ed): Surgical Treatment of Metastatic Cancer. JB Lippincott, Philadelphia, 1987, pp 165-222.
2852. Wright, DE and Drouin, P: Cisplatin-induced myasthenic syndrome. Clinical Pharmacokinetics 1:76-78, 1982.
2853. Wright, DH, Hise, JH, Bauserman, SC, et al: Intracranial granulocytic sarcoma: CT, MR and angiography. J Comput Assist Tomogr 16:487-489, 1992.
2854. Wyllie, AH: Apoptosis (The 1992 Frank Rose Memorial Lecture). Br J Cancer 67:205-208, 1993.
2855. Yaar, I, Ron, E, Modan, B, et al: Long-lasting cerebral functional changes following moderate dose x-radiation treatment to the scalp in childhood: An electroencephalographic power spectral study. J Neurol Neurosurg Psychiatry 45:166-169, 1982.
2856. Yadin, E, Bruno, L, Micalizzi, M, et al: An animal model to detect learning deficits following treatment of the immature brain. Studies using radiation and methotrexate. Childs Brain 10:273-280, 1983.
2857. Yaegashi, H and Takahashi, T: Encasement and other deformations of tumor-embedded host arteries due to loss of medial smooth muscles. Morphometric and three-dimensional reconstruction studies on some human carcinomas. Cancer 65:1097-1103, 1990.
2858. Yamazaki, T, Harigaya, T, Noguchi, O, et al: Calcified miliary brain metastases with mitochondrial inclusion bodies. J Neurol Neurosurg Psychiatry 56:110-111, 1993.
2859. Yanovski, JA, Packer, RJ, Levine, JD, et al: An animal model to detect the neuropsychological toxicity of anticancer agents. Med Pediatr Oncol 17:216-221, 1989.
2860. Yap, H-Y, Blumenschein, GR, Yap, BS, et al: High-dose methotrexate for advanced breast cancer. Cancer Treat Rep 63:757-761, 1979.
2861. Yap, H-Y, Tashima, CK, Blumenschein, GR, et al:

Diabetes insipidus and breast cancer. Arch Intern Med 139:1009-1011, 1979.
2862. Yap, H-Y, Yap, B-S, Rasmussen, S, et al: Treatment for meningeal carcinomatosis in breast cancer. Cancer 50:219-222, 1982.
2863. Yap, H-Y, Yap, B-S, Tashima, CK, et al: Meningeal carcinomatosis in breast cancer. Cancer 42:283-286, 1978.
2864. Yeung, WT, Lee, T, Del Maestro, RF, et al: Effect of steroids on iopamidol blood-brain transfer constant and plasma volume in brain tumors measured with X-ray computed tomography. J Neurooncol 18:53-60, 1994.
2865. Yim, YS, Mahoney, DH, Jr, and Oshman, DG: Hemiparesis and ischemic changes of the white matter after intrathecal therapy for children with acute lymphocytic leukemia. Cancer 67:2058-2061, 1991.
2866. Yoneda, Y, Alsina, MM, Watatani, K, et al: Dependence of a human squamous carcinoma and associated paraneoplastic syndromes on the epidermal growth factor receptor pathway in nude mice. Cancer Res 51:2438-2443, 1991.
2867. Yorke, ED, Fuks, Z, Norton, L, et al: Modeling the development of metastases from primary and locally recurrent tumors: Comparison with a clinical data base for prostatic cancer. Cancer Res 53:2987-2993, 1993.
2868. Yoshida, TK, Shimizu, K, Koulousakis, A, et al: Intrathecal chemotherapy with ACNU in a meningeal gliomatosis rat model. J Neurosurg 77:778-782, 1992.
2869. Yoss, RE, Corbin, KB, MacCarty, CS, et al: Significance of symptoms and signs in localization of involved root in cervical disk protrusion. Neurology 7:673-683, 1957.
2870. Young, DF and Posner, JB: Nervous system toxicity of the chemotherapeutic agents. In Vinken, PJ and Bruyn, GW (eds): Handbook of Clinical Neurology, vol 39. North-Holland, Amsterdam, 1980, pp 91-130.
2871. Young, DF, Posner, JB, Chu, F, et al: Rapid-course radiation therapy of cerebral metastases: Results and complications. Cancer 4:1069-1076, 1974.
2872. Young, GB, Bolton, CF: Septic encephalopathy: What significance in patients with sepsis? Journal of Critical Illness 7:668-682, 1992.
2873. Young, GB, Bolton, CF, Archibald, YM, et al: The electroencephalogram in sepsis-associated encephalopathy. J Clin Neurophysiol 9:145-152, 1992.
2874. Young, GB, Bolton, CF, Austin, TW, et al: The encephalopathy associated with septic illness. Clin Invest Med 13:297-304, 1990.
2875. Young, LS, Armstrong, D, Blevins, A, et al: *Nocardia asteroides* infection complicating neoplastic disease. Am J Med 50:356-367, 1971.
2876. Young, RF, Post, EM, and King, GA: Treatment of spinal epidural metastases. Randomized prospective comparison of laminectomy and radiotherapy. J Neurosurg 53:741-748, 1980.
2877. Young, RSK and Zalneraitis, EL: Marantic endocarditis in children and young adults: Clinical and pathological findings. Stroke 12:635-639, 1981.
2877a. Younger, DS, Rowland, LP, Latov, N, et al: Lymphoma, motor neuron diseases, and anyotrophic lateral sclerosis. Ann Neurol 29:78-86, 1991.
2878. Yousem, DM, Patrone, PM, and Grossman, RI: Leptomeningeal metastases: MR evaluation. J Comput Assist Tomogr 14:255-261, 1990.
2879. Yu, YL, Lau, YN, Woo, E, et al: Cryptococcal infection of the nervous system. Q J Med 66:87-96, 1988.
2880. Yuh, WT, Nguyen, HD, Gao, F, et al: Brain parenchymal infection in bone marrow transplantation patients: CT and MR findings. AJR 162:425-430, 1994.
2881. Yuh, WTC, Engelken, JD, Muhonen, MG, et al: Experience with high-dose gadolinium MR imaging in the evaluation of brain metastases. AJNR 13:335-354, 1992.
2882. Yutani, C, Matsuda, Y, Murao, S, et al: Necrotizing myopathy as a remote effect of gastric cancer accompanied with Hashimoto's thyroiditis. Acta Pathol Jpn 28:165-174, 1978.
2883. Zacharski, LR, Henderson, WG, Rickles, FR, et al: Effect of warfarin anticoagulation on survival in carcinoma of the lung, colon, head and neck and prostate: Final report of VA Cooperative Study #75. Cancer 53:2046-2052, 1984.
2884. Zagoren, JC, Seelig, M, Bornstein, MB, et al: The evolution of cellular degeneration in dorsal root ganglia exposed to doxorubicin in tissue culture. J Neuropathol Exp Neurol 43:384-394, 1984.
2885. Zagzag, D, Miller, DC, Cangiarella, J, et al: Brainstem glioma after radiation therapy for acute myeloblastic leukemia in a child with Down's syndrome. Possible pathogenic mechanisms. Cancer 70:1188-1193, 1992.
2886. Zaheer, W, Friedland, ML, Cooper, EB, et al: Spontaneous regression of small cell carcinoma of lung associated with severe neuropathy. Cancer Invest 11:306-309, 1993.
2886a. Zalutsky, MR, McLendon, RE, Garg, PK, et al: Radioimmunotherapy of neoplastic meningitis in rats using an α-particle-emiting immunoconjugate. Cancer Res 54:4719-4725, 1994.
2887. Zandman-Goddard, G, Matzner, Y, Konijn, AM, et al: Cerebrospinal fluid ferritin in malignant CNS involvement. Cancer 58:1346-1349, 1986.
2888. Zappia, RJ, Smith, ME, and Gay, AJ: Prostatic carcinoma metastatic to optic nerve and choroid. Association with changes resembling papilledema. Arch Ophthalmol 87:642-645, 1972.
2889. Zaret, BS and Cohen, RA: Reversible valproic acid–induced dementia: a case report. Epilepsia 27(3):234-240, 1986.
2890. Zec, N, Donovan, JW, Aufiero, TX, et al: Seizures in a patient treated with continuous povidone-iodine mediastinal irrigation. Letter to the Editor. N Engl J Med 326:1784, 1992.
2891. Zeidman, I and Buss, JAM: Transpulmonary passage of tumor cell emboli. Cancer Res 12:731-733, 1952.
2892. Zeman, W and Samorajski, T: Effects of irradiation on the nervous system. In Berdjis, CC (ed): Pathology of Irradiation. Williams & Wilkins Company, Baltimore, 1971, pp 213-277.
2893. Zeromski, J: Immunological findings in sensory

carcinomatous neuropathy. Application of peroxidase labeled antibody. Clin Exp Immunol 6:633-637, 1970.
2894. Zevallos, M, Chan, PY, Munoz, L, et al: Epidural spinal cord compression from metastatic tumor. Int J Radiat Oncol Biol Phys 13:875-878, 1987.
2895. Zhang, RD, Price, JE, Fujimaki, T, et al: Differential permeability of the blood–brain barrier in experimental brain metastases produced by human neoplasms implanted into nude mice. Am J Pathol 141:1115-1124, 1992.
2896. Zhang, RD, Price, JF, Schackert, G, et al: Malignant potential of cells isolated from lymph node or brain metastases of melanoma patients and implications for prognosis. Cancer Res 51:2029-2035, 1991.
2897. Ziegler, J, Gliedman, P, Fass, D, et al: Brain metastases from ovarian cancer. J Neurooncol 5:211-215, 1987.
2897a. Zijlstra, EJ, Taphoorn, MJB, Barkhof, F, et al: Radiotherapy response of cerebral metastases quantified by serial MR imaging. J Neurooncol 21:171-176, 1994.
2898. Zilkha, A and Diaz, AS: Computed tomography in the diagnosis of superior sagittal sinus thrombosis. J Comput Assist Tomogr 4:124-126, 1980.
2899. Zimm, S, Wampler, GL, Stablein, D, et al: Intracerebral metastases in solid tumor patients. Natural history and results of treatment. Cancer 48:384-394, 1981.
2900. Zimmerman, RA: Imaging of intracranial infections. In Scheld, WM, Whitley, RJ, and Durack, DT (eds): Infections of the Central Nervous System. Raven Press, New York, 1991, pp 887-908.
2901. Zito, G and Kadis, GN: Multiple vertebral hemangiomas resembling metastases with spinal cord compression. Arch Neurol 37:247-248, 1980.
2902. Zochodne, DW, Bolton, CF, Wells, GA, et al: Critical illness polyneuropathy. A complication of sepsis and multiple organ failure. Brain 110:819-842, 1987.
2903. Zochodne, DW, Cairncross, JG, Arce, FP, et al: Astrocytoma following scalp radiotherapy in infancy. Can J Neurol Sci 11:475-478, 1984.
2904. Zochodne, DW, Ramsay, DA, Salv, V, et al: Acute necrotizing myopathy of intensive care: Electrophysiological studies. Muscle Nerve 17:285-292, 1994.
2905. Zonderman, AB, Costa, PT, Jr, and McCrae, RR: Depression as a risk for cancer morbidity and mortality in a nationally representative sample. JAMA 262:1191-1195, 1989.
2906. Zovickian, J and Youle, RJ: Efficacy of intrathecal immunotoxin therapy in an animal model of leptomeningeal neoplasia. J Neurosurg 68:767-774, 1988.
2907. Zunkeler, B, Carson, RE, Olson, J, et al: Unpublished material, 1994.

INDEX

An "f" following a page number indicates a figure; a "t" indicates a table.

ISBN 0-8036-0006-2
90000>
EAN
9 780803 600065